NAPLEX®

2015
STRATEGIES, PRACTICE, & REVIEW
with 2 Practice Tests

NAPLEX®
2015
STRATEGIES, PRACTICE, & REVIEW
with 2 Practice Tests

BOOK + ONLINE

Amie McCord Brooks, PharmD, FCCP, BCPS

Cynthia Sanoski, BS, PharmD, FCCP, BCPS

Emily Hajjar, PharmD, BCPS, BCACP, CGP

Brian R. Overholser, PharmD, FCCP

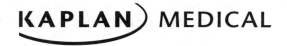

Published by Kaplan Publishing, a division of Kaplan, Inc.
395 Hudson Street
New York, NY 10014

Printed in the United States of America

Retail ISBN: 978-1-61865-796-1
10 9 8 7 6 5 4 3 2 1

Course ISBN: 978-1-62523-182-6 | Course Item Number: NP5001P
10 9 8 7 6 5 4 3 2 1

Kaplan Publishing books are available at special quantity discounts to use for sales promotions, employee premiums, or educational purposes. For more information or to purchase books, please call the Simon & Schuster special sales department at 866-506-1949.

About the Authors

Amie McCord Brooks, PharmD, FCCP, BCPS, is an associate professor of pharmacy practice at the St. Louis College of Pharmacy and a clinical pharmacy specialist in ambulatory care at St. Louis County Department of Health. Dr. Brooks is the program director for a PGY1 residency program, a board-certified pharmacotherapy specialist, and a fellow of the American College of Clinical Pharmacy. She received her Doctor of Pharmacy degree from the St. Louis College of Pharmacy and completed her pharmacy residency training at the Jefferson Barracks VA Medical Center in St. Louis, Missouri. Her research interests include clinical pharmacy services, diabetes, resistant hypertension, and collaborative practice.

Cynthia Sanoski, BS, PharmD, FCCP, BCPS, is the chair of the department of pharmacy practice at the Jefferson School of Pharmacy at Thomas Jefferson University. Dr. Sanoski received her Doctor of Pharmacy degree from Ohio State University, and subsequently completed a 2-year fellowship in cardiovascular pharmacotherapy at the University of Illinois at Chicago. She is also a board-certified pharmacotherapy specialist and a fellow of the American College of Clinical Pharmacy. Dr. Sanoski serves as an instructor with Kaplan Medical, teaching NAPLEX review courses for graduating pharmacy students across the country.

Emily Hajjar, PharmD, BCPS, BCACP, CGP, is associate professor in the Jefferson School of Pharmacy at Thomas Jefferson University in Philadelphia, Pennsylvania. Dr. Hajjar earned her PharmD at Duquesne University. She completed a pharmacy practice residency at the University of Rochester Medical Center in Rochester, New York, a geriatric pharmacy specialty residency at the Minneapolis Veteran's Affairs Medical Center, and a geriatric pharmacotherapy-epidemiology fellowship at the University of Minnesota, College of Pharmacy. Dr. Hajjar provides clinical services to the Jefferson Family and Community Medicine Senior Center Practice and the Kimmel Cancer Center Senior Adult Oncology and Outpatient Palliative Care clinics. Her research interests include geriatric pharmacotherapy and polypharmacy.

Brian R. Overholser, PharmD, FCCP, is associate professor of pharmacy practice in the College of Pharmacy at Purdue University and Adjunct Associate Professor in the Division of Clinical Pharmacology at the Indiana University School of Medicine in Indianapolis, Indiana. Dr. Overholser earned his PharmD and conducted his postdoctoral research in pharmacokinetics and pharmacodynamics at Purdue University. His primary teaching responsibilities include courses in pharmacokinetics, pharmacodynamics, and pharmacogenetics at both Purdue and Indiana University. Dr. Overholser's research program is focused on elucidating the pathological regulation that increases the susceptibility of arrhythmias in patients with heart failure.

The authors wish to thank the following test item writers: LeAnn C. Boyd, PharmD, BCPS, CDE; Elizabeth Langan, MD; Amy Egras, PharmD, BCPS; Stacey Thacker, PharmD; and Arneka Tillman, PharmD candidate, Xavier University College of Pharmacy.

The authors also wish to thank the following individuals for serving as expert reviewers: Rebecca Bragg, PharmD, BCPS, Assistant Professor St. Louis College of Pharmacy; and Ashley H. Vincent, PharmD, BCACP, BCPS, Clinical Assistant Professor, Purdue University College of Pharmacy. The authors would also like to acknowledge the contributions of Karen Nagel, BS Pharm, PhD, and Steven T. Boyd, PharmD, BCPS, CDE.

Table of Contents

PART ONE

Overview

How to Use This Book

Congratulations! You've taken the first step to prepare yourself for the NAPLEX®. This book contains the information you want and need to do your best.

The authors are proud to release the 2015 edition of this NAPLEX® review book, which incorporates readers' feedback. The edition has been updated throughout with current drug information and Top 200 drugs as determined by the authors.

REVIEW STRUCTURE

This content of this book is designed to provide a concentrated and concise review of the competency areas tested on the exam. This book is not intended to replace standard textbooks in pharmacy. Rather, it should serve as a primary tool in the weeks and months prior to taking the exam. Since it is not practical to re-read textbooks, you will need a resource that will provide concise, focused review. This book fills that need.

Kaplan suggests that areas in which you feel weakest should be studied first; in this way, you can spend additional review time on difficult concepts.

This book covers all of the areas tested on the NAPLEX® and features an efficient time-management tool to ensure adequate preparation. Each chapter includes a *suggested study time*, prepared by the authors. These are only suggested rates; certainly, the study rate will vary based on your own level of comfort with the subject matter. By gauging yourself, however, you will be able to practice for test day, when your time on the computer will be limited.

The review is arranged by disease states, focusing on the following:

- Definitions of the disease
- Diagnosis
- Signs and symptoms
- Guidelines
- Guidelines summary

- Medication charts
- Storage & administration pearls
- Patient education pearls

Each chapter also contains a few practice questions, allowing you to apply the information you have just reviewed.

PRACTICE TESTS

The NAPLEX® is a computer-adaptive examination consisting of 185 questions. To assist you in preparing for the test-taking experience, this book offers two complete practice examinations of 185 questions each. One practice exam, along with answer explanations, is included in the text of this book. A second test is available online.

Practice Test 1 should be taken prior to the beginning of your study period. Then, use the results to identify areas of strength and weakness and to tailor an individualized study plan. For example, if you score below average on questions related to oncology therapeutics, plan to spend some additional days studying this subject. Likewise, if cardiovascular therapeutics was the area in which you scored the highest, you may want to leave this section for last.

Both practice tests should be taken in quiet areas—dedicate 4 hours and 15 minutes for each test. It is advisable to take the practice exam somewhere with limited distractions, such as a library. The goal is to simulate examlike conditions and to obtain data that will help structure an effective study plan.

As you work through the items, pay particular attention to the explanations. Often, studying the explanations is one of the most valuable study resources. Note that for difficult questions, explanations have been provided that explain the reasoning for not choosing the incorrect answer choices. Use this information to understand the rationale behind eliminating each distracter. The online companion to this book includes animated flashcards to help you with self-assessment on the material prior to the final practice test.

Finally, take Practice Test 2 a week or two prior to your exam date. Test 2 should be taken once the majority of your study has been completed. Test 2 is provided as an online companion to this book and also contains 185 unique questions. Our intention—and our hope—is that this book will be an integral part of your preparation for the NAPLEX®.

ACCESSING THE ONLINE COMPANION:

kaptest.com/booksonline

As owner of this guide, you are entitled to get more practice online. Log on to kaptest.com/booksonline to access the second full-length practice test.

Just as in the book, the 185-question practice test includes detailed answer explanations. Access to online NAPLEX® practice material is free of charge to purchasers of this book. You'll be asked for a specific password derived from the text in this book, so have your book handy when you log on.

Best of luck to you on your journey toward a successful career as a pharmacist!

For Any Test Changes or Late-Breaking Developments

kaptest.com/publishing

The material in this book is up-to-date at the time of publication. However, the NABP® may have instituted changes in the test after this book was published. Be sure to carefully read the materials you receive when you register for the test. If there are any important late-breaking developments—or any changes or corrections to the Kaplan test preparation materials in this book—we will post that information online at kaptest.com/publishing.

Introduction and Test-Taking Strategies

WHAT IS THE NAPLEX®?

NAPLEX stands for North American Pharmacist Licensure Examination. The NAPLEX is issued by the National Association of Boards of Pharmacy (NABP®) and is utilized by the boards of pharmacy as part of their assessment of competence to practice pharmacy. NABP represents each of the 50 states in the United States, the District of Columbia, and the five major U. S. territories. South Africa, New Zealand, Australia, and Canada also utilize the NAPLEX for licensure.

These boards of pharmacy have a mandate to protect the public from unsafe and ineffective pharmacy care, and each board has been given responsibility to regulate the practice of pharmacy in its respective state. In fact, the NAPLEX is often referred to as "The Boards" or "State Boards."

Each state requires applicants to take and pass the NAPLEX in order to obtain a license to practice as a registered pharmacist. The NAPLEX has only one purpose: to determine if it is safe for you to begin practicing as an entry-level pharmacist.

To take the NAPLEX, you must meet the eligibility requirements of the board of pharmacy from which you seek licensure. The board will determine your eligibility in accordance with the jurisdiction's requirements. If you are determined to be eligible, the board will notify NABP of your eligibility. Once that happens, a letter will be issued to you by Pearson VUE, the test administrator, with information about how to schedule your testing appointment.

CONTENT AND STRUCTURE

The NAPLEX is a computer-adaptive test that consists of 185 multiple-choice questions. Of these, 150 questions will be used to calculate your test score. The remaining 35 items serve as experimental questions and do not affect your score.

The NAPLEX is not a test of achievement or intelligence, nor is it designed for pharmacists with years of experience. The questions do not involve high-tech clinical pharmacy or equipment. Note, too, that you will not be tested on all the content you were taught in pharmacy school.

Many of the questions on the NAPLEX are asked in a scenario-based format (i.e., patient profiles with accompanying test questions). To properly analyze and answer the questions, you must refer to the information provided in the patient profile. Other questions are answered solely from the information provided in the question.

There is also a combined-response type question, otherwise called the K question. This type of question includes three Roman-numeral choices. For example:

Ideally, Lovastatin affects blood lipids by which of the following?

    I. Increasing HDLs
   II. Decreasing LDLs
  III. Decreasing triglycerides

The standard response format is typically:

  (A) I only
  (B) III only
  (C) I and II only
  (D) II and III only
  (E) I, II, and III

K questions can seem confusing if you haven't tackled them before. These are actually a series of true/false questions packaged together. For each question, focus on whether each of the three given statements (I, II, and III) is true or false.

Over the past few years, the number of K questions has been declining on the NAPLEX, and they are being replaced by questions in various other formats. These other formats on the NAPLEX include the following:

  (1)   multiple choice
  (2)   multiple response
  (3)   constructed response
  (4)   ordered response
  (5)   hot-spot

Each format is described with examples in the sections that follow. Note that the examples provided are to demonstrate the question structure rather than to stress NAPLEX content.

Multiple-Choice Format

The multiple-choice format has been used historically on the NAPLEX and remains a mainstay of the exam. An example of a multiple-choice question is provided:

Which of the following is most likely a symptom of digoxin overdose and toxicity?

(A) Ototoxicity
(B) Hepatotoxicity
(C) Visual disturbances
(D) Renal failure
(E) Dizziness

Multiple-Response Format

The multiple-response format is likely designed to replace the traditional K-style questions on the NAPLEX. The premise of these questions is very similar to K questions, but more options are available. Similar to the K questions, these can be broken down into a series of true and false statements. The test-taker's goal is to identify all the true statements. An example multiple-response question is provided:

Which of the following could alter a patient's response to warfarin? (Select **ALL** that apply.)

(A) Increased intake of charred meats
(B) New prescription for amiodarone
(C) Increased intake of vitamin D
(D) Acute hepatic failure
(E) New prescription for fexofenadine

Constructed-Response Format

The constructed-response format is simply a fill-in-the-blank style of question. Although the NABP has not given much guidance regarding the use of these questions, the examples they have provided have largely been calculation questions answered to the nearest whole number. In the examples provided by the NABP, the units of the final answer have been stated in the question, as in the constructed-response example here:

The "Sig" for a prednisone prescription is "25 mg today, 10 mg bid for 2 days, 5 mg bid for 3 days, then 5 mg qd for 1 week." How many 5-mg tablets should be dispensed?

(Answer must be numeric; round the final answer to the nearest **WHOLE** number.)

Ordered-Response Format

The ordered-response format is designed for the test taker to assign ranks to an unordered list of options. The NABP has listed a sample question in this format to rank topical corticosteroids from highest to lowest potencies. Another example of an ordered-response question is provided:

Rank the following HMG-CoA reductase inhibitors from highest to lowest potency. (**ALL** options must be used.)

Unordered Options   **Ordered Response**

Atorvastatin 20 mg

Fluvastatin 20 mg

Pravastatin 40 mg

Rosuvastatin 20 mg

Hot-Spot Format

The hot-spot format is designed for the test taker to identify the correct portion of a diagram that is related to the question presented. The NABP NAPLEX-MPJE registration guide presents a sample question in this format. The question displays a diagram of the HIV life cycle and asks the test taker to identify the portion of the life cycle during which maraviroc exerts its mechanism of action. Another example of a hot-spot question is provided here:

Using the diagram below, identify where on a ventricular action potential ibutilide would exert the greatest effect. (Select the TEXT response, and left-click the mouse. To change your answer, move the cursor, select alternate TEXT response and click.)

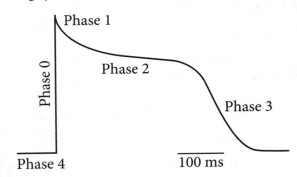

HOW IS THE NAPLEX SCORED, AND WHAT SCORE DO YOU NEED TO PASS?

Your NAPLEX score is a scaled score, not a number-correct score or a percentile score. The scoring scale ranges from 0 to 150. **The minimum passing score is 75.** The algorithms for determining your scaled score are highly confidential and are not released to the public.

Candidates who fail to answer at least 162 of the 185 questions will not receive any score. Since the computer format requires that you answer every question on the screen, the only way you could answer only 162 would be to stop short before the end of the exam. If you complete at least 162 questions but fewer than 185, you will receive a penalty, and your score will be adjusted to reflect the number of questions that remained unanswered. It is certainly in your best interest to answer all questions presented.

NABP will forward your NAPLEX score to the board of pharmacy from which you are seeking licensure. NABP **does not** provide scores to candidates, and score results **are not** released at the test center.

WHAT IF YOU FAIL THE NAPLEX?

First of all, it's unlikely you will fail. Be positive! Currently, the passage rate is approximately 93%. Candidates who receive a failing score on the NAPLEX will automatically be provided with a diagnostic report that indicates their relative performance in each major competency area. The board of pharmacy will notify the candidates of the NAPLEX results and diagnostic report.

THE CAT FORMAT

What Is a CAT?

A computer-adaptive test (CAT) is quite different from a paper-and-pencil test. Each CAT is assembled interactively based on the accuracy of the candidate's response to the questions. This ensures that the questions you are answering are not "too hard" or "too easy" for your skill level. Your first question may be relatively easy; that is, below the level of minimum competency. If you answer that question correctly, the computer will likely select a slightly more difficult question. If you answer the first question incorrectly, the computer may select a slightly easier question. By continuing to do this as you answer questions, the computer is able to calculate your level of competence. Despite this relatively simple-to-understand format, do not try to interpret how well you are performing based on the level of difficulty of the questions that you are being presented. The NAPLEX may not present easier questions immediately following an incorrect answer. Furthermore, the experimental questions may be intermingled. Therefore, although general understanding of the CAT format may serve you well, you will not be able to predict your performance based on that alone.

Because the CAT presents questions on the basis of your responses to previous questions, **you may not change an answer once you have confirmed an answer choice. Likewise, you may not go back to review a question once you have moved on to the next question.** You must answer **all** questions in the order in which they are presented, and you may not skip a question.

In a CAT, the questions are adapted to your ability level. The computer selects questions that represent all areas of pharmacy, as defined by the NAPLEX test plan and by the level of item difficulty. Each question is self-contained, so all of the information you need to answer a question is presented on the computer screen. This difficulty-level determination will then be used to calculate your score.

Strategies for Success with a CAT

1. There is a timer at the top of the computer screen to help you pace yourself. You can hide it if it distracts you—but since the test is timed, you might find it helpful for pacing. You have **4 hours and 15 minutes** to complete all 185 questions.

2. There is a 10-minute break at the 2-hour time point. Make sure to take that break! You need to rest your brain. And while the average candidate takes 2.5 to 3 hours to complete the exam, there are no bonus points for finishing early.

3. It is possible that questions involving mathematical calculations will be weighted more heavily than other questions. Spend extra time solving them, but try to limit yourself to a maximum of 5 or 6 minutes each, if time is a concern.

4. If a question calls for a calculation or a certain mechanism, scratch a rough image. Having a crude diagram to look at, rather than having to imagine it from the computer screen, will help you to see what you're dealing with. Such notes also often stimulate more recall.

5. Look for key words in questions. Words such as "most likely" may help you eliminate some choices even when you don't have comprehensive recall—the most likely choice is probably the one that is most familiar as you review the choices.

6. You cannot cross off an answer choice and banish it from your sight (it's on a computer screen, after all), so you have to be disciplined about not reconsidering choices you've already eliminated.

NAPLEX REGISTRATION

The NAPLEX is administered year-round on business days. There are several steps in registering for the exam. As of this printing, the fee for the exam is $505. (Also, be sure to check with your local board of pharmacy for its fees.)

- **First Step:**
  - Contact the board of pharmacy in the state in which you want to be licensed. The state board will issue paperwork and instructions that determine your eligibility, and will notify the NABP. You will then be issued an authorization to test (ATT), as well as other documents, including:
    - » Test authorization number
    - » Expiration date
    - » Range of dates during which you can take the NAPLEX
- **Second Step:**
  - Once you receive your authorization packet from the NABP, you can call or register online at Pearson VUE to choose your testing center to schedule your test date. You will need your ATT information to schedule a testing date.
  - For more information about registration, go to:
    - » NABP   http://www.nabp.net
    - » Pearson VUE   http://www.pearsonvue.com/

TAKING THE EXAM

There is no time limit for each individual question; however, you have a total of 4 hours and 15 minutes to complete the exam. This does not include the beginning tutorial or the 10-minute break given after the first 2 hours of testing.

Remember, every question counts. There is no warm-up time, so it is important for you to be ready to answer questions correctly from the very beginning. Concentration is also key. You need to give your best thinking to each question.

ON THE DAY OF THE EXAM

1. Arrive at the test center at least 30 minutes before your scheduled testing time to allow for check-in. If you arrive late, you may be required to forfeit your appointment. **If you forfeit your appointment, your testing fee will not be refunded.**

2. Bring two forms of identification: a picture ID that includes your signature and a second form of ID. You will be required to show these IDs for entry. Your thumbprint will also be required when you enter the testing room.

3. You will be provided with laminated note boards, which may be replaced as needed during testing. You will not be allowed to take your own scratch paper or pencil into the testing room.

4. An on-screen, five-function calculator can be activated during the test administration for your use. You may also request a hand-held, five-function calculator from the test administrator.

5. The seating time for the exam is 4 hours and 15 minutes with a 10-minute mandatory break after approximately 2 hours of testing time. Any voluntary breaks will be subtracted from your testing time.

NAPLEX BLUEPRINT

The questions on the NAPLEX involve integrated pharmacy content. The NAPLEX Competency Statements provide a blueprint of the topics covered on the exam. Reviewing these statements will assist you in preparation for the exam.

- **Competence Area 1:** Assess Pharmacotherapy to Assure Safe and Effective Therapeutic Outcomes (about 56% of exam)

- **Competence Area 2:** Assess Safe and Accurate Preparation and Dispensing of Medications (33% of exam)

- **Competence Area 3:** Assess, Recommend, and Provide Healthcare Information that Promotes Public Health (about 11% of exam)

For specific subcategories under each competence areas, go to **www.nabp.net**.

TEST-TAKING STRATEGIES

As you review each chapter in this book, it is important to focus on your own areas of weakness. To help you do so, keep the following in mind:

Key Steps toward Preparedness

- Assess your strengths and weaknesses. Review your weakest subjects first. The best way to identify your weaknesses is through practice exams.
- Focus heavily on the Top 200 drugs by unit. Use the online flashcard component that accompanies this book and spend extra time reviewing the Top 200. These are important.
- Practice calculations to increase your confidence.
- Schedule extra time before your testing date to revisit your weaker areas.
- Complete the practice test under real exam conditions.
- Order and complete the Pre-NAPLEX exam, available from NABP.
- When you review the practice exams, make sure you understand why your incorrect answer choices were incorrect.
- Be sure you understand why you missed a question. Did you simply forget a fact? Choose your answer too quickly? Misunderstand the question? Miss an important clue within the question? Finally, do you keep making the same mistakes over and over? If so, it is important to spend more time on those areas.

Guessing

During the exam, there are sure to be some questions that stump you. For those, just narrow down the choices and take your best guess. You don't want to spend too much time analyzing a question you do not know and then run out of time toward the end of the exam. Remember, you cannot simply leave a question blank, so in some shape or form, you'll have to take your best guess.

Keep in mind that 35 experimental questions are not calculated into your score, so if you answer a few questions incorrectly, it's possible that they won't be scored at all.

When you just don't know the answer: narrow the answer choices to two likely choices, then use the "upper, then lower" decision rule to select one of them. This rule means you alternate your guess, using the upper choice the first time you are stuck, then the lower choice the next time you are stuck. This technique helps keep you moving forward.

Positive Attitude

The most important decision you can make in your studying process is to have a positive attitude, especially on test day. Remember this:

- The odds are on your side; around 93% of pharmacy graduates pass the NAPLEX.
- This is a minimal competency exam.
- You spent a minimum of 6 years in school to become a pharmacist. If you did that, you can conquer this exam!

You **are** prepared, and this book is a tool to increase your confidence.

Part Two

Review of Therapeutics

Cardiovascular Disorders

1

This chapter covers the following diseases:

- **Hypertension**
- **Dyslipidemia**
- **Heart failure**
- **Antiarrhythmic drugs**
- **Antithrombotic drugs**
- **Ischemic heart disease**
- **Acute pharmacologic management of STEMI**

The text also provides an overview of the antiarrhythmic drugs and antithrombotic drugs commonly used in clinical practice.

 Suggested Study Time: **2.5 hours**

HYPERTENSION

Definitions

Hypertension (HTN) is defined as a systolic blood pressure (SBP) >140 mmHg, a diastolic blood pressure (DBP) >90 mmHg, or any patient requiring antihypertensive therapy. Most patients with HTN have primary (essential) HTN (due to an unknown cause, likely genetic), while less than 10% have secondary HTN (due to chronic kidney disease [CKD], pheochromocytoma, Cushing's syndrome, or medications [nonsteroidal anti-inflammatory drugs (NSAIDs), corticosteroids, cyclosporine, tacrolimus, estrogens, erythropoietin, venlafaxine, sympathomimetics, cocaine]).

Diagnosis

- Average of ≥2 blood pressure (BP) measurements ≥140/90 mmHg

Signs and Symptoms

- Can develop target organ damage with chronic, uncontrolled HTN:
  - Cardiac
    - » Angina, myocardial infarction (MI), history of coronary revascularization (e.g., percutaneous coronary intervention [PCI], coronary artery bypass graft [CABG] surgery), left ventricular hypertrophy (LVH), left ventricular (LV) dysfunction (i.e., heart failure with reduced ejection fraction [HFrEF])
  - Cerebrovascular
    - » Stroke, transient ischemic attack (TIA)
  - Renal
    - » CKD
  - Ophthalmologic
    - » Retinopathy, blindness
  - Vascular
    - » Peripheral arterial disease (PAD)

Guidelines

James PA, Oparil S, Carter BL, et al. 2014 evidence-based guideline for the management of high blood pressure in adults: report from the panel members appointed to the Eighth Joint National Committee (JNC 8). *JAMA* 2014;311:507–520.

Rosendorff C, Black HR, Cannon CP, et al; American Heart Association Council for High Blood Pressure Research; American Heart Association Council on Clinical Cardiology; American Heart Association Council on Epidemiology and Prevention. Treatment of hypertension in the prevention and management of ischemic heart disease: a scientific statement from the American Heart Association Council for High Blood Pressure Research and the Councils on Clinical Cardiology and Epidemiology and Prevention. *Circulation* 2007;115:2761–2788.

Kidney Disease: Improving Global Outcomes (KDIGO) Blood Pressure Work Group. KDIGO clinical practice guideline for the management of blood pressure in chronic kidney disease. *Kidney Int Suppl* 2012:337–414.

American Diabetes Association. Standards of medical care in diabetes—2014. *Diabetes Care* 2014;(37 suppl 1):S14–80.

Guidelines Summary

- General population <60 yr: <140/90 mmHg (JNC 8 guidelines)
- General population ≥60 yr: <150/90 mmHg (JNC 8 guidelines)

- CKD
  - <140/90 mmHg (JNC 8 guidelines)
  - Urine albumin excretion <30 mg/day: <140/90 mmHg (KDIGO guidelines)
  - Urine albumin excretion ≥30 mg/day: <130/80 mmHg (KDIGO guidelines)
- Diabetes mellitus (DM)
  - <140/90 mmHg (JNC8 guidelines)
  - <140/80 mmHg (American Diabetes Association guidelines)
- Known coronary artery disease (CAD) or CAD equivalent (e.g., carotid artery disease, peripheral arterial disease, abdominal aortic aneurysm), 10-year Framingham risk score ≥10%, stable/unstable angina (UA), or MI: <130/80 mmHg (American Heart Association guidelines)
- Lifestyle modifications: weight loss (goal body mass index [BMI] 18.5–24.9 kg/m^2), diet rich in fruits, vegetables, and low-fat dairy products with ↓ saturated and total fat, ↓ sodium (Na$^+$) intake (≤2.4 g/day), ↑ physical activity (30 minutes most days of the week), moderation of alcohol use (≤1 ounce of ethanol/day), smoking cessation
- Pharmacologic therapy:
  - Initial antihypertensive drug selection (JNC8 guidelines):
    » Nonblack patients (with or without DM): Thiazide diuretic, angiotensin-converting enzyme inhibitor (ACEI), angiotensin II receptor blocker (ARB), and/or calcium channel blocker (CCB)
    » Black patients (with or without DM): Thiazide diuretic and/or CCB
    » CKD (regardless of race or presence of DM): ACEI or ARB (alone or in combination with other drug class)
    » NOTE: β-blockers are no longer considered first-line therapy for patients with HTN without specific comorbidities (see below)
  - Presence of other comorbidities may warrant selection of other agents as first-line antihypertensive therapy (based on guidelines for each of these conditions):
    » HFrEF: Diuretic, ACEI, β-blocker (carvedilol, metoprolol succinate, or bisoprolol), ARB, aldosterone receptor antagonist (ARA), hydralazine/isosorbide dinitrate (for black patients)
    » Post-MI: β-blocker, ACEI (or ARB)
    » High coronary disease risk: ACEI (or ARB), thiazide diuretic, CCB
    » Recurrent stroke prevention: ACEI, diuretic
  - Approaches for initiation and titration of antihypertensive therapy:
    » Initiate one antihypertensive drug → Titrate to maximum dose to achieve goal BP → If goal BP not achieved, add second antihypertensive drug → Titrate dose of second drug to maximum → If goal BP still not achieved, add third antihypertensive drug
      – Avoid concomitant use of ACEI and ARB

» Initiate one antihypertensive drug → If goal BP not achieved, add second antihypertensive drug before maximum dose of initial drug achieved → If goal BP not achieved, titrate doses of both drugs up to maximum → If goal BP still not achieved, add third antihypertensive drug

– Avoid concomitant use of ACEI and ARB

» Initiate two antihypertensive drugs at same time (avoid concomitant use of ACEI and ARB) → If goal BP not achieved, titrate doses of both drugs up to maximum → If goal BP still not achieved, add third antihypertensive drug

– Initial two-drug approach should be considered when: BP >160 mmHg and/or DBP >100 mmHg **OR** SBP is >20 mmHg and/or DBP is >10 mmHg above goal

Diuretics

Generic	Brand	Dose	Contra-indications	Primary Side Effects	Key Monitoring	Pertinent Drug Interactions	Med Pearl	Top 200
Thiazide Diuretics – inhibit Na$^+$ reabsorption in the distal convoluted tubule								
Chlorothiazide	Diuril	500–2,000 mg/day	Sulfa allergy	• Hypokalemia • Hypomagnesemia • Hyponatremia • Hypercalcemia • Hyperglycemia • Hyperuricemia • Photosensitivity	• BP • Electrolytes • Blood urea nitrogen (BUN)/serum creatinine (SCr) • Blood glucose • Uric acid	• May ↑ risk of lithium toxicity • May ↓ effect of antidiabetic agents • NSAIDs ↓ antihypertensive effects	• Often used as 1st-line therapy for HTN • Synergistic effect with other antihypertensives • Not effective (except metolazone) when CrCl <30 mL/min; use loop diuretics • Have ceiling dose (unlike loop diuretics)	No
Chlorthalidone	Thalitone	12.5–100 mg/day						Yes
Hydrochlorothiazide	Microzide	12.5–50 mg/day						Yes
Indapamide	Only available generically	1.25–5 mg/day						No
Metolazone	Zaroxolyn	2.5–5 mg/day						Yes

Loop Diuretics – inhibit Na$^+$ reabsorption in the ascending limb of loop of Henle (should only be used for HTN in patients with renal insufficiency [maintain efficacy when CrCl <30 mL/min], severe edema, or HF) (see HF section for further details)

Potassium-Sparing Diuretics – inhibit Na$^+$ reabsorption in the collecting ducts

Generic	Brand	Dose	Contra-indications	Primary Side Effects	Key Monitoring	Pertinent Drug Interactions	Med Pearl	Top 200
Amiloride	Only available generically	5–10 mg/day	• Hyperkalemia • CKD	Hyperkalemia	• BP • Potassium (K$^+$) • BUN/SCr	Use with K$^+$ supplements, ACEIs, ARBs, ARAs, or NSAIDs may ↑ risk of hyperkalemia	• Not used often as monotherapy (weak antihypertensives) • Often used with hydrochlorothiazide to ↓ K$^+$ loss	No
Triamterene	Dyrenium	50–100 mg/day						No

Combination products:
Triamterene/hydrochlorothiazide (Dyazide, Maxzide)
Amiloride/hydrochlorothiazide (only available generically)

Aldosterone Receptor Antagonists – have similar mechanism of action to K$^+$-sparing diuretics (also block the effects of aldosterone) (not used often for HTN) (see HF section for further details)

Combination products:
Spironolactone/hydrochlorothiazide (Aldactazide)

β-Blockers

Mechanism of action – ↓ cardiac output (CO) by negative inotropic (↓ contractility) and negative chronotropic (↓ heart rate [HR]) effects

- Cardioselective – bind more to β_1 than β_2 receptors (at low doses); less likely to cause bronchoconstriction or vasoconstriction at low doses (safer to use in patients with asthma, chronic obstructive pulmonary disease [COPD], PAD, or DM); cardioselectivity may be lost at higher doses
  - Bisoprolol, atenolol, metoprolol, betaxolol, acebutolol, nebivolol (BAMBAN)
- Intrinsic sympathomimetic activity (ISA) – have partial β-receptor agonist activity
  - Carteolol, acebutolol, pindolol, penbutolol (CAPP)
- Lipophilic vs. hydrophilic – lipophilic (propranolol, metoprolol, carvedilol, labetalol, pindolol, nebivolol) more likely to cause central nervous system (CNS) side effects (e.g., depression, fatigue) than hydrophilic (atenolol)

Generic	Brand	Dose	Contraindications	Primary Side Effects	Key Monitoring	Pertinent Drug Interactions	Med Pearl	Top 200
Cardioselective:								
Acebutolol	Sectral	200–1,200 mg/day	• ≥2nd degree heart block (in absence of pacemaker) • HF (except metoprolol succinate or bisoprolol)	• Bradycardia/heart block • HF exacerbation • Bronchospasm • Cold extremities • Fatigue • ↓ exercise tolerance • Depression • Glucose intolerance • Mask hypoglycemia (in patients with DM)	• BP • HR • S/S HF • Blood glucose (in patients with DM)	Use with other negative chronotropes (e.g., digoxin, verapamil, diltiazem, or clonidine) may ↑ risk of bradycardia	Abrupt discontinuation may cause angina, MI, or hypertensive emergency; need to taper over 2 wks	No
Atenolol	Tenormin	25–100 mg/day						Yes
Betaxolol	Kerlone	5–20 mg/day						No
Bisoprolol	Zebeta	2.5–20 mg/day						No
Metoprolol	• Tartrate: Lopressor (2 × daily) • Succinate: Toprol XL (1 × daily)	25–400 mg/day						Yes
Nebivolol	Bystolic	5–40 mg/day						Yes
Nonselective:								
Carvedilol	• Coreg • Coreg CR	Immediate-release (IR): 12.5–50 mg/day (in two divided doses) Controlled-release (CR): 20–80 mg/day (1 × daily)	• ≥2nd degree heart block (in absence of pacemaker) • HF (except carvedilol)	Same as with selective β-blockers	Same as with selective β-blockers	Same as with selective β-blockers	• Same as with selective β-blockers • Labetalol and carvedilol also have α_1-blocking properties	Yes
Labetalol	Trandate	200–2,400 mg/day						No
Nadolol	Corgard	20–320 mg/day						No
Pindolol	Only available generically	5–60 mg/day						No
Propranolol	• Inderal • Inderal LA • InnoPran XL	80–640 mg/day (IR given 2–3 × daily; extended-release [ER] given 1 × daily)						Yes
Timolol	Only available generically	20–60 mg/day						No

Combination products:
Atenolol/chlorthalidone (Tenoretic)
Bisoprolol/hydrochlorothiazide (Ziac)
Nadolol/bendroflumethiazide (Corzide)
Propranolol/hydrochlorothiazide (Inderide)
Metoprolol tartrate/hydrochlorothiazide (Lopressor HCT)
Metoprolol succinate/hydrochlorothiazide (Dutoprol)

Angiotensin-Converting Enzyme Inhibitors

Mechanism of action – inhibit angiotensin-converting enzyme and prevent the conversion of angiotensin I to angiotensin II → vasodilation; ↓ aldosterone production; also inhibit degradation of bradykinin

Generic	Brand	Dose	Contraindications	Primary Side Effects	Key Monitoring	Pertinent Drug Interactions	Med Pearl	Top 200
Benazepril	Lotensin	5–40 mg/day	• Pregnancy • History of angioedema or renal failure with prior use • Hyperkalemia • Bilateral renal artery stenosis	• Hyperkalemia • Renal insufficiency • Cough (dry) • Angioedema	• BP • BUN/SCr • K+	• Use with ARBs, K+ supplements, K+-sparing diuretics, ARAs, or NSAIDs may ↑ risk of hyperkalemia • May ↑ risk of lithium toxicity	• Captopril has shortest duration of action • Enalapril also available as oral solution (Epaned) and injection (enalaprilat) • If patient has intolerable dry cough, may switch to ARB • Hyperkalemia and renal insufficiency also likely to occur with ARBs (risk of angioedema cross-sensitivity with ARBs controversial)	Yes
Captopril	Capoten	12.5–450 mg/day						No
Enalapril	Vasotec	2.5–40 mg/day						Yes
Fosinopril	Only available generically	5–80 mg/day						Yes
Lisinopril	Prinivil, Zestril	2.5–40 mg/day						Yes
Moexipril	Univasc	3.75–30 mg/day						No
Perindopril	Aceon	4–16 mg/day						No
Quinapril	Accupril	10–80 mg/day						Yes
Ramipril	Altace	1.25–20 mg/day						Yes
Trandolapril	Mavik	0.5–4 mg/day						Yes

Combination products:

Benazepril/amlodipine (Lotrel)
Benazepril/hydrochlorothiazide (Lotensin HCT)
Captopril/hydrochlorothiazide (only available generically)
Enalapril/hydrochlorothiazide (Vaseretic)
Fosinopril/hydrochlorothiazide (only available generically)
Lisinopril/hydrochlorothiazide (Prinzide, Zestoretic)
Moexipril/hydrochlorothiazide (Uniretic)
Quinapril/hydrochlorothiazide (Accuretic)
Trandolapril/verapamil (Tarka)

Angiotensin II Receptor Blockers

Mechanism of action – inhibit the binding of angiotensin II to the angiotensin type 1 (AT_1) receptor → vasodilation, ↓ aldosterone production; no effect on bradykinin

Generic	Brand	Dose	Contraindications	Primary Side Effects	Key Monitoring	Pertinent Drug Interactions	Med Pearl	Top 200
Azilsartan	Edarbi	40–80 mg/day	Same as for ACEIs	• Same as for ACEIs (except no cough) • Sprue-like enteropathy (olmesartan)	Same as for ACEIs	• Use with ACEIs, K^+ supplements, K^+-sparing diuretics, ARAs, or NSAIDs may ↑ risk of hyperkalemia • May ↑ risk of lithium toxicity	Hyperkalemia and renal insufficiency also likely to occur with ACEIs (risk of angioedema cross-sensitivity with ACEIs is controversial)	No
Candesartan	Atacand	4–32 mg/day						No
Eprosartan	Teveten	400–800 mg/day						No
Irbesartan	Avapro	75–300 mg/day						Yes
Losartan	Cozaar	25–100 mg/day						Yes
Olmesartan	Benicar	20–40 mg/day						Yes
Telmisartan	Micardis	20–80 mg/day						Yes
Valsartan	Diovan	80–320 mg/day						Yes

Combination products:
Azilsartan/chlorthalidone (Edarbyclor)
Candesartan/hydrochlorothiazide (Atacand HCT)
Eprosartan/hydrochlorothiazide (Teveten HCT)
Irbesartan/hydrochlorothiazide (Avalide)
Losartan/hydrochlorothiazide (Hyzaar)
Olmesartan/amlodipine (Azor)
Olmesartan/amlodipine/hydrochlorothiazide (Tribenzor)
Olmesartan/hydrochlorothiazide (Benicar HCT)
Telmisartan/amlodipine (Twynsta)
Telmisartan/hydrochlorothiazide (Micardis HCT)
Valsartan/amlodipine (Exforge)
Valsartan/hydrochlorothiazide (Diovan HCT)
Valsartan/amlodipine/hydrochlorothiazide (Exforge HCT)

Renin Inhibitor

Mechanism of action – inhibits renin and prevents the conversion of angiotensinogen to angiotensin I, which then ↓ production of angiotensin II

Generic	Brand	Dose	Contraindications	Primary Side Effects	Key Monitoring	Pertinent Drug Interactions	Med Pearl	Top 200
Aliskiren	Tekturna	150–300 mg/day	• Pregnancy • History of ACEI- or ARB-induced angioedema • Hyperkalemia • Bilateral renal artery stenosis	• Headache • Dizziness • Diarrhea • May also cause hyperkalemia and renal insufficiency	• BP • BUN/SCr • K^+	• Use with ACEIs, ARBs, K^+ supplements, K^+-sparing diuretics, ARAs, or NSAIDs may ↑ risk of hyperkalemia or renal impairment • Itraconazole or cyclosporine may ↑ effects; avoid concurrent use • May ↓ effects of furosemide	• Use with caution in patients with CrCl <30 mL/min • Avoid taking with high-fat meals • Avoid use with ARB or ACEI in patients with diabetes mellitus or moderate renal impairment	Yes

Combination products:
Aliskiren/amlodipine (Tekamlo)
Aliskiren/amlodipine/hydrochlorothizide (Amturnide)
Aliskiren/hydrochlorothiazide (Tekturna HCT)

Calcium Channel Blockers

Generic	Brand	Dose	Contra-indications	Primary Side Effects	Key Monitoring	Pertinent Drug Interactions	Med Pearl	Top 200
Mechanism of action – bind to L-type channels in heart and coronary/peripheral arteries to block inward movement of calcium (Ca^{2+}) → vascular smooth-muscle relaxation (vasodilation); all (except for amlodipine and felodipine) have negative inotropic effects (↓ contractility) • Dihydropyridines (DHPs) – more selective to vasculature; more potent vasodilators; have no effect on cardiac conduction • Non-DHPs – cause less peripheral vasodilation than DHPs; have negative chronotropic properties (↓ HR)								
DHPs:								
Amlodipine	Norvasc	2.5–10 mg/day	None	• Reflex tachycardia • Headache • Flushing • Peripheral edema • Gingival hyperplasia • HF exacerbation (except amlodipine and felodipine)	• BP • HR • S/S HF	• CYP3A4 substrate • CYP3A4 inhibitors may ↑ effects • CYP3A4 inducers may ↓ effects	• Sublingual nifedipine should not be used → may ↑ risk of MI, death • Do not use grapefruit juice • Nicardipine also available as injection	Yes
Felodipine	Plendil	2.5–20 mg/day						Yes
Isradipine	Only available generically	5–10 mg/day						No
Nicardipine	• Cardene • Cardene SR	60–120 mg/day (IR given 3 × daily; sustained-release [SR] given 2 × daily)						No
Nifedipine	• Adalat CC • Afeditab CR • Nifediac CC • Nifedical XL • Procardia XL	30–180 mg/day						Yes
Nisoldipine	Sular	ER: 10–40 mg/day Geomatrix: 17–34 mg/day						No
Non-DHPs:								
Diltiazem	• Cardizem CD • Cardizem LA • Cartia XT • Dilacor XR • Taztia XT • Tiazac	120–540 mg/day	• ≥2nd degree heart block (in absence of pacemaker) • Systolic HF	• Bradycardia/heart block • Constipation • Peripheral edema • Gingival hyperplasia • HF exacerbation	Same as for DHPs	• Same as for DHPs • Use with other negative chronotropes (e.g., digoxin, β-blockers, or clonidine) may ↑ risk of bradycardia • May ↑ effect/ toxicity of CYP3A4 substrates • May ↑ risk of digoxin toxicity	Do not use grapefruit juice	Yes
Verapamil	• Calan • Calan SR • Isoptin SR • Verelan • Verelan PM	120–360 mg/day (IR given 2–3 × daily, SR given 1–2 × daily)						Yes

α₁-Receptor Antagonists

Mechanism of action – block the α₁ receptor on peripheral blood vessels → arterial and venous vasodilation

Generic	Brand	Dose	Contraindications	Primary Side Effects	Key Monitoring	Pertinent Drug Interactions	Med Pearl	Top 200
Doxazosin	Cardura	1–16 mg/day	Should not be used with phosphodiesterase (PDE)-5 inhibitors (e.g., sildenafil, tadalafil, vardenafil) → ↑ risk of hypotension	• Orthostatic hypotension • Reflex tachycardia • Peripheral edema • Headache • Drowsiness	• BP • HR	↑ risk of hypotension with PDE-5 inhibitors (avoid concurrent use)	• Take dose at bedtime to minimize risk of orthostatic hypotension • ALLHAT trial → 25% ↑ in cardiovascular events with doxazosin • Also used for benign prostatic hyperplasia	Yes
Prazosin	Minipress	1–20 mg/day						No
Terazosin	Only available generically	1–20 mg/day						Yes

Central α₂-Receptor Agonists

Mechanism of action – stimulate α₂ receptors in brain → ↓ sympathetic outflow (release of norepinephrine) → ↓ BP and HR

Generic	Brand	Dose	Contraindications	Primary Side Effects	Key Monitoring	Pertinent Drug Interactions	Med Pearl	Top 200
Clonidine	• Catapres • Catapres-TTS	Oral: 0.2–2.4 mg/day Transdermal: 0.1–0.3 mg weekly		• Sedation • Orthostatic hypotension • Depression • Peripheral edema • Dry mouth • Bradycardia • Hepatitis (methyldopa)	• BP • HR • Liver function tests (LFTs) (methyldopa)	Use with other negative chronotropes (e.g., digoxin, verapamil, diltiazem, or β-blockers) may ↑ risk of bradycardia	• Clonidine patch should be applied once weekly • Abrupt discontinuation (especially in presence of β-blockers) may cause angina, MI, or hypertensive emergency; need to taper over 2 wks • When starting clonidine patch, overlap with oral for 2–3 days, then discontinue oral • Should not be used as first-line therapy • Clonidine also available as epidural injection (for pain) • Methyldopa safe to use in pregnant women with HIV	Yes
Methyldopa	Only available generically	250–1,000 mg/day	Methyldopa: Liver disease					No

Direct Vasodilators

Generic	Brand	Dose	Contra-indications	Primary Side Effects	Key Monitoring	Pertinent Drug Interactions	Med Pearl	Top 200
Mechanism of action – ↑ cyclic GMP → arterial vasodilation								
Hydralazine	Only available generically	25–300 mg/day	• Acute MI • Aortic dissection	• Reflex tachycardia • Orthostatic hypotension • Peripheral edema • Lupus-like syndrome (hydralazine) • Hirsutism (minoxidil)	• BP • HR • S/S lupus (e.g., stabbing chest pain, joint pain, fever, rash)	None	• Should not be used as 1st-line therapy • Minoxidil is usually absolutely last-line therapy (because of side effects) • Hydralazine also available as injection • Minoxidil also available as topical solution/foam	No
Minoxidil	Only available generically	2.5–100 mg/day						No

Storage and Administration Pearls

- When initiating antihypertensive drug therapy in the elderly, initiate at a low dose and slowly titrate to achieve goal BP ("start low and go slow").

Patient Education Pearls

- Diuretics should be taken in the morning to avoid nocturia. Patients receiving diuretics should wear sunscreen and protective clothing. Also, they should report any episodes of muscle cramps, as this may be a symptom of hypokalemia or hypomagnesemia.
- Patients receiving K^+-sparing diuretics, ARAs, ACEIs, ARBs, or aliskiren should avoid excessive intake of foods high in K^+ (e.g., green leafy vegetables, potatoes, apricots, bananas, dates, oranges, avocados) and K^+-containing salt substitutes.
- α_1-receptor antagonists should be taken at bedtime to minimize the risk of developing orthostatic hypotension.
- Patients receiving α_1-receptor antagonists, α_2-receptor agonists, or direct vasodilators should rise slowly from a sitting position.
- Patients receiving ACEIs or ARBs should call 911 immediately if he/she experiences lip, tongue, or facial swelling or has difficulty breathing.
- ACEIs, ARBs, and aliskiren should be avoided in pregnant patients. Antihypertensive drugs that can be safely used in pregnancy include methyldopa, labetalol, or CCBs.

DYSLIPIDEMIA

Definitions

Dyslipidemia can refer to any lipid disorder including ↑ total cholesterol (TC), low-density lipoprotein cholesterol (LDL-C), and triglycerides (TGs), and ↓ high-density lipoprotein cholesterol (HDL-C). Dyslipidemia can predispose patients to the development of cardiovascular disease, cerebrovascular disease, or PAD. While most forms of dyslipidemia are due to genetic factors, certain drugs may also cause elevated lipid concentrations, including β-blockers, diuretics, corticosteroids, isotretinoin, protease inhibitors, cyclosporine, and estrogens.

Diagnosis

- Fasting lipid profile should be obtained in adults ≥20 years every 5 years.
- The Friedewald LDL equation (applies if TG <400 mg/dL) is LDL = TC – (HDL-C + TG/5).
- Factors that need to be considered when evaluating whether or not a patient is a candidate for statin therapy:
  - Presence of clinical atherosclerotic cardiovascular disease (ASCVD)
    - » Acute coronary syndromes (ACS), history of MI, stable/unstable angina, coronary or other arterial revascularization, stroke/TIA, or PAD
  - Age
  - LDL-C level
  - Presence of DM
  - 10-year ASCVD risk
    - » Do NOT need to estimate risk in patients with ASCVD or LDL-C ≥190 mg/dL
    - » Do NOT need to calculate on exam; however, should know implications of various risk categories

Signs and Symptoms

- Most patients with dyslipidemias are asymptomatic until a significant degree of atherosclerosis occurs.
- Complications of dyslipidemias may include MI, stroke, PAD, erectile dysfuction, and sudden cardiac death.

Guidelines

Stone NJ, Robinson JG, Lichtenstein AH, et al. 2013 ACC/AHA guideline on the treatment of blood cholesterol to reduce atherosclerotic cardiovascular risk in adults: a report of the American College of Cardiology/American Heart Association Task Force on Practice Guidelines. *Circulation* 2014;129(25 suppl 2):S1–45.

Guidelines Summary

- Achievement of specific LDL-C goals is *no longer* recommended in the most recent dyslipidemia guidelines.
- Four groups most likely to benefit from statin therapy are listed here:
  - Clinical ASCVD (secondary prevention)
  - LDL-C ≥190 mg/dL (primary prevention)
  - Age 40–75 yr with DM **AND** LDL-C 70–189 mg/dL (primary prevention)

- Age 40–75 yr without clinical ASCVD or DM, and with LDL-C 70–189 mg/dL and 10-yr ASCVD risk ≥7.5%
- Heart-healthy lifestyle habits should be encouraged for all patients.
- Pharmacologic therapy:
  - Statin therapy recommendations for four major benefit groups:

Major Benefit Groups	Statin Therapy Recommendations
Clinical ASCVD	• Age ≤75 yr → High-intensity statin therapy • Age >75 yr **OR** if not a candidate for high-intensity statin therapy → Moderate-intensity statin therapy
LDL-C ≥190 mg/dL	High-intensity statin therapy (moderate-intensity if not candidate for high-intensity therapy)
Age 40–75 yr with DM **AND** LDL-C 70–189 mg/dL	• 10-yr ASCVD risk <7.5% → Moderate-intensity statin therapy • 10-yr ASCVD risk ≥7.5% → High-intensity statin therapy
Age 40–75 yr without clinical ASCVD or DM, and with LDL-C 70–189 mg/dL and 10-yr ASCVD risk ≥7.5%	Moderate–high intensity statin therapy

- High- versus moderate-intensity statin therapy
  - » High-intensity: ↓ LDL-C by ≥50%
    - Atorvastatin 40–80 mg daily
    - Rosuvastatin 20–40 mg daily
  - » Moderate-intensity: ↓ LDL-C by 30–<50%
    - Atorvastatin 10–20 mg daily
    - Rosuvastatin 5–10 mg daily
    - Simvastatin 20–40 mg daily
    - Pravastatin 40–80 mg daily
    - Lovastatin 40 mg daily
    - Fluvastatin XL 80 mg daily
    - Fluvastatin 40 mg twice daily
    - Pitavastatin 2–4 mg daily
- Nonstatin therapy can be considered in selected high-risk patients (clinical ASCVD, LDL-C ≥190 mg/dL, or age 40–75 yr with DM and LDL-C 70–189 mg/dL) who are/have:
  - » Less than anticipated response to statin therapy
  - » Unable to tolerate a less than recommended intensity of statin therapy
  - » Completely intolerant to statin therapy

Lipid-Lowering Effects of Various Drug Classes

Drug Class	Effect on LDL-C	Effect on HDL-C	Effect on TGs
Bile acid resins	↓ 15–30%	↑ 3–5%	↑ 1–10%
Niacin	↓ 5–25%	↑ 15–35%	↓ 20–50%
Fibric acid derivatives	↓/↑ 5–20%	↑ 10–20%	↓ 20–50%
Statins	↓ 18–55%	↑ 5–15%	↓ 7–30%
Cholesterol absorption inhibitors	↓ 15–20%	↑ 1%	↓ 8%

Bile Acid Resins

Mechanism of action – bind bile acids in intestines, forming insoluble complex that is excreted in feces → ↓ in bile acids causes liver to convert cholesterol into bile acids, which then ↓ cholesterol stores → ↑ demand for cholesterol in liver → upregulation of LDL receptors → ↑ LDL-C clearance from bloodstream

Generic	Brand	Dose	Contra-indications	Primary Side Effects	Key Monitoring	Pertinent Drug Interactions	Med Pearl	Top 200
Cholestyramine	• Prevalite • Questran	4–24 g/day	Complete biliary obstruction	• Constipation • Bloating • Abdominal pain • Nausea/vomiting (N/V) • Flatulence • ↑ TGs	Lipid panel	Bind to and ↓ absorption of many drugs (e.g., warfarin, digoxin, thiazides, levothyroxine)	• Used to ↓ LDL-C • Can be used in patients with liver disease • Do not use in patients with ↑ TGs • Colesevelam has fewer gastrointestinal (GI) side effects and drug interactions	No
Colesevelam	Welchol	3.75 g/day						Yes
Colestipol	Colestid	• Granules: 5–30 g/day • Tablets: 2–16 g/day						No

Niacin

Mechanism of action – ↓ production of very low density lipoproteins (VLDL) in liver → ↓ synthesis of LDL-C

Generic	Brand	Dose	Contra-indications	Primary Side Effects	Key Monitoring	Pertinent Drug Interactions	Med Pearl	Top 200
Niacin	Niaspan; also available as over-the-counter (OTC) product	500–3,000 mg/day	• Hepatic dysfunction • Active gout • Active peptic ulcer disease	• Flushing/itching • Nausea • Orthostatic hypotension • ↑ LFTs • Myopathy • Hyperuricemia • Hyperglycemia	• Lipid panel • LFTs • Creatine kinase (CK) (if muscle aches) • Uric acid • Blood glucose (if patient has DM)	None significant	• Used to ↓ LDL-C, ↓ TGs, and ↑ HDL-C • Most effective drug for ↑ HDL-C • Do not ↑ dose by >500 mg in 4-week period • Avoid use of OTC SR products (↑ risk of hepatotoxicity)	Yes

Combination products: Niacin/lovastatin (Advicor)   Niacin/simvastatin (Simcor)

Fibric Acid Derivatives

Mechanism of action – ↑ activity of lipoprotein lipase → ↑ catabolism of VLDL → ↓ TGs

Generic	Brand	Dose	Contra-indications	Primary Side Effects	Key Monitoring	Pertinent Drug Interactions	Med Pearl	Top 200
Fenofibrate	• Antara • Fenoglide • Fibricor • Lipofen • Lofibra, Tricor • Triglide	43–200 mg/day (depending on brand)	• Hepatic dysfunction • Severe renal dysfunction • Gallbladder disease	• Nausea/vomiting/diarrhea (N/V/D) • Abdominal pain • ↑ LFTs • Myopathy	• Lipid panel • LFTs • CK (if muscle aches)	• Avoid using gemfibrozil with statins (↑ risk of myopathy) • ↑ effects of warfarin and sulfonylureas • ↓ cyclosporine levels	• Used to ↓ TGs and/or ↑ HDL-C • Gemfibrozil should not be used with statins → ↑ risk of myopathy • Fenofibrate preferred with statins • Adjust dose in renal insufficiency	Yes
Gemfibrozil	Lopid	1,200 mg/day						Yes

Omega-3 Fatty Acids (Fish Oil)

Mechanism of action – ↓ production of TGs in the liver

Generic	Brand	Dose	Contraindications	Primary Side Effects	Key Monitoring	Pertinent Drug Interactions	Med Pearl	Top 200
Icosapent ethyl	Vascepa	4 g/day	Fish allergy	Arthralgia	Lipid panel	May ↑ risk of bleeding with antithrombotic agents	• Used to ↓ TGs • Minimal effect on LDL-C	No
Omega-3-Acid Ethyl Esters	• Epanova • Lovaza • Omtryg • Also available as OTC product	• 2–4 g/day • Omtryg: 4.8 g/day	Fish allergy	• Belching ("fishy taste") • Dyspepsia	Lipid panel	May ↑ risk of bleeding with antithrombotic agents	• Used to ↓ TGs • May ↑ LDL-C	Yes

HMG-CoA Reductase Inhibitors (Statins)

Mechanism of action – inhibit HMG-CoA reductase → prevent the conversion of HMG-CoA to mevalonate (rate-limiting step in cholesterol synthesis)

Generic	Brand	Dose	Contraindications	Primary Side Effects	Key Monitoring	Pertinent Drug Interactions	Med Pearl	Top 200
Atorvastatin	Lipitor	10–80 mg/day	• Hepatic dysfunction • Pregnancy (Pregnancy Category X) • Concomitant use with cyclosporine (pitavastatin) • Concomitant use with strong CYP3A4 inhibitors (simvastatin and lovastatin) • Concomitant use with gemfibrozil, cyclosporine or danazol (simvastatin)	• ↑ LFTs • Myopathy • N/V • Constipation	• Lipid panel • LFTs • CK (if muscle aches)	• Atorvastatin, lovastatin, rosuvastatin, and simvastatin are CYP3A4 substrates; CYP3A4 inhibitors may ↑ risk of side effects; may ↑ effects of warfarin • Fluvastatin and pitavastatin are CYP2C9 substrates; may ↑ effects of warfarin • Pravastatin not metabolized by CYP enzymes	• Most effective drugs for ↓ LDL-C • Lower maximum dosage of simvastatin and lovastatin when used with amiodarone, dronedarone, verapamil, amlodipine, diltiazem, lomitapide, ranolazine, or niacin • Adjust rosuvastatin dose if CrCl <30 mL/min • Lower maximum dosage of rosuvastatin when used with cyclosporine, lopinavir/ritonavir, or atazanavir/ritonavir • Lower maximum dosage of pitavastatin when used with erythromycin or rifampin • Adjust pitavastatin dose if CrCl 15–60 mL/min	Yes
Fluvastatin	Lescol, Lescol XL	20–80 mg/day						No
Lovastatin	• Altoprev • Mevacor	20–80 mg/day						Yes
Pitavastatin	Livalo	1–4 mg/day						No
Pravastatin	Pravachol	10–80 mg/day						Yes
Simvastatin	Zocor	10–40 mg/day						Yes
Rosuvastatin	Crestor	5–40 mg/day						Yes

Combination products: Atorvastatin/amlodipine (Caduet) Atorvastatin/ezetimibe (Liptruzet) Simvastatin/ezetimibe (Vytorin)

Cholesterol Absorption Inhibitor

Mechanism of action – prevents absorption of cholesterol from small intestine

Generic	Brand	Dose	Contraindications	Primary Side Effects	Key Monitoring	Pertinent Drug Interactions	Med Pearl	Top 200
Ezetimibe	Zetia	10 mg/day	None	• Headache • Diarrhea	Lipid panel	• Cyclosporine and fibrates may ↑ effects • ↑ cyclosporine levels • ↑ effects of warfarin	• Used to ↓ LDL-C • Can add to statin to further ↓ LDL-C or if dose-limiting side effects occur with statin	Yes

Microsomal Triglyceride Transfer Protein (MTP) Inhibitor

Generic	Brand	Dose	Contraindications	Primary Side Effects	Key Monitoring	Pertinent Drug Interactions	Med Pearl	Top 200
Lomitapide	Juxtapid	5–60 mg/day	• Pregnancy (Pregnancy Category X) • Concomitant use with moderate or strong CYP3A4 inhibitors • Hepatic dysfunction	• ↑ LFTs • N/V/D	• Lipid panel • LFTs	• CYP3A4 inhibitors may ↑ risk of side effects • May ↑ effects of warfarin • May ↑ risk of side effects with simvastatin and lovastatin (limit statin dose) • May ↑ effect/toxicity of P-glycoprotein substrates	• Used to ↓ LDL-C in patients with homozygous familial hypercholesterolemia • Has REMS program • Lower maximum dosage when used with amiodarone, amlodipine, atorvastatin, cyclosporine, fluoxetine, or oral contraceptives	No

Storage and Administration Pearls

- Bile acid resins
  - Cholestyramine available as powder; colestipol available as granules and tablets; colesevelam available as tablets
  - Should be administered with meals
  - Powder can be mixed in applesauce, pudding, oatmeal, Jell-O, etc. to improve its palatability (do not mix in carbonated beverages)
  - Give other medications 1 hour *before* or 4 hours *after* cholestyramine or colestipol
- Niacin: Give at bedtime (so flushing reaction can occur while patient is sleeping)
- Fibric acid derivatives: Can be administered with meals to ↓ GI effects
- Statins: IR lovastatin administered with meals; ER lovastatin administered at bedtime
- Most statins administered in the evening (at bedtime)—most hepatic cholesterol production occurs during the night (~2 A.M.); atorvastatin, rosuvastatin, and pitavastatin administered in the morning or evening
- Lomitapide: Administer ≥2 hours after evening meal (giving with food may ↑ GI effects)
- After initiating lipid-lowering therapy, lipid profile reassessed in 6 weeks to determine if any changes in therapy are needed.

Patient Education Pearls

- Fiber/fiber supplements may help minimize GI side effects associated with bile acid resins.
- Any episodes of muscle pain/aches or dark urine should be reported.
- Flushing reaction associated with niacin may be minimized by taking aspirin (325 mg) or an NSAID at least 30 minutes before dose, taking with food, slowly titrating the dose, and avoiding alcohol or hot beverages. Tolerance usually develops.
- Statins and lomitapide should be avoided if the patient is pregnant (Category X).

HEART FAILURE

Definition

HF is a condition in which the heart is unable to pump out enough blood (CO) to meet the metabolic demands of the body. The decrease in CO leads to the activation of numerous compensatory mechanisms, which attempt to improve CO. There are two types of HF: HF with reduced ejection fraction (HFrEF) (previously known as systolic HF) (pumping function/contractility impaired; left ventricular ejection fraction [LVEF] ≤40%) or HF with preserved ejection fraction (HFpEF) (previously known as diastolic HF) (impaired ability to relax, which leads to underfilling; normal LVEF [>40%]). The majority of HF cases are due to either CAD or HTN. A number of drugs can also precipitate or worsen HF by causing negative inotropic effects (e.g., β-blockers, CCBs [except amlodipine and felodipine], antiarrhythmics [except amiodarone and dofetilide], itraconazole, terbinafine), causing Na^+ and water retention (e.g., corticosteroids, NSAIDs, thiazolidinediones), causing vasoconstriction (e.g., sympathomimetics), or acting as a direct cardiotoxin (e.g., anthracyclines, cyclophosphamide, trastuzumab).

Diagnosis

- Diagnosis is primarily based on the patient's physical exam findings in conjunction with the past medical history and results from laboratory and diagnostic tests.
- Echocardiogram provides information regarding LV function and can reflect whether the patient has HFrEF or HFpEF.
- B-type natriuretic peptide (BNP) concentration can also be obtained to help differentiate between acute HF and other causes of dyspnea (e.g., pneumonia, bronchitis, COPD, pulmonary embolus) (>500 pg/mL in patients with acute decompensated HF [ADHF]).

Signs and Symptoms

- Signs and symptoms of left-sided HF (reflect pulmonary congestion)
  - Symptoms: Dyspnea, orthopnea, paroxysmal nocturnal dyspnea, cough
  - Signs: Rales (usually bibasilar), pulmonary edema, pleural effusion, S_3 gallop
- Signs and symptoms of right-sided HF (reflect systemic congestion)
  - Symptoms: Anorexia, N/V, constipation, abdominal pain, bloating
  - Signs: Jugular venous distention, (+) hepatojugular reflux, ascites, peripheral edema, hepatomegaly, splenomegaly

Classification of HF

New York Heart Association (NYHA) Functional Classification	American College of Cardiology/ American Heart Association Staging System
• Functional class I = Patients have LV dysfunction but no physical limitations; lack symptoms with ordinary physical activity ("well compensated") • Functional class II = Slight limitation of physical activity; symptoms with ordinary physical activity (e.g., walking two blocks) • Functional class III = Marked limitation of physical activity; minimal activity (e.g., activities of daily living) causes symptoms • Functional class IV = Unable to carry on physical activity without discomfort; symptoms at rest	• Stage A = At high risk for development of HF but have no structural heart disease or symptoms of HF. Includes patients with HTN, DM, and CAD • Stage B = Structural heart disease (e.g., LVH, previous MI, LV systolic dysfunction, or valvular heart disease) but no symptoms of HF (NYHA class I symptoms) • Stage C = Structural heart disease with current or previous symptoms of HF (NYHA class I, II, III, or IV symptoms) • Stage D = Refractory symptoms of HF at rest despite maximal medical therapy (often hospitalized) (end-stage HF) (NYHA class IV symptoms)

Guidelines

Heart Failure Society of America, Lindenfeld J, Albert NM, et al. HFSA 2010 Comprehensive Heart Failure Practice Guideline. J Card Fail 2010;16(6):e1–194.

Yancy CW, Jessup M, Bozkurt B, et al; American College of Cardiology Foundation; American Heart Association Task Force on Practice Guidelines. 2013 ACCF/AHA guideline for the management of heart failure: a report of the American College of Cardiology Foundation/American Heart Association Task Force on Practice Guidelines. *J Am Coll Cardiol* 2013;62(16):e147–239.

Guidelines Summary

The goals of therapy are to relieve symptoms, improve quality of life, improve survival, reduce hospitalizations, and slow the progression of disease.

- Nonpharmacologic therapy: Regular low-intensity physical activity, ↓ Na$^+$ (≤3 g/day), ↓ fluid intake (<2 L/day), weight loss (if obese), alcohol restriction, and smoking cessation
- Pharmacologic therapy:
  - Stage A: Modify risk factors and control HTN, DM, CAD, and dyslipidemia; ACEI or ARB in patients with risk factors for vascular disease
  - Stage B: ACEI + β-blocker
  - Stage C: ACEI + β-blocker + diuretic
    - » Other drugs to be considered:
      - – ARA: NYHA class II-IV patients who are already receiving ACEI (or ARB) and β-blocker; NYHA class II patients should have history of

prior cardiovascular hospitalization or ↑ BNP level to be considered for ARA therapy

- ARBs: Patients who cannot tolerate an ACEI due to intractable cough; symptomatic patients who are receiving ACEI and β-blocker and cannot tolerate or have a contraindication to an ARA

- Digoxin: Patients who remain symptomatic despite optimal therapy with ACEI (or ARB), β-blocker, and diuretic

- Hydralazine/isosorbide dinitrate: Patients with intolerance or contraindications (renal insufficiency, hyperkalemia) to ACEI or ARB; African-American patients with NYHA class III or IV symptoms who remain symptomatic despite optimal therapy with ACEI (or ARB) and β-blocker

- Stage D: Chronic positive inotrope therapy (e.g., dobutamine, milrinone), mechanical circulatory support (e.g., LV assist device), heart transplant, end-of-life care/hospice

Medication Charts

Loop Diuretics

Mechanism of action – inhibit Na$^+$ reabsorption in the ascending limb of loop of Henle; ↓ preload

Generic	Brand	Dose	Contra-indications	Primary Side Effects	Key Monitoring	Pertinent Drug Interactions	Med Pearl	Top 200
Bumetanide	Only available generically	0.5–10 mg/day	Sulfa allergy	• Hypocalcemia • Hypokalemia • Hypomagnesemia • Hyponatremia • Hyperglycemia • Hyperuricemia • Metabolic alkalosis • Azotemia	• BP • Electrolytes • BUN/SCr • Blood glucose • Uric acid • Jugular venous pressure • Urine output • Weight (↓ by 0.5–1 kg/day initially)	• May ↑ risk of lithium toxicity • May ↑ risk of ototoxicity with aminoglycosides • May ↓ effect of antidiabetic agents • NSAIDs ↓ effects	• ↓ symptoms; effect on mortality unknown • If initial dose inadequate, double dose, dose 2x daily, add metolazone, or use IV • Similar side effects as thiazides (except loops cause hypocalcemia) • BUN/SCr ratio >20:1 → dehydration (prerenal azotemia) • Furosemide PO dose = 2x IV dose	No
Furosemide	Lasix	20–600 mg/day						Yes
Torsemide	Demadex	10–200 mg/day						No

ACE Inhibitors

- See HTN monograph for further details
- Medication pearls specific to their use in HF:
  - ↓ mortality; ↓ preload and afterload
  - Strive to achieve target dose, if possible (titrate dose to symptoms, not BP)

Drug	Initial Dose	Target Dose
Captopril	6.25 mg TID	50 mg TID
Enalapril	2.5 mg BID	10 mg BID
Lisinopril	2.5 mg daily	40 mg daily
Ramipril	1.25 mg daily	10 mg daily
Trandolapril	1 mg daily	4 mg daily
Fosinopril	5 mg daily	40 mg daily
Quinapril	5 mg BID	20 mg BID
Perindopril	2 mg daily	16 mg daily

β-Blockers

Generic	Brand	Dose	Contraindications	Primary Side Effects	Key Monitoring	Pertinent Drug Interactions	Med Pearl	Top 200
Mechanism of action – ↓ activation of the sympathetic nervous system; slows and potentially reverses detrimental effects (e.g., ventricular remodeling) of catecholamines								
Bisoprolol	Zebeta	1.25–10 mg/day Target dose: 10 mg daily	• Symptomatic bradycardia • ≥2nd-degree heart block (in absence of pacemaker) • SBP <85 mmHg • Severe asthma • Decompensated HF	See HTN section	• BP • HR • S/S HF • Weight	Carvedilol may ↑ digoxin levels	• ↓ mortality • Metoprolol succinate (not tartrate) approved for HF	No
Carvedilol	• Coreg • Coreg CR	IR: 6.25–100 mg/day (in two divided doses) Target dose: <85 kg = 25 mg BID; >85 kg = 50 mg BID CR: 10–80 mg/day (1x daily) Target dose: 80 mg daily					• Patient should be fairly euvolemic before starting • Strive to achieve target dose, if possible • Dose can be doubled every 2–4 wks to achieve target dose (unless side effects) • Manage worsening HF by ↑ diuretic dose • If hypotension occurs, may ↓ dose of ACEI, ARB, or other vasodilator (more common with carvedilol) • If bradycardia occurs, ↓ dose • Abrupt discontinuation may cause worsening HF	Yes
Metoprolol succinate	Toprol XL	12.5–200 mg/day Target dose: 200 mg daily						Yes

Digoxin

Generic	Brand	Dose	Contra-indications	Primary Side Effects	Key Monitoring	Pertinent Drug Interactions	Med Pearl	Top 200
Mechanism of action – inhibits Na$^+$/K$^+$ ATPase pump → ↑ intracellular Ca^{2+} → ↑ myocardial contractility; also ↓ neurohormonal activation								
Digoxin	Lanoxin	0.125–0.25 mg/day (loading doses not necessary in HF)	≥2nd-degree heart block (in absence of pacemaker)	• Bradycardia/heart block • S/S digoxin toxicity (visual disturbances, N/V, confusion, anorexia, arrhythmias)	• HR • Electrolytes (predisposed to toxicity if hypokalemia, hypomagnesemia, or hypercalcemia) • BUN/SCr • Digoxin concentrations	• Amiodarone, dronedarone, quinidine, verapamil, and clarithromycin may ↑ levels • Antacids may ↓ levels (separate by 1–2 hours) • Use with other negative chronotropes (e.g., β-blockers, verapamil, diltiazem, or clonidine) may ↑ risk of bradycardia	• Improves symptoms, ↓ hospitalizations; no effect on mortality • Used to ↑ contractility in HFrEF and to ↓ HR in atrial fibrillation (AF) • Abrupt discontinuation may cause worsening HF • ↓ dose by 50% when starting amiodarone or dronedarone • Adjust dose in patients with renal dysfunction • Target level: 0.5–0.9 ng/mL (↑ mortality if >0.9 ng/mL)	Yes

Aldosterone Receptor Antagonists

Mechanism of action – inhibit the effects of aldosterone → ↓ remodeling and Na+/water retention
- Spironolactone is nonselective ARA (also blocks androgen and progesterone receptors → associated with endocrine side effects)
- Eplerenone is selective ARA (not associated with endocrinologic side effects)

Generic	Brand	Dose	Contraindications	Primary Side Effects	Key Monitoring	Pertinent Drug Interactions	Med Pearl	Top 200
Eplerenone	Inspra	25–50 mg/day	• K+ >5 mEq/L • SCr >2.5 mg/dL (men) or >2 mg/dL (women) (or CrCl ≤30 mL/min) • Concomitant ACEI **and** ARB use • Also for eplerenone: Use of strong CYP3A4 inhibitors (e.g., ritonavir, ketoconazole, itraconazole, nefazodone, clarithromycin, nelfinavir)	• Hyperkalemia • Also for spironolactone: Gynecomastia, breast tenderness, menstrual changes, hirsutism	• BP • K+ • BUN/SCr	Use with ACEIs, ARBs, K+ supplements, or NSAIDs may ↑ risk of hyperkalemia	• ↓ mortality • Should consider discontinuing or ↓ dose of K+ supplements • Eplerenone tends to be used in patients who develop endocrine side effects (i.e., gynecomastia) with spironolactone	No
Spironolactone	Aldactone	12.5–25 mg/day						No

Angiotensin II Receptor Blockers

- See HTN monograph for further details
- Medication pearls specific to their use in HF:
  - Only candesartan, losartan, or valsartan recommended for the management of HF (only candesartan and valsartan approved for HF)
  - Should not be considered equivalent or superior to ACEIs

Hydralazine/Isosorbide Dinitrate

Mechanism of action:
- Hydralazine – causes arterial vasodilation (↓ afterload)
- Isosorbide dinitrate – causes venous vasodilation (↓ preload)

Generic	Brand	Dose	Contra-indications	Primary Side Effects	Key Monitoring	Pertinent Drug Interactions	Med Pearl	Top 200
Hydralazine	Only available generically	40–300 mg/day	None	• Headache • Dizziness • Reflex tachycardia • Peripheral edema (hydralazine) • Lupus-like syndrome (hydralazine)	• BP • HR	None	• ↓ mortality (when used together) • Combination often used in patients who cannot tolerate ACEIs or ARBs due to renal insufficiency, hyperkalemia, or angioedema • Do not use hydralazine alone (↑ mortality)	No
Isosorbide dinitrate	Isordil	30–120 mg/day						Yes

Combination product:
Hydralazine/isosorbide dinitrate (BiDil) – approved for African-American patients with NYHA class III or IV HF due to LV systolic dysfunction (LVEF ≤40%) who are receiving an ACEI (or ARB) and a β-blocker (can also use individual products together if there are financial concerns)

Intravenous Drugs for Treatment of ADHF

Drug	Mechanism of Action	Primary Side Effects	Med Pearl
Vasodilators			
Nitroglycerin (NTG)	• Venous vasodilation → ↓ preload • Can cause arterial vasodilation at higher doses	Hypotension, tachycardia, headache, tolerance	• Especially useful in patients with myocardial ischemia • Tolerance can develop (overcome by ↑ infusion rate)
Nitroprusside	Arterial and venous vasodilation → ↓ preload and afterload	Hypotension, N/V, cyanide/ thiocyanate toxicity (risk ↑ if infusion >24 hours)	Avoid in patients with renal dysfunction
Nesiritide (Natrecor)	• BNP • Arterial and venous vasodilation → ↓ preload and afterload	Hypotension, headache	Infusion should not be titrated more frequently than every 3 hours
Positive Inotropes			
Dopamine	• 0.5–3 mcg/kg/min → Stimulates dopamine receptors → ↑ urine output • 3–10 mcg/kg/min → Stimulates β₁ receptors → ↑ CO, ↑ HR • >10 mcg/kg/min → Stimulates α₁ receptors → ↑ BP	Arrhythmias, tachycardia, myocardial ischemia, N/V	Avoid in patients with myocardial ischemia
Dobutamine	β₁ and β₂ receptor agonist and weak α₁ receptor agonist → ↑ CO and vasodilation	Arrhythmias, tachycardia, myocardial ischemia, hypokalemia, tremor	• Avoid in patients with myocardial ischemia • Should not be used in patients receiving chronic β-blocker therapy • Tolerance can develop
Milrinone	PDE III inhibitor → ↑ CO and vasodilation	Hypotension, arrhythmias	• Can be used in patients receiving chronic β-blocker therapy, or in those not responding to or tolerating dobutamine • Tolerance does not develop • Use lower initial dose in patients with renal dysfunction

Storage and Administration Pearls

- Captopril should be administered at least 1 hour *before* or 2 hours *after* meals.
- Carvedilol should be administered with food to minimize the risk of orthostatic hypotension.
- Nitroprusside infusions should be protected from light.

Patient Education Pearls

- If a patient is taking >1 dose of diuretic each day, the last dose should be taken before 5 P.M. to minimize nocturia.
- Patients should weigh themselves daily (first thing in the morning after urinating) and should contact their healthcare provider if they gain more than 3–5 lb in a week.
- Patients receiving diuretics should wear sunscreen and protective clothing. Also, they should report any episodes of muscle cramps, as this may be a symptom of hypokalemia or hypomagnesemia.
- A patient who is receiving ARAs, ACEIs, or ARBs should avoid excessive intake of foods high in K^+ (e.g., green leafy vegetables, potatoes, apricots, bananas, dates, oranges, avocados) and K^+-containing salt substitutes.
- A patient who is receiving ACEIs or ARBs should call 911 immediately if he/she experiences lip, tongue, or facial swelling or is having difficulty breathing.
- ACEIs and ARBs should be avoided in patients who are pregnant.
- Patients should not stop their β-blocker or digoxin therapy abruptly, as this may cause a sudden worsening of HF symptoms.

ANTIARRHYTHMIC DRUGS

Class IA

Generic	Brand	Dose	Contra-indications	Primary Side Effects	Key Monitoring	Pertinent Drug Interactions	Med Pearl	Top 200
Mechanism of action – Na$^+$ channel blockers; slow conduction velocity, prolong refractoriness, ↓ automaticity								
Disopyramide	• Norpace • Norpace CR • Only available generically	400–1,600 mg/day	• HF • ≥2nd-degree heart block (in absence of pacemaker) • Long QT syndrome	• Dry mouth • Urinary retention • Blurred vision • Constipation • HF exacerbation • Hypotension • Torsades de pointes (TdP)	• Electrocardiogram (ECG) (QTc interval, QRS duration) • BP • S/S HF • Electrolytes • Disopyramide concentrations	• CYP3A4 inhibitors and anticholinergics may ↑ risk of side effects • CYP3A4 inducers may ↓ effects • ↑ risk of TdP with other drugs that prolong QT interval	• Used for atrial and ventricular arrhythmias • Therapeutic range: 2–5 mcg/mL • Adjust dose in renal dysfunction	No
Procainamide	Only available generically	IV: *Loading dose:* 15–17 mg/kg over 25–60 min *Maintenance dose:* 1–4 mg/min continuous infusion	• ≥2nd-degree heart block (in absence of pacemaker) • Long QT syndrome	• Lupus-like syndrome • TdP • Hypotension • Agranulocytosis	• ECG (QTc interval, QRS duration) • BP • S/S lupus (e.g., stabbing chest pain, joint pain, rash) • Procainamide/ N-acetylprocainamide (NAPA) concentrations • Complete blood count (CBC) with differential • Electrolytes	↑ risk of TdP with other drugs that prolong QT interval	• Used for atrial and ventricular arrhythmias • Therapeutic range: 4–10 mcg/mL (procainamide); 15–25 mcg/mL (NAPA); 10–30 mcg/mL (total) • Use with caution, if at all, in renal insufficiency	No
Quinidine	Only available generically	• Sulfate: 800–2,400 mg/day • Gluconate: 648–2,916 mg/day	• ≥2nd-degree heart block (in absence of pacemaker) • Long QT syndrome • Use of ritonavir	• Diarrhea • Stomach cramps • TdP • Hypotension • Cinchonism (tinnitus, blurred vision, headache) • Thrombocytopenia	• ECG (QTc interval, QRS duration) • BP • Quinidine concentrations • CBC with differential • LFTs • Electrolytes	• CYP3A4 inhibitors may ↑ risk of side effects • CYP3A4 inducers may ↓ effects • ↑ risk of digoxin toxicity • May ↑ toxicity of CYP3A4 and CYP2D6 substrates • ↑ risk of TdP with other drugs that prolong QT interval	• Used for atrial and ventricular arrhythmias • Therapeutic range: 2–5 mcg/mL • Administer with food to minimize GI effects	No

■ Avoid all Class IA antiarrhythmics in patients with structural heart disease (i.e., HF, CAD, left ventricular hypertrophy, valvular disease)

Class IB

Mechanism of action – Na$^+$ channel blockers; little effect on conduction velocity, shorten refractoriness, ↓ automaticity

Generic	Brand	Dose	Contraindications	Primary Side Effects	Key Monitoring	Pertinent Drug Interactions	Med Pearl	Top 200
Lidocaine	Xylocaine	IV: *Loading dose:* 1–1.5 mg/kg, up to 3 mg/kg (total) *Maintenance dose:* 1–4 mg/min	≥2nd-degree heart block (in absence of pacemaker)	CNS toxicity (dizziness, blurred vision, slurred speech, confusion, paresthesias, seizures)	• ECG (QRS duration) • BP • Neurologic exam • Lidocaine concentrations (if duration of therapy >24 hours)	Amiodarone may ↑ risk of toxicity	• Used only for ventricular arrhythmias • Therapeutic range: 1.5–5 mcg/mL • Use lower infusion rate in elderly, HF or hepatic dysfunction	No
Mexiletine	Only available generically	600–1,200 mg/day	Same as for lidocaine	• CNS toxicity (same as lidocaine) • N/V	• ECG (QRS duration) • BP • LFTs • Neurologic exam	• ↑ risk of theophylline toxicity • CYP1A2 and CYP2D6 inhibitors may ↑ risk of toxicity	• Used only for ventricular arrhythmias • Take with food to minimize GI effects • ↓ dose in HF or hepatic dysfunction	No

- Class IB antiarrhythmics do not cause TdP

Class IC

Generic	Brand	Dose	Contraindications	Primary Side Effects	Key Monitoring	Pertinent Drug Interactions	Med Pearl	Top 200
Mechanism of action – Na⁺ channel blockers (most potent); markedly slow conduction velocity, no effect on refractoriness, ↓ automaticity; propafenone also has nonselective β-blocking properties								
Flecainide	Only available generically	*Loading dose (for AF conversion):* 200–300 mg × 1 dose *Maintenance dose:* 100–400 mg/day	• ≥2nd-degree heart block (in absence of pacemaker) • History of MI • HF	• Dizziness • Tremor • HF exacerbation • Ventricular tachycardia (VT)	• ECG (QRS duration) • Echocardiogram (at baseline to evaluation LV function) • Electrolytes	• ↑ risk of digoxin toxicity	• Used for atrial and ventricular arrhythmias • Adjust dose in renal dysfunction	No
Propafenone	• Rythmol • Rythmol SR	IR: *Loading dose (for AF conversion):* 450–600 mg × 1 *Maintenance dose:* 450–900 mg/day (in three divided doses) SR: *Maintenance dose:* 450–950 mg/day (in two divided doses)	• ≥2nd-degree heart block (in absence of pacemaker) • Bradycardia • Bronchospastic disorders • HF • History of MI	• Bradycardia/heart block • HF exacerbation • Bronchospasm • Taste disturbances • VT	• ECG (QRS duration, PR interval) • BP • HR • Echocardiogram (at baseline to evaluation LV function) • Electrolytes	• ↑ risk of digoxin toxicity • ↑ effects of warfarin • Use with other negative chronotropes (e.g., β-blockers, digoxin, verapamil, diltiazem, or clonidine) may ↑ risk of bradycardia	• Used for atrial and ventricular arrhythmias	No

■ Avoid Class IC antiarrhythmics in patients with structural heart disease

■ Class IC antiarrhythmics do not cause TdP

Class II

(See medication chart in HTN section for discussion on β-blockers)

Class III

Mechanism of action – K+ channel blockers; no effect on conduction velocity or automaticity; amiodarone and dronedarone also have Na+-channel blocking, β-blocking, and CCB properties; sotalol also has nonselective β-blocking properties

Generic	Brand	Dose	Contraindications	Primary Side Effects	Key Monitoring	Pertinent Drug Interactions	Med Pearl	Top 200
Amiodarone	• Cordarone • Pacerone	Loading dose (IV): *Stable VT:* 150 mg over 10 min *Pulseless VT / ventricular fibrillation:* 300 mg IV push *AF:* 5 mg/kg over 30–60 min Loading dose (PO): *Ventricular arrhythmias:* 1,200–1,600 mg/day *Atrial arrhythmias:* 800–1200 mg/day until 10 g total Maintenance dose: IV: 1 mg/min × 6 hrs, then 0.5 mg/min PO: 100–400 mg/day	≥2nd-degree heart block (in absence of pacemaker)	IV: • Hypotension • Bradycardia/heart block • Phlebitis PO: • Hypo-/hyper-thyroidism • Pulmonary fibrosis • Bradycardia/heart block • Corneal microdeposits • Optic neuritis • N/V • ↑ LFTs • Ataxia • Paresthesias • Photosensitivity • Blue-gray skin discoloration	• ECG (QTc interval, QRS duration, PR interval) • BP • HR • Chest x-ray (baseline; then every 12 months) • Pulmonary function tests (if symptoms) • Thyroid function tests (TFTs) (baseline; then every 6 months) • LFTs (baseline; then every 6 months) • Ophthalmologic exam (baseline if significant visual abnormalities; then if symptoms develop)	• Inhibits CYP1A2, CYP2C9, CYP2D6, and CYP3A4 • CYP3A4 substrate • ↑ risk of digoxin toxicity (↓ digoxin dose by 50%) • ↑ effects of warfarin (↓ warfarin dose by 30%) • Use with other negative chronotropes (e.g. β-blockers, digoxin, verapamil, diltiazem, or clonidine) may ↑ risk of bradycardia • May ↑ cyclosporine or phenytoin levels • May ↑ risk of side effects of simvastatin and lovastatin	• Used for atrial and ventricular arrhythmias • Safe to use in HF • Half-life = 40–60 days • If pulmonary fibrosis or blurred vision occur, discontinue therapy • If TFTs abnormal, treat thyroid disorder • If ↑ LFTs occur, ↓ amiodarone dose • Take with food to minimize GI effects	Yes

Class III *(cont'd)*

Generic	Brand	Dose	Contraindications	Primary Side Effects	Key Monitoring	Pertinent Drug Interactions	Med Pearl	Top 200
Dronedarone	Multaq	400 mg 2 × daily with meals	• Permanent AF • NYHA class IV HF or NYHA class II–III HF with recent decompensation requiring hospitalization or referral to specialized HF clinic • ≥2nd-degree heart block (in absence of pacemaker) • Bradycardia • Concurrent use of strong CYP3A4 inhibitors (e.g., ketoconazole, itraconazole, voriconazole, cyclosporine, telithromycin, clarithromycin, nefazodone, ritonavir) or strong CYP3A4 inducers (e.g., rifampin, phenobarbital, phenytoin, carbamazepine, St. John's wort) • Concurrent use of other drugs that prolong QT interval • QTc interval ≥500 msec • PR interval >280 msec • Severe hepatic impairment • Liver or lung toxicity related to previous amiodarone use • Pregnancy	• N/V/D • ↑ SCr • Bradycardia • ↑ LFTs • New-onset or worsening HF	• ECG (QTc interval, PR interval) • HR • SCr • S/S HF • LFTs	• Inhibits CYP2D6 and CYP3A4 • CYP3A4 substrate • May ↑ toxicity of CYP3A4 and CYP2D6 substrates • CYP3A4 inhibitors may ↑ risk of side effects • CYP3A4 inducers may ↓ effects • ↑ risk of digoxin toxicity (↓ digoxin dose by 50% or consider discontinuing) • Use with other negative chronotropes (e.g. β-blockers, digoxin, verapamil, diltiazem, or clonidine) may ↑ risk of bradycardia • ↑ effects of dabigatran (↓ dose of dabigatran to 75 mg BID if CrCL 30–50 mL/min) • May ↑ risk of side effects of simvastatin and lovastatin	• Used only for atrial arrhythmias • Structurally related to amiodarone (does not have iodine component); less likely to cause organ toxicities; also has shorter half-life	No

Class III *(cont'd)*

Generic	Brand	Dose	Contraindications	Primary Side Effects	Key Monitoring	Pertinent Drug Interactions	Med Pearl	Top 200
Dofetilide	Tikosyn	• 500 mcg 2 × daily (if CrCl >60 mL/min) • Adjust dose if CrCl ≤60 mL/min	• CrCl <20 mL/min • QTc interval >440 msec • Hypokalemia/ hypomagnesemia • Use of verapamil, ketoconazole, cimetidine, trimethoprim, prochlorperazine, hydrochlorothiazide, dolutegravir, megestrol, or other drugs that prolong QT interval	TdP	• ECG (QTc interval) • SCr • Electrolytes	↑ risk of TdP with other drugs that prolong QT interval	• Used only for atrial arrhythmias • Adjust dose based on renal function and QT interval • Must be initiated in hospital • Safe to use in HF	No
Ibutilide	Corvert	IV: 1 mg over 10 min; repeat × 1, if needed	• QTc interval >440 msec • Hypokalemia/ hypomagnesemia • Concurrent use of other drugs that prolong QT interval	TdP	• ECG (QTc interval) • Electrolytes	↑ risk of TdP with other drugs that prolong QT interval	Used only for atrial arrhythmias	No
Sotalol	Betapace, Betapace AF, Sorine	• 160–640 mg/day (in 2 divided doses) • Extend dosing interval if CrCl ≤60 mL/min	• ≥2nd-degree heart block (in absence of pacemaker) • Concurrent use of other drugs that prolong QT interval • CrCl <40 mL/min (for AF) • Long QT syndrome • HF	• TdP • Bradycardia/ heart block • Bronchospasm • HF exacerbation	• ECG (QTc interval, PR interval) • HR • SCr • Electrolytes	• ↑ risk of TdP with other drugs that prolong QT interval • Use with other negative chronotropes (e.g., β-blockers, digoxin, verapamil, diltiazem, or clonidine) may ↑ risk of bradycardia	• Used for atrial and ventricular arrhythmias • Adjust dosing interval in renal dysfunction	No

Class IV Antiarrhythmics

(See medication chart in HTN section for discussion on CCBs)

KAPLAN MEDICAL

ANTITHROMBOTIC DRUGS

Warfarin (Coumadin)

- Commonly prescribed for patients with a variety of conditions where clotting is a risk, such as AF, to prevent the formation of thrombi.
- Mechanism of action: Interferes with the synthesis of the vitamin K-dependent clotting factors of the liver (II, VII, IX, and X) as well as protein C and S
  - Regular monitoring of the PT/INR is necessary.

- Contraindications: Pregnancy (Category X), recent surgery
- Side effects: Bleeding, skin necrosis (especially with Protein C deficiency), purple toe syndrome
- Drug interactions:

Increased Anticoagulant Effect	Decreased Anticoagulant Effect
Alcohol (acute ingestion), amiodarone, azole antifungals, cephalosporins, cimetidine, corticosteroids, dronedarone, fluoroquinolones, lovastatin, macrolides, omeprazole, penicillins, simvastatin, sulfonamides, thyroid hormones	Alcohol (chronic ingestion), barbiturates, carbamazepine, cholestyramine, phenytoin, rifampin, St. John's wort, vitamin K

- Antidote: Vitamin K
- Dosing:
  - Must be individualized
  - The full effect of a specific warfarin dose (or dosage change) is not seen for 72–96 hours (3–4 days). A good rule to follow is that 50% of warfarin's effect will be evident after 1 day, 25% more (75% total) on day 2 and 25% more (100% total effect) on days 3–4.
  - The INR obtained "today" is a reflection of the last 3 doses.
  - Continually monitor for trends related to changes in the INR.
  - Review all medications (new and existing) that may have been added or changed.
  - Consider the possibility of drug-drug interactions with warfarin.
  - Monitor for signs/symptoms of bleeding (labs and physical).

Dabigatran (Pradaxa)

- Indicated for:
  - Prevention of stroke and systemic embolism in patients with AF
  - Treatment of deep vein thrombosis (DVT) and pulmonary embolism (PE)
  - Prevention of recurrent DVT and PE

- Considered as an alternative to warfarin
- Mechanism of action: Direct thrombin inhibitor (oral)
- Contraindications: Active bleeding
- Side effects: Bleeding, dyspepsia
- Drug interactions:
  - P-gp → ↑ anticoagulant effects
    - » AF: ↓ dabigatran dose to 75 mg BID when used with dronedarone or keto-conazole if CrCl 30–50 mL/min; avoid if CrCl <30 mL/min
    - » DVT treatment/prevention: Avoid concomitant use if CrCl <50 ml/min
  - Rifampin → ↓ anticoagulant effects (avoid concomitant use)
- Antidote: None available
- Recommended dose:
  - AF
    - » CrCl >30 mL/min: 150 mg BID
    - » CrCl 15–30 mL/min: 75 mg BID
    - » CrCl <15 mL/min: NOT recommended
  - Treatment/prevention of recurrent DVT/PE
    - » CrCl >30 mL/min: 150 mg BID
    - » CrCl <30 mL/min: No dosing recommendations

Rivaroxaban (Xarelto)

- Indicated for:
  - Prevention of stroke and systemic embolism in patients with AF
  - Prevention of venous thromboembolism (VTE) in patients undergoing hip or knee replacement surgery
  - Treatment of DVT and PE
  - Prevention of recurrent DVT and PE
- Mechanism of action: Factor Xa inhibitor (oral)
- Contradications:
  - Active bleeding
  - CrCl <30 mL/min (postoperative VTE prophylaxis and DVT/PE treatment)
  - CrCl <15 mL/min (AF)
- Side effects: Bleeding
- Drug interactions:
  - Avoid concomitant use with COMBINED P-gp and strong CYP3A4 inhibitors (e.g., ketoconazole, itraconazole, ritonavir, indinavir, conivaptan)
  - Avoid concomitant use with COMBINED P-gp and strong CYP3A4 inducers (e.g., carbamazepine, phenytoin, rifampin, St. John's wort)

- Antidote: None available
- Recommended dose:
  - Postoperative VTE prophylaxis: 10 mg daily (× 35 days for hip replacement; × 12 days for knee replacement)
  - AF
    - » CrCl >50 mL/min: 20 mg daily with evening meal
    - » CrCl 15–50 mL/min: 15 mg daily with evening meal
  - DVT/PE treatment: 15 mg BID with food × 21 days, then 20 mg daily with food
  - Prevention of DVT/PE recurrence: 20 mg daily with food

Apixaban (Eliquis)

- Indicated for:
  - Prevention of stroke and systemic embolism in patients with AF
  - Prevention of VTE in patients undergoing hip or knee replacement surgery
  - Treatment of DVT and PE
  - Prevention of recurrent DVT and PE
- Mechanism of action: Factor Xa inhibitor (oral)
- Contraindications: Active bleeding
- Side effects: Bleeding
- Drug interactions:
  - Concomitant use with strong dual inhibitors of P-gp and CYP3A4 (e.g., ketoconazole, itraconazole, ritonavir, clarithromycin) → ↓ apixaban dose to 2.5 mg BID (avoid use if patient already receiving this dose)
  - Avoid concomitant use with strong dual inducers of P-gp and CYP3A4 (e.g., carbamazepine, phenytoin, rifampin, St. John's wort)
- Antidote: None available
- Recommended dose:
  - AF
    - » 5 mg BID
    - » If patient has ≥2 of the following (age ≥80 yr, weight ≤60 kg, SCr ≥1.5 mg/dL) → ↓ dose to 2.5 mg BID
    - » If patient on hemodialysis → 5 mg BID; ↓ dose to 2.5 mg BID if patient ≥80 yr or weight ≤60 kg
  - Postoperative VTE prophylaxis: 2.5 mg BID (×35 days for hip replacement; ×12 days for knee replacement)
  - Treatment of DVT/PE: 10 mg BID ×7 days, then 5 mg BID
  - Prevention of recurrent DVT/PE: 2.5 mg BID after at least 6 months of treatment for DVT/PE

ISCHEMIC HEART DISEASE

Definitions

Ischemic heart disease (IHD) is characterized by a lack of oxygen resulting from in-adequate perfusion of the myocardium, which is often due to narrowing or blockage in a coronary artery. Patients with IHD may present with chronic stable angina, vasospastic angina (variant or Prinzmetal's angina), or an acute coronary syndrome (ACS). ACS can include UA, non–ST-segment-elevation MI (NSTEMI), or ST-segment–elevation MI (STEMI). An ACS is precipitated by rupture of an atherosclerotic plaque, followed by formation of a thrombus at the site of plaque rupture. In NSTEMI, the thrombus tends to contain more platelets than fibrin ("white clot") and does not completely occlude the vessel. In STEMI, the thrombus contains more fibrin and red blood cells than platelets ("red clot") and completely occludes the vessel.

This section reviews the management of NSTEMI and STEMI.

Diagnosis

- If ischemic-like chest pain persists for at least 20 minutes, ACS should be suspected.
  - An ECG should be performed and serial cardiac enzymes (troponin, CK-MB) should be obtained.

Findings	UA	NSTEMI	STEMI
Cardiac enzymes (troponin, CK-MB)	Negative	Positive	Positive
ECG changes	ST-segment depression, T-wave inversion, or no ECG changes (any changes are usually transient)	ST-segment depression, T-wave inversion, or no ECG changes	ST-segment elevation

Signs and Symptoms

- Chest pain/pressure (substernal, crushing) that may radiate to the left arm, jaw, shoulders, and back are common symptoms.
- Other symptoms include dyspnea, diaphoresis, N/V.
- When compared to chronic stable angina, pain in ACS may be more severe, occur at rest, occur more frequently, be precipitated by less exertion, and be refractory to sublingual NTG.
- Patients may also present with signs/symptoms of HF or with arrhythmias.

Guidelines

Anderson JL, Adams CD, Antman EM, et al; American College of Cardiology Foundation /American Heart Association Task Force on Practice Guidelines. 2012 ACCF/AHA focused update incorporated into the ACCF/AHA 2007 guidelines for the management of patients with unstable angina/non-ST-elevation myocardial infarction: a report of the American College of Cardiology Foundation/American Heart Association Task Force on Practice Guidelines. *Circulation* 2013;127(23):e663–828.

American College of Emergency Physicians; Society for Cardiovascular Angiography and Interventions, O'Gara PT, Kushner FG, Ascheim DD, et al. 2013 ACCF/AHA guideline for the management of ST-elevation myocardial infarction: a report of the American College of Cardiology Foundation/American Heart Association Task Force on Practice Guidelines. *J Am Coll Cardiol* 2013;61(4):e78–140.

ACUTE PHARMACOLOGIC MANAGEMENT OF UA/NSTEMI

Anti-Ischemic and Analgesic Therapy

Morphine

- Can be given to patients who continue to have chest discomfort despite the use of NTG or have recurrence of chest pain despite the use of other anti-ischemic therapies
- Dose: 2–4 mg IV every 5–30 minutes as needed for pain

NTG

- Can be given to patients with ongoing chest discomfort (0.4 mg sublingually every 5 min × 3 doses); following these doses, give IV NTG within the initial 48 hours if patients continue to have ischemia, or if they present with HF or are hypertensive
- Dose: 5–10 mcg/min continuous infusion; can be titrated up to 100 mcg/min for relief of symptoms
- Adverse effects: Reflex tachycardia, hypotension, headache

β-Blockers

- Oral β-blockers: Given within the first 24 hours to patients who **do not** have signs/ symptoms of HF, risk factors for developing cardiogenic shock (age >70 years, SBP <120 mmHg, HR >110 beats per minute (bpm) or <60 bpm, or prolonged duration since presenting with UA/NSTEMI), PR interval >0.24 sec, ≥2nd-degree heart block, or severe reactive airway disease
- IV β-blockers can be used as an alternative

CCBs

- A non-DHP CCB (verapamil or diltiazem) can be used alternatively if the patient has a contraindication to β-blocker therapy and does not have evidence of LV dysfunction
- A long-acting non-DHP CCB can be used in patients who have recurrent ischemia despite being on a β-blocker and nitrate therapy

ACEIs

- Should be given within the first 24 hours to patients with pulmonary congestion or LVEF ≤40%, provided they are not hypotensive (SBP <100 mmHg) or have contraindications
- Can also be useful if given within the first 24 hours to patients without pulmonary congestion or LVEF ≤40%, provided they are not hypotensive (SBP <100 mmHg) or have contraindications
- An ARB can be used alternatively in patients who cannot tolerate ACEIs

Antiplatelet Therapy

Aspirin

- All patients should receive 160–325 mg (non–enteric-coated) at the onset of chest pain (should be chewed and swallowed).
- Patients experiencing UA/NSTEMI should continue to receive the following aspirin regimens (based on whether or not they received a stent):

Procedure	Indefinite Therapy
No stent	75–162 mg daily
Bare-metal stent (BMS)	81 mg daily
Drug-eluting stent (DES)—Sirolimus-eluting	81 mg daily
DES—Paclitaxel-eluting	81 mg daily

Clopidogrel (Plavix)

- Prodrug; must be converted via CYP2C19 to active drug
- This is an alternative to aspirin in patients who are allergic or have a major GI intolerance to aspirin.
- The following loading and maintenance doses should be given (**with** aspirin):
  - Early invasive strategy (PCI ± stent)
    - » Loading dose = 600 mg × 1
    - » Maintenance dose = 75 mg daily
  - Conservative (medical) strategy
    - » Loading dose = 300 mg × 1
    - » Maintenance dose = 75 mg daily

- Clopidogrel should be continued (**with** aspirin) for the following durations of time:
  - BMS: Up to 12 months
  - DES (sirolimus or paclitaxel): At least 12 months
  - No stent: Up to 12 months
- Discontinue ≥5 days before CABG

Prasugrel (Effient)

- Prodrug
- Alternative to clopidogrel in patients with ACS managed with PCI
- Achieves faster inhibition of platelet aggregation than clopidogrel
- Administered as a loading dose of 60 mg prior to PCI, followed by maintenance dose of 10 mg daily (↓ dose to 5 mg daily in patients <60 kg)
- Not recommended for patients ≥75 years unless they have DM or history of MI (↑ risk of bleeding) or in patients with prior history of stroke or TIA
- Prasugrel should be continued (**with** aspirin) for the following duration of time:
  - BMS: Up to 12 months
  - DES: At least 12 months
- Discontinue ≥7 days before CABG

Ticagrelor (Brilinta)

- NOT a thienopyridine
  - Reversibly binds the P2Y12 receptor
  - Does not require conversion to an active metabolite (NOT a prodrug)
- Alternative antiplatelet in patients with ACS managed medically or with PCI
- Administered as a loading dose of 180 mg prior to PCI, followed by maintenance dose of 90 mg BID (dose of aspirin during maintenance therapy should not exceed 100 mg/day)
- Should be continued (**with** aspirin) for the following duration of time:
  - BMS: Up to 12 months
  - DES: At least 12 months
  - No stent: Up to 12 months
- Discontinue ≥5 days before CABG

Glycoprotein IIb/IIIa Receptor Blockers (GPBs)

- PCI planned: Clopidogrel (or prasugrel or ticagrelor) and/or GPB (eptifibatide or tirofiban) can be initiated prior to angiography. Do not need GPB if bivalirudin + 300 mg loading dose of clopidogrel (given ≥6 hours before angiography) are used.
- Conservative strategy: Adding eptifibatide or tirofiban to clopidogrel or ticagrelor can be considered (especially if patient has recurrent ischemia and requires angiography).

Anticoagulant Therapy

- PCI planned: Unfractionated heparin (UFH), enoxaparin, fondaparinux, or bivalirudin should be added to antiplatelet therapy.
- Conservative strategy: UFH, enoxaparin, or fondaparinux should be added to antiplatelet therapy.

ACUTE PHARMACOLOGIC MANAGEMENT OF STEMI

Anti-Ischemic and Analgesic Therapy

Morphine, NTG, β-Blockers, ACEIs

- Same recommendations as for UA/NSTEMI

Antiplatelet Therapy

Aspirin

- Same recommendations as for UA/NSTEMI

Clopidogrel

- This is an alternative to aspirin in patients who are allergic or have a major GI intolerance to aspirin.
- The following loading and maintenance doses should be given:
  - Patients undergoing primary PCI:
    - » Loading dose = 600 mg × 1
    - » Maintenance dose = 75 mg daily
  - Patients receiving fibrinolytic therapy and patients who do not receive reperfusion therapy:
    - » Loading dose = 300 mg × 1 (no loading dose in patients age ≥75 years)
    - » Maintenance dose = 75 mg daily
- Clopidogrel should be continued (**with** aspirin) for the following durations of time:
  - BMS or DES: 12 months
  - No stent: At least 14 days (can be considered for up to 1 year)
- Discontinue ≥ 5 days before CABG

Prasugrel

- Same recommendations as for UA/NSTEMI

Ticagrelor

- Same recommendations as for UA/NSTEMI

GPBs

- Can be used if patient undergoing primary PCI

Fibrinolytic Therapy

- Should be used in patients presenting to a hospital without the capability to perform PCI or cannot perform PCI within 120 minutes of first medical contact ("door-to-balloon" time)
- Should be initiated within 30 minutes of presenting to the hospital ("door-to-needle" time)

Anticoagulant Therapy

- Fibrinolytic administered: UFH, enoxaparin, or fondaparinux can be used; should be continued for up to 8 days; UFH should only be used if the treatment duration is <48 hours because of risk for heparin-induced thrombocytopenia (HIT) with prolonged therapy.
- Primary PCI: UFH or bivalirudin can be used.

SECONDARY PREVENTION OF MI

- **Aspirin:** See recommendation above regarding dosing and duration of therapy.
- **Clopidogrel, prasugrel, or ticagrelor:** See recommendations above in respective NSTEMI and STEMI sections regarding dosing and duration of therapy.
- **β-blockers:** Continue indefinitely.
- **ACEIs:** Should be given and continued indefinitely in all patients; ARB can be used in patients intolerant of ACEIs.
- **ARAs:** Should be given to patients with LVEF ≤40% receiving optimal ACEI and β-blocker therapy who have DM or HF.
- **Statins:** Should be given and continued indefinitely in all patients.

Glycoprotein IIb/IIIa Receptor Blockers

Mechanism of action – block the glycoprotein IIb/IIIa receptor on platelets to prevent the binding of fibrinogen → Inhibit platelet aggregation

Generic	Brand	Dose	Contra-indications	Primary Side Effects	Key Monitoring	Pertinent Drug Interactions	Med Pearl
Abciximab	ReoPro	*Loading dose*: 0.25 mg/kg IV bolus *Maintenance dose*: 0.125 mcg/kg/min (max of 10 mg/min); continue for 12 hr after PCI	• Active bleeding • Prior stroke within past 30 days or any hemorrhagic stroke • History of intracranial neoplasms or aneurysm • Thrombocytopenia • BP >180/110 mmHg • Dialysis-dependent (for eptifibatide)	• Bleeding • Thrombocytopenia	• CBC • Prothrombin time (PT)/activated partial thromboplastin time (aPTT) • Activated clotting time (ACT) (with PCI) • S/S bleeding • SC (baseline)	Anticoagulants and other antiplatelets may ↑ risk of bleeding	• Abciximab preferred over others in NSTEMI only if there is no significant delay to PCI (otherwise, eptifibatide or tirofiban preferred) • Adjust maintenance dose infusion of tirofiban and eptifibatide in renal dysfunction
Eptifibatide	Integrilin	*Loading dose*: 180 mcg/kg IV bolus × 2 (given 10 min apart) *Maintenance dose*: 2 mcg/kg/min; continue for 18–24 hr after PCI					
Tirofiban	Aggrastat	NSTEMI: *Loading dose*: 0.4 mcg/kg/min × 30 min *Maintenance dose*: 0.1 mcg/kg/min; continue for 18–24 hr after PCI STEMI (with PCI): *Loading dose*: 25 mcg/kg IV bolus *Maintenance dose*: 0.1 mcg/kg/min; continue for up to 18 hr after PCI					

Anticoagulants

Generic	Brand	Dose	Contra-indications	Primary Side Effects	Key Monitoring	Pertinent Drug Interactions	Med Pearl
Mechanism of action: • UFH: Potentiates the action of antithrombin III, which inactivates the clotting factors, IIa (thrombin), IXa, Xa, XIa, and XIIa, and ultimately prevents the conversion of fibrinogen to fibrin • Enoxaparin: Low molecular-weight heparin; similar mechanism as UFH, but primarily inhibits factor Xa • Fondparinux: Selective inhibitor of factor Xa • Bivalirudin: Direct thrombin inhibitor							
UFH	None	*Loading dose:* 60 units/kg IV bolus (max = 4,000 units) *Maintenance dose:* 12 units/kg/hr (max = 1,000 units/hr)	• Active bleeding • History of HIT • Recent stroke	• Bleeding • Thrombocytopenia (UFH and LMWH)	• PT/aPTT (only for UFH) • CBC • Anti-Xa levels (for enoxaparin) (consider in obese or renal dysfunction) • S/S bleeding	Antiplatelets and other anticoagulants may ↑ risk of bleeding	• If platelets <100,000 or ↓ by >50% from baseline, test for HIT; discontinue UFH and start direct thrombin inhibitor (e.g., argatroban) • Protamine can be used to reverse effects
Enoxaparin	Lovenox	*Loading dose:* 30 mg IV × 1 *Maintenance dose:* 1 mg/kg SC every 12 hr					• ↓ enoxaparin dose to 1 mg/kg every 24 hr if CrCl <30 mL/min • Should not use in patients with suspected HIT • Protamine only partially reverses effects
Fondaparinux	Arixtra	2.5 mg SC daily	• Active bleeding • CrCl <30 mL/min				For STEMI, can give initial dose IV
Bivalirudin	Angiomax	*Loading dose:* 0.1 mg/kg IV bolus *Maintenance dose:* 0.25 mg/kg/hr	Active bleeding		• PT/aPTT • ACT		Can also be used during PCI in patients with HIT

Fibrinolytic Agents

Mechanism of action – activate and convert plasminogen into plasmin, which then degrades fibrin (lyses the clot) to form fibrin degradation products

Generic	Brand	Dose	Contra-indications	Primary Side Effects	Key Monitoring	Pertinent Drug Interactions	Med Pearl
Reteplase (rPA)	Retavase	10 units IV × 2 doses (separated by 30 min)	• Active bleeding • Any history of intracranial hemorrhage • Known intracranial neoplasm or arteriovenous malformation • Suspected aortic dissection • Significant closed head or facial trauma within 3 months	Bleeding	• CBC • ECG (for signs of reperfusion) • S/S bleeding	Antiplatelets and other anticoagulants may ↑ risk of bleeding	tPA also approved for treatment of acute ischemic stroke and pulmonary embolism
Tenecteplase (TNK)	TNKase	All doses given as IV bolus: • <60 kg: 30 mg • 60–69.9 kg: 35 mg • 70–79.9 kg: 40 mg • 80–89.9 kg: 45 mg • ≥90 kg: 50 mg					
Tissue plasminogen activator (tPA)	Alteplase	15 mg IV bolus, then 0.75 mg/kg (max = 50 mg) over 30 min, then 0.5 mg/kg (max = 35 mg) over 60 min					

Learning Points

- **HTN**
  - For patients with stage 1 HTN who do not have a compelling indication, a thiazide diuretic should be considered 1st-line therapy. If these patients have stage 2 HTN, two antihypertensives should be started initially, one of which should be a thiazide diuretic. If patients have a compelling indication, antihypertensive agent(s) that can also be used to treat this disease state should be initiated.

- **Dyslipidemia**
  - For all patients (except for those with TG >500 mg/dL), the primary objective of therapy is achieving their individualized LDL-C goal.
  - Statins are the most effective drugs for ↓ LDL-C.
  - Niacin is the most effective drug for ↑ HDL-C.
  - Myopathy and ↑ LFTs are potential side effects of niacin, fibric acid derivatives, and statins.

- **Heart Failure**
  - ACEIs, β-blockers, ARAs, and hydralazine/isosorbide dinitrate have been shown to ↓ mortality in patients with systolic HF.
  - β-blockers should not be initiated in patients who have evidence of fluid overload (peripheral or pulmonary); patients should be relatively euvolemic before starting β-blocker therapy.
  - ARBs can be used in patients who develop intolerable cough from ACEI therapy. Hyperkalemia and renal insufficiency can be associated with both ACEIs and ARBs. If patients are unable to tolerate ACEIs or ARBs because of hyperkalemia or renal insufficiency, hydralazine/isosorbide dinitrate can be used as an alternative.

- **Antiarrhythmic Drugs**
  - Know which antiarrhythmic drugs belong in which class and their basic mechanism of action (e.g., Na^+-channel blocker)
  - Dosages of disopyramide, procainamide, flecainide, sotalol, and dofetilide must be adjusted in patients with renal dysfunction.
  - Amiodarone and dofetilide are the antiarrhythmics of choice in patients with AF who have HF.
  - Dronedarone should not be used in patients with severe HF.
  - Class IA and IC antiarrythmics should be avoided in patients with structural heart disease.
  - Lidocaine and mexiletine are only effective for ventricular arrhythmias.

- Amiodarone has a large volume of distribution and a very long half-life. It can be associated with toxicities that affect just about every organ system in the body. Chest x-ray should be performed annually while TFTs and LFTs should be evaluated every 6 months. Pulmonary function tests can be performed if patient complains of symptoms, such as shortness of breath or cough. An ophthalmologic exam can be performed if patient complains of visual changes.

- **Ischemic Heart Disease**
  - Fibrinolytic drugs should only be used for STEMI.
  - For patients undergoing PCI and receiving a DES, clopidogrel, prasugrel, or ticagrelor should be administered for at least 12 months.
  - Know examples of GPBs, LMWHs, factor Xa inhibitors, direct-thrombin inhibitors, and fibrinolytic drugs.
  - Drugs used for the secondary prevention of MI include aspirin, statins, β-blockers, ACEIs, clopidogrel/prasugrel/ticagrelor, and ARAs.

PRACTICE QUESTIONS

1. Which of the following drugs may be associated with bradycardia?

    I.   Bisoprolol
    II. Clonidine
    III. Amlodipine

    (A) I only
    (B) III only
    (C) I and II only
    (D) II and III only
    (E) I, II, and III

2. A patient has been on simvastatin 80 mg PO at bedtime for 3 weeks and is now complaining of muscle pain. Which of the following laboratory tests should be obtained?

    (A) Blood glucose
    (B) Creatine kinase
    (C) Complete blood count
    (D) Simvastatin blood concentration
    (E) Thyroid function tests

3. Which of the following is/are potential side effects of nitroglycerin?

    I.   Arrhythmias
    II. Headache
    III. Tachycardia

    (A) I only
    (B) III only
    (C) I and II only
    (D) II and III only
    (E) I, II, and III

4. Which of the following drugs is/are considered positive inotropes?

    I.   Nesiritide
    II. Hydralazine
    III. Dobutamine

    (A) I only
    (B) III only
    (C) I and II only
    (D) II and III only
    (E) I, II, and III

5. Which of the following drugs antagonize both β_1 and β_2 receptors at low doses?

   (A) Atenolol
   (B) Bisoprolol
   (C) Carvedilol
   (D) Metoprolol
   (E) Nebivolol

6. Which of the following statements regarding niacin is/are TRUE?

   I. It is also available over-the-counter.
   II. Patients should be advised to take acetaminophen 30 minutes before each dose.
   III. It can increase a patient's risk for developing hypoglycemia.

   (A) I only
   (B) III only
   (C) I and II only
   (D) II and III only
   (E) I, II, and III

7. Which of the following drugs has been shown to improve survival in patients with HFrEF?

   I. Enalapril
   II. Carvedilol
   III. Digoxin

   (A) I only
   (B) III only
   (C) I and II only
   (D) II and III only
   (E) I, II, and III

8. Which of the following oral antithrombotic agents is/are approved for the treatment of DVT and PE?

   I. Dabigatran
   II. Rivaroxaban
   III. Apixaban

   (A) I only
   (B) III only
   (C) I and II only
   (D) II and III only
   (E) I, II, and III

9. Nitroglycerin is available in which of the following formulations?

    I.   Injection
    II. Sublingual tablets
    III. Topical ointment

    (A) I only
    (B) III only
    (C) I and II only
    (D) II and III only
    (E) I, II, and III

10. Which of the following drugs is considered a class IV antiarrhythmic?

    (A) Dofetilide
    (B) Diltiazem
    (C) Flecainide
    (D) Metoprolol
    (E) Procainamide

ANSWERS

1. C

Both bisoprolol and clonidine decrease atrioventricular (AV) nodal conduction, and therefore may cause bradycardia and/or heart block. Thus, choice (C) is correct. The non-DHP CCBs (i.e., verapamil, diltiazem) also decrease AV nodal conduction and can cause bradycardia. However, the DHP CCBs, including amlodipine, have no effect on AV nodal conduction. Instead, these drugs can actually cause reflex tachycardia.

2. B

For a patient on a statin who complains of muscle pain, a creatine kinase should be obtained. Therefore, choice (B) is correct.

3. D

Nitroglycerin could potentially cause headaches and tachycardia, so choice (D) is correct. Nitroglycerin does not cause cardiac arrhythmias.

4. B

Dobutamine stimulates β_1 receptors in the heart and increases myocardial contractility and is therefore considered a positive inotrope. Nesiritide is an arterial and venous vasodilator, while hydralazine is a direct arterial vasodilator. While these drugs may increase CO, they do so by decreasing afterload and not by increasing myocardial contractility. Therefore, choice (B) is correct.

5. C

Carvedilol (C) is a nonselective β-blocker, antagonizing both the β_1 and β_2 receptors. Atenolol (A), bisoprolol (B), metoprolol (D), and nebivolol (E) are all considered cardioselective β-blockers (i.e., selectively block β_1 receptors), especially at low doses.

6. A

Niacin is available as a prescription product as well as an over-the-counter product (I). To prevent niacin-induced flushing, patients should be counseled to take either an aspirin or an NSAID 30 minutes before each dose because this adverse reaction is mediated by prostaglandins. Acetaminophen (II) does not antagonize the effects of prostaglandins and would not reduce the incidence of niacin-induced flushing. Niacin has been associated with hyperglycemia, not hypoglycemia (III).

7. **C**

ACEIs (I), certain β-blockers (carvedilol, metoprolol succinate, and bisoprolol) (II), ARAs, and isosorbide/dinitrate have all been associated with a reduction in mortality in patients with HFrEF. Although the use of digoxin (III) has been shown to reduce symptoms in patients with HFrEF, it has not been associated with a reduction in mortality.

8. **E**

All three of the novel oral anticoagulants—dabigatran (I), rivaroxaban (II), and apixaban (III)—are currently approved by the Food and Drug Administration for the treatment of DVT and PE.

9. **E**

Nitroglycerin is currently available as an IV injection (I), sublingual tablet (II), and topical ointment (III). This drug is also available as a sublingual spray, transdermal patch, and rectal ointment (for chronic anal fissures).

10. **B**

The non-DHP CCBs—verapamil and diltiazem (B)—are considered class IV antiarrhythmics. Dofetilide (A) is primarily a K^+ channel blocker and is considered a class III antiarrhythmic. Flecainide (C) and procainamide (E) are Na^+ channel blockers and are considered class I antiarrhythmics, with flecainide designated a class Ic antiarrhythmic and procainamide class Ia. β-blockers (i.e., metoprolol [D]) are considered class II antiarrhythmics.

2

Infectious Diseases

This chapter reviews various antibiotic agents, including antibacterial, antifungal, and antiviral agents. A brief overview of the recommended pharmacologic treatments of the following infections is also provided:

- **Urinary tract infections**
- **Pneumonia**
- **Meningitis**
- **Otitis media**
- **Sexually transmitted diseases**
- **Skin and soft tissue infections**
- **Invasive fungal infections**
- **Human immunodeficiency virus**
- **Tuberculosis**

 Suggested Study Time: **4 hours**

PRINCIPLES OF ANTIBIOTIC THERAPY

Factors to Consider When Selecting Antibiotic Therapy

- Identity/susceptibility of bacteria
    - Important to know which bacteria may be causing the infection
        - » Can begin empiric antibiotic therapy without knowing the actual identity (or sensitivities) of the organism; select antibiotic(s) (usually broad-spectrum) based on the organism(s) *most* likely to cause a particular infection
        - » Once organism (and sensitivities) are identified, can adjust/narrow antibiotic therapy, as needed, to cover this organism

- Site of infection
  - Especially important for meningitis, UTIs, prostatitis, and osteomyelitis
    - » Only certain antibiotics can penetrate into these areas to target the infection; these drugs may need to be used at higher doses, especially for meningitis, prostatitis, and osteomyelitis
- Patient allergies
- Concomitant medications
  - May need to be concerned with potential drug interactions when selecting an antibiotic
- Hepatic and renal function
  - May need to adjust antibiotic dosages if hepatic or renal dysfunction present
- Past medical history
  - Certain antibiotics may need to be avoided in particular disease states (e.g., seizure disorders)
- Patient age
  - Some antibiotics are contraindicated in pediatric patients
- Pregnancy/breastfeeding
  - Some antibiotics are contraindicated in these patients

URINARY TRACT INFECTIONS

Common Organisms

Community-Acquired	Nosocomial (Hospital-Acquired)
• *E. coli* • *Staphylococcus saprophyticus* • *Klebsiella pneumoniae* • *Proteus mirabilis*	• *E. coli* • *Pseudomonas aeruginosa* • *Klebsiella pneumoniae* • *Proteus mirabilis* • *Enterobacter* spp. • *Staphylococcus aureus* • Fungus (e.g., *Candida*)

Diagnosis

- Confirmed by urinalysis
  - Bacteruria: $>10^2$ cfu/mL
  - Pyuria: >5–10 white blood cells (WBCs)/mm^3
  - Nitrite-positive
  - Leukocyte esterase–positive
  - Casts (may be present in pyelonephritis)

Signs and Symptoms

- Lower UTI (cystitis)
  - Dysuria
  - Urgency
  - Frequency
  - Nocturia
  - Suprapubic pressure/pain
- Upper UTI (pyelonephritis)
  - All of the above symptoms, *plus*
  - Flank pain
  - Fever
  - Nausea/vomiting (N/V)
- Complicated UTI factors
  - Male
  - Elderly
  - Pregnancy
  - Children
  - Nosocomial
  - Recent use of antibiotics
  - Diabetes
  - Immunosuppressed
  - Catheterized

Guidelines

Gupta K, Hooton TM, Naber KG, et al; Infectious Diseases Society of America; European Society for Microbiology and Infectious Diseases. International clinical practice guidelines for the treatment of acute uncomplicated cystitis and pyelonephritis in women: a 2010 update by the Infectious Diseases Society of America and the European Society for Microbiology and Infectious Diseases. *Clin Infect Dis* 2011;52:e103–20.

Guidelines Summary

Acute Uncomplicated Cystitis

First-line therapy	Nitrofurantoin 100 mg PO BID × 5 days
Second-line therapy	Trimethoprim/sulfamethoxazole (TMP/SMX) 160/800 mg (double-strength [DS]) PO BID × 3 days
Third-line therapy	Fosfomycin 3 g PO × 1 dose

- *Alternative agents:*
  - Fluoroquinolone (FQ) x 3 days
    - » Only use when other agents cannot be used
  - β-lactams (i.e., amoxicillin-clavulanate, cefdinir, cefaclor, cefpodoxime) x 3–7 days
    - » Avoid unless other agents are not appropriate

Acute Pyelonephritis (outpatient therapy)

- First-line therapy:
  - Ciprofloxacin 500 mg PO BID x 7 days
  - Cipro XR 1 g PO daily x 7 days
  - Levofloxacin 750 mg PO daily x 5 days
- Second-line therapy: TMP/SMX DS PO BID x 14 days

+/–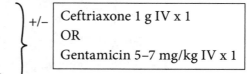

| Ceftriaxone 1 g IV x 1 |
| OR |
| Gentamicin 5–7 mg/kg IV x 1 |

- Third-line therapy: Oral β-lactam (i.e., amoxicillin-clavulanate) x 10–14 days AND one-time dose of ceftriaxone 1 g IV or gentamicin 5–7 mg/kg IV

Acute Pyelonephritis (inpatient therapy)

- IV FQ
- Aminoglycoside +/- IV ampicillin
- IV extended-spectrum cephalosporin or penicillin +/- aminoglycoside
- IV carbapenem (e.g., imipenem/cilastatin)

Complicated UTIs

- Duration of therapy: 10–14 days

PNEUMONIA

Common Organisms

Community-Acquired	Hospital-Acquired (occurs ≥48 hours after admission)
• *Mycoplasma pneumoniae*	• *Staphylococcus aureus*
• *Streptococcus pneumoniae*	• *Pseudomonas aeruginosa*
• *Haemophilus influenzae*	• *Klebsiella pneumoniae*
• *Chlamydia pneumoniae*	• *Enterobacter*
• *Legionella pneumophila*	• *E. coli*
• *Moraxella catarrhalis*	• *Acinetobacter spp.*
• *Viruses*	• *Serratia spp.*
	• *Anaerobes*

Diagnosis

- Symptoms and ausculatory findings consistent with pneumonia, plus an infiltrate on chest x-ray
- Diagnosis can often be made on history and physical exam findings

Signs and Symptoms

- Fever, chills, dyspnea, cough (may or may not be productive), rigors, pleuritic pain
- Physical examination:
  - Tachypnea
  - Tachycardia
  - Dullness to percussion
  - Inspiratory crackles
  - ↓ breath sounds over affected area
- Laboratory findings
  - ↑ WBCs
- Infiltrate on chest x-ray

Guidelines

Mandell LA, Wunderink RG, Anzueto A; Infectious Diseases Society of America; American Thoracic Society. Infectious Diseases Society of America/American Thoracic Society consensus guidelines on the management of community-acquired pneumonia in adults. *Clin Infect Dis* 2007;44(suppl 2):S27–72.

American Thoracic Society; Infectious Diseases Society of America. Guidelines for the management of adults with hospital-acquired, ventilator-associated, and health care–associated pneumonia. *Am J Respir Crit Care Med* 2005;171(4):388–416.

Guidelines Summary

Diagnosis	Treatment	Duration
Community-acquired (ambulatory)	*Previously healthy and no antibiotic therapy in past 3 months:* Macrolide (clarithromycin or azithromycin) **OR** Doxycycline	≥5 days
	With comorbidities (see below)[1] at risk for drug-resistant Streptococcus pneumoniae or antibiotic use in past 3 months: FQ (moxifloxacin, gemifloxacin, or levofloxacin) **OR** Macrolide (or doxycycline) *plus* one of the following: • High-dose amoxicillin • Amoxicillin/clavulanate • Cephalosporin (ceftriaxone, cefuroxime, or cefpodoxime)	
Community-acquired (hospitalized)	*Moderate:* FQ (moxifloxacin, gemifloxacin, or levofloxacin) **OR** Macrolide (or doxycycline) *plus* one of the following: • Ampicillin • Ceftriaxone • Cefotaxime	
	Severe: FQ (moxifloxacin, gemifloxacin, or levofloxacin) **OR** Azithromycin *plus* one of the following: • Ampicillin/sulbactam • Ceftriaxone • Cefotaxime	
Hospital-acquired	*Hospitalized <5 days and no risk factors for multidrug-resistant (MDR) organisms (see below) (select one of the following drugs):[2]* • 3rd-generation cephalosporin (ceftriaxone or cefotaxime) • FQ (ciprofloxacin, moxifloxacin, or levofloxacin) • Ampicillin/sulbactam • Ertapenem	8 days (14 days if due to *Pseudomonas*)
	Hospitalized ≥5 days or risk factors for MDR organisms (see below)[2]: FQ (ciprofloxacin or levofloxacin) **OR** Aminoglycoside *plus* one of the following: • Ceftazidime or cefepime • Imipenem/cilastatin or meropenem • Piperacillin/tazobactam	

[1] *Comorbidities: Chronic obstructive pulmonary disease (COPD), diabetes, chronic renal failure, chronic liver failure, heart failure (HF), cancer, asplenia, immunosuppressed*

[2] *Risk factors for MDR organisms: Recent antibiotic therapy (in last 90 days), hospitalized ≥5 days, ↑ resistance in environment, nursing home resident, chronic dialysis, home infusion therapy, immunosuppressed*

MENINGITIS

Common Organisms

Age Group	Most Common Organisms
<1 mo	• *Streptococcus agalactiae* (Group B Strep) • *E. coli* • *Listeria monocytogenes* • *Klebsiella* spp.
1–23 mo	• *Streptococcus pneumoniae* • *Neisseria meningitidis* • Group B Strep • *Haemophilus influenzae* • *E. coli*
2–50 yr	• *Neisseria meningitidis* • *Streptococcus pneumoniae*
>50 yr	• *Streptococcus pneumoniae* • *Neisseria meningitidis* • Group B Strep

Diagnosis

- Confirmed by analysis of cerebrospinal fluid (CSF)
  - Bacterial meningitis: ↓ glucose, ↑ protein, ↑ WBCs
  - Gram stain can help identify organism

Signs and Symptoms

- Symptoms
  - Fever, chills
  - Headache, photophobia
  - Nuchal rigidity
  - N/V
  - Altered mental status
  - Petechiae/purpura (*Neisseria meningitidis*)
- Signs
  - Brudzinski's sign (flexion of hips and knees upon flexing the neck)
  - Kernig's sign (pain develops when the knee is extended after flexing the hip to 90 degrees)
  - Bulging fontanelle (children)

Guidelines

Tunkel AR, Hartman BJ, Kaplan SL, et al. Practice guidelines for the management of bacterial meningitis. *Clin Infect Dis* 2004;39:1267–84.

Guidelines Summary

Empiric Treatment

Age Group	Treatment
<1 mo	Ampicillin + aminoglycoside **OR** Ampicillin + cefotaxime
1–23 mo	Third-generation cephalosporin (cefotaxime or ceftriaxone) + vancomycin
2–50 yr	Third-generation cephalosporin (cefotaxime or ceftriaxone) + vancomycin
>50 yr	Third-generation cephalosporin (cefotaxime or ceftriaxone) + vancomycin + ampicillin

- Dexamethasone may be considered as adjunctive therapy for the following:
  - Infants and Children: *H. influenzae* meningitis
  - Adults: *Streptococcus pneumonia* meningitis

OTITIS MEDIA

Definitions

- Acute otitis media (AOM): Rapid onset of signs/symptoms of inflammation and effusion (fluid) in the middle ear
- Otitis media with effusion (OME): Fluid and inflammation in the middle ear *without* evidence of signs/symptoms of acute infection
- Recurrent AOM: ≥3 episodes of AOM within previous 6 months **OR** 4 episodes of AOM within previous 12 months (with ≥1 episode within previous 6 months)

Common Organisms

- *Streptococcus pneumoniae*
- *Haemophilus influenzae*
- *Moraxella catarrhalis*

Diagnosis

- Key elements in diagnosis of AOM:
  - Acute (<48 hr) onset of signs/symptoms

- Middle ear inflammation and erythema of tympanic membrane
- Presence of middle ear effusion
  » Leads to bulging of tympanic membrane → May lead to perforation and drainage (otorrhea)

Signs and Symptoms

- Otalgia
  - May be demonstrated by:
    » Holding/tugging/rubbing of ear
    » Excessive crying
    » Fever
    » Changes in sleep or behavior pattern
- Otoscopic findings:
  - Middle ear effusion
  - Tympanic membrane → Bulging and erythematous

Guidelines

Lieberthal AS, Carroll AE, Chonmaitree T, et al. The diagnosis and management of acute otitis media. *Pediatrics* 2013;131(3):e964–99.

Guidelines Summary

Initial Management of Uncomplicated AOM

Age	Otorrhea with AOM	Unilateral or Bilateral AOM with Severe Symptoms	Bilateral AOM without Otorrhea	Unilateral AOM without Otorrhea
6 months–2 years	Antibiotic therapy	Antibiotic therapy	Antibiotic therapy	Antibiotic therapy **OR** additional observation
≥2 years	Antibiotic therapy	Antibiotic therapy	Antibiotic therapy **OR** additional observation	Antibiotic therapy **OR** additional observation

Recommended Antibiotic Therapy for Management of Uncomplicated AOM

	First-Line Therapy	Alternative Therapy
Initial Immediate or Delayed Treatment	Amoxicillin (high-dose) 80–90 mg/kg/day PO in 2 divided doses **OR** *If history of amoxicillin use in past 90 days, concurrent purulent conjunctivitis, or history of recurrent AOM unresponsive to amoxicillin:* Amoxicillin-clavulanate (high-dose) 90 mg/kg/day + 6.4 mg/kg/day of clavulanate in 2 divided doses	*If penicillin allergy:* Cefdinir **OR** Cefuroxime **OR** Cefpodoxime **OR** Ceftriaxone × 1 or 3 days
Treatment After 48–72 Hours of Failure of Initial Antibiotic Treatment	Amoxicillin-clavulanate (high-dose) 90 mg/kg/day + 6.4 mg/kg/day of clavulanate po in 2 divided doses **OR** Ceftriaxone 50 mg IM or IV for 3 days	Ceftriaxone × 3 days **OR** Clindamycin

Duration of Therapy

Age/Characteristic of Symptoms	Duration
<2 yr or severe symptoms	10 days
2–5 yr with mild–moderate symptoms	7 days
≥6 yr with mild–moderate symptoms	5–7 days

SEXUALLY TRANSMITTED DISEASES

Causative Organisms

Disease	Organisms
Chlamydia	*Chlamydia trachomatis*
Gonorrhea	*Neisseria gonorrhoeae*
Syphilis	*Treponema pallidum*

Diagnosis

- Chlamydia: Test performed on urine swab or endocervical/vaginal/male urethral swab
- Gonorrhea: Gram-stained smears or culture (endocervical/vaginal/male urethral/urine specimen)
- Syphilis: Dark field examination and direct fluorescent antibody stains of exudates
  - Serologic testing
    - » Nontreponemal: Venereal Disease Research Laboratory (VDRL) slide test, rapid plasma regain (RPR) test; can be used for screening

» Treponemal: Fluorescent treponemal antibody absorbed (FTA-ABS), *T. pallidum* particle agglutination (TP-PA); can be used to confirm diagnosis

Signs and Symptoms

- Chlamydia
  - Penile/vaginal discharge, dysuria
  - May also be asymptomatic
- Gonorrhea
  - Penile/vaginal discharge, dysuria, urinary frequency
  - May also be asymptomatic
- Syphilis
  - Primary (10–90 days after exposure): Presence of chancre
  - Secondary (2–8 wk after development of primary stage): Variety of rashes/lesions, flu-like symptoms, and lymphadenopathy
  - Latent (positive serologic test but no clinical manifestations)
  - Tertiary: Cardiovascular (e.g., aortic insufficiency) and neurologic abnormalities (e.g., deafness, blindness, dementia, paresis)

Guidelines

Workowski KA, Berman S; Centers for Disease Control and Prevention (CDC). Sexually transmitted diseases treatment guidelines, 2010. *MMWR Recomm Rep* 2010;59(RR-12):1–110.

Guidelines Summary

Disease	Treatment
Chlamydia	Azithromycin 1 g PO × 1 dose **OR** Doxycycline 100 mg PO q12h × 7 days
Gonorrhea	Ceftriaxone 250 mg IM × 1 dose **PLUS** Treatment for chlamydia (if not ruled out)
Syphilis	*Primary, secondary, or early latent syphilis (<1 yr in duration):* • Benzathine penicillin G 2.4 million units IM × 1 dose *Late latent syphilis (>1 yr in duration), latent syphilis of unknown duration, or tertiary syphilis (not neurosyphilis):* • Benzathine penicillin G 2.4 million units IM once weekly × 3 weeks *Neurosyphilis:* • Aqueous penicillin G 3–4 million units IV or as continuous infusion q4h × 10–14 days

SKIN AND SOFT TISSUE INFECTIONS

Common Organisms

- Community-acquired SSTIs
  - *Staphylococcus aureus* (especially methicillin-resistant *Staphylococcus aureus* [MRSA])
  - Group A streptococci (*Streptococcus pyogenes*)
- Nosocomial SSTIs
  - Gram-negative organisms (e.g., *Pseudomonas aeruginosa, E. coli*)
  - Anaerobes

Diagnosis

- Purulent SSTIs
  - Abscess: Collection of pus within the dermis and deeper skin tissues
    » Painful, tender, fluctuant red nodules accompanied by a pustule and surrounded by rim of erythematous swelling
  - Furuncle: Infection of the hair follicle ("boil"); pus extends into subcutaneous tissue
    » Inflammatory nodules with overlying pustules through which hair emerges
  - Carbuncle: Adjacent furuncles coalesce to form a single pus-filled mass
- Nonpurulent SSTIs
  - Cellulitis: Affects epidermis and dermis; may spread within superficial fascia
  - Erysipelas: Form of cellulitis that tends to be limited to upper dermis
  - Necrotizing fasciitis: Severe, life-threatening infection of subcutaneous tissue that results in progressive destruction of superficial fascia and subcutaneous fat

Signs and Symptoms

- Purulent SSTIs
  - Pus-filled, erythematous lesion(s)
  - Systemic signs/symptoms of infection uncommon
- Nonpurulent SSTIs
  - Rapidly spreading areas of erythema, swelling, tenderness, and warmth
  - Lymph nodes may become swollen
  - Systemic signs/symptoms of infection more common

Guidelines

Stevens DL, Bisno AL, Chambers HF, et al. Practice guidelines for the diagnosis and management of skin and soft tissue infections: 2014 update by the Infectious Diseases Society of America. *Clin Infect Dis* 2014;59(2):e10–52.

Guidelines Summary

Infection	Empiric Treatment
Purulent SSTIs	
Mild	Incision and drainage; no antibiotics
Moderate (with systemic signs of infection*)	Incision and drainage **PLUS** antibiotics: TMP/SMX **OR** Doxycycline
Severe (failed incision and drainage plus PO antibiotics **OR** have systemic signs of infection,* **OR** are immunocompromised)	Incision and drainage **PLUS** antibiotics: Vancomycin **OR** Daptomycin **OR** Linezolid **OR** Telavancin **OR** Ceftaroline **OR** Dalbavancin **OR** Oritavancin **OR** Tedizolid
Nonpurulent SSTIs	
Mild	Penicillin VK **OR** Cephalosporin (PO) **OR** Dicloxacillin **OR** Clindamycin (PO)
Moderate (with systemic signs of infection*)	Penicillin (IV) **OR** Ceftriaxone **OR** Cefazolin **OR** Clindamycin (IV)

Infection	Empiric Treatment
Non Purulent SSTIs (cont'd)	
Severe (failed PO antibiotics **OR** signs of systemic infection*, **OR** immunocompromised **OR** signs of deeper infection [e.g., bullae, skin sloughing, hypotension, evidence of organ dysfunction])	Emergent surgical inspection/debridement **PLUS** antibiotics: Vancomycin **AND** Piperacillin/tazobactam

* Signs of systemic infection: Temperature >38°C, heart rate >90 beats/minute, respiratory rate >24 breaths/minute, WBCs >12,000 cells/µL or <400 cells/µL

Invasive Fungal Infections

Drugs of Choice for Selected Invasive Fungal Infections

Organism	Disease	First-Line Therapy	Duration
Candida albicans, C. glabrata, C. krusei, C. tropicalis	Candidemia	*Nonneutropenic:* Fluconazole **OR** Echinocandin *Neutropenic:* Echinocandin **OR** Lipid amphotericin B	14 days after first negative blood culture
	Urinary candidiasis	Treat only if symptomatic or high-risk: Fluconazole	14 days
Blastomyces dermatitidis	Pulmonary blastomycosis	*Mild to moderate:* Itraconazole *Moderately severe to severe:* Amphotericin B × 1–2 wks, then itraconazole × 6–12 months	6–12 months
	Disseminated blastomycosis	*Mild to moderate:* Itraconazole *Moderately severe to severe:* Amphotericin B × 1–2 wks, then itraconazole × 12 months	*Mild to moderate:* 6–12 mo *Moderately severe to severe:* 12 mo
	Immunosuppressed	Amphotericin B × 1–2 wks, then itraconazole × 12 mo	12 mo
Aspergillus fumigatus, A. flavus, A. niger	Pulmonary aspergillosis	Voriconazole	Not well defined; treat until resolution/ stabilization of all clinical and radiographic signs/ symptoms

Drugs of Choice for Selected Invasive Fungal Infections *(cont'd)*

Organism	Disease	First-Line Therapy	Duration
Coccidioides immitis	Pulmonary coccidioidomycosis	Amphotericin B or high-dose fluconazole	1 year
	Disseminated (nonmeningeal) coccidioidomycosis	Fluconazole or itraconazole	Prolonged (may be lifelong)
	Disseminated (meningeal) coccidioidomycosis	Fluconazole	Prolonged (may be lifelong)
Histoplasma capsulatum	Pulmonary histoplasmosis	*Mild to moderate:* Symptoms <4 wks: No treatment Symptoms >4 wks: Itraconazole *Moderately severe to severe:* Amphotericin B × 1–2 wks, then itraconazole × total of 12 wks	*Mild to moderate:* 6–12 wks *Moderately severe to severe:* 12 wks
Cryptococcus neoformans	Cryptococcal meningoencephalitis (in HIV-infected patients)	*Induction:* Amphotericin B + flucytosine *Consolidation:* Fluconazole	*Induction:* ≥2 wks *Consolidation:* ≥8 wks

Medication Charts: Antibacterial Agents

Penicillins (β-Lactams)

Mechanism of action – inhibit bacterial cell wall synthesis; bactericidal

Generic	Brand	Dose/Dosage Forms	Spectrum of Activity	Contra-indications	Primary Side Effects	Pertinent Drug Interactions	Med Pearl	Top 200
Natural Penicillins								
Penicillin G	Pfizerpen	• 2–4 million units IV q4–6h • Injection	• Strep. viridans • Strep. pyogenes • Strep. pneumoniae (↑ resistance) • Mouth anaerobes	Allergy to penicillins, cephalosporins, or carbapenems	• Hypersensitivity reaction (rash, hives, dyspnea, throat swelling) • N/V/D • Interstitial nephritis • Hemolytic anemia (with prolonged administration)	• Probenecid may ↑ effects (may be used for this purpose) • May ↓ effects of oral contraceptives	• Adjust dose in renal dysfunction • Penicillin G benzathine or procaine used for syphilis; benzathine also used for Strep throat	No
Penicillin G benzathine	Bicillin LA	• 1.2–2.4 million units IM at specified intervals • Injection						No
Penicillin G procaine	Wycillin	• 1.2–4.8 million units IM/day at specified intervals • Injection					• Take penicillin VK 1 hour before or 2 hours after meals	No
Penicillin VK	Veetids	• 250–500 mg PO q6h • Solution, tabs						Yes
Penicillinase-Resistant Penicillins								
Dicloxacillin	Only available generically	• 125–500 mg PO q6h • Caps	• Staph aureus (methicillin-sensitive, MSSA) • Streptococcus	Same as natural penicillins	Same as natural penicillins	Same as natural penicillins	• No need to adjust dose in renal dysfunction (cleared by biliary excretion) • Take dicloxacillin 1 hour before or 2 hours after meals • Patients on nafcillin (IV) can be switched to dicloxacillin (PO)	No
Nafcillin	Only available generically	• 500 mg–2 g IV q4–6h • Injection						No
Oxacillin	Only available generically	• 250 mg–2 g IV q4–6h • Injection						No

Penicillins (β-Lactams) *(cont'd)*

Generic	Brand	Dose/Dosage Forms	Spectrum of Activity	Contra-indications	Primary Side Effects	Pertinent Drug Interactions	Med Pearl	Top 200
Aminopenicillins								
Amoxicillin	Moxatag	• Immediate-release (IR): 250–500 mg PO q8h or 500–875 mg PO q12h • Extended release (ER): 775 mg PO daily • Caps, suspension, chewable tabs, tabs (ER and IR)	• *Strep pneumoniae* • *H. influenzae* • *E. coli* • *Proteus mirabilis* • *Salmonella* • *Shigella*	Same as natural penicillins	Same as natural penicillins	Same as natural penicillins	• Amoxicillin can be used in three-drug regimen for *H. pylori* • Adjust dose in renal dysfunction • Take ampicillin 1 hour before or 2 hours after meals	Yes
Ampicillin	Only available generically	• 250–500 mg PO q6h • 250 mg–2 g IV q4–6h • Caps, injection, suspension						No
Aminopenicillins + β-Lactamase Inhibitors								
Amoxicillin-clavulanate	Augmentin	• IR: 250–500 mg PO q8h or 500–875 mg PO q12h • ER: 2,000 mg PO q12h • Chewable tabs, suspension, tabs (ER and IR)	• β lactamase-producing *Staph. aureus* (MSSA), *H. influenzae, M. catarrhalis, E. coli,* and *K. pneumoniae* • Anaerobes	Same as natural penicillins	Same as natural penicillins	Same as natural penicillins	• Adjust dose in renal dysfunction • Patients on ampicillin sulbactam (IV) can be switched to amoxicillin-clavulanate (PO) • Good anaerobic coverage	Yes
Ampicillin-sulbactam	Unasyn	• 1.5–3 g IV q6h • Injection						No
Antipseudomonal Penicillins + β-Lactamase Inhibitors								
Piperacillin-tazobactam	Zosyn	• 3.375 IV q6h or 4.5 g IV q6–8h • Injection	• Same as amoxicillin-clavulanate and ampicillin-sulbactam	Same as natural penicillins	Same as natural penicillins	Same as natural penicillins	• Adjust dose in renal dysfunction • Primarily used for *Pseudomonas* infections	No
Ticarcillin-clavulanic acid	Timentin	• 3.1 g IV q4–6h • Injection	• *Pseudomonas aeruginosa*				• Good anaerobic coverage • Contain Na$^+$ (use with caution in volume-overloaded patients)	No

Cephalosporins (β-Lactams)

Generic	Brand	Dose/Dosage Forms	Spectrum of Activity	Contraindications	Primary Side Effects	Pertinent Drug Interactions	Med Pearl	Top 200
Mechanism of action – inhibit bacterial cell wall synthesis; bactericidal • As drugs move from 1st through 4th generation, ↑ activity against Gram (−) organisms and ↓ activity against Gram (+) organisms								
First-Generation								
Cefadroxil	Only available generically	• 500 mg–1 g PO q12h • Caps, suspension, tabs	• *Staph. aureus* • *Staph. epidermidis* • *Strep. pyogenes* • *Strep. pneumoniae* • *E. coli* • *P. mirabilis* • *K. pneumoniae*	Allergy to penicillins, cephalosporins, or carbapenems (up to 10% risk of cross-sensitivity)	Same as natural penicillins	Same as natural penicillins	• Adjust dose in renal dysfunction	No
Cefazolin	Ancef	• 250 mg–1 g IV q8h • Injection					• Patients on cefazolin (IV) can be switched to cephalexin (PO)	No
Cephalexin	Keflex	• 250–500 mg PO q6h • Caps, suspension, tabs					• Cefazolin often used for surgical prophylaxis	Yes
Second-Generation								
Cefaclor	Only available generically	• 250–500 mg PO q8h • Caps, ER tabs, suspension	• Gram (+) activity similar to 1st-generation agents • Same Gram (−) activity as 1st-generation agents, but with added activity against *Acinetobacter, Citrobacter, Enterobacter, Neisseria, Serratia,* and *H. influenzae* • Anaerobic activity (cefotetan and cefoxitin only)	Same as 1st-generation agents	• Same as natural penicillins • Bleeding/bruising (with cefotetan and cefoxitin)	• Same as natural penicillins • Disulfiram-like reaction may occur if alcohol is used during treatment with cefotetan • Cefotetan and cefoxitin may ↑ effects of warfarin	• Adjust dose in renal dysfunction • Take cefaclor ER tabs and cefuroxime suspension with food to ↑ absorption	No
Cefotetan	Only available generically	• 1–2 g IV q12h • Injection						No
Cefoxitin	Mefoxin	• 1–2 g IV q6–8h • Injection						No
Cefprozil	Only available generically	• 250–500 mg q12–24h • Suspension, tabs						No
Cefuroxime	• Ceftin • Zinacef	• 250–500 mg PO q12h • 500 mg–1.5 g IV q8h • Injection, suspension, tabs						No

Cephalosporins (β-Lactams) *(cont'd)*

Generic	Brand	Dose/Dosage Forms	Spectrum of Activity	Contraindications	Primary Side Effects	Pertinent Drug Interactions	Med Pearl	Top 200
Third-Generation								
Cefdinir	Only available generically	• 300 mg PO q12h or 600 mg PO daily • Caps, suspension	• Limited Gram (+) activity • More extensive Gram (−) activity vs. 2nd-generation agents • *Pseudomonas aeruginosa* (ceftazidime only)	• Same as 1st-generation agents • Ceftriaxone should be avoided in neonates (↑ risk of hyperbilirubinemia, kernicterus)	Same as natural penicillins	• Same as natural penicillins • Antacids and iron may ↓ absorption of cefdinir	• Adjust dose for all, except cefoperazone and ceftriaxone, in renal dysfunction • Take cefpodoxime and cefditoren tabs with food to ↑ absorption • Take ceftibuten suspension 2 hours before or 1 hour after meals • Ceftriaxone often used for meningitis and STDs	Yes
Cefditoren	Spectracef	• 200–400 mg PO q12h • Tabs				• Antacids and H₂ antagonists may ↓ absorption of cefpodoxime • Ceftriaxone may cause precipitation if given with Ca²⁺-containing solutions		No
Cefixime	Suprax	• 400 mg PO daily • Caps, suspension, chewable tabs, tabs						No
Cefpodoxime	Only available generically	• 100–400 mg PO q12h • Suspension, tabs						No
Cefotaxime	Claforan	• 1–2 g IV q8h • Injection						No
Ceftazidime	• Fortaz • Tazicef	• 1–2 g IV q8–12h • Injection						No
Ceftibuten	Cedax	• 400 mg PO daily • Caps, suspension						No
Ceftriaxone	Rocephin	• 1–2 g IV daily • Injection						No
Fourth-Generation								
Cefepime	Maxipime	• 1–2 g IV q8–12h • Injection	• Gram (+) activity better than 3rd-generation agents • More extensive Gram (−) activity vs. 3rd-generation agents • *Pseudomonas aeruginosa*	Same as 1st-generation agents	Same as natural penicillins	Same as natural penicillins	Adjust dose in renal dysfunction	No

Cephalosporins (β-Lactams) *(cont'd)*

Generic	Brand	Dose/Dosage Forms	Spectrum of Activity	Contraindications	Primary Side Effects	Pertinent Drug Interactions	Med Pearl	Top 200
Fifth-Generation								
Ceftaroline	Teflaro	• 600 mg IV q12h • Injection	• *Staph. aureus* (MSSA and MRSA [for skin infections only]) • *Strep. pyogenes* • *Strep. pneumoniae* • *Klebsiella* • *E. coli* • *H. influenzae*	Same as 1st-generation agents	Same as natural penicillins	Same as natural penicillins	Adjust dose in renal dysfunction	No

Carbapenems (β-Lactams)

Generic	Brand	Dose/Dosage Forms	Spectrum of Activity	Contraindications	Primary Side Effects	Pertinent Drug Interactions	Med Pearl	Top 200
Mechanism of action – inhibit bacterial cell wall synthesis; bactericidal								
Doripenem	Doribax	• 500 mg IV q8h • Injection	• Broad-spectrum (active against Gram (+), Gram (–), and anaerobic organisms) • All, except ertapenem, are active against *Pseudomonas aeruginosa*	Allergy to penicillins, cephalosporins, or carbapenems	• Same as natural penicillins • Seizures (esp. in patients with renal dysfunction or history of seizure disorder)	• Same as natural penicillins • May ↓ valproic acid levels	• Adjust dose in renal dysfunction • Risk of seizures is highest with imipenem/cilastatin	No
Ertapenem	Invanz	• 1 g IV daily • Injection						No
Imipenem-cilastatin	Primaxin	• 250 mg–1 g IV q6–12h • Injection						No
Meropenem	Merrem	• 500 mg–1 g IV q8h • Injection						No

Monobactam (β-Lactam)

Mechanism of action – inhibit bacterial cell wall synthesis; bactericidal

Generic	Brand	Dose/Dosage Forms	Spectrum of Activity	Contra-indications	Primary Side Effects	Pertinent Drug Interactions	Med Pearl	Top 200
Aztreonam	• Azactam • Cayston	• 500 mg–2 g IV q6–12h • Injection, nebulizer solution	Only effective against Gram (–) organisms, including *Pseudomonas aeruginosa*	None	Same as natural penicillins	None	• Can be used in patients allergic to penicillins, cephalosporins, or carbapenems • Adjust dose in renal dysfunction • Cayston used for cystic fibrosis patients (*Pseudomonas*)	No

Aminoglycosides

Generic	Brand	Dose/Dosage Forms	Spectrum of Activity	Contra-indications	Primary Side Effects	Pertinent Drug Interactions	Med Pearl	Top 200
Mechanism of action – inhibit bacterial protein synthesis by binding to the 30S subunit of the bacterial ribosome; bactericidal								
Amikacin	Only available generically	• 15 mg/kg IV q24h or 5–7.5 mg/kg IV q8h • Injection	• Primarily used for Gram (–) organisms (E. coli, Klebsiella, P. mirabilis, Enterobacter, Acinetobacter, Serratia, Pseudomonas aeruginosa) • Provide synergistic activity against Staph., Strep., or Enterococcus when used with penicillins or vancomycin	None	• Nephrotoxicity • Ototoxicity (both related to dose and duration of therapy; may be reversible)	• May ↑ effects of neuromuscular blocking agents • ↑ risk of nephrotoxicity when used with amphotericin B, loop diuretics, tacrolimus, cyclosporine, or cisplatin	• Bactericidal effect is concentration–dependent • Target serum concentrations (for traditional dosing): • Amikacin: Peak = Life-threatening infections: 25–40 mcg/mL; serious infections: 20–25 mcg/mL; urinary tract infections: 15–20 mcg/mL; Trough <8 mcg/mL (The American Thoracic Society [ATS] recommends trough levels of <4–5 mcg/mL for patients with hospital-acquired pneumonia)	No
Gentamicin	Gentak	• 5–7 mg/kg IV q24h or 1–2.5 mg/kg IV q8–12h • Injection, ophthalmic ointment/solution, topical cream/ointment						No
Neomycin	Only available generically	• 500 mg–2 g PO q6–8h • Tabs, oral solution	• Streptomycin and amikacin active against Mycobacteria • Neomycin used as prep for bowel surgery or for hepatic encephalopathy				• Tobramycin and gentamicin: Peak = 4–10 mcg/mL, depending on the infection; Trough = 0.5–2 mcg/mL for serious infections; <1 mcg/mL for hospital-acquired pneumonia • Target serum concentrations (for extended-interval dosing) (peaks not routinely monitored):	No
Streptomycin	Only available generically	• 15 mg/kg/day IM • Injection						No
Tobramycin	TOBI	• 5–7 mg/kg IV q24h or 1–2.5 mg/kg IV q8–12h • Injection, nebulizer solution, ophthalmic ointment/solution					• Amikacin: Trough <8 mcg/mL (The ATS recommends trough levels of <4–5 mcg/mL for patients with hospital-acquired pneumonia) • Tobramycin and gentamicin: Trough = 0.5–2 mcg/mL for serious infections, <1 mcg/mL for hospital-acquired pneumonia • TOBI used for cystic fibrosis patients (Pseudomonas)	No

Macrolides and Ketolides

Mechanism of action – inhibit bacterial protein synthesis by binding to the 50S subunit of the bacterial ribosome; bacteriostatic

Macrolides

Generic	Brand	Dose/Dosage Forms	Spectrum of Activity	Contraindications	Primary Side Effects	Pertinent Drug Interactions	Med Pearl	Top 200
Azithromycin	• AzaSite • Zithromax • Zmax	• 250–500 mg PO/IV q24h • Zmax: 2 g PO x 1 • Injection, ophthalmic solution, suspension (IR and ER), tabs	• Gram (+) organisms (esp. *Streptococcus*); azithromycin and clarithromycin have better activity against *Streptococcus* than erythromycin	QT interval prolongation or concurrent use with other drugs that prolong QT interval (azithromycin, clarithromycin, and erythromycin)	• Prolonged QT interval (azithromycin, clarithromycin, and erythromycin) • N/V/D • Phlebitis (erythromycin IV)	• Clarithromycin and erythromycin are major substrates and inhibitors of CYP3A4 (azithromycin less affected by CYP interactions) • CYP3A4 inhibitors may ↑ risk of side effects of clarithromycin and erythromycin	• Azithromycin ER suspension is not interchangeable with IR formulations • 400 mg erythromycin ethylsuccinate (EES) = 250 mg erythromycin base or stearate • Azithromycin, clarithromycin, and erythromycin are good alternatives when patients allergic to penicillins • Take with food to ↓ gastrointestinal (GI) effects	Yes
Clarithromycin	Biaxin	• IR: 250–500 mg PO q12h • ER: 1,000 mg PO q24h • Suspension, tabs (IR and ER)	• Gram (–) organisms • Atypical organisms (e.g., *Chlamydia pneumoniae, Legionella, Mycoplasma pneumoniae*)			• CYP3A4 inducers may ↓ effects of clarithromycin and erythromycin • Clarithromycin and erythromycin may ↑ effect/toxicity of CYP3A4 substrates • ↑ risk of torsade de pointes (TdP) with other drugs that prolong QT interval (azithromycin, clarithromycin, and erythromycin)	• Clarithromycin can be used in three-drug regimen for *H. pylori* • Erythromycin can be used for diabetic gastroparesis and acne • Take ER azithromycin suspension 1 hour before or 2 hours after meals • Take ER clarithromycin tabs with food to ↑ absorption	Yes
Erythromycin	• E.E.S • EryPed • Ery-Tab • Erythrocin • PCE	• 250–500 mg PO q6h • 500 mg–1 g IV q6h • Caps, injection, ophthalmic ointment, suspension, tabs, topical gel/ ointment/solution	• Azithromycin and clarithromycin active against *Mycobacteria* • Fidaxomicin active against *Clostridium difficile*			• Clarithromycin, azithromycin, and erythromycin may ↑ effects of warfarin • Clarithromycin, azithromycin, and erythromycin may ↑ risk of digoxin toxicity		No
Fidaxomicin	Dificid	• 200 mg PO q12h • Tabs					• Azithromycin or erythromycin preferred in pregnancy • Fidaxomicin used to treat *Clostridium difficile*	No

Macrolides and Ketolides *(cont'd)*

Generic	Brand	Dose/Dosage Forms	Spectrum of Activity	Contraindications	Primary Side Effects	Pertinent Drug Interactions	Med Pearl	Top 200
Ketolide								
Telithromycin	Ketek	• 800 mg PO q24h • Tabs	• Greater activity (vs. macrolides) against resistant *Strep. pneumoniae* and *H. influenzae* • Atypical organisms	• History of hepatitis or jaundice with previous use of telithromycin or macrolides • Myasthenia gravis • QT interval prolongation • Concurrent use with other drugs that prolong QT interval	• N/V/D • ↑ LFTs / hepatitis • Visual disturbances (double vision, blurred vision, trouble focusing) • Loss of consciousness • Prolonged QT interval	• CYP3A4 inhibitors may ↑ risk of side effects • CYP3A4 inducers may ↓ effects • May ↑ effect/toxicity of CYP3A4 substrates • May ↑ effects of warfarin • May ↑ risk of digoxin toxicity • ↑ risk of TdP with other drugs that prolong QT interval	• Monitor LFTs and vision • Adjust dose in renal dysfunction	No

Tetracyclines

Mechanism of action – inhibit bacterial protein synthesis by binding to the 30S subunit of the bacterial ribosome; bacteriostatic

Generic	Brand	Dose/Dosage Forms	Spectrum of Activity	Contraindications	Primary Side Effects	Pertinent Drug Interactions	Med Pearl	Top 200
Demeclocycline	• Only available generically	• 150 mg PO q6h or 300 mg PO q12h • Tabs	• Gram (+) organisms • Gram (−) organisms • Atypical organisms	Children ≤8 yr and pregnant or breast-feeding women (may cause permanent teeth discoloration and impaired teeth/bone growth)	• N/V/D • Photosensitivity • Phlebitis (IV) • Vertigo (minocycline)	• Absorption ↓ with antacids, dairy products, and products containing iron, magnesium, aluminum, calcium, or zinc (separate by 2 hr) • CYP3A4 inhibitors may ↑ risk of side effects • CYP3A4 inducers may ↓ effects • May ↑ effect/toxicity of CYP3A4 substrates • May ↑ effects of warfarin • May ↓ effects of oral contraceptives	• Good alternative for patients allergic to penicillin • Demeclocycline also used to treat syndrome of inappropriate antidiuretic hormone secretion (SIADH) • Tetracycline can be used in four-drug regimen for *H. pylori* • All except demeclocycline can be used for acne • Doxycycline is drug of choice for Lyme disease • Take demeclocycline and tetracycline 1 hour before or 2 hours after meals • Do not use after expiration date (can cause Fanconi syndrome) • Adjust dose for all, except doxycycline, in renal dysfunction	No
Doxycycline	• Doryx • Vibramycin	• 100 mg IV/PO q12h • Caps, delayed-release caps/tabs, injection, suspension, syrup, tabs						Yes
Minocycline	• Minocin • Solodyn	• 100 mg PO q12h • Injection, caps, tabs (IR and ER)						Yes
Tetracycline	Only available generically	• 250–500 mg PO q6–12h • Caps						No

Glycylcyclines

Mechanism of action – inhibit bacterial protein synthesis by binding to the 30S subunit of the bacterial ribosome (mechanism similar to tetracyclines); bacteriostatic

Generic	Brand	Dose/Dosage Forms	Spectrum of Activity	Contraindications	Primary Side Effects	Pertinent Drug Interactions	Med Pearl	Top 200
Tigecycline	Tygacil	• 100 mg IV x 1, then 50 mg IV q12h • Injection	• Gram (+) organisms (MSSA, MRSA, vancomycin-sensitive *Enterococcus faecalis*) • Gram (−) organisms (*E. coli, Enterobacter, H. influenzae, Klebsiella, Legionella*)	Children ≤8 yr and pregnant/breast-feeding women (may cause permanent teeth discoloration and impaired teeth/bone growth)	• N/V/D • Infusion site reaction • Photosensitivity • Hepatotoxicity • Pancreatitis	May ↑ effects of warfarin	• Indicated for complicated skin/skin structure infections, complicated intraabdominal infections, and community-acquired pneumonia • Structurally similar to tetracyclines	No

Glycylcyclines *(cont'd)*

Mechanism of action – Inhibits bacterial cell wall synthesis; bactericidal

Generic	Brand	Dose/Dosage Forms	Spectrum of Activity	Contra-indications	Primary Side Effects	Pertinent Drug Interactions	Med Pearl	Top 200
Telavancin	Vibativ	• 10 mg/kg IV q24h • Injection	Gram (+) organisms (MSSA, MRSA, vancomycin-sensitive *Enterococcus faecalis, Streptococcus*)	Pregnancy	• Hypersensitivity reactions • Insomnia • Headache • Renal dysfunction • Red-man syndrome • Metallic taste • N/V/D • QT interval prolongation	↑ risk of nephro-toxicity when used with amphotericin B, loop diuretics, tacrolimus, cyclosporine, or cisplatin	• Indicated for complicated skin/skin structure infections and hospital-acquired and ventilator-associated pneumonia • Adjust dose in renal dysfunction • Monitor renal function • If red-man syndrome occurs, ↓ infusion rate • May interfere with PT, INR, aPTT	No
Vancomycin	Vancocin	• 125–250 mg PO q6h • 500 mg–1 g q12h • Caps, injection	• Gram (+) organisms (MSSA, MRSA) • *Clostridium difficile*	None	• Red-man syndrome (flushing, hypotension, erythema, pruritus) • Nephrotoxicity • Ototoxicity	↑ risk of nephro-toxicity when used with amphotericin B, loop diuretics, tacrolimus, cyclosporine, or cisplatin	• Bactericidal effect is time-dependent • Adjust dose in renal dysfunction • Often used in patients with penicillin allergy • Use PO (NOT IV) to treat *Clostridium difficile* (PO not effective for any other type of infection) • If red-man syndrome occurs, ↓ infusion rate • Target serum concentrations (peaks not routinely monitored); Trough = 5–10 mcg/mL	No

Oxazolidinones

Generic	Brand	Dose/Dosage Forms	Spectrum of Activity	Contra-indications	Primary Side Effects	Pertinent Drug Interactions	Med Pearl	Top 200
Mechanism of action – inhibit bacterial protein synthesis by binding to bacterial 23S ribosomal RNA of the 50S subunit of the bacterial ribosome; bacteriostatic								
Linezolid	Zyvox	• 400–600 mg IV/PO q12h • Injection, suspension, tabs	Gram (+) organisms (vancomycin-resistant *Enterococcus faecium* [VRE], MRSA, resistant *Strep. pneumoniae*)	• Concurrent or recent (within 2 wk) use of MAO inhibitors (MAOI) • Patients with uncontrolled hypertension, pheochromocytoma, thyrotoxicosis, and/or taking sympathomimetic agents (e.g., pseudoephedrine), vasopressor agents (e.g., epinephrine), or dopaminergic agents (e.g., dopamine) • Concurrent use of selective serotonin reuptake inhibitors, tricyclic antidepressants, serotonin 5-HT1 receptor agonists (triptans), meperidine or buspirone	• N/V/D • Headache • Myelosuppression (more common if therapy >2 wk) • Peripheral/optic neuropathy (more common if therapy >4 wk) • Seizures	• Avoid taking with foods or beverages with high tyramine content (may ↑ risk of hypertensive crises) • Use with serotonergic agents may ↑ risk of serotonin syndrome; avoid concurrent use • Use with adrenergic agents (e.g., dopamine, epinephrine) may ↑ risk of hypertensive crises • Use with tramadol may ↑ risk of seizures • Use with insulin or oral hypoglycemic agents may ↑ risk of hypoglycemia	• Indicated for nosocomial/community-acquired pneumonia, skin/skin structure infections, and VRE • Weak MAOI • Monitor CBC weekly if therapy >2 wk	Yes
Tedizolid	Sivextro	200 mg IV/PO q24h × 6 days; Injection, tabs	Gram (+) organisms (MSSA, MRSA, *Enterococcus faecalis*, *Streptococcus*)	None	• N/V/D • Headache • Dizziness	Unknown (recently approved drug)	• Indicated for skin/skin structure infections/weak MAOI	No

Streptogramin

Generic	Brand	Dose/Dosage Forms	Spectrum of Activity	Contra-indications	Primary Side Effects	Pertinent Drug Interactions	Med Pearl	Top 200
Mechanism of action – inhibit bacterial protein synthesis by binding to the 50S subunit of the bacterial ribosome; bactericidal								
Quinupristin-dalfopristin	Synercid	• 7.5 mg/kg IV q8–12h • Injection	Gram (+) organisms (MSSA and *Strep. pyogenes*)	None	• N/V/D • Infusion site reactions (pain, phlebitis) • Muscle/joint pain • ↑ bilirubin	May ↑ effect/toxicity of CYP3A4 substrates	• Indicated for complicated skin/skin structure infections • Flush line with D5W before and after infusion • If infusion reaction occurs, can ↑ volume of diluent or administer via central line	No

Fluoroquinolones

Mechanism of action – inhibit bacterial DNA topoisomerase and gyrase → inhibit bacterial DNA replication; bactericidal

Generic	Brand	Dose/Dosage Forms	Spectrum of Activity	Contraindications	Primary Side Effects	Pertinent Drug Interactions	Med Pearl	Top 200
Besifloxacin	Besivance	• 1 drop TID • Ophthalmic solution	• Gram (+) organisms (levofloxacin, gemifloxacin, and moxifloxacin have greatest activity against *Streptococcus*) • Gram (−) organisms • Ciprofloxacin active against *Pseudomonas aeruginosa*	• Children <18 yr and pregnant/breast-feeding women (may cause impaired bone growth) • Concurrent use with other drugs that prolong QT interval	• N/D • Photosensitivity • Tendinitis/tendon rupture • Hyper-/hypoglycemia • Peripheral neuropathy • Seizures • Prolonged QT interval	• Absorption ↓ with antacids, dairy products, and products containing iron, magnesium, aluminum, calcium, or zinc (separate by 2 hours) • Use with corticosteroids may ↑ risk of tendon rupture • Use with nonsteroidal anti-inflammatory drugs (NSAIDs) may ↑ risk of seizures		No
Ciprofloxacin	• Cetraxal • Cipro • Cipro XR • Ciloxan	• IR: 250–750 mg PO q12h • ER: 500 mg–1 g PO q24h • IV: 200–400 mg IV q8–12h • Injection, ophthalmic ointment/solution, suspension, tabs (ER and IR), otic solution				• Ciprofloxacin and ofloxacin may ↑ effects of CYP1A2 substrates • Ciprofloxacin may ↓ phenytoin levels	• Ciprofloxacin ER and IR tabs are not interchangeable • Adjust dose for all, except moxifloxacin, in renal dysfunction • Take levofloxacin oral solution 1 hour before or 2 hours after meals • Patients with diabetes should monitor their blood glucose more frequently • Ophthalmic preparations used to treat bacterial conjunctivitis	Yes
Gatifloxacin	Zymaxid	• 1 drop q2h while awake on day 1, then 1 drop 2–4 times/day while awake • Ophthalmic solution	• Atypical organisms					No
Gemifloxacin	Factive	• 320 mg PO q24h • Tabs				• May ↑ effects of warfarin		No
Levofloxacin	• Levaquin • Quixin	• 250–750 mg IV/PO q24h • Injection, ophthalmic solution, solution, tabs				• May ↑ effects of antidiabetic agents • ↑ risk of TdP with other drugs that prolong QT interval		Yes
Moxifloxacin	• Avelox • Moxeza • Vigamox	• 400 mg IV/PO q24h • Injection, ophthalmic solution, tabs						Yes
Ofloxacin	• Floxin • Ocuflox	• 200–400 mg PO q12h • Ophthalmic solution, otic solution, tabs						No

Sulfonamides

Generic	Brand	Dose/Dosage Forms	Spectrum of Activity	Contraindications	Primary Side Effects	Pertinent Drug Interactions	Med Pearl	Top 200
Mechanism of action – inhibit incorporation of para-aminobenzoic acid (PABA) into DNA → inhibit folic acid production and bacterial growth; bacteriostatic								
TMP/SMX	• Bactrim • Septra • Sulfatrim	• 1 double-strength tab PO q12h • 10–20 mg/kg/day of TMP IV in divided doses • Injection, suspension, tabs	• Gram (+) organisms (including MSSA, MRSA) • Gram (−) organisms • SMX/TMP is 1st-line drug to treat/prevent *Pneumocystis jiroveci* pneumonia (PJP)	• Sulfa allergy • Porphyria • Megaloblastic anemia • Infants and pregnant/breast-feeding women (↑ risk of kernicterus) • G6PD deficiency	• N/V/D • Rash • Stevens-Johnson syndrome • Photosensitivity • Folate deficiency • Hypoglycemia (in patients with diabetes)	• May ↑ effects/toxicity of methotrexate • May ↑ effects of warfarin • May ↑ effects of antidiabetic agents	• Instruct patients to take with a full glass of water (to prevent crystalluria) • Adjust dose in renal dysfunction	Yes

Cyclic Lipopeptide

Generic	Brand	Dose/Dosage Forms	Spectrum of Activity	Contra-indications	Primary Side Effects	Pertinent Drug Interactions	Med Pearl	Top 200
Mechanism of action – bind to bacterial cell membranes and cause rapid depolarization → inhibit protein, DNA, and RNA synthesis; bactericidal								
Daptomycin	Cubicin	• 4–6 mg/kg IV q24h • Injection	Gram (+) organisms (MSSA, MRSA, vancomycin-sensitive *Enterococus faecalis*)	None	• Nausea/diarrhea • Infusion site reactions • Myopathy/rhabdomyolysis • Peripheral neuropathy	Use with statins may ↑ risk of myopathy; consider discontinuing statin therapy throughout treatment	• Monitor creatine kinase levels weekly • Adjust dose in renal dysfunction • Indicated for complicated skin/skin structure infections and *Staph. aureus* bloodstream infections	No

Glycopeptides

Generic	Brand	Dose/Dosage Forms	Spectrum of Activity	Contra-indications	Primary Side Effects	Pertinent Drug Interactions	Med Pearl	Top 200
Dalbavancin	Dalvance	1,000 mg IV × 1, then 500 mg IV 1 wk later; injection	Gram (+) organisms (MSSA, MRSA, *Streptococcus*)	None	• Hypersensitivity reactions • Headache • N/D • Red-man syndrome	None	• Indicated for skin/skin structure infections • Adjust dose in renal dysfunction • If red-man syndrome occurs, ↓ infusion rate	No
Oritavancin	Orbactiv	• 1,200 mg IV ×1 • Injection	Gram (+) organisms (MSSA, MRSA, vancomycin-sensitive *Enterococcus faecalis*, *Streptococcus*)	Use of heparin × 48 hr after administration	• Hypersensitivity reactions • Headache • N/V/D • Red-man syndrome	May ↑ effects of warfarin	• Indicated for skin/skin structure infections • If red-man syndrome occurs, ↓ infusion rate • May interfere with PT, INR, aPTT	No

Miscellaneous Antibacterial Agents

Generic	Brand	Dose/Dosage Forms	Spectrum of Activity	Contra-indications	Primary Side Effects	Pertinent Drug Interactions	Med Pearl	Top 200
Mechanism of action – inhibits bacterial protein synthesis by binding to the 50S subunit of the bacterial ribosome; bacteriostatic								
Chloramphenicol	Only available generically	• 12.5–25 mg/kg IV q6h • Injection	• Gram (+) organisms (VRE) • Gram (−) organisms	Neonates (↑ risk of gray-baby syndrome)	• N/V/D • Myelosuppression (anemia, leukopenia, thrombocytopenia, aplastic anemia) • Gray-baby syndrome (vomiting, lethargy, respiratory depression, death) • Optic neuritis	• Phenobarbital and rifampin may ↓ effects • May ↑ effects of warfarin and phenytoin	• Only used for life-threatening infections • Monitor CBC frequently • Target serum concentrations: Peak = 15–25 mcg/mL; Trough = 5–10 mcg/mL	No
Mechanism of action – inhibits bacterial protein synthesis by binding to the 50S subunit of the bacterial ribosome; bacteriostatic								
Clindamycin	• Cleocin • Clindesse • Evoclin	• 150–450 mg PO q6h • 300–900 mg IV q8h • Caps, injection, solution, topical foam/gel/lotion/ pledgets/solution, vaginal cream/ suppository	• Gram (+) organisms • Anaerobes	History of pseudo-membranous colitis or ulcerative colitis	• N/V/D • Pseudomembranous colitis (*Clostridium difficile*) (highest incidence)	None significant	• Also used for acne (topical) • Patients using intravaginally should avoid intercourse (↓ efficacy of condoms and diaphragms)	Yes
Mechanism of action – interferes with bacterial DNA synthesis; bactericidal								
Metronidazole	• Flagyl • Metrogel • Noritate • Vandazole	• 250–500 mg PO q8–12h • 500 mg IV q8–12h • Caps, injection, tabs (ER and IR), topical cream/gel/lotion, vaginal gel	Anaerobes	Pregnancy (1st trimester)	• N/D • Confusion • Dizziness • Peripheral neuropathy • Metallic taste	• Disulfiram-like reaction may occur if alcohol is used during treatment • May ↑ effects of warfarin and lithium • Phenobarbital and phenytoin may ↓ effects • Cimetidine may ↑ effects	• Can be used in four-drug regimen for *H. pylori* • Drug of choice for *Clostridium difficile* • Take ER tabs 1 hour before or 2 hours after meals	Yes

Medication Charts: Antifungal Agents

Azole Antifungals

Mechanism of action – inhibit synthesis of ergosterol (essential component of fungal cell membrane)
- Imidazoles: butoconazole, clotrimazole, econazole, ketoconazole, miconazole, oxiconazole, sulconazole, tioconazole
- Triazoles: fluconazole, itraconazole, terconazole, posaconazole, voriconazole

Generic	Brand	Dose/Dosage Forms	Spectrum of Activity	Contra-indications	Primary Side Effects	Pertinent Drug Interactions	Med Pearl	Top 200
Fluconazole	Diflucan	• 100–800 mg IV/PO q24h • Injection, tabs, suspension	• *Candida* spp. • *Coccidioides* spp. • *Histoplasma* spp. • *Cryptococcus* spp. • *Aspergillus* spp. (only itraconazole)	None	• Headache • N/V/D • Abdominal pain • Rash • ↑ LFTs • Prolonged QT interval	• May ↑ effect/toxicity of CYP2C9, CYP2C19, and CYP3A4 substrates • Rifampin may ↓ effects • ↑ risk of TdP with other drugs that prolong QT interval	• Adjust dose in patients with renal dysfunction • Conversion from IV to PO is 1:1 • Monitor LFTs	Yes
Itraconazole	• Sporanox • Onmel	• 100–400 mg/day PO • Caps, solution, tabs		• Concurrent use of dofetilide, ergot alkaloids, lovastatin, midazolam, pimozide, quinidine, simvastatin, or triazolam • HF	• Nausea • Abdominal pain • Rash • ↑ LFTs • Prolonged QT interval	• CYP3A4 inhibitors may ↑ risk of side effects • CYP3A4 inducers may ↓ effects • May ↑ effect/toxicity of CYP3A4 substrates • ↑ risk of digoxin toxicity • Absorption ↓ with antacids, H₂ antagonists, and proton pump inhibitors (acidic environment required for absorption) (separate by 2 hr) • ↑ risk of TdP with other drugs that prolong QT interval	• Caps and solution cannot be used interchangeably (bioavailability of solution > caps) • Potent negative inotrope • Monitor LFTs	No
Ketoconazole	Nizoral	• 200–400 mg PO q24h • Rx: Topical cream/gel/shampoo/aerosol, tabs • OTC: shampoo		• Concurrent use of ergot alkaloids • Hepatic dysfunction	• N/V • Gynecomastia • Sexual dysfunction • ↑ LFTs • Prolonged QT interval	Same as itraconazole	• May ↓ testosterone levels • Monitor LFTs	Yes

Azole Antifungals *(cont'd)*

Generic	Brand	Dose/Dosage Forms	Spectrum of Activity	Contra-indications	Primary Side Effects	Pertinent Drug Interactions	Med Pearl	Top 200
Posaconazole	Noxafil	• 100–800 mg/day PO • Injection, suspension, tabs	• *Candida* spp. • *Coccidioides* spp. • *Histoplasma* spp. • *Cryptococcus* spp. • *Aspergillus* spp.	Concurrent use of ergot alkaloids, quinidine, or pimozide	• Headache • N/V • Rash • Prolonged QT interval • ↑ LFTs	• May ↑ effect/toxicity of CYP3A4 substrates • ↑ risk of TdP with other drugs that prolong QT interval	• Must be taken with full meal to ↑ absorption • Monitor LFTs	No
Voriconazole	Vfend	• *Loading dose:* 6 mg/kg IV q12h for 24 hr • *Maintenance dose:* 3–4 mg/kg IV q12h; 100–300 mg PO q12h • Injection, suspension, tabs		Concurrent use of pimozide, quinidine, long-acting barbiturates, carbamazepine, ergot alkaloids, rifampin, rifabutin, ritonavir (≥800 mg/day), efavirenz (≥800mg/day), St. John's wort, or sirolimus	• Visual disturbances (transient) (blurred vision, photophobia, altered perception of color) • Rash • Photosensitivity • ↑ LFTs • Hallucinations • N/V • Prolonged QT interval	• May ↑ effect/toxicity of CYP2C9, CYP2C19, and CYP3A4 substrates • CYP2C9 and CYP2C19 inducers may ↓ effects • May ↑ efavirenz levels • Efavirenz may ↓ effects • ↑ risk of TdP with other drugs that prolong QT interval	• ↓ dose of cyclosporine by 50% • When using with efavirenz, ↑ voriconazole dose and ↓ efavirenz dose • ↑ dose of voriconazole when using with phenytoin • Use PO when CrCl <50 mL/min (diluent in IV can accumulate) • Take PO 1 hour before or after meals • Monitor LFTs and vision	No

Echinocandins

Mechanism of action – inhibit synthesis of 1,3-β-d-glucan (essential component of fungal cell wall)

Generic	Brand	Dose/Dosage Forms	Spectrum of Activity	Contra-indications	Primary Side Effects	Pertinent Drug Interactions	Med Pearl	Top 200
Anidulafungin	Eraxis	• 100–200 mg IV on day 1, then 50–100 mg IV q24h • Injection	• *Candida* spp. • *Aspergillus* spp.	None	• N/V • Headache • Hypokalemia • Rash	None	Monitor LFTs	No
Caspofungin	Cancidas	• 70 mg IV on day 1, then 50 mg IV q24h • Injection			• Fever • ↑ LFTs • Phlebitis	• Rifampin, carbamazepine, dexamethasone, efavirenz, nevirapine, and phenytoin may ↓ effects • May ↓ tacrolimus levels • Cyclosporine may ↑ risk of side effects	• ↑ dose of caspofungin to 70 mg/day when used with rifampin, carbamazepine, dexamethasone, efavirenz, nevirapine, or phenytoin • Adjust dose in moderate hepatic dysfunction • Monitor LFTs	No
Micafungin	Mycamine	• 50–150 mg IV q24h • Injection				None	Monitor LFTs	No

Amphotericin B

Mechanism of action – bind to ergosterol in cell membrane → produce a channel in cell membrane (↑ permeability) → allow K^+ and Mg^{2+} to leak out of cell ("leaky membrane") → cell death

Generic	Brand	Dose/Dosage Forms	Spectrum of Activity	Contra-indications	Primary Side Effects	Pertinent Drug Interactions	Med Pearl	Top 200
Amphotericin B desoxycholate	Fungizone	• Test dose of 1 mg IV should be given over 20–30 min (monitor patient for 2–4 hr before starting infusion) • 0.5–1.5 mg/kg/day IV • Injection	• *Candida* spp. • *Coccidioides* spp. • *Blastomyces* spp. • *Histoplasma* spp. • *Cryptococcus* spp. • *Aspergillus* spp.	None	• Nephrotoxicity (less common with lipid-based formulations) • Infusion reactions (fever, chills, hypotension, nausea, tachypnea) • Phlebitis • Electrolyte disturbances (i.e., hypokalemia, hypomagnesemia)	↑ risk of nephrotoxicity when used with aminoglycosides, loop diuretics, tacrolimus, cyclosporine, or cisplatin	• May premedicate with acetaminophen, NSAIDs, diphenhydramine, and/or corticosteroid to prevent infusion reactions (give 30–60 min before infusion); meperidine may be used for rigors • Infusion reactions less common with lipid-based formulations (amphotericin B deoxycholate > ABLC > L-Amb) • Infusion reactions ↓ after first few doses • Sodium loading (500 mL of 0.9% NaCl before and after infusion) may ↓ risk of nephrotoxicity with amphotericin B desoxycholate • Monitor BUN, SCr, potassium, and magnesium	No
Amphotericin B lipid complex (ABLC)	Abelcet	• 5 mg/kg IV q24h • Injection						No
Liposomal amphotericin B (L-AmB)	AmBisome	• 3–6 mg/kg IV q24h • Injection						No

Other Antifungals

Generic	Brand	Dose/Dosage Forms	Spectrum of Activity	Contra-indications	Primary Side Effects	Pertinent Drug Interactions	Med Pearl	Top 200
Mechanism of action – similar to amphotericin B								
Nystatin	Mycostatin	• Suspension: 400,000–600,000 units 4 times/day • Topical: Apply 2–3 times daily • Topical cream/ointment/powder, suspension, tabs	*Candida* spp.	None	• N/V/D • Abdominal pain	None	Suspension should be swished and swallowed	Yes
Mechanism of action – inhibits squalene epoxidase → inhibits synthesis of ergosterol								
Terbinafine	Lamisil	• PO: 250 mg q24h • Topical: Apply 1–2 times daily • Rx: Granules, tabs, topical solution • OTC: Topical cream/gel/solution	*Trichophyton* spp.	• Liver disease • CrCl <50 mL/min	• Headache • N/V/D • ↑ LFTs	• May ↑ effect/toxicity of CYP2D6 substrates • May ↓ cyclosporine levels	• Oral used for onychomycosis or tinea capitis (scalp ringworm); topical used for tinea pedis (athlete's foot), tinea corporis (ringworm), or tinea cruris (jock itch) • Give for 6 wks for fingernail infection; 12 wks for toenail infection • Monitor LFTs	Yes
Mechanism of action – inhibit fungal protein synthesis								
Tavaborole	Kerydin	Apply once daily × 48 wk; topical solution	*Trichophyton* spp.	None	Application reactions	None	Indicated for onychomycosis	No

Other Antifungals *(cont'd)*

Generic	Brand	Dose/Dosage Forms	Spectrum of Activity	Contra-indications	Primary Side Effects	Pertinent Drug Interactions	Med Pearl	Top 200
Mechanism of action – enters fungal cell wall → converted into 5-fluorouracil, which interferes with fungal RNA and protein synthesis								
Flucytosine	Ancobon	• 25–37.5 mg/kg PO q6h (administered with amphotericin B) • Caps	*Candida* spp. *Cryptococcus* spp.	None	• Confusion • Hallucinations • Ataxia • Headache • N/V/D • ↑LFTs • Renal dysfunction • Bone marrow depression	None	• Should not be used as monotherapy • Adjust dose in patients with renal dysfunction • Monitor LFTs, BUN/SCr, and CBC • Flucytosine concentrations: Peak: 50–100 mcg/mL; Trough: 25–50 mcg/mL	No
Mechanism of action – inhibits fungal cell mitosis								
Griseofulvin	• Grifulvin V • Gris-PEG	• Microsize: 500–1,000 mg/day PO • Ultramicrosize: 375 mg/day PO • Microsize: Suspension, tabs • Ultramicrosize: Tabs	*Trichophyton* spp.	• Liver disease • Porphyria	• Rash/hives • N/V/D • Headache • Confusion • Photosensitivity	• Barbiturates may ↓ effects • May ↓ effects of cyclosporine and warfarin	• Monitor LFTs • Use with alcohol may cause disulfiram reaction • Administer with high-fat meal to ↑ absorption	No

Medication Charts: Antiviral Agents

Drugs for Treatment of Herpes Simplex Virus and Varicella-Zoster Virus

Mechanism of action – inhibit viral DNA polymerase → inhibit replication of viral DNA

Generic	Brand	Dose/Dosage Forms	Spectrum of Activity	Contra-indications	Primary Side Effects	Pertinent Drug Interactions	Med Pearl	Top 200
Acyclovir	Zovirax, Sitavig	• *Genital herpes (initial episode):* 200 mg PO 5 times/day × 7–10 days 5 mg/kg IV q8h × 5–7 days • *Herpes labialis (cold sores):* 400 mg PO 5 times/day × 5 days • *Varicella (chickenpox):* 800 mg PO q6h × 5 days 10 mg/kg IV q8h × 7 days • *Herpes zoster (shingles):* 800 mg PO 5 times/day × 7–10 days 10 mg/kg IV q8h × 7 days • Caps, injection, suspension, tabs, buccal tabs, topical cream/ointment	• Herpes simplex virus (HSV)-1 (herpes labialis) and HSV-2 (genital herpes) • Varicella zoster virus (causes chickenpox and shingles)	None	• N/V/D • Headache • Phlebitis (IV acyclovir) • Renal dysfunction (IV acyclovir) • Seizures (esp. in patients with renal dysfunction)	None	• Adjust dose for all, except penciclovir, in renal dysfunction • To avoid renal damage with IV acyclovir (can crystallize), infuse slowly and keep patient hydrated • Sitavig is a buccal tab for treatment of recurrent cold sores	Yes
Famciclovir (prodrug of penciclovir)	Famvir	• *Genital herpes (initial episode):* 250 mg PO q8h × 7–10 days • *Cold sores:* 1,500 mg PO × 1 • *Herpes zoster:* 500 mg PO q8h × 7 days • Tabs						Yes
Penciclovir	Denavir	*Cold sores:* • Apply q2h while awake × 4 days • Topical cream						No
Valacyclovir (prodrug of acyclovir)	Valtrex	• *Genital herpes (initial episode):* 1 g PO q12h × 10 days • *Genital herpes (recurrence):* 500 mg PO q12h × 3 days • *Cold sores:* 2 g PO q12h × 1 day • *Herpes zoster:* 1 g PO q8h × 7 days • Tabs						Yes

Drugs for Treatment of Cytomegalovirus

Generic	Brand	Dose/Dosage Forms	Spectrum of Activity	Contraindications	Primary Side Effects	Pertinent Drug Interactions	Med Pearl	Top 200
Mechanism of action – inhibit replication of viral DNA								
Cidofovir	Only available generically	• 5 mg/kg IV once weekly × 2 wk, then q2 wk • Injection	• Cytomegalovirus • HSV (foscarnet) • Acute herpetic keratitis (ophthalmic ganciclovir)	• SCr >1.5 mg/dL, CrCl ≤55 mL/min, or proteinuria • Use of other nephrotoxic drugs within 7 days	• Nephrotoxicity • Neutropenia • Metabolic acidosis • ↓ intraocular pressure • Uveitis/iritis	Use of antiretroviral drugs may ↑ risk of side effects	• Monitor BUN/SCr • To minimize renal damage, administer 1 L of 0.9% NaCl before and after each infusion; also give 2 g of probenecid 3 hr before each infusion and then 1 g at 2 hr and 8 hr after each infusion • If SCr ↑ by 0.3–0.4 mg/dL above baseline, ↓ dose to 3 mg/kg; if SCr ↑ by ≥0.5 mg/dL, discontinue • Advise patients to use effective contraception	No
Foscarnet	Foscavir	• 60 mg/kg IV q8h or 90 mg/kg IV q12h × 14–21 days, then 90–120 mg/kg IV q24h • Injection		None	• Nephrotoxicity • N/V • Anemia • Electrolyte disturbances • Genital sores • Seizures	• ↑ risk of renal dysfunction when used with other nephrotoxic drugs • Zidovudine may ↑ risk of anemia	• Adjust dose in renal dysfunction • Monitor BUN/SCr • To minimize renal damage, administer 1 L of 0.9% NaCl with each infusion • Rapid infusion associated with seizures and arrhythmias	No
Ganciclovir	• Cytovene • Zirgan	• 5 mg/kg IV q12h × 14–21 days, then either 5 mg/kg/day IV 7 times/wk or 6 mg/kg/day IV 5 times/wk • 1 drop 5 times/day until ulcer heals, then 1 drop 3 times/day/7 days • Injection, ophthalmic gel		• Neutropenia • Thrombocytopenia • Anemia	• Myelosuppression • Fever • Rash • Phlebitis (IV) • ↑ LFTs • Nephrotoxicity • Seizures • N/V/D	• ↑ risk of myelosuppression when used with other immunosuppressive drugs • ↑ risk of renal dysfunction when used with other nephrotoxic drugs • May ↑ effects/toxicity of zidovudine	• Adjust dose in renal dysfunction • Advise patients to use effective contraception during treatment and for at least 90 days after treatment • Take valganciclovir with food	No
Valganciclovir (prodrug of ganciclovir)	Valcyte	• 900 mg PO q12h × 21 days, then 900 mg PO q24h • Tabs, solution						No

Drugs for Treatment of Influenza

Mechanism of action – inhibit the enzyme (neuraminidase) responsible for releasing the newly formed mature virus from the host cell

Generic	Brand	Dose/Dosage Forms	Spectrum of Activity	Contra-indications	Primary Side Effects	Pertinent Drug Interactions	Med Pearl	Top 200
Oseltamivir	Tamiflu	• *Prophylaxis:* 75 mg PO q24h × 7–10 days (6 wk for community outbreak) • *Treatment:* 75 mg PO q12h × 5 days • Caps, suspension	• Influenza A and B • H1N1 influenza	None	• N/V/D • Headache • Rash • Neuropsychiatric events (e.g., confusion, delirium, hallucinations, self-injury)	None	• For prophylaxis, initiate therapy within 2 days of contact with infected person • For treatment, initiate therapy within 2 days of onset of symptoms • Adjust dose in renal dysfunction • ↓ flu severity and duration by ~ 1 day • Can be used in children ≥1 yr (prophylaxis) or ≥2 wk (treatment)	No
Zanamivir	Relenza	• *Prophylaxis:* 2 inhalations q24h × 7–10 days (28 days for community outbreak) • *Treatment:* 2 inhalations q12h × 5 days • Powder for oral inhalation		Asthma/COPD	• Bronchospasm • Cough • Headache • N/D • Rash • Neuropsychiatric events (e.g., confusion, delirium, hallucinations, self-injury)		• For prophylaxis, initiate therapy within 1.5 days (5 days in community setting) of contact with infected person • For treatment, initiate therapy within 2 days of onset of symptoms • ↓ flu severity and duration by ~ 1 day • Can be used in children ≥5 yr (prophylaxis) or ≥7 yr (treatment)	No

HUMAN IMMUNODEFICIENCY VIRUS

Definitions

HIV is a human retrovirus that infects lymphocytes and other cells that bear the CD4 surface protein. Infection leads to CD4 T-cell depletion, impaired cell-mediated immunity, and polyclonal B-cell activation. Over time, this immune system dysfunction leads to acquired immune deficiency syndrome (AIDS) and illnesses such as opportunistic infections and malignancies.

Diagnosis

- The Centers for Disease Control and Prevention (CDC) recommends routine HIV screening for adults, adolescents and pregnant women in healthcare settings in the United States.
- Persons at a high risk for HIV infection should be screened for HIV at least annually:
  - Healthcare workers, intravenous drug users, men who have sex with men, hemophiliacs, sexual partners of persons living with HIV, commercial sex workers and their partners, persons with a history of sexually transmitted infections, and persons with multiple sex partners or those with a history of unprotected sexual encounters
- Pregnant women should receive HIV testing during the routine panel of prenatal screening tests.
- Laws requiring informed consent for HIV testing vary depending upon the state. Most states have adopted the "opt-out" testing strategy recommended by the CDC. This strategy notifies a patient that HIV screening will be taking place unless the patient declines.
- Screening for HIV is performed with an enzyme-linked immunosorbent assay (ELISA) test. Positive results must always be confirmed with a Western blot.

Signs and Symptoms

Acute HIV infection most commonly presents with a "flu-like" illness that resolves within 2–4 weeks. After acute infection, patients may remain symptom-free for 8–9 years or more. As the virus continues to multiply and destroy immune cells, the patient may develop chronic symptoms such as:

- Swollen lymph nodes, diarrhea, weight loss, rash, fever, cough, and shortness of breath

When a patient's CD4 cell count declines to <200 cells/mm^3, the immune system is significantly compromised and the patient is at an increased risk for opportunistic infections such as:

- Oropharyngeal candidiasis, *Pneumocystis jirovecii* pneumonia, *Toxoplasma gondii*, *Cryptococcus neoformans*, and *Mycobacterium avium intracellulare*

Guidelines

Panel on Antiretroviral Guidelines for Adults and Adolescents. Guidelines for the use of antiretroviral agents in HIV-1-infected adults and adolescents. Department of Health and Human Services. May 1, 2014; 1–285. Available at http://www.aidsinfo.nih.gov/ContentFiles/AdultandAdolescentGL.pdf.

Panel on Opportunistic Infections in HIV-Infected Adults and Adolescents. Guidelines for the prevention and treatment of opportunistic infections in HIV-infected adults and adolescents: recommendations from the Centers for Disease Control and Prevention, the National Institutes of Health, and the HIV Medicine Association of the Infectious Diseases Society of America. July 8, 2013; 1–417. Available at http://aidsinfo.nih.gov/contentfiles/lvguidelines/adult_oi.pdf.

Guidelines Summary

For the NAPLEX®, you should make learning the names of the medications and their respective classes a priority. Below are some helpful learning tips:

- Memorize the non-nucleoside reverse transcriptase inhibitors (NNRTIs)
  - Efavirenz, nevirapine, etravirine, rilpivirine
- All protease inhibitors (PIs) end in "-navir"
  - Examples: Darunavir, atazanavir, ritonavir
- There are only three integrase inhibitors: Dolutegravir, raltegravir, elvitegravir (only available as combination product)
- There is only one fusion inhibitor: Enfuvirtide
- There is only one CCR5 inhibitor: Maraviroc
- The remaining agents are nucleoside reverse transcriptase inhibitors (NRTIs)
  - Examples: Tenofovir, emtricitabine, abacavir, lamivudine, zidovudine, didanosine, stavudine

For the NAPLEX®, know the indications for initiating an antiretroviral regimen in treatment-naïve patients:

- CD4 cell count <500 cells/mm^3
- An AIDS-defining illness or history of an opportunistic infection
- HIV-associated nephropathy
- Hepatitis B co-infection that requires treatment

- Pregnancy
- HIV-associated dementia
- Acute HIV infection

For the NAPLEX®, know the signature side effects for the major drug classes (NNRTIs, NRTIs, and PIs) and know the seven antiviral regimens that are recommended for starting therapy in treatment-naïve patients:

- Tenofovir + emtricitabine + efavirenz
- Tenofovir + emtricitabine + raltegravir
- Tenofovir + emtricitabine + darunavir + ritonavir
- Tenofovir + emtricitabine + atazanavir + ritonavir
- Dolutegravir + abacavir + lamivudine (only for patients who are HLA-B 5701 negative)
- Dolutegravir + tenofovir + emtricitabine
- Elvitegravir + cobicistat + tenofovir + emtricitabine

Below is a summary of acceptable initial combination regimens for antiretroviral naïve patients:

- NNRTI-based regimen: 1 NNRTI + 2 NRTIs
- PI-based regimen: PI (boosted with ritonavir) + 2 NRTIs
- Integrase inhibitor-based regimen: Integrase inhibitor + 2 NRTIs

Drugs of Choice

Prophylaxis of First-Episode Opportunistic Infections in Patients with HIV

Opportunistic Infection	Indication	First-Line Therapy
Pneumocystis jiroveci pneumonia (PJP)	CD4 count <200 cells/mm^3 **OR** Oropharyngeal candidiasis **OR** History of AIDS-defining illness	TMP/SMX 1 DS tablet PO daily **OR** TMP/SMX 80/400 mg (single-strength [SS]) PO daily
Toxoplasma gondii encephalitis	Toxoplasma IgG (+) with CD4 count <100 cells/mm^3	TMP/SMX 1 DS tablet PO daily
Mycobacterium avium complex (MAC) disease	CD4 count <50 cells/mm^3	Azithromycin 1200 mg PO 1 × weekly **OR** Clarithromycin 500 mg PO BID **OR** Azithromycin 600 mg PO 2 × weekly

Treatment and Secondary Prophylaxis of AIDS-Associated Opportunistic Infections

Opportunistic Infection	First-Line Therapy/Duration
PJP	*Treatment:* TMP/SMX (IV/PO) ± corticosteroids* × 21 days *Secondary Prophylaxis:* TMP/SMX 1 DS tablet PO daily **OR** TMP/SMX 1 SS tablet PO daily
Toxoplasma gondii encephalitis	*Treatment:* Pyrimethamine (PO) + sulfadiazine (PO) + leucovorin[†] (PO) × ≥6 wks *Secondary Prophylaxis:* Pyrimethamine + sulfadiazine + leucovorin[†]
MAC disease	*Treatment:* Clarithromycin (or azithromycin) (PO) + ethambutol (PO) × ≥12 months *Secondary Prophylaxis:* Clarithromycin (or azithromycin) + ethambutol
Mucocutaneous candidiasis	*Treatment:* Oropharyngeal: Fluconazole (PO) **OR** clotrimazole (troche) **OR** miconazole (buccal) × 7–14 days Esophageal: Fluconazole (IV/PO) **OR** itraconazole (PO) × 14–21 days *Secondary Prophylaxis:* Usually not recommended unless patients have frequent or severe recurrences
Cryptococcal meningitis	*Treatment:* Induction: Lipid amphotericin B (IV) + Flucytosine (PO) × ≥2 wks Consolidation: Fluconazole (IV/PO) × ≥8 wks *Secondary Prophylaxis:* Fluconazole (PO)
Cytomegalovirus retinitis	*Treatment:* Ganciclovir (or foscarnet) (via intravitreal injection) × 1–4 doses over 7–10 days + valganciclovir (PO) × 14–21 days *Secondary Prophylaxis:* Valganciclovir (PO)

*Indications for adjunctive corticosteroid therapy for PJP include PaO_2 <70 mmHg (room air) **OR** alveolar-arterial O_2 gradient >35 mmHg.

[†]Leucovorin reduces the risk of bone marrow suppression associated with pyrimethamine.

Non-Nucleoside Reverse Transcriptase Inhibitors (NNRTIs)

Generic	Brand	Dose	Contraindications	Primary Side Effects	Key Monitoring	Pertinent Drug Interactions	Med Pearl	Top 200
Mechanism of action – binds to an allosteric site on reverse transcriptase that results in a conformational change to the enzyme's active site								
Efavirenz	Sustiva	600 mg PO QHS on an empty stomach	None	• Rash • ↑ LFTs • Dyslipidemia • Drowsiness • Dizziness • Insomnia • Abnormal vivid dreaming • Agitation	LFTs	• 3A4 substrate • Inhibits: 3A4, 2C9 • Induces: 3A4, 2B6	Can cause a false positive cannabinoid or benzodiazepine screening test	No
Etravirine	Intelence	200 mg PO BID with food	None	• Rash • ↑ LFTs	LFTs	• 3A4, 2C9, 2C19 substrate • Inhibits: 2C9, 2C19 • Induces: 3A4	May disperse tabs in water	No
Nevirapine	Viramune	200 mg PO daily × 2 weeks, then 200 mg BID or 400 mg (XR) daily thereafter	None	• Rash • ↑ LFTs	LFTs	• 3A4 substrate • Inhibits: 3A4, 2D6, 1A2 • Induces: 3A4, 2B6	• Risk of hepatotoxicity in men and women with CD4 count >400 and 250 cells/mm^3, respectively • Hepatotoxicity often associated with a rash • Also available as oral suspension	No
Rilpivirine	Edurant	25 mg PO daily with food	None	• Rash • ↑ LFTs	LFTs	• 3A4 substrate • Not expected to induce or inhibit CYP enzymes	• Requires at least a 500-calorie meal • ↑ virologic failure with high baseline HIV RNA (>100,000 copies/mL)	No

Nucleoside Reverse Transcriptase Inhibitors (NRTIs)

Mechanism of action – triphosphate moiety competes with natural substrates for incorporation into proviral DNA that is developed by reverse transcriptase

Generic	Brand	Dose	Contraindications	Primary Side Effects	Key Monitoring	Pertinent Drug Interactions	Med Pearl	Top 200
Abacavir	Ziagen	300 mg PO BID or 600 mg PO daily	Discontinue drug promptly and do not rechallenge in patients with hypersensitivity	Hypersensitivity reaction	Hypersensitivity symptoms: fever, rash, N/V/D, malaise, fatigue, cough	None	• Perform HLA-B*5701 test prior: only use if negative • Also available as oral solution	No
Didanosine	Videx EC	≥60 kg: 400 mg PO daily <60 kg: 250 mg PO daily	None	• Peripheral neuropathy • Pancreatitis • Diarrhea • Nausea • Optic neuritis	None	Tenofovir ↑ levels (avoid combination)	• Administer on an empty stomach • Do not crush or open • Also available as oral solution	No
Emtricitabine	Emtriva	200 mg PO daily	None	• N/V • Hyperpigmentation of palms/soles	None	None	• Also active against hepatitis B • Also available as oral solution	No
Lamivudine	Epivir	150 mg PO BID or 300 mg PO daily	None	• N/V/D	None	None	• Also active against hepatitis B • Also available as oral solution	No
Stavudine	Zerit	≥60 kg: 40 mg PO BID <60 kg: 30 mg PO BID	None	• Peripheral neuropathy • Pancreatitis • Lipoatrophy	None	Additive risk of pancreatitis with concurrent didanosine	Also available as oral solution	No
Tenofovir	Viread	300 mg PO daily	None	• Renal insufficiency • Fanconi syndrome • ↓ bone mineral density	SCr	↓ atazanavir levels	• Also active against hepatitis B • Also available as oral powder	No
Zidovudine	Retrovir	300 mg PO BID	Concurrent ribavirin due to additive toxicity	• Anemia • Neutropenia • Headache • Nausea	CBC with differential	None	• First antiretroviral for HIV • Also available as IV and oral	No

Protease Inhibitors (PIs)

Mechanism of action – inhibits HIV protease enzyme from processing the gag-pol polyprotein precursor, thereby preventing development and maturation of new HIV particles

Generic	Brand	Dose	Contraindications	Primary Side Effects	Key Monitoring	Pertinent Drug Interactions	Med Pearl	Top 200
Atazanavir	Reyataz	• Therapy naïve: 300 mg PO daily + ritonavir 100 mg PO daily **OR** 400 mg PO daily (if unable to tolerate ritonavir) • Therapy experienced: 300 mg PO daily + ritonavir 100 mg PO daily	None	• Indirect hyperbilirubinemia • PR prolongation • Dyslipidemia (greater with ritonavir) • Hepatotoxicity • GI upset • Hyperglycemia • Fat maldistribution • Cholelithiasis • Nephrolithiasis • Rash	• LFTs • Bilirubin • Lipids	• 3A4 inhibitor and substrate • ↑ Tenofovir levels	• Acid dependent absorption; follow guidelines for using in combination with PPIs, H$_2$ blockers and antacids • Must be taken with food	No
Darunavir	Prezista	• Therapy naïve or therapy experienced (with no darunavir mutations): 800 mg PO daily + ritonavir 100 mg PO daily • Therapy experienced (with ≥1 darunavir mutation): 600 mg PO BID + ritonavir 100 mg PO BID	None	• Dyslipidemia • Rash • Hepatotoxicity • GI upset • Hyperglycemia • Fat maldistribution	• LFTs • Lipids	• 3A4 inhibitor and substrate • ↑ Atorvastatin and rosuvastatin levels	• Must be taken with food • Also available as oral suspension • Use with caution in patients with sulfa allergy	No
Fosamprenavir	Lexiva	• Therapy naïve: 1,400 mg PO BID OR 1,400 mg PO daily + ritonavir 100–200 mg PO daily OR 700 mg PO BID + ritonavir 100 mg PO BID • Therapy experienced: 700 mg PO BID + ritonavir 100 mg PO BID	None	• Dyslipidemia • Rash • Hepatotoxicity • GI upset • Hyperglycemia • Fat maldistribution • Nephrolithiasis	• LFTs • Lipids	• 3A4 inhibitor and substrate • Separate administration from H$_2$ blockers	• Also available as oral suspension	No
Indinavir	Crixivan	800 mg PO BID + ritonavir 100–200 mg PO BID	None	• Dyslipidemia • Hepatotoxicity • GI upset • Nephrolithiasis • Indirect hyperbilirubinemia • Hyperglycemia • Fat maldistribution	• LFTs • Lipids • Bilirubin	3A4 inhibitor and substrate	Patients are advised to drink six 8 oz glasses of water per day	No

Protease Inhibitors (PIs) *(cont'd)*

Generic	Brand	Dose	Contraindications	Primary Side Effects	Key Monitoring	Pertinent Drug Interactions	Med Pearl	Top 200
Lopinavir/ Ritonavir	Kaletra	• Lopinavir 400 mg/ritonavir 100 mg PO BID **OR** • Lopinavir 800 mg/ ritonavir 200 mg PO daily	None	• Dyslipidemia • Pancreatitis • Hepatotoxicity • GI upset • Hyperglycemia • Fat maldistribution • PR prolongation • QT prolongation	• LFTs • Lipids	3A4 substrate and inhibitor	• Also available as oral solution • Recommended PI for pregnant women (BID dosing only)	No
Nelfinavir	Viracept	1250 mg PO BID	Concurrent use of PPIs	• Diarrhea • Dyslipidemia • Hepatotoxicity • Hyperglycemia • Fat maldistribution	• LFTs • Lipids	• 3A4 and 2C19 substrate • 3A4 inhibitor	• Administer with food • May disperse in water • Also available as oral powder	No
Ritonavir	Norvir	100 mg–200 mg to boost other PIs	None	• Dyslipidemia • Hepatotoxicity • GI upset • Hyperglycemia • Fat maldistribution	• LFTs • Lipids	• 3A4, 2D6 substrate and inhibitor • 1AC, 2C9, and 3A4 inducer	• Only used for boosting • Administer with food • Also available as oral solution (43% alcohol)	No
Saquinavir	Invirase	1000 mg PO BID + ritonavir 100 mg PO BID	Concurrent use of class IA or class III antiarrhythmics	• PR prolongation • QT prolongation • Dyslipidemia • Hepatotoxicity • GI upset • Hyperglycemia • Fat maldistribution	• LFTs • Lipids	3A4 substrate and inhibitor	• Administer with food	No
Tipranavir	Aptivus	500 mg PO BID + ritonavir 200 mg PO BID	None	• Hepatotoxicity • Rash • Dyslipidemia • Hyperglycemia • Fat maldistribution	• LFTs • Lipids	• 3A4 substrate • 2D6 inhibitor • Separate dosing from antacids	• Also available as oral solution	No

Integrase Inhibitors

Generic	Brand	Dose	Contraindications	Primary Side Effects	Key Monitoring	Pertinent Drug Interactions	Med Pearl	Top 200
Mechanism of action – inhibits integration of proviral DNA into host CD4 T-cell genome								
Dolutegravir	Tivicay	Therapy naïve or therapy experienced, integrase inhibitor naïve: 50 mg PO daily	None	• Hypersensitivity reaction • Insomnia • Headache	None	• Efavirenz • Fosamprenavir/ritonavir • Tipranavir/ritonavir and rifampin ↓ levels (↑dose to 50 mg PO BID)	Primarily metabolized via UGT1A1 glucuronidation	No
Elvitegravir	Only available in combination with cobicistat, tenofovir, and emtricitabine (Stribild)	1 tab PO daily	CrCl <70 mL/min	• GI upset • Renal insufficience • ↓ Bone mineral density	SCr	• Elvitegravir: 3A4 substrate, 2C9 inducer • Cobicistat: 2D6 substrate, 2D6 and 3A4 inhibitor	Administer with food	No
Raltegravir	Isentress	400 mg PO BID	None	• Nausea • Headache • Diarrhea • ↑ CPK • Muscle weakness • Rhabdomyolysis • Rash	None	Rifampin ↓ levels (↑ dose to 800 mg PO BID)	• No CYP450 metabolism; only UGT1A1 glucuronidation • Also available as packet for oral suspension	No

CCR5 Inhibitor

Generic	Brand	Dose	Contraindications	Primary Side Effects	Key Monitoring	Pertinent Drug Interactions	Med Pearl	Top 200
Mechanism of action – acts as an antagonist for the CCR5 receptor, a chemokine coreceptor that can facilitate HIV entry into CD4 T-cells								
Maraviroc	Selzentry	300 mg PO BID	None	• Abdominal pain • Cough • Dizziness • Musculoskeletal symptoms • Rash • Hepatotoxicity • Orthostatic hypotension	LFTs	• 3A4 substrate • ↑ dose to 600 mg PO BID with strong 3A4 inducers • ↓ dose to 150 mg PO BID with strong 3A4 inhibitors	Hepatotoxicity may be preceded by systemic hypersensitivity reaction (rash, eosinophilia)	No

Fusion Inhibitor

Generic	Brand	Dose	Contraindications	Primary Side Effects	Key Monitoring	Pertinent Drug Interactions	Med Pearl	Top 200
Mechanism of action – blocks conformational changes in gp41 on the surface of HIV that are required for HIV fusion with CD4 cell membranes								
Enfuvirtide	Fuzeon	90 mg SC BID	None	Local injection site reactions (pain, erythema, induration, nodules and cysts, pruritus, ecchymosis)	Injection sites	None	Only HIV medication available as SC injection	No

Combination Products: See individual drug components for important points

Brand	Components	Dosing
Atripla	Efavirenz, tenofovir, emtricitabine	1 tablet PO daily
Combivir	Lamivudine, zidovudine	1 tablet PO BID
Complera	Rilpivirine, tenofovir, emtricitabine	1 tablet PO daily
Epzicom	Abacavir, lamivudine	1 tablet PO daily
Stribild	Elvitegravir, cobicistat, emtricitabine, tenofovir	1 tablet PO daily
Triumeq	Dolutegravir, abacavir, lamivudine	1 tablet PO daily
Trizivir	Abacavir, lamivudine, zidovudine	1 tablet PO BID
Truvada	Emtricitabine, tenofovir	1 tablet PO daily

KAPLAN MEDICAL

TUBERCULOSIS

Definitions

TB is a communicable infection disease caused by *Mycobacterium tuberculosis*. It can produce a silent, latent infection, as well as an active disease state. Although TB is far less common today in the United States, it remains the most prevalent infection on the planet. Effective therapy for *Mycobacterium tuberculosis* infections require combination chemotherapy designed to prevent the emergence of resistant organisms. Increased resistance to the conventional antituberculous agents has led to the use of more complex regimens.

Diagnosis

- Diagnosis relies on skin testing with the tuberculin purified protein derivative (PPD).
- PPD should be performed on high-risk patients.
  - High-risk patients include HIV-infected, hospital employees, nursing home staff and residents, workers in prisons, immigrants, and healthcare students.
- The intracutaneous PPD injection should produce a small, raised, blanched wheal. This test should be read by an experienced professional in 48 to 72 hours.
  - Measured area >5 mm is considered positive for HIV-infected persons, recent contact of a person with TB disease, persons with fibrotic changes on chest radiograph consistent with prior TB, patients with organ transplants, and persons who are immunosuppressed for other reasons.
  - Measured area >10 mm is considered positive for recent immigrants from high-prevalence countries, injection drug users, residents and employees of high-risk congregate settings, mycobacteriology laboratory personnel, persons with clinical conditions that place them at high risk, children <4 years of age, and infants, children, and adolescents exposed to adults in high-risk categories.
  - Measured area >15 mm is considered positive for any person, including persons with no known risk factors for TB.
- After a positive PPD skin test, a diagnostic test must be performed to rule out active disease.
  - Confirmatory diagnosis is performed with chest radiographs and microbiologic examination or sputum.
  - A total of three sputum samples should be collected and sent for acid-fast bacillus testing.

Signs and Symptoms

TB can present with generalized symptoms of weight loss, malaise, fever, and night sweats. As the disease progresses, the patient may develop a persistent cough, which is often productive of sputum. Frequently, the onset of TB is insidious and the diagnosis may not be considered until a chest radiograph is performed.

Guidelines

Blumberg HM, Burman WJ, Chaisson RE, et al; American Thoracic Society, Centers for Disease Control and Prevention and the Infectious Diseases Society. American Thoracic Society/Centers for Disease Control and Prevention/Infectious Diseases Society of America: treatment of tuberculosis. *Am J Respir Crit Care Med* 2003;167:603–62.

Guidelines Summary

The overall goals for treatment of TB are: (*1*) To cure the individual patient, and (*2*) to minimize the transmission of *Mycobacterium tuberculosis* to other persons.

- Risk factors
  - Location of birth (New York, New Jersey, California, Florida, and Texas account for 92% of cases)
  - Close contact (>40 hours per week) with TB patients
  - Increase in age
  - Race and ethnicity: Hispanics, African Americans, and Asian Pacific Islanders
- Successful treatment of TB has benefits for both the individual patient and the community in which the patient resides.
- Prescribing physician responsibility for treatment completion is a fundamental principle in TB control.
- Treatment of patients with TB is most successful within a comprehensive framework that addresses both clinical and social issues of relevance to the patient.
- It is strongly recommended that patient-centered care be the initial management strategy, regardless of the source of supervision. This strategy should always include an adherence plan that emphasizes directly observed therapy (DOT).
- Patients with TB caused by drug-susceptible organisms usually are treated initially with a four-drug regimen (rifampin, isoniazid, pyrazinamide, and ethambutol [RIPE]) followed by a two-drug continuation phase (rifampin and isoniazid).

Tuberculosis

Generic	Brand	Dose	Contra-indications	Primary Side Effects	Key Monitoring	Pertinent Drug Interactions	Med Pearl	Top 200
Mechanism of action — inhibits mycolic acid synthesis resulting in disruption of the bacterial cell wall								
Isoniazid	Only available generically	• Latent: 5 mg/day (max = 300 mg) PO daily × 6–9 mo **OR** 15 mg/kg (max = 900 mg) PO weekly × 6–9 mo • Active: multiple scenarios	• Liver disease • Previous severe reactions (drug fever, chills, arthritis)	• Depression • Flushing • Jaundice	• LFTs • Sputum cultures	• 2C19, 2D6 inhibitor	• Severe and sometimes fatal hepatitis may occur within 3 months of treatment • Drinking alcohol not recommended during treatment • Pyridoxine should be administered to prevent peripheral neuropathy	No
Mechanism of action — inhibits bacterial RNA synthesis by binding to the beta subunit of DNA-dependent RNA polymerase, blocking RNA transcription								
Rifampin	Rifadin	• PO/IV: 10 mg/kg/day (max = 600 mg/day)	Concurrent use of Fosamprenavir, saquinavir/ritonavir	• Numbness • Flu-like syndrome • Rash • Discoloration of urine • Neutropenia/leukopenia	• LFTs • CBC • Sputum cultures • Chest x-ray	1AC, 2C19, 2C9,3A4 inducer	May cause red/orange discoloration of bodily fluids	No
Mechanism of action — kills mycobacteria replicating in macrophages; exact mechanism is not known								
Pyrazinamide	Only available generically	• 40–55 kg: 1000 mg/day • 56–75 kg: 1500 mg/day • 76–90 kg: 2000 mg/day (max dose)	• Acute gout • Liver disease	• Malaise • Anorexia • Hepatotoxicity	• LFTs • Uric acid levels • Sputum cultures • Chest x-ray	None	Typically used for the first 2 months of therapy	No
Mechanism of action — suppresses mycobacteria multiplication by interfering with RNA synthesis								
Ethambutol	Myambutol	• PO: 15–25 mg/kg/day (max = 1,600 mg/day)	Optic neuritis	• Myocarditis • Headache • Gout • Hepatotoxicity	• Baseline and periodic (monthly) visual testing • LFTs	Aluminum hydroxide ↓ absorption (separate by 4 hours)	Optic neuritis manifests as ↓ red–green color perception, ↓ visual field	No

LEARNING POINTS

- Compliance is a must with antiretroviral therapy. If a patient is going to stop the prescribed regimen, all the antiretrovirals must be stopped at the same time to prevent resistance.
- Patients receiving antibiotics should complete the entire course of therapy.
- Be aware of the patient's allergies when selecting antibiotic therapy (especially penicillin and sulfa allergies).
- Know agents to treat unique organisms:
  - MRSA: Vancomycin, linezolid, tigecycline, daptomycin, telavancin, ceftaroline
  - *Pseudomonas aeruginosa*: Piperacillin/tazobactam, ticarcillin/clavulanic acid, aztreonam, aminoglycosides, ciprofloxacin, ceftazidime, cefepime, carbapenems (except ertapenem)
  - Anaerobes: Metronidazole, clindamycin, piperacillin/tazobactam, ticarcillin/clavulanic acid, cefoxitin, cefotetan, carbapenems
- Know important/notable side effects and drug interactions of antibiotics:
  - Which ones cause nephrotoxicity?
  - Which ones are associated with QT interval prolongation?
  - Which ones cause myelosuppression?
  - Which ones are associated with a disulfiram reaction?
  - Which ones should be avoided with antacids or products containing di-/trivalent cations?
  - Which ones cause photosensitivity?
- Given an active case of TB, the clinician must ensure DOT to reduce bacterial resistance and exposure to other patients.
- Isoniazid is currently the drug of choice for a positive PPD and in combination-treatments for TB.

PRACTICE QUESTIONS

1. Which of the following medications should NOT be given to a 1-year-old child?

    (A) Amoxicillin
    (B) Cefuroxime
    (C) Clindamycin
    (D) Penicillin
    (E) Tetracycline

2. Which of the following medications would be appropriate for the treatment of *Pseudomonas aeruginosa*?

    (A) Ampicillin
    (B) Cefepime
    (C) Ceftriaxone
    (D) Erythromycin
    (E) Clindamycin

3. A patient admitted to the hospital is diagnosed with aspergillosis. Which of the following antimicrobial agents would be most appropriate to initiate in this patient?

    (A) Nystatin
    (B) Tigecycline
    (C) Chloramphenicol
    (D) Acyclovir
    (E) Caspofungin

4. Patients taking which of the following antimicrobial agents should be counseled to wear sunscreen because of the risk of photosensitivity?

    I. Cleocin
    II. Biaxin
    III. Factive

    (A) I only
    (B) III only
    (C) I and II only
    (D) II and III only
    (E) I, II, and III

5. Which of the following drugs used in the treatment of tuberculosis can cause orange-red discoloration of a patient's urine?

   (A) Isoniazid
   (B) Ethambutol
   (C) Rifampin
   (D) Pyrazinamide
   (E) Streptomycin

6. A woman diagnosed with an STD picks up her antibiotic prescription at her local pharmacy. The pharmacist counsels her that she should not drink alcoholic beverages while taking this medication because it may lead to an unpleasant reaction. Which of the following antibiotics has been prescribed for this patient?

   (A) Azithromycin
   (B) Cefixime
   (C) Doxycycline
   (D) Metronidazole
   (E) Penicillin VK

7. An 85-year-old female patient has been hospitalized with an infection. She has a CrCl of 25 mL/min. Which of the following antibiotics does NOT need to be dose-adjusted in this patient?

   (A) Ceftriaxone
   (B) Gentamicin
   (C) Meropenem
   (D) Piperacillin-tazobactam
   (E) Vancomycin

8. Which of the following antibiotics is the first-line treatment for *Pneumocystis jiroveci* pneumonia?

   (A) Acyclovir
   (B) Azithromycin
   (C) Ciprofloxacin
   (D) Fluconazole
   (E) Trimethoprim-sulfamethoxazole

9. Which of the following is an acceptable antiviral regimen for a treatment-naïve patient with HIV?

   (A) Abacavir + didanosine + zidovudine
   (B) Efavirenz + nevirapine + emtricitabine
   (C) Darunavir + ritonavir + atazanavir
   (D) Tenofovir + emtricitabine + raltegravir
   (E) Dolutegravir + tipranavir + stavudine

10. Acyclovir is available in which of the following formulations?

      I. Injection
     II. Topical ointment
   III. Transdermal patch

(A) I only
(B) III only
(C) I and II only
(D) II and III only
(E) I, II, and III

ANSWERS

1. E

Tetracycline should not be given to children younger than 9 years of age, as it can cause enamel hypoplasia or permanent tooth discoloration, therefore choice (E) is correct. The other medications can be administered safely to children.

2. B

Cefepime, a 4th-generation cephalosporin, is the only antibiotic listed that would treat an infection caused by *Pseudomonas aeruginosa*; therefore, choice (B) is correct.

3. E

Aspergillosis is a serious fungal infection. Both caspofungin and nystatin (A) are considered antifungal agents; however, nystatin is used topically (as an oral suspension for thrush or as topical cream/ointment/powder) for local infections caused by *Candida* spp. Caspofungin is administered intravenously and can be used for the treatment of aspergillosis; thus, choice (E) is correct. Tigecycline (B) and chloramphenicol (C) are used for bacterial infections. Acyclovir (D) is an antiviral agent.

4. B

Fluoroquinolones are associated with an increased risk of photosensitivity. Therefore, patients receiving Factive (gemifloxacin) should be counseled to wear sunscreen during the course of therapy. Neither Cleocin (clindamycin) nor Biaxin (clarithromycin) is associated with photosensitivity.

5. C

Rifampin (C) can cause an orange-red discoloration of all bodily fluids (e.g., tears, saliva, urine). Rifabutin can also cause this discoloration of bodily fluids. Isoniazid (A), ethambutol (B), pyrazinamide (D), and streptomycin (E) do not cause discoloration of the urine.

6. D

Metronidazole should not be taken with alcohol as this may lead to a disulfiram-like reaction, which can manifest as severe flushing, headache, nausea, vomiting, or chest and abdominal pain. Although patients generally should not take any of their medications with alcohol, the concomitant use with metronidazole can lead specifically to this very unpleasant reaction; therefore, answer (D) is correct.

7. **A**

Ceftriaxone (A) is eliminated via both biliary and renal excretion. Therefore, the dose of this antibiotic does not need to be adjusted in patients with renal dysfunction. The dose of gentamicin (B), meropenem (C), piperacillin-tazobactam (D), and vancomycin (E) would all need to be adjusted in this patient with a CrCl of 25 mL/min.

8. **E**

TMP/SMX (E) is the drug of choice for the treatment of *Pneumocystis jiroveci* pneumonia, provided that the patient does not have a sulfa allergy. Alternative medications, including dapsone, pentamidine, or atovaquone, can be used for the treatment of this opportunistic infection in patients with a sulfa allergy.

9. **D**

The regimen consisting of tenofovir + emtricitabine + raltegravir (D) is an acceptable approach for management of a treatment-naïve patient with HIV because it contains 2 NRTIs (tenofovir and emtricitabine) and an integrase inhibitor (raltegravir). Other acceptable antiviral regimens include those that contain 1 NNRTI + 2 NRTIs or PI (preferably boosted with ritonavir) + 2 NRTIs. Choice (A) contains 3 NRTIs (abacavir + didanosine + zidovudine). Choice (B) contains 2 NNRTIs (efavirenz and nevirapine) + 1 NRTI (emtricitabine). Choice (C) contains 3 PIs (darunavir + ritonavir + atazanavir). Choice (E) contains an integrase inhibitor (dolutegravir), a PI (tipranavir), and a NRTI (stavudine). None of these four regimens is acceptable for the management of a treatment-naïve patient with HIV.

10. **C**

Acyclovir is available as an IV injection (I) and as a topical ointment (II). This drug is also available as a capsule, tablet, oral suspension, buccal tablet, and topical cream. Acyclovir is not available as a transdermal patch (III).

Pulmonary Disorders

3

This chapter covers the following diseases:

- **Asthma**
- **Chronic obstructive pulmonary disease**
- **Smoking Cessation**

 Suggested Study Time: **45 minutes**

ASTHMA

Definitions

Asthma is a disease of the airways characterized by airway inflammation and broncho-constriction of the smooth muscles. This hyperactivity is due to a wide variety of stimuli or triggers. The hallmark features of asthma include airflow obstruction that is reversible, bronchial hyperresponsiveness, and airway inflammation. The hyperactivity and inflammation lead to obstruction of the airways, cough, dyspnea, chest tightness, and wheezing. The inflammatory cell infiltration mainly consists of neutrophils (especially in sudden-onset, fatal asthma exacerbations, and in patients who smoke), eosinophils, lymphocytes, mast cell activation, and epithelial cell injury and is called remodeling.

Diagnosis

To diagnose asthma, a patient has to have episodes of airway obstruction or airway hyperresponsiveness and at least partially reversible airway obstruction, all alternative diagnoses excluded.

- Pulmonary function tests (PFTs) provide an objective means to diagnose asthma.

- PFTs are measured using spirometry and demonstrate an obstructive pattern of decreases in expiratory flow rates.

- Spirometry measures FVC and FEV1.
- FVC is the volume of air forcibly exhaled from the point of maximal inspiration; FEV1 is the volume of aired exhaled during the first second.
- The guidelines recommend that spirometry measurements of FEV1, FVC, and FEV1/FEV are used before and after the patient inhales a short-acting bronchodilator to assess bronchodilation. Improvements are defined as an increase of FEV1 by more than 12%, which is diagnostic of asthma.

Signs and Symptoms

- Shortness of breath
- Wheezing
- Chest tightness
- Coughing
- Worsening of symptoms at night
- Triggers: pollen, dust, chemicals, changes in weather, perfumes, smoke, heartburn, mold, exercise
- Nasal polyps

Guidelines

National Heart, Lung and Blood Institute, National Asthma Education and Prevention Program, Expert Panel Report 3: Guidelines for the Diagnosis and Management of Asthma—Full Report, 2007. http://nhlbi.nih.gov/guidelines/asthma/asthsumm.pdf.

Global Initiative for Asthma Pocket Guide for Asthma Management and Prevention. http://www.ginasthma.org/local/uploads/files/GINA_Pocket2013_May15.pdf.

Guidelines Summary

There are four components to asthma management:

- Measurement of assessment and monitoring
- Controlling environmental factors and comorbid conditions
- Education for asthma care
- Pharmacologic therapy

The goals of therapy are as follows:

- Patient education is a must.
- Daily usage of peak flow meter will provide an objective FEV1.

- Implementation of an action plan:
  - Green zone ("I feel good"), yellow zone ("I do not feel good"), red zone ("I feel awful")
  - Green zone = FEV1 >80% of personal best
  - Yellow zone = FEV1 >50–80% of personal best
  - Red zone = FEV1 <50% of personal best
- Attempt to identify triggers:
  - Consider subcutaneous allergen immunotherapy.
  - Management of gastrointestinal reflux disease (GERD) can greatly improve symptoms.
  - Avoid aspirin therapy due to prostaglandin inhibition; can cause bronchoconstriction.
  - Smoking cessation is recommended.
  - Consider clean home, dust, plastic case over mattress.
  - Identify frequency of symptoms and nighttime awakenings.
  - Identify use of short-acting beta-2 agonists and lung function.
    - » Ensure adherence with medications.
    - » Ensure proper inhaler technique.
    - » Use a stepwise approach to treatment.
    - » Long-term medications should include anti-inflammatory mechanism.

Asthma

Mechanism of action – glucocorticoid receptor agonist with an affinity for the receptor resulting in anti-inflammatory and immunosuppressive properties, and antiproliferative actions

Generic	Brand	Dose	Contra-indications	Primary Side Effects	Key Monitoring	Pertinent Drug Interactions	Med Pearl	Top 200
Fluticasone	• Flovent Diskus • Flovent HFA	88–440 mcg BID	Primary treatment of acute bronchospasm	• Throat irritation • Cough • Oral candidiasis • Upper respiratory tract infection • Sinusitis	• FEV1 • Peak flow • Other PFTs • HPA axis suppression	• Cobicistat (component of Stribild) • Ritonavir	• HFA formulation • Most potent corticosteroid	Yes
Budesonide	• Pulmicort • Respules	180–720 mcg BID					Respules are the only nebulized corticosteroid	Yes
Mometasone	Asmanex	110–880 mcg/day					True once daily	No
Beclomethasone	QVAR	40–320 mcg BID					HFA formulation	Yes
Flunisolide	Aerospan	160–320 mcg BID					AeroBid(M) has a mint flavor	No
Ciclesonide	Alvesco	80 mcg BID (max = 640 mcg/day)					Drug is a solution aerosol so no shaking is required	No

Mechanism of action – long-acting beta-2 agonists

Generic	Brand	Dose	Contra-indications	Primary Side Effects	Key Monitoring	Pertinent Drug Interactions	Med Pearl	Top 200
Salmeterol	Serevent Diskus	*Diskus:* 50 mcg/puff (max = 2 puffs/day)	• Use as an acute bronchodilator • Presence of tachyarrhythmias	• Headache • Hypertension • Dizziness • Chest pain • Throat irritation	• FEV1 • Peak flow • Other PFTs	• Cobicistat (component of Stribild) • Ritonavir	Long-acting beta-2 agonists may increase the risk of asthma-related deaths; should be used only in adjunct therapy with inhaled corticosteroids	No
Formoterol	• Foradil aerolizer • Perforomist	• *DPI:* 12 mcg/capsule (max = 2 puffs/day) • 20 mcg BID				None		No

Mechanism of action – prevents the mass cells from releasing histamine and leukotrienes

Generic	Brand	Dose	Contra-indications	Primary Side Effects	Key Monitoring	Pertinent Drug Interactions	Med Pearl	Top 200
Cromolyn neb & inhaler	Gastrocom	20–80 mg/day	Primary treatment for acute bronchospasms	• Cough and irritation • Unpleasant taste • Increase in sneezing	Pulmonary function tests	None	• Safety is the primary advantage of this drug class • May take 4–6 weeks for full benefit • Approved to >2 yr of age	No

Asthma *(cont'd)*

Generic	Brand	Dose	Contra-indications	Primary Side Effects	Key Monitoring	Pertinent Drug Interactions	Med Pearl	Top 200
Mechanism of action – IgG monoclonal antibody which inhibits IgE receptor on mast cells and basophils.								
Omalizumab	XOLAIR	SC 150–375 mg every 2–4 wk, based on weight and serum IgE	Acute bronchospasms	• Pain and bruising of injection sites • Anaphylaxis has been reported • Neuromuscular pain	Be prepared for anaphylaxis	None	Do not administer more than 150 mg per injection site	No
Mechanism of action – selective leukotriene-receptor antagonist of leukotrienes D4 and E4								
Montelukast	Singulair	4–10 mg/HS	Hypersensitivity	• Headache • Rare Churg-Strauss syndrome		CYP450 2C9 inhibitors and inducers	Approved as young as 1 year of age	Yes
Zafirlukast	Accolate	10–20 mg BID		• Elevations in LFTs • Headache	Must be taken on empty stomach	• Warfarin • Pimozide • CYP450 2C9 inhibitors and inducers	Must be taken on empty stomach	No
Mechanism of action – 5-lipoxygenase inhibitor limits neutrophil and monocyte aggregation								
Zileuton	• Zyflo • Zyflo CR	• IR: 600 mg QID • CR: 1,200 mg BID	Acute liver disease	• Elevations in LFTs • Headache	• LFT baseline every 2 months • Peak flow	CYP450 inhibitor: 1A2	• QID dose is disadvantage for IR • CR should be taken with food	No
Mechanism of action – methylxanthine causes bronchodilation by increasing tissue concentrations of cyclic adenine monophosphate								
• Theophylline • Liquid, sustained-release tabs & caps	• Theo-24 • Theocron • Elixophyllin	10 mg/kg/day up to 600 mg/day	Allergy to corn-derived dextrose	• Tachycardia • N/V • CNS stimulation • Theophylline toxicity: persistent, repetitive vomiting	• Serum range: 10–20 mcg/mL • Serum levels <20 mcg/mL have few side effects	CYP450: inhibits 1A2, 3A4	Dosage adjustments should be in small increments (maximum: 25%); elderly patients should be started on 25% reduction in the adult dose	Yes
Aminophylline	Only available generically	Diagnosis- and age-dependent	Hypersensitivity to theophylline and ethylendiamine	• Tachycardia • Tremor • CNS stimulation	• Vital signs • In&Outs • Serum theophylline concentrations • CNS effects	CYP1A2, CYP3A4	IV only	No

Asthma *(cont'd)*

Generic	Brand	Dose	Contra-indications	Primary Side Effects	Key Monitoring	Pertinent Drug Interactions	Med Pearl	Top 200
Mechanism of action – relaxes bronchial smooth muscle by acting on beta-2 receptors								
Albuterol	• Ventolin HFA • Proventil HFA • Pro Air HFA	MDI: 90 mcg/ puff Neb: 2.5 mg/ 3 mL	Hypersensitivity	• Dose-dependent • Angina, atrial fibrillation, arrhythmias, chest discomfort, cough, tremor	• FEV1 • Peak flow • Blood pressure • Heart rate	Nonselective beta-adrenergic blockers decrease albuterol's effect	Excessive use can increase risk of death; nebulizer is compatible with budesonide, cromolyn, ipratropium	Yes
Levalbuterol	Xopenex, Xopenex HFA	MDI: 45 mcg/ puff 200 puffs/canister Neb: 0.63/3 mL		• Tremor • Rhinitis • Tachycardia			• Prime the inhaler by releasing 4 actuations prior to use • Fewer cardiac side effects	Yes
Combination		• See above for individual interactions • Synergistic effects are likely with combination products • Maximum dose of Advair is 1 puff BID; dosages: 100/50, 200/50, 500/50						
Fluticasone/ salmeterol	• Advair Diskus • Advair HFA							Yes
Formoterol/ budesonide	Symbicort							Yes
Mometasone/ formoterol	Dulera							No

Storage and Administration Pearls

- Metered-dose inhaler (MDI) requires hand coordination and proper technique.
- Dry powder inhaler (DPI) is breath-actuated and requires less coordination.
- Spacer with non–breath-actuated MDIs and mouth washing and spitting after inhalation decreases local side effects.
- Hydrofluoroalkane (HFA) is an earth-friendly alternative to CFCs.
- Aminophylline is incompatible with phenytoin.

Patient Education Pearls

- Using a spacer with inhaled corticosteroids allows for better deposition into the lungs and helps to prevent thrush.
- Patient should rinse and spit to avoid thrush from inhaled corticosteroids.
- Adherence is a must with all asthma medications.

CHRONIC OBSTRUCTIVE PULMONARY DISEASE

Definitions

Chronic obstructive pulmonary disease (COPD) is characterized by persistent and largely irreversible airflow obstruction causing dyspnea, which does not fluctuate like asthma. Airflow obstruction is generally progressive and associated with abnormal inflammatory responses of lungs to noxious particles and gases. It is a disease entity with a spectrum of manifestation depending on the lung region affected. Chronic bronchitis affects the larger airways; emphysema affects the smaller airways, called alveolar sacs.

Diagnosis

If COPD is suspected, perform spirometry because diagnosis has to be confirmed with spirometry. FEV1 is the forced expiratory volume in 1 second. This percent is gathered from using spirometry and aids in determining the severity of COPD.

- History of cigarette smoking is a factor.
- α_1-antitrypsin deficiency in nonsmokers is a factor.
- Nocturnal symptoms are unusual.
- Chest x-ray often shows low and flattened diaphragms.
- FEV1 and all measurements of expiration airflow are reduced.
- FEV1 is the standard way to assess clinical course for response to therapy.
- FEV1/FVC <0.70 confirms diagnosis of airflow limitation that is not reversible.

Signs and Symptoms

- Cough with mucus
- Dyspnea and dyspnea on exertion
- FEV_1/FVC ratio <0.70
- Chest tightness
- Wheezing
- Tachypnea
- Pursed lip breathing
- Hyperinflation of the lungs
- Use of accessory muscles for breathing

Classification of Airflow Severity

- GOLD I—Mild COPD: FEV1 ≥80% predicted.
- GOLD II—Moderate COPD: 50% ≤FEV1 <80% predicted.
- GOLD III—Severe COPD: 30% ≤FEV1 <50% predicted.
- GOLD IV—Very severe COPD: FEV1 <30% predicted.

Classification of COPD Exacerbation Risk

- Group A: Mild to moderate airflow limitation, low risk of exacerbation
- Group B: Mild to moderate airflow limitation, low risk of exacerbation with more symptoms that group A
- Group C: Severe to very severe airflow limitation, high risk of exacerbation
- Group D: Severe to very severe airflow limitation, high risk of exacerbation with more symptoms than group C

Guidelines

American College of Physicians 2008. www.acp.com.

Global Initiative for Chronic Obstructive Lung Disease. Global Strategy for the Diagnosis, Management, and Prevention of Chronic Obstructive Pulmonary Disease. 2010.

National Heart, Lung and Blood Institute, Expert Panel Report 3: Global Initiative for Chronic Obstructive Lung Disease (GOLD). www.goldcopd.org.

Guidelines Summary

- **Global Initiative for Chronic Obstructive Lung Disease (GOLD)**
  - Spirometry should be used to diagnose airway obstruction in symptomatic patients >40 years old.

- Smoking cessation should be encouraged for all patients who smoke.
- Inhaled bronchodilator therapy, prescribed either as needed or scheduled, is the mainstay of treatment for COPD.
- May combine bronchodilators from different classes to improve efficacy.
- Inhaled corticosteroids may be used to prevent exacerbations.
- Consider influenza and pneumococcal vaccines.
- Oral corticosteroids may be used to prevent exacerbations.
- Antibiotics may be given if the patient has increased dyspnea, sputum production, and sputum purulence.

Drugs for COPD

Generic	Brand	Dose	Contra-indications	Primary Side Effects	Key Monitoring	Pertinent Drug Interactions	Med Pearl	Top 200
Mechanism of action – partial α4β2 nicotinic receptor agonist; prevents nicotine stimulation of mesolimbic dopamine system								
Varenicline	Chantix	0.5–2 mg/day	Hypersensitivity	• Insomnia • Headache • Abnormal dreams • Nausea • Suicidal ideation	Psychiatric symptoms of depression/ suicide/agitation	None	Start 1 week prior to target stop day with 0.5 mg/day	Yes
Mechanism of action – inhibits neuronal uptake of norepinephrine and dopamine								
Bupropion	Zyban	150–300 mg/day	• Seizure disorder • Anorexia/bulimia • Use of MAOI within 14 days	• Tachycardia • Headache • Insomnia • Dry mouth	• Body weight • Mental status for depression • Suicidal ideation	• CYP450 2D6 inhibitor • Tamoxifen • MAOI • Tnioridazine	Can be co-administered with nicotine replacement patches	Yes
Mechanism of action – supplements nicotine which exhibits primary effects via autonomic ganglia stimulation								
Nicotine	• Commit • NicoDerm • Nicorette	• Gum: max 24 pieces/day • Inhaler: max 16 cartridges/day • Patch: 1 patch per day • Lozenge: 2–4 mg (max = 20/day) • Spray: (max = 80 sprays/day)	• Smoking or chewing tobacco • Post-myocardial infarction • Life-threatening arrhythmias • Worsening angina	• Headache • Mouth or throat irritation • Dyspepsia • Cough	• HR • BP • Nicotine toxicity (severe headache, dizziness, mental confusion)		Antidepressant medications may increase suicidal behavior in young adults	No
Mechanism of action – long-acting beta2-adrenergic agonist; relaxes bronchial smooth muscle								
Indacaterol	Arcapta Neohaler	75 mcg daily	Monotherapy in the treatment of asthma	• Cough • Headache • Nasopharyngitis	• PFTs • HR	Nonselective beta-blockers	Not approved for the treatment of asthma	No
Mechanism of action – long-acting beta2-agonist								
Arformoterol	Brovana	15 mcg BID	Monotherapy in the treatment of asthma	• Chest pain • Pain • Diarrhea • Flu-like syndrome	• PFTs • HR	Nonselective beta-blockers	Available as nebulizer solution	No

Drugs for COPD *(cont'd)*

Mechanism of action – inhibits phosphodiesterase-4 leading to an accumulation of cyclic AMP

Mechanism of action – blocks acetylcholine at the parasympathetic sites in bronchial smooth muscle, causing bronchodilation

Generic	Brand	Dose	Contra-indications	Primary Side Effects	Key Monitoring	Pertinent Drug Interactions	Med Pearl	Top 200
Roflumilast	Daliresp	500 mcg/day	• Hepatic impairment (Child-Pugh class B or C)	• Diarrhea • Weight loss • Nausea	• Weight • LFTs	• Cimetidine • CYP3A4 inducers • Ciprofloxacin • Rifampin	Not indicated for relieving acute bronchospasms or for use as monotherapy of COPD	No
Ipratropium	• Atrovent • Atrovent HFA • Combivent (ipratropium & albuterol)	• MDI: 17 mcg/puff (max = 12 puffs/24 hrs) • Neb: 0.25 mg/mL	• Hypersensitivity • Peanuts allergy (due to soya lecithin) • Does not apply to Atrovent HFA	• Upper respiratory tract infection • Palpitation • Xerostomia • Pharyngeal irritation	• FEV1 • Peak flow • Other pulmonary function tests	CYP450 – substrate 2D6, 3A4	• Not recommended for initial treatment of acute episode of bronchospasm • Anticholinergic side effects are possible. Be careful in BPH, narrow-angle glaucoma, and myasthenia gravis	Yes
Tiotropium	Spiriva	DPI: 18 mcg/puff (max = 1 puff/day)	• Contains lactose					Yes
Aclidinium	Tudorza Pressair	400 mcg inhalation BID		• Headache • Nasopharyngitis • Diarrhea	PFTs	• Avoid use with other anticholinergic inhalers • Potassium		No
Umeclidinium	Incruse Ellipta					Unknown (newly approved drug)		No
Combination								
Ipratropium/ Albuterol	Combivent Respimat	400 mcg inhalation BID		• Headache • Nasopharyngitis • Diarrhea	PFTs	• Avoid use with other anticholinergic inhalers • Potassium		No
Umeclidinium/ Vilanterol	Anoro Ellipta	62.5 mg/25 mcg; 1 inhalation daily	Hypersensitivity to umeclindinium or milk protein	• Pharyngitis • Limb, muscle, chest pain • Sinusitis	PFTs	• Avoid use with other anticholinergic inhalers • Potassium	Discard inhaler 6 weeks after opening foil pack	No
Fluticasone/ Vilanterol	Breo Ellipta	100 mcg/25 mcg; 1 inhalation daily	Hypersensitivity to components or milk protein	• Nasopharyngitis • URI • Arthralgia • HTN • Peripheral edema	• PFTs • BP • BMD	• Cobicistat • Nonselective beta blockers • Pimecrolimus • Tacrolimus		No

STORAGE AND ADMINISTRATION PEARLS

- Nicotrol inhaler: Protect from light.
- Tiotropium: Do not store capsules in Handihaler device. Capsules should be used within 2 days of removal from blister pack.
- Umeclidinium/vilanterol: Discard inhaler 6 weeks after opening foil pack.

Patient Education Pearls

- For improved outcomes, it is important to have consistent and regular interventions with the patient regarding smoking cessation education.
- When working with patient to stop smoking, it is recommended to use the 5 As: Ask, Advise, Assess, Assist, Arrange.

SMOKING CESSATION

Definitions

The dependence on tobacco is a chronic disease that often requires repeated intervention and multiple attempts to quit. Tobacco dependence is both physiological and psychological, so treatment interventions must be prepared to target both. Informing patients about the dangers of tobacco use is critical, as is educating patients about treatment options available.

Diagnosis

Patients are not always forthcoming about their use of tobacco, so it is important to assess patients' use status in every interaction possible.

Guidelines

Tobacco Use and Dependence Guideline Panel. Treating Tobacco Use and Dependence: 2008 Update. Rockville (MD): US Department of Health and Human Services; 2008 May.

Guidelines Summary

- The model for treatment and intervention of tobacco use and dependence is summarized by the "5 A's":
  - **ASK.** Identify and document tobacco use status for every patient and every visit.
  - **ADVISE.** Urge every tobacco user to quit in a strong and personalized manner.
  - **ASSESS.** Evaluate if your patient is willing to make a quit attempt.
  - **ASSIST.** For patients willing to make a quit attempt, offer treatment options and additional counseling; for those not willing, use motivational strategies to promote quitting.

- **ARRANGE.** Schedule follow-ups with those patients willing to make a quit attempt; for those not willing to make an attempt, address willingness to quit at the next visit.

- Tobacco dependence is a chronic disease that often requires repeated intervention and multiple attempts to quit. Effective treatments exist that can significantly increase rates of long-term abstinence.

- It is essential that health care providers consistently identify and document tobacco use status and treat every tobacco user seen in a health care setting.

- Tobacco dependence treatments are effective across a broad range of populations. Clinicians should encourage every patient willing to make a quit attempt to use the counseling treatments and medications recommended.

- Brief tobacco dependence treatment is effective. Clinicians should offer every patient who uses tobacco at least the brief treatments shown to be effective.

LEARNING POINTS

- Inhaled corticosteroids are the primary treatment for asthma. They prevent remodeling, improve symptoms, and prevent exacerbations as compared to the other medications.

- Peak flow meters are crucial to the maintenance of asthma. Peak flow meters should be used to determine a patient's personal best and used every morning to identify an early exacerbation.

- All patients with asthma should have a short-acting bronchodilator for rescue therapy.

- Smoking cessation will help slow the progression of COPD and is the most important intervention when dealing with patients who have COPD.

PRACTICE QUESTIONS

1. What is Zyflo's mechanism of action?

   (A) Selective leukotriene-receptor antagonist of leukotrienes D4 and E4
   (B) 5-lipoxygenase inhibitor limits neutrophil and monocyte aggregation
   (C) Methylxanthine causes bronchodilation by increasing tissue concentrations of cyclic adenine monophosphate
   (D) Relaxes bronchial smooth muscle by stimulating beta-2 receptors

2. The device used to measure forced vital capacity is called a

   (A) tonometer.
   (B) optomyometer.
   (C) sphygmomanometer.
   (D) spirometer.
   (E) gonioscope.

3. QVAR is indicated for which of the following scenarios?

   I. Asthma
   II. COPD
   III. Smoking cessation

   (A) I only
   (B) III only
   (C) I and II only
   (D) II and III only
   (E) I, II, and III

4. Which of the following have the same active ingredient?

   I. Flonase
   II. Flovent
   III. Veramyst
   (A) I only
   (B) III only
   (C) I and II only
   (D) II and III only
   (E) I, II, and III

5. Patient counseling that includes the need for the patient to rinse his or her mouth and spit after use is applicable to which medication?

   (A) Breo Ellipta
   (B) Arcapta Neohaler
   (C) Xopenex HFA
   (D) Servent Diskus

6. Which of the following should be used in combination with an inhaled corticosteroid in the treatment of asthma?

    (A) Budesonide
    (B) Cromolyn
    (C) Formoterol
    (D) Levalbuterol

7. Which of the following should be monitored for varenicline?

        I. Constipation
       II. Blood pressure
      III. Suicidal ideation

    (A) I only
    (B) III only
    (C) I and II only
    (D) II and III only
    (E) I, II, and III

ANSWERS

1. **B**

The challenging aspect of this question is that Zyflo is classified as a leukotriene modifier (A), like Accolate or Singulair, but the two have different mechanisms of action. Zyflo's mechanism is an inhibitor of 5-lipoxygenase versus an antagonist at the receptor. Choice (C) is the mechanism of theophylline and choice (D) is the mechanism of albuterol.

2. **D**

A spirometer is a gasometer used for measuring respiratory gases, so (D) is correct. A tonometer (A) determines pressure or tension within the eye. An optomyometer (B) is an instrument for determining the relative power of the extrinsic muscles of the eye. A sphygmomanometer (C) measures arterial blood pressure. A gonioscope (E) measures the lens angle in relationship to the eye.

3. **A**

QVAR is an inhaled corticosteroid that is indicated only for the maintenance and pro-phylactic treatment of asthma, so (A) is the only correct answer.

4. **E**

Flonase, Flovent, and Veramyst all have the same active ingredient—fluticasone—so (E) is correct.

5. **A**

Breo Ellipta contains fluticasone, which is an inhaled corticosteroid. Counseling for inhaled corticosteroids should include having the patient rinse his or her mouth with water and spit it out to reduce the risk of thrush or hoarseness. The other medications listed do not contain an inhaled corticosteroid and therefore do not require the patient to rinse his or her mouth after use.

6. **C**

Formoterol is a long-acting beta-2 agonist that needs to be administered in conjunc-tion with an inhaled corticosteroid. Use of long-acting beta-2 agonists without the use of an inhaled corticosteroid has been associated with increased risk of asthma-related deaths. Budesonide is an inhaled corticosteroid and should not be used with another inhaled corticosteroid. Cromolyn and levalbuterol do not need to be administered with an inhaled corticosteroid, although they often are.

7. **B**

Suicidal ideation and other psychiatric symptoms such as depression, agitation, and insomnia have been associated with varenicline. Patients should be monitored for these symptoms at regular intervals while they are taking varenicline for smoking cessation therapy. Constipation and blood pressure alterations generally are not seen with varenicline use and do not need to be monitored.

Endocrine Disorders

4

This chapter covers the following diseases:

- **Diabetes mellitus**
- **Hypothyroidism**
- **Hyperthyroidism**
- **Polycystic ovarian syndrome**

 Suggested Study Time: **40 minutes**

DIABETES MELLITUS

Definition—Type 1

Diabetes mellitus (DM) type 1 accounts for fewer than 10% of all cases of diabetes, occurs in younger persons, and is caused by insulin deficiency that results from an immune-mediated destruction of the pancreatic-islet beta cells. Exogenous insulin is required to control blood glucose, prevent diabetic ketoacidosis (DKA), and preserve life. A transient period of insulin independence ("honeymoon phase") or reduced insulin requirement may occur early in the course of type 1 DM.

Definition—Type 2

Diabetes mellitus type 2 accounts for more than 90% of all DM. Most commonly diagnosed in adults, type 2 DM is increasing in prevalence in younger age groups. Obesity, insulin resistance, and relative insulin deficiency are characteristic findings.

Diagnosis

- Impaired fasting glucose (IFG) is defined by a fasting plasma glucose between 100 and 125 mg/dL and is indicative of prediabetes.

- Impaired glucose tolerance (IGT) is defined by a 2-hour oral glucose tolerance test plasma glucose between 140 and 199 mg/dL and is indicative of prediabetes.
- A1c 5.7% to 6.4% is considered "increased risk for diabetes."
- Diagnostic test results:
  - A1c $\geq$ 6.5%
  - Plasma glucose of $\geq$126 mg/dL after an overnight fast (and/or)
  - Symptoms of diabetes and random plasma glucose $\geq$200 mg/dL (and/or)
  - Oral glucose tolerance test indicating a plasma glucose of $\geq$200 mg/dL 2 hours after a 75-g glucose load.
  - Confirmation requires a second positive test on a subsequent day (any of the above).

Signs and Symptoms

- Polyuria is a symptom, which is characterized by excessive excretion of urine
- Polyphagia is a symptom, which is characterized by excessive eating
- Polydipsia is a symptom, which is characterized by excessive thirst that is relatively prolonged
- Weight loss is due to excretion of glucose in the urine when blood sugars exceed 180 mg/dL. The excretion of glucose results in loss of calorie retention. In addition, the excessive polyuria leads to polyphagia and polydipsia.

Diabetes Complications

- Retinopathy—Diabetic retinopathy is caused by damage to blood vessels in the eye over a long period of the disease. There are two stages of retinopathy: non-proliferative, in which blood vessel leakage in the eye leads to macular edema; and proliferative, in which abnormal blood vessels form in the eye. The growth of these vessels can lead to vitreous hemorrhage and retinal detachment, both of which can cause blindness.
- Neuropathy—Neuropathies are common in patients with diabetes and can lead to pain and other complications. There are two main types of neuropathies: distal polyneuropathy, in which demyelination in sensory nerves causes numbness, tingling, and paresthesias as these nerves lose function; and autonomic neuropathy, in which the functions of the sympathetic and parasympathetic nervous systems are lost. Examples of autonomic neuropathies include gastroparesis, orthostatic hypotension, and erectile dysfunction.
- Nephropathy—Nephropathy occurs in patients with diabetes as a result of dysfunction in the glomeruli of the kidney. The symptoms of this disease are preceded by a period of hyperfiltration, followed by glomerular changes that cause proteinuria. As the damage progresses, proteinuria worsens until end-stage renal failure is reached, accompanied by massive proteinuria.

- Atherosclerosis—Diabetes is a major risk factor for atherosclerosis and subsequent cardiovascular diseases, including myocardial infarctions, strokes, and peripheral arterial disease.

Guidelines

American Diabetes Association. *Diabetes Care*, no. 37 (Suppl 1) (2014): http://care.diabetesjournals.org.

American Association of Clinical Endocrinologists. *Endocrine Practice*, no. 17 (Suppl 2) (March/April 2011): www.aace.com/publications/guidelines.

Guidelines Summary

- American Diabetes Association (ADA) Goals
  - Preprandial glucose 70–130 mg/dL
  - Postprandial glucose <180 mg/dL
  - A1c <7%
  - Blood pressure 140/80 mmHg
  - Goals should be individualized
- American Association of Clinical Endocrinologists (AACE) Guidelines
  - Preprandial glucose <110 mg/dL
  - Postprandial glucose <140 mg/dL
  - A1c <6.5%

Patient education is integral to successful management of diabetes. Diabetes education should be conducted through an interdisciplinary approach.

Dietary education should focus on medical nutrition therapy provided by a registered dietician.

Exercise should include 150 min/week of moderate intensity aerobic activity or 75 min/week of vigorous aerobic activity.

- Insulin replacement is necessary in type 1 DM and is generally initiated at 0.5–1 units/kg/day.
  - Analog-based basal bolus regimen (50% basal, 50% bolus [divided into three meals]), or
  - Human insulin–based split-mixed regimen (70% AM; 50% PM [each dose 2/3 NPH to 1/3 Regular])
- Insulin regimens are adjusted based upon patient response (self-monitored blood glucose [SMBG]).

- Metformin is first-line therapy for patients with type 2 DM unless contraindicated.
- Second-line options include insulin, sulfonylureas, DPPIV inhibitors, GLP1 agonists, and thiazolidinediones.
- Second-line selection is made based upon patient-specific considerations of efficacy needed, risk of hypoglycemia/weight gain, other side effects, and cost.
- SGLT2 inhibitors are the newest class of medications. They are not addressed in current guidelines, but they would be reasonable options for third-line treatment.

Treatment Algorithm

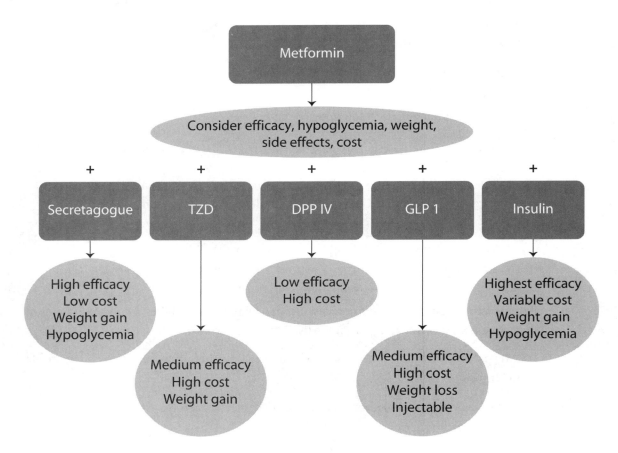

KAPLAN MEDICAL

Drugs for Diabetes (Insulin)

Generic	Brand	Onset	Peak	Duration	Comments	Top 200
Rapid acting					• Hypoglycemia is the most common side effect. It is defined as blood sugar <70 mg/dL and must be treated as soon as recognized.	
Aspart	NovoLog	5–15 min	30–90 min	<5 hrs		Yes
Lispro	Humalog	5–15 min	30–90 min	<5 hrs	• Insulin dosage is individually based due to sensitivity; 0.5–1.0 units/kg/day for the average non-obese patient.	Yes
Glulisine	Apidra	5–15 min	30–90 min	<5 hrs	• Duration of action is prolonged in renal failure.	No
Short-acting						
Regular	Humulin R (OTC)	30–60 min	2–3 hrs	5–8 hrs		Yes
Intermediate, Basal						
NPH (Neutral Protamine Hagedorn)	Humulin N (OTC)	2–4 hrs	4–10 hrs	10–16 hrs		Yes
Long-acting, basal						
Glargine	Lantus	2–4 hrs	No peak	20–24 hrs		Yes
Detemir	Levemir	3–8 hrs	No peak	6–24 hrs		Yes
Premixed						
75% Lispro protamine /25% lispro	Humalog Mix 75/25	5–15 min	Dual	10–16 hrs		No
50% Lispro protamine / 50% lispro	Humalog Mix 50/50	5–15 min	Dual	10–16 hrs		No
50% Aspart protamine / 50% aspart	NovoLog Mix 50/50	5–15 min	Dual	10–16 hrs		No
70% Insulin aspart protamine / 30% aspart	NovoLog Mix 70/30	5–15 min	Dual	10–16 hrs		No
70% NPH / 30% regular	70/30 (OTC)	30–60 min	Dual	10–16 hrs		No

• OTC insulin is available without a prescription.
• Rapid-acting insulin should be given at time of meal ingestion, no more than 15 minutes from eating.
• Regular insulin should be given 30 minutes prior to meal due to delayed onset of action.

Drugs for Diabetes (Oral)

Generic	Brand	Dose & Max	Contra-indications	Primary Side Effects	Key Monitoring	Pertinent Drug Interactions	Med Pearl	Top 200
Sulfonylureas, first generation – stimulate insulin release from the pancreatic beta cells								
Tolbutamide	• Apo-tolbutamide • Orinase	0.5–3 g	• Type 1 DM • Sulfa allergy	• Hypoglycemia • Weight gain	Fasting plasma glucose and A1c at 3 months	• Cimetidine may increase hypoglycemia effects (CYP450) • Chronic ethanol ingestion may decrease hypoglycemic effect	Response plateaus after half maximum dose	No
Acetohexamide	Dymelor	0.25 mg–1.5 g						No
Tolazamide	Tolinase	0.1–1 g						No
Chlorpropamide	Diabinese	0.1–0.5 g	CrCl <50 mL/min					No
Sulfonylureas, second generation – stimulate insulin release from the pancreatic beta cells								
Glyburide	• Micronase • DiaBeta	1.25–20 mg	• Type 1 DM • Sulfa allergy	• Hypoglycemia • Weight gain	Fasting plasma glucose and A1c at 3 months	• Cimetidine may increase hypoglycemia effects (CYP450) • Chronic ethanol ingestion may decrease hypoglycemic effect	• Response plateaus after half maximum dose • Administer with meals	Yes
Glipizide	• Glucotrol • Glucotrol XL	2.5–40 mg						Yes
Glimepiride	Amaryl	1–8 mg						Yes
Meglitinides – stimulates insulin release from the pancreatic beta cells								
Repaglinide	Prandin	1–16 mg (0.5–4 mg taken BID-QID)	Type 1 DM	• Hypoglycemia • Weight gain	Postprandial plasma glucose and A1c	• Decrease effect by CYP3A4, CYP2C8/9 inducers • Increase effect by CYP3A4 inhibitors	Faster acting and shorter duration than the traditional sulfonylureas, and recommended for postprandial blood sugars	No
Amino acid derivative – stimulates insulin release from the pancreatic beta cells								
Nateglinide	Starlix	180–360 mg (60–120 mg taken TID)	Type 1 DM	• Hypoglycemia • Weight gain	Postprandial plasma glucose and A1c	• Decrease effect by CYP3A4, CYP2C8/9 inducers • Increase effect by CYP3A4 inhibitors	Faster acting than the traditional sulfonylureas, and recommended for postprandial blood sugars	No

Drugs for Diabetes (Non-Insulin)

Generic	Brand	Dose & Max	Contra-indications	Primary Side Effects	Key Monitoring	Pertinent Drug Interactions	Med Pearl	Top 200
Biguanide – decreases hepatic glucose production, decreases intestinal absorption of glucose, improves insulin sensitivity								
Metformin	• Glucophage • Glucophage XR	500 mg–2.550 g	• SCr ≥1.5 male • SCr ≥1.4 female • Lactic acidosis • Contraindicated in severe heart failure, renal failure, radiographic dyes	GI intolerance (flatulence and diarrhea); lactic acidosis	• Serum creatinine • Fasting plasma glucose • A1c every 3 months	Cimetidine increases peak metformin plasma and whole blood concentration by 60%	Lactic acidosis black box warning.	Yes
Alpha-glucosidase inhibitors – inhibit pancreatic alpha-amylase and alpha-glucosidases, block carbohydrate hydrolysis to glucose								
Acarbose	Precose	75–300 mg (divided TID)	• Cirrhosis • Inflammatory bowel disease • Intestinal obstruction	• Abdominal pain and diarrhea • Flatulence	• LFTs q3 months × 1 year • Postprandial blood sugars and A1c	Hypoglycemia risk when given with sulfonylureas or insulin	• Must treat hypoglycemia with simple carbo-hydrate such as glucose • Administer with food	No
Miglitol	Glyset	75–300 mg (divided TID)			• Postprandial blood sugars and A1c			No
Thiazolidinediones – PPAR-gamma activator, which improves insulin sensitivity								
Rosiglitazone	Avandia	2–8 mg	• History of liver disease • Unstable heart failure • Previous MI • Osteopenial osteoporosis	Fluid retention and hepatotoxicity	Monitor LFTs, baseline and periodically	• Decrease effect by CYP3A4, CYP2C8 inducers • Decrease effect by CYP2C8 inhibitors	• Available only via REMS program • Rosi: potential link to an increase in cardiovascular events; controversial	No
Pioglitazone	Actos	15–45 mg	• History of bladder cancer			Decrease effect by CYP3A4, CYP2C8 inducers	• Pio: thought to have a better lipid profile	Yes
Amylinomimetic – Amylin cosecreted with insulin reduces postprandial blood sugars, prolonging gastric emptying, reducing postprandial glucagon secretion, and caloric intake through centrally mediated appetite suppression								
Pramlintide	Symlin	15–120 mcg	• Gastroparesis • Hypoglycemia unawareness	• Nausea from delayed gastric emptying • Severe hypoglycemia	• Hypoglycemia • Blood sugars and A1c	• May delay absorption of other drugs due to increased gastric emptying time • Pramlintide: must reduce dose of insulin by 50% when starting	• Administer medications 1 hour prior to the use of pramlintide and exenatide • Adjunctive treatment *with* insulin	No

Drugs for Diabetes (Non-Insulin) *(cont'd)*

Generic	Brand	Dose & Max	Contra-indications	Primary Side Effects	Key Monitoring	Pertinent Drug Interactions	Med Pearl	Top 200
GLP-1 inhibitors – glucagon-like peptide which increases insulin secretion, increases B-cell growth/replication, slows gastric emptying, decreases food intake								
Exenatide	BYETTA	5–10 mcg SC BID	• CrCl <30 mL/min • Pancreatitis	• Nausea • Hypoglycemia • Decreased appetite	• Renal function • Blood sugars and A1c • Pancreatitis • Hypoglycemia • Thyroid tumors	• Delays gastric emptying so it may impact absorption of concomitantly administered medications • Administer other medications 1 hour prior	Acute pancreatitis	Yes
	Bydureon	2 mg SC/week						No
Liraglutide	Victoza	0.6–1.8 mg SC injection daily	• Pancreatitis • CrCl <30 mL/min • Family Hx of medullary thyroid carcinoma • Multiple endocrine neoplasia syndrome	• Headache • N • D • Antiliraglutide antibody formation				No
Albiglutide	Tanzeum	30–50 mg SC once weekly		• Nausea • Headache • Decreased appetite • Local injection site reactions	• Blood sugars • A1c • Pancreatitis • Thyroid tumors		• Reconstituted prior to injection, must be injected within 8 hours of reconstitution • Administered without regard to meals	No
Dipeptidyl-peptidase 4 inhibitors – prolong the active incretin levels of GLP and GIP								
Sitagliptin	Januvia	25–100 mg	Type 1 DM	• Headache • Nasopharyngitis	• Renal function • Blood sugars and A1c	May increase digoxin concentration	• 100 mg dose is preferred unless patient has renal impairment • CrCl <30 mL/min, 25 mg/day • CrCl <30–50 mL/min, 50 mg/day	Yes
Saxagliptin	Onglyza	5 mg/day	Type 1 DM	• URI • UTI • Headache • Peripheral edema	A1C, absolute lymphocyte counts when clinically indicated	Coadministration with strong CYP3A4/5 inhibitors; these increase saxagliptins concentration and dose is decreased to 2.5 mg/day	• CrCl ≤50 mL/min, 2.5 mg once a day	No

Drugs for Diabetes (Non-Insulin) *(cont'd)*

Generic	Brand	Dose & Max	Contra-indications	Primary Side Effects	Key Monitoring	Pertinent Drug Interactions	Med Pearl	Top 200
Linagliptin	Tradjenta	5 mg/day	Type 1 DM	• Nasopharyngitis • Arthralgia • D • Hyperuricemia • Headache	Blood sugars and A1c	Loop and thiazide diuretics may decrease hypoglycemic effects	No renal dose adjustment	No
Alogliptin	Nesina	25 mg/day (adjust for renal and hepatic insufficiency)	Type 1 DM	• URI • Headache • Increased ALT	• Blood sugars and A1c • Creatinine and LFTs at baseline, then clinically as indicated		• CrCl <30 mL/min, 6.25 mg/day • CrCl 30–60 mL/min, 12.5 mg/day	No
Sodium-glucose cotransporter 2 (SGLT2) inhibitors – reduce reabsorption of filtered glucose from tubular lumen, increasing glucosuria								
Canagliflozin	Invokana	100–300 mg daily	CrCl <30 mL/min, ESRD/HD	Genitourinary infections (especially in females), dehydration, hyperkalemia, hypotension	A1c, blood glucose, renal function, blood pressure	• Diuretics (enhanced diuretic effect may lead to dehydration) • Potassium supplementation	Administer before first meal of the day	No
Dapagliflozin	Farxiga	5–10 mg daily						No

Drugs for Diabetes (Non-Insulin) *(cont'd)*

Generic	Brand	Dose & Max	Contra-indications	Primary Side Effects	Key Monitoring	Pertinent Drug Interactions	Med Pearl	Top 200
Combination								
Sitagliptin/ metformin	Janumet	• See above for individual interactions • Synergistic effects are likely with combination products • Maximum dose of metformin is 2,000 mg in combination products • Maximum dose for immediate release metformin is 2,550 mg per day						Yes
Glyburide/ metformin	Glucovance							Yes
Rosiglitazone/ metformin	Avandamet							No
Rosiglitazone/ glimepiride	Avandaryl							No
Pioglitazone/ metformin	Actos Plus							No
Glipizide/ metformin	Metaglip							No
Alogliptin/ metformin	Kazano							No
Alogliptin/ pioglitazone	Oseni							No
Linagliptin/ metformin	Jentadueto							No
Saxagliptin/ metformin	Kombiglyze XR							No
Repaglinide/ metformin	Prandimet							No
Pioglitazone/ glimepiride	Duetact							No

Storage and Administration Pearls

- Unopened containers of insulin should be stored in the refrigerator.
- If not refrigerated, use within 28 days and protect from heat and light.
- Do not freeze insulin or other injectable products.
- Once opened or in use, vials or pens may be stored in refrigerator or at room temperature for up to 28 days (42 days for detemir).
- IV infusion: Must be kept stable for 24 hours at room temperature.
- Weekly exenatide and albiglutide must be reconstituted prior to injection.
- Detemir's storage life is 42 days outside of refrigerator.

Patient Education Pearls

- A patient who is on alpha-glucosidase inhibitors must use a simple sugar to treat hypoglycemia anytime.
- Rotate insulin injection sites.
- Mixing rule: "Clear, then cloudy" is the rule. It still applies to NPH (cloudy), regular (clear), fast-acting (clear).
- The exceptions: Never mix detemir or glargine (clear) with anything.
- May take several weeks to see the full effect of thiazolidinediones.

HYPOTHYROIDISM

Definitions

Primary hypothyroidism accounts for more than 90% of cases. It is due to actual disease of the thyroid itself and not from a feedback or hypothalamus issue. Hashimoto's disease is the most common cause and may be associated with Addison's disease (chronic adrenocortical insufficiency) and other endocrine deficits.

Diagnosis

Plasma thyroid-stimulating hormone (TSH) is the best initial diagnostic test. A TSH that is markedly elevated (>20 mcgU/mL) confirms the diagnosis.

Signs and Symptoms

- Most symptoms are nonspecific and develop gradually.
- Typical symptoms are cold intolerance, fatigue, weight gain, dry skin, somnolence, poor memory, and depression.

- Atypical symptoms are constipation, menorrhagia, myalgias, and hoarseness.
- Physical exam will often show slow tendon reflexes, bradycardia, and facial and periorbital edema.
- Myxedema coma (acute, severe hypothyroidism) decreased mental status, non-pitting edema, hypothermia

Guidelines

American Association of Clinical Endocrinologists/American Thyroid Association. *Endocrine Practice* vol. 18 no. 6 (Nov/Dec 2012): www.aace.com/publications/guidelines.

Guidelines Summary

The treatment and management of chronic thyroiditis and clinical hypothyroidism must be tailored to the individual patient. Many clinical endocrinologists treat the goiter of chronic thyroiditis with levothyroxine, even in patients with normal levels of TSH, and all physicians will treat clinical hypothyroidism with levothyroxine replacement therapy.

- Thyroid stimulating hormone (TSH) is the primary marker for medication monitoring. Because thyroid hormone functions on a negative feedback loop, elevated levels indicate hypothyroid state and low levels indicate hyperthyroid state.
- Initial dose of levothyroxine is 1.7 mcg/kg/day. Adjust doses in 10–25 mcg/day increments based upon clinical response. Half-life of levothyroxine is approximately 1 week. TSH monitoring and dose adjustments occur at 4–8 week intervals.

Drugs for Hypothyroidism

Generic	Brand	Dose	Contra-indications	Primary Side Effects	Key Monitoring	Pertinent Drug Interactions	Med Pearl	Top 200
Mechanism of action — T4 is converted to T3 and exerts many metabolic effects through control of DNA transcription and protein synthesis								
Levothyroxine (T4)	• Synthroid • Levoxyl • Unithroid	• Inj. powder: 0.2 and 0.5 mg • Tab: 25–300 mcg	• Recent myocardial infarction or thyrotoxicosis • Uncorrected adrenal insufficiency	• Angina • Anxiety • Alopecia • LFTs increased • Tachycardia	• TSH • T3 • T4 • Free T4 • Heart rate • Blood pressure • Weight • Levothyroxine half-life ~1 week, so monitor TSH at 4–8 week intervals	Some drugs will decrease absorption: cholestyramine, aluminum-containing, sucralfate, Kayexalate, phenytoin, carbamazepine, rifampin may decrease levothyroxine levels	• T4: not the active compound; must be converted to T3 to become active • Thyroid treatment: used to augment depression treatment • Narrow therapeutic index drug • Often involved in drug errors	Yes
Liothyronine (T3)	Cytomel	• Inj. powder: 10 mcg/mL • Tab: 5–100 mcg						No
Desiccated thyroid T4 (80%) T3 (20%)	• Armour • Thyroid	Tab: 15–120 mg per day (0.25–2g)	• Hypersensitivity to beef or pork • Recent myocardial infarction or thyrotoxicosis • Uncorrected adrenal insufficiency				• Same as above • Origin: hog, cow, sheep • 80% T4 and 20% T3 is to mimic natural physiologic production	Yes
Liotrix	Thyrolar	5–50 mcg	• Uncorrected adrenal cortical insufficiency • Untreated thyrotoxicosis				Liotrix is LT4/LT3 which is T4:T3 ratio; this ratio is 4:1	No

Storage and Administration Pearls

- Levothyroxine: Administered on an empty stomach
- Levothyroxine tabs: Protect from light and moisture
- Levothyroxine injection at room temperature (59–86°F)
  - IV solution not mixed with other IV infusion solutions
  - Dilute vial with 5 mL of normal saline and inject immediately

Patient Education Pearls

- Thyroid supplementation is ineffective and potentially toxic for weight reduction (in euthyroid patients).
- TSH will be rechecked 4–8 weeks following dose change.

HYPERTHYROIDISM

Definitions

Hyperthyroidism includes Graves' disease, which causes most cases of hyperthyroidism, especially in young patients. This autoimmune disorder may cause exophthalmos (protrusion of the eyes) and pretibial myxedema (nodules and plaques on skin). Toxic multinodular goiter is a common cause. Other causes can be drug-induced by amiodarone or radiographic contrast media and thyroid adenomas.

Diagnosis

- Plasma TSH is the best initial diagnostic test. The TSH will be markedly suppressed (<0.1 mcg/mL).

Signs and Symptoms

- Typical symptoms: Heat intolerance, insomnia, weight loss, weakness, palpitations, oligomenorrhea, and anxiety
- Sinus tachycardia, atrial fibrillation, and exacerbation of coronary artery disease
- Brisk tendon reflexes, fine tremor, proximal weakness, stare, and eyelid lag
- Thyroid storm: Presents as an acute life-threatening exaggeration of usual hyperthyroid symptoms

Guidelines

American Association of Clinical Endocrinologists/American Thyroid Association. *Endocrine Practice* vol. 17 no. 3 (May/June 2011): www.aace.com/publications/guidelines.

Guidelines Summary

Three types of therapy are available for Graves' disease: (*1*) Surgical intervention, (*2*) antithyroid drugs, and (*3*) radioactive iodine.

- In the United States, radioactive iodine is currently the treatment of choice for Graves' disease. Many clinical endocrinologists prefer an ablative dose of radioactive iodine, but some prefer use of a smaller dose in an attempt to render the patient euthyroid. Ablative therapy with radioactive iodine yields quicker resolution of the hyperthyroidism than does small-dose therapy, and thereby minimizes potential hyperthyroid-related morbidity.

- Although thyroidectomy for Graves' disease was frequently used in the past, it is now uncommonly performed in the United States unless coexistent thyroid cancer is suspected.

- Antithyroid medications methimazole and propylthiouracil have been used since the 1940s and are prescribed in an attempt to achieve a remission. The remission rates are variable, and relapses are frequent. Patients in whom remission is most likely to be achieved are those with mild hyperthyroidism and small goiters. Antithyroid drug treatment is not without the risk of adverse reactions, including minor rashes, and, in rare instances, agranulocytosis and hepatitis.

Drugs for Hyperthyroidism

Mechanism of action – inhibits synthesis of thyroid hormones by blocking the oxidation of iodine in the thyroid gland

Generic	Brand	Dose	Contra-indications	Primary Side Effects	Key Monitoring	Pertinent Drug Interactions	Med Pearl	Top 200
Propylthiouracil (PTU)	Only available generically	• Initial: 300–600 mg daily divided by TID or QID • Maintenance: 50–300 mg daily • (max = 1,200 mg daily)	Hypersensitivity	• Minor: therapy may still continue • Benign transient leukopenia (WBC <4,000/mm³, most common) • Pruritic maculopapular rashes, arthralgias, fevers	• WBC with differential • Granulocyte <250/mm³ (most severe) • LFT • TSH	Increase activity of anticoagulants	• Clinical improvement approx. 4–8 weeks • PTU is an error-prone abbreviation • Tapering doses may start once clinical improvement seen	No
Methimazole (MMI)	Tapazole	• Initial: 30–60 mg TID • Maintenance: 5–30 mg daily • (max = 120 mg daily)	Hypersensitivity	• Greater frequency in higher doses and in children • Rashes may be treated with antihistamines • Severe side effect require discontinuation • Fever, malaise, gingivitis, sore throat, oropharyngeal infections • Aplastic anemia, lupus-like syndrome, polymyositis (rhabdomyolysis), GI intolerance, hepatotoxicity, hepatitis, hypoprothrombinemia, death	• T3 • T4	• CYP450 inhibitor • Moderate: CPY2D6 • Weak: CPY3A4, CPY1A2	• Alternate thioamide may be used, but cross-sensitivity is 50% • Correction of hyperthyroidism may alter disposition of beta-blockers, digoxin, and theophylline • PTU preferred in pregnancy	No

KAPLAN) MEDICAL

Storage and Administration Pearls

- Methimazole: Protect from light.
- On the NAPLEX and in the work force, PTU is an error-prone abbreviation and is not recommended for use on prescription pads, verbally, or within your computer system.

Patient Education Pearls

- If the patient is pregnant or is thinking about getting pregnant, it is recommended that she avoid taking propylthiouracil and methimazole; they cross the placenta and are found in breast milk. PTU is preferred over methimazole in pregnancy.

POLYCYSTIC OVARIAN SYNDROME

Definitions

Polycystic ovarian syndrome (PCOS) is a metabolic disorder involving infertility, hirsutism, obesity, and amenorrhea. The fundamental defect of PCOS is unknown but is thought to be from adrenal androgen excess of obesity, which results in enhanced extraglandular formation of estrogen. The dysfunctional uterine bleeding is usually due to estrogen excess.

Diagnosis

- History and physical examination, including the onset and duration of various signs of androgen excess; menstrual history; family history of diabetes and cardiovascular disease; lifestyle factors; evaluation of blood pressure, body mass index, and waist-hip ratio; and presence of acne, hirsutism, androgenic alopecia, and acanthosis nigricans
- Laboratory tests, including documentation of biochemical hyperandrogenemia (total testosterone and/or bioavailable or free testosterone); exclusion of other causes of hyperandrogenism, such as thyroid dysfunction, hyperprolactinemia, nonclassical congenital adrenal hyperplasia, and Cushing's syndrome; evaluation for metabolic abnormalities; and fasting lipid and lipoprotein level
- Optional tests to consider:
  - Ultrasound evaluation of ovaries
  - Gonadotropin determinations
  - Fasting insulin levels
  - 24-hour urine test

Signs and Symptoms

- Infertility: Inability to become pregnant
- Hirsutism: Caused by excess androgen levels
- Obesity: BMI > 29 kg/m^2
- Anovulation: Lack of ovulation; however, the woman may experience withdrawal bleeding after progestogen administration

Guidelines

American College of Obstetricians and Gynecologists, Medical Specialty Society. (December 2002). http://www.acog.org.

Guidelines Summary

Treatment is based on a symptoms approach for anovulation, amenorrhea, ovulation induction, and hirsutism.

Anovulation and Amenorrhea

- Combination oral contraceptives are often used to regulate or restore irregular or absent menses.
- Weight-reduction programs are important, and they affect and improve insulin resistance.
- Progestin, including medroxyprogesterone acetate, is often used to induce menses.
- Insulin-sensitizing agents, including metformin, pioglitazone, and rosiglitazone, are used to reduce insulin resistance.

Ovulation Induction

- Lifestyle modifications, especially weight loss, will assist with ovulation induction.
- Clomiphene citrate is used to induce ovulation for up to 6 months.
- Ovarian drilling with laser or diathermy can be considered but is not recommended.
- Insulin-sensitizing agents, such as metformin and thiazolidinediones, can induce ovulation.

Hirsutism

- Oral contraceptives can reduce hair growth.
- Antiandrogens, including spironolactone, flutamide, and insulin-sensitizing agents, and eflornithine can be used to reduce hair growth.
- Mechanical hair removal, such as shaving, plucking, waxing, depilatory creams, electrolysis, and laser vaporization, can also be used.

Drugs for Polycystic Ovarian Syndrome

Generic	Brand	Dose	Contraindications	Primary Side Effects	Key Monitoring	Pertinent Drug Interactions	Med Pearl	Top 200
Mechanism of action – inhibits secretion of pituitary gonadotropins, which prevents follicular maturation and ovulation; causes endometrial thinning								
Medroxyprogesterone	Provera	Amenorrhea: 5–10 mg × 10 days	• History of deep venous thrombosis, pulmonary embolism • Pregnancy	• Headaches • Weight changes • Edema • Menstrual irregularities	• Pregnancy should be ruled out • Symptoms of migraine	• CYP450 • Induces CYP3A4	Long-term use can lead to loss of bone mineral density	Yes
Mechanism of action – Enclomiphene is less potent in inducing ovulation; however, it is rapidly absorbed to be metabolized, allowing for the more potent zuclomiphene to act. Zuclomiphene – inhibits normal estrogen negative feedback, which results in release of luteinizing hormone (LH) and FSH; more potent than enclomiphene								
Clomiphene citrate* – zuclomiphene (38%) – enclomiphene (62%)	Clomid	50–100 mg daily for 5 days	• Liver disease • Abnormal uterine bleeding • Ovarian cysts • Uncontrolled thyroid or adrenal dysfunction • Pregnancy category X	• Ovarian enlargement • Hot flashes • Breast discomfort • Nausea • Bloating	• Pregnancy test • Menstrual cycle	• Ospemifene	Dosages of 150 mg or greater do not improve symptoms for PCOS	No
Mechanism of action – competes with aldosterone receptor sites in the distal tubules								
Spironolactone	Aldactone	50–200 mg	• Acute renal failure • Hyperkalemia • Pregnancy category D	• Gynecomastia (men) • Hyperkalemia • Nausea, cramping	• BP • Renal function • Potassium	May reduce the inotropic (contraction) effect of digoxin and mitotane.	Needs to be renally adjusted	Yes
Mechanism of action – nonsteroidal antiandrogen that inhibits androgen uptake or inhibits binding to androgen in target tissue								
Flutamide	Eulexin	125–250 mg	• Severe hepatic impairment • Pregnancy category D	• Gynecomastia • Hot flashes • Breast tenderness • Galactorrhea • Libido decreased	LFTs monthly for 4 months, then periodically	• CYP450 • Inhibits CYP1A2	Boxed warning for liver failure within 3 months of taking flutamide	No

Drugs for Polycystic Ovarian Syndrome *(cont'd)*

Generic	Brand	Dose	Contraindications	Primary Side Effects	Key Monitoring	Pertinent Drug Interactions	Med Pearl	Top 200
Mechanism of action – inhibitor of 5-alpha reductase which results in the inhibition of the conversion of testosterone to dihydrotestosterone								
Finasteride	• Proscar • Propecia	1–5 mg/day	Pregnancy category X Hirsutism	• Impotence • Ejaculation disturbances • Decreased libido • Orthostatic hypotension	Absolute need for dual forms of birth control	• CYP450 • Substrate CYP3A4	• Category X in pregnancy (abnormalities of external male genitalia were reported in animal studies) • High-alert medication	Yes
Mechanism of action – inhibits ornithine decarboxylase (ODC), the rate-limiting enzyme in biosynthesis of putrescine, spermin, and spermidine (rapid dividing cell most susceptible)								
Eflornithine	VANIQA	• Cream (facial hair) • Apply BID	Hypersensitivity	• Acne • Pruritus • Alopecia • Stinging	CBC and platelets (systemic only)	Cream could interact with other creams; wait to apply until skin is dry	• Do not wash affected area for 8 hours following application • Onset of action 4–8 weeks	No

Storage and Administration Pearls

- Finasteride needs to be protected from light.
- Spironolactone needs to be protected from light.

Patient Education Pearls

- Prolonged use of medroxyprogesterone contraception injection may result in a loss of bone mineral density (BMD).

LEARNING POINTS

- The basic diagnoses for type 1 and type 2 DM are identical. However, patients with type 2 will go undiagnosed for as long as 10 years, whereas type 1 is usually diagnosed within 6 months. As a result, it is important to consider and assess risk factors for type 2 DM.
- For the NAPLEX, it is important that you understand the different mechanisms of action of the diabetes medications to ensure you can catch duplication of actions within the patient's drug profile.
- Hypothyroidism and hyperthyroidism have opposite side effects (i.e., somnolence with hypothyroid; insomnia with hyperthyroidism).
- PCOS has become more common as obesity rates have risen and as more women want to become pregnant.
- Remember, many women with diabetes may have PCOS and may be placed on an insulin sensitizer such as a glitazone. As a result, it is important to counsel the patient on an increased risk for ovulation if her uterus is still intact.

PRACTICE QUESTIONS

1. Patients with overactive thyroid may present with which of the following symptoms?

    (A) Weight loss
    (B) Heat intolerance
    (C) Heart palpitations
    (D) Goiter
    (E) All of the above

2. A patient comes to the pharmacy and tells you that her blood sugars were 126 and 127 mg/dL fasting on two occasions. She wants some advice because her doctor didn't have time to talk with her. What is the main point you will be addressing with this woman?

    (A) This patient does not have diabetes because the doctor did the same test.
    (B) This patient has diabetes but it's not bad and will not need medication.
    (C) This patient has diabetes but does not need education; she should just watch what she eats and exercise more.
    (D) This patient doesn't have diabetes but might develop it soon.
    (E) This patient has diabetes, needs a formal diabetes education class, and is likely a candidate for a medication called metformin.

3. How many days can a Humalog stay out of the refrigerator and be considered safe to administer?

    (A) 1 day
    (B) 28 days
    (C) 56 days
    (D) 90 days
    (E) 180 days

4. A 62-year-old woman (5'2", 180 lb) with type 2 diabetes, history of medullary thyroid carcinoma, osteopenia, and stage 3 chronic kidney disease (CrCl = 45 mL/min) presents for routine follow-up. Current medications include metformin 1 g BID, lisinopril 10 mg PO daily, calcium carbonate/vitamin D 600/400 BID, and aspirin 81 mg PO daily. Labs today include A1c 7.6%, AST 20 IU/L, ALT 22 IU/L and K 4.2 mEq/L. Which of the following is the most appropriate recommendation?

    (A) Initiate Bydureon 2 mg SC once each week.
    (B) Initiate pioglitazone 30 mg PO once daily.
    (C) Initiate insulin glargine 40 units once daily.
    (D) Initiate sitagliptin 50 mg PO daily.

5. Which of the following medications is contraindicated in a patient with heart failure?

    (A) Exenatide
    (B) Sitagliptin
    (C) Glimepiride
    (D) Pioglitazone

6. Which of the following medications is most likely to cause hypoglycemia?

    (A) Metformin
    (B) Glipizide
    (C) Sitagliptin
    (D) Exenatide

7. Which of the following mechanisms most accurately describes the action of exenatide?

    (A) Mimics glucagon-like peptide-1
    (B) Inhibits gluconeogenesis in the liver
    (C) Inhibits the dipeptidyl peptidase IV enzyme
    (D) Increases insulin sensitivity in the periphery

8. A 65-year-old woman (5'2", 182 lb) with hypertension, heart failure (NHYA Class I), and history of pancreatitis is newly diagnosed with type 2 diabetes. Medications include lisinopril 20 mg PO daily, carvedilol 6.25 mg PO BID, and aspirin 81 mg PO daily. Serum laboratory results today include A1c 8.3%, creatinine 1.5 mg/dL, ALT 35 IU/L, and BNP 20 pg/mL. A prescription is written for metformin. Which of the following statements is the best evaluation of this therapy?

    (A) Appropriate drug; no contraindications present
    (B) Inappropriate drug; contraindicated due to pancreatitis
    (C) Inappropriate drug; contraindicated due to heart failure
    (D) Inappropriate drug; contraindicated due to renal function

9. A 72-year-old man with hypothyroidism is treated with levothyroxine 88 mcg PO daily for 6 weeks. His TSH returns at 18 mIU/L (normal range 0.4–4 mIU/L). Which of the following is the most appropriate recommendation?

    (A) Increase levothyroxine dose to 100 mcg PO daily, recheck TSH in 2 weeks.
    (B) Increase levothyroxine dose to 100 mcg PO daily, recheck TSH in 6 weeks.
    (C) Decrease levothyroxine dose to 75 mcg PO daily, recheck TSH in 2 weeks.
    (D) Decrease levothyroxine dose to 75 mcg PO daily, recheck TSH in 6 weeks.

10. Which of the following is an appropriate patient education to provide for a patient on oral levothyroxine?

   (A) Take medication after a high-fat meal.
   (B) Take medication on an empty stomach.
   (C) Take medication without regard to meals.
   (D) Take medication with a glass of milk.

ANSWERS

1. E

Weight loss, heat intolerance, heart palpitations, and goiter are all commonly seen symptoms with hyperthyroid disorders. Other common symptoms include nervousness, emotional lability, bowel frequency, irregular menses, and increased appetite.

2. E

This patient has diabetes and needs a formal diabetes education class. The newest guidelines suggest starting all eligible patients on metformin at the time of diagnosis. Choice (A) is not correct because this woman does have diabetes—her fasting blood sugar was verified and was ≥126 mg/dL. Although the doctor caught the disease early, the patient still needs to seek formal education as this will lead to the best management.

3. B

Most unopened insulin preparations are stable at normal temperatures for 28 days. They should not be used if frozen or exposed to temperature greater than 98.6°F. Once opened (in use), vials may be stored in the refrigerator or for up to 28 days at room temperature.

4. D

Sitagliptin 50 mg PO daily is an appropriate agent to lower the A1c as needed and at an appropriate dose for renal function (30–50 mL/min = 50 mg daily). Bydureon (A) would be inappropriate for this patient due to the history of medullary thyroid carcinoma. Pioglitazone (B) would not be a good choice due to its potential to decrease bone mineral density; this patient has osteopenia. Although insulin glargine (C) would be an appropriate option, the dose of 40 units daily is too high for a starting dose.

5. D

Pioglitazone is contraindicated in a patient with heart failure. Thiazolidinediones have a side effect profile that includes fluid retention/edema and have demonstrated increases in heart failure exacerbations. The class should be avoided in patients with heart failure, especially NYHA classes III and IV.

6. B

Sulfonylureas such as glipizide have the greatest risk of hypoglycemia among the listed agents. Metformin (A) does not cause hypoglycemia as monotherapy. Although sitagliptin (C) and exenatide (D) can cause hypoglycemia, the risk is significantly lower than with secretagogues.

7. **A**

Exenatide is a glucagon-like peptide agonist that, by mimicking this incretin hormone, results in glucose-dependent insulin secretion, slowed gastric emptying, and diminished glucagon secretion postprandially.

8. **D**

Metformin is contraindicated in female patients with serum creatinine ≥1.4 mg/dL and males with serum creatinine ≥1.5 mg/dL. Pancreatitis (B) is not a contraindication to the use of metformin. Decompensated heart failure (C) is a contraindication to the medication, but this patient's heart failure is currently compensated (NYHA class I).

9. **B**

The TSH elevation indicates that the patient remains hypothyroid and requires a higher dose of levothyroxine. The half-life of levothyroxine is ~1 week; therefore, TSH levels are checked at 4–8 weeks to allow medication to reach steady state.

10. **B**

Levothyroxine is best and most consistently absorbed when taken on an empty stomach. Taking it with a high-fat meal (A), other food (C), or milk (D) would decrease absorption.

Neurological Disorders

5

This chapter covers the following disease states:

- **Multiple sclerosis**
- **Epilepsy**
- **Parkinson's disease**
- **Migraine headache**
- **Alzheimer's disease**

 Suggested Study Time: **55 minutes**

MULTIPLE SCLEROSIS

Definitions

Multiple sclerosis (MS) is a disease of the central nervous system (CNS) characterized by inflammation within the brain and spinal cord that results in areas of plaque formation and sclerosis and leads to neurological symptoms. The basic pathophysiological defect in MS is the demyelinization of the sheath surrounding the neurons in the CNS.

Diagnosis

The diagnosis of MS is based primarily on clinical presentation and requires two or more episodes of neurologic symptoms that: (*1*) cannot be attributed to another cause, (*2*) represent distinct areas of CNS involvement, and (*3*) occur at least 3 months apart. The McDonald criteria are often used to diagnose MS. These criteria do require two lesions separated by 3 months but allow for the use of magnetic resonance imaging (MRI) and cerebrospinal fluid analysis to be used as identification of a second attack. MRI is a useful tool for confirming diagnosis of MS because it is highly selective for MS lesions.

Signs and Symptoms

- The most common symptoms of early MS include weakness/numbness of limbs and visual disturbances. The clinical presentation of MS varies among patients and is classified as relapsing-remitting, primary progressive, or secondary progressive.

- Relapsing-remitting MS is most common (85%) and is characterized by frequent symptomatic episodes of ≥24 hours' duration followed by periods of remission of at least 30 days. During remission, residual symptoms and increasing clinical deficit are common.

- Primary progressive MS occurs in ~10% of patients and consists of persistently progressive disease from the time of disease onset that does not include remissions or relapses. This classification is associated with a poor prognosis.

- Secondary progressive MS occurs in about 5% of patients and consists of few exacerbations, no permanent disability, and gradual worsening of neurological symptoms. Many patients originally classified as relapsing-remitting may be reclassified as secondary progressive during the course of illness.

Guidelines

Medical Advisory Board of the National Multiple Sclerosis Society (2008). Disease Management Consensus Statement Regarding the Use of Disease Modifying Agents. Expert Opinion Paper. http://www.nationalmssociety.org.

Medical Advisory Board of the National Multiple Sclerosis Society. Recommendations Regarding Corticosteroids in the Management of Multiple Sclerosis Expert Opinion Paper. 2008. http://www.nationalmssociety.org.

Guidelines Summary

The clinical management of MS should include consideration of treatment for acute exacerbations, retarding disease process, and alleviating ongoing symptoms related to the disease.

Disease-modifying drugs (DMDs) are used to alter the disease process, and treatment with interferon beta or glatiramer should be initiated as soon as possible after diagnosis in patients with relapsing disease. Therapies should be continued indefinitely except in the case of intolerable side effects, clear lack of benefit, or new therapy considerations.

Natalizumab may be considered if a patient cannot tolerate or has a poor response to another MS medication. Mitoxantrone may be considered for patients with secondary-progressive MS or those with a worsening course.

Acute exacerbations — The cornerstone of therapy for acute exacerbations is intravenous (IV) corticosteroids. Methylprednisolone is most commonly used at 50–100 mg/day for 3 to 10 days. Oral prednisone may also be considered, but there is not strong evidence for this route. Although corticosteroids have been shown to be very effective in the treatment of acute exacerbations, they do not alter the disease process.

Altering disease process — DMDs are the therapy of choice in altering the MS disease process. There are currently eight approved DMDs: interferon-β1a (Avonex and Rebif), interferon-β1b (Betaseron and Extavia), glatiramer acetate (Copaxone), natalizumab (Tysabri), mitoxantrone (Novantrone), dalfampridine (Ampyra), dimethyl fumarate (Tecfidera), teriflunomide (Aubagio), and fingolimod (Gilenya).

- The interferon agents and glatiramer acetate are considered first-line DMDs, whereas natalizumab is reserved for patients who do not respond to those therapies.
- Dimethyl fumarate is approved for relapsing MS, and its place in therapy is not fully known.
- Teriflunomide is approved for relapsing MS. Its place in therapy is yet to be determined, and it carries at black box warning for hepatotoxicity.
- Mitoxantrone is the only available agent that is approved to treat worsening relapsing-remitting MS and progressive MS.
- Patients are generally treated with one DMD at a time, but worsening disease can be treated with combination DMD + mitoxantrone pulse therapy.

Disease-Modifying Drugs

Generic	Brand	Dose & Max	Contra-indications	Primary Side Effects	Key Monitoring Parameters	Pertinent Drug Interactions	Med Pearls	Top 200
Disease-Modifying Drugs								
Mechanism of action – interferon β: anti-inflammatory and immunomodulatory effects are exerted through binding of interferon to human cell-surface receptors and subsequent decreased T-cell production of pro-inflammatory cytokines, decreased production of pro-inflammatory lymphocytes, and increased production of anti-inflammatory lymphocytes								
Interferon-β1a	• Avonex intramuscular (IM) injection • Rebif subcutaneous (SC) injection	30 mcg IM 1 × week 8.8 mcg sub-Q TIW–44 mcg 3 × week sub-Q	• Hypersensitivity to interferon beta or human albumin • Allergy to interferons	Flu-like symptoms (fever, chills, fatigue, muscle aches); injection site reactions; mild anemia; thrombocytopenia; liver damage; depression	• Liver transaminases periodically • Response to therapy • Presence of adverse effects • Periodic complete blood count (CBC)		• Acetaminophen or NSAIDs can decrease flu-like symptoms • Neutralizing antibodies may develop, rendering the drug less efficacious	No
Interferon-β1b	• Betaseron SC injection • Extavia SC injection	0.25 mg sub-Q every other day	• Hypersensitivity to interferon beta or human albumin • Allergy to interferons	Flu-like symptoms (fever, chills, fatigue, muscle aches); injection site reactions; mild anemia; thrombocytopenia; liver damage; depression	• Liver transaminases periodically • Response to therapy • Presence of adverse effects • Periodic CBC		• Acetaminophen or NSAIDs can decrease flu-like symptoms • Neutralizing antibodies may develop, rendering the drug less efficacious	No
Mechanism of action – glatiramer acetate: influences immature CD4 cells to become less inflammatory, thereby suppressing demyelination and preventing nerve fiber damage								
Glatiramer acetate	Copaxone SC injection	20 mg sub-Q daily or 40 mg sub-Q 3 × week	Hypersensitivity to the drug or to mannitol	Injection site reactions; postinjection reaction (chest pain, palpitations)	Response to therapy	None known	Does not produce neutralizing antibodies	No
Mechanism of action – fingolimod, decreases central inflammation by binding to sphingosine 1-phosphate receptors								
Fingolimod	Gilenya	0.5 mg PO once daily	• MI • Unstable angina • TIA/CVA • Class III/IV or decompensated • AV block/SSS • QTC interval ≥500 msec • Concurrent use with class Ia or III antiarrhythmic	Bradycardia, hypertension, immunosuppression, macular edema, dyspnea, elevated liver enzymes, diarrhea, headache, back pain, flu-like syndrome, HF	• HR • BP • CBC • ECG • Ophthalmologic exam • Decrease in relapse rate	Class IA and class III antiarrhythmics (may result in bradyarrhythmias), live vaccines, QTC-prolonging agents	Zoster vaccination prior to administration	No

Disease-Modifying Drugs *(cont'd)*

Generic	Brand	Dose & Max	Contra-indications	Primary Side Effects	Key Monitoring Parameters	Pertinent Drug Interactions	Med Pearls	Top 200
Mechanism of action – natalizumab: monoclonal antibody inhibits pro-inflammatory interactions within vascular endothelial cells and parenchymal brain cells								
Natalizumab	Tysabri IV infusion	300 mg IV infusion every 4 wks	• Hypersensitivity • Current or history of PML	• Infusion reactions are common (rash, drowsiness, fever, chills, hypotension, nausea, shortness of breath); headache, fatigue, urinary tract infection, joint pain, abdominal discomfort • Rare, potentially fatal ADE – progressive multifocal leukoencephalopathy (PML)	MRI at baseline, 3 mos, 6 mos; liver enzymes periodically	Other DMDs increase risk of PML	• Reserved for patients who have not responded to other DMDs; should be used as monotherapy *only*; combining with other DMDs increases risk of PML • Available only through a restrictive prescribing program – TOUCH	No
Mechanism of action – mitoxantrone decreases migration of T cells into the CNS by arresting the cell cycle and interfering with DNA repair and RNA synthesis								
Mitoxantrone	Novantrone IV infusion	12 mg/m² IV infusion every 3 mos; max = cumulative dose of 140 mg/m²	Hypersensitivity	Cardiac toxicity (heart failure, decreased LVEF); nausea; leukopenia; alopecia; menstrual irregularities; urinary and respiratory infections	• LVEF at baseline and prior to each IV infusion • Periodic CBC • LFTs	• Natalizumab (combination increases risk of PML) • Live vaccines	• Black box warning on cardiac risks and need for frequent LVEF monitoring • Discontinue therapy if LVEF <50% or with clinically significant decline	No
Mechanism of action – broad spectrum potassium channel blocker; increases action potential in demyelinated axons								
Dalfampridine	Ampyra	10 mg PO BID	• History of seizures • Moderate-severe renal impairment (CrCl <50 mL/min) • Hypersensitivity	Urinary tract infections, dizziness, insomnia, headache, back pain, nausea, constipation, balance disturbance, MS relapse, paresthesia, seizures	• Renal function periodically • Response to therapy	None known (limited data available)	• Indicated to improve walking in patients with MS • Risk of seizure is dose-dependent	No

Disease-Modifying Drugs *(cont'd)*

Mechanism of action – dimethyl fumarate; activate nuclear factor–like 2 (Nrf 2) pathway, decreasing inflammatory response to oxidative stress

Generic	Brand	Dose & Max	Contra-indications	Primary Side Effects	Key Monitoring Parameters	Pertinent Drug Interactions	Med Pearls	Top 200
Dimethyl fumarate	Tecfidera	120 mg–240 mg PO BID	None	• Dermatitis • Irritation of mucous membranes • Flushing • Elevated LFTs, lymphopenia • N/V	CBC at baseline and annually	Live vaccines may have decreased effectiveness and increased adverse effects	Place in therapy not fully known, indicated for relapsing MS	No

Mechanism of action – teriflunomide; inhibits pyrimidine synthesis, decreasing proliferation and inflammation

Generic	Brand	Dose & Max	Contra-indications	Primary Side Effects	Key Monitoring Parameters	Pertinent Drug Interactions	Med Pearls	Top 200
Teriflunomide	Aubagio	7–14 mg PO once daily	• Severe hepatic impairment • Pregnancy • Women of childbearing age without adequate contraception	Elevated liver transaminases, headache, alopecia, nausea, diarrhea, neutropenia, influenza, hypophosphatemia	CBC (periodic), LFTs monthly for first 6 months, serum K and creatinine monthly for first 6 months, TB and pregnancy tests prior to initiation	Leflunomide, natalizumab, pimecrolimus, tacrolimus, tofacitinib, BCG, live vaccines (all category X; avoid combination)	Black box warning for liver failure	No

Storage and Administration Pearls

- Interferon β1a, interferon β1b, glatiramer acetate, natalizumab, and mitoxantrone should be refrigerated to 2–8°C (36–46°F). These products should not be frozen and should be protected from light.
- Interferon β1 products and glatiramer acetate are available in prefilled syringes.
- Interferon β1 products and glatiramer acetate can be self-administered. Natalizumab and mitoxantrone are administered via IV infusion by qualified healthcare professionals.

Patient Education Pearls

- For self-injectable therapies:
  - Use the auto-injector supplied by the manufacturer (when available).
  - Apply ice to the injection site prior to injection.
  - Allow the medication to reach room temperature prior to injection.
  - Rotate injection sites.
- For those newly initiated on therapy, a Natalizumab medication guide should be provided. Both patient and provider must be enrolled in TOUCH prescribing program.
- Dimethyl fumarate should not be crushed or chewed. It may irritate mucous membranes on contact.
- Teriflunomide requires a reliable form of contraception.

EPILEPSY

Definitions

Epilepsy is a symptom of disturbed electrical activity within the brain. Epilepsy is a general term that encompasses a wide variety of symptomatic presentations that include periodic and recurrent seizures with or without convulsions. Seizures are classified as partial, generalized, or status epilepticus.

Partial seizures begin in one hemisphere of the brain and result in symptoms that are asymmetrical. Partial seizures can be classified as simple (no impairment of consciousness), complex (with impaired consciousness), or secondarily generalized (partial onset which becomes generalized).

Generalized seizures are bilateral/symmetrical in symptoms and can be classified as absence, myoclonic, clonic, tonic, tonic-clonic, atonic, or infantile spasms. The most common types are absence and tonic-clonic.

Diagnosis

The diagnosis of epilepsy is based on comprehensive history and physical, electroencephalography (EEG), and brain imaging by computed tomography (CT) scan or MRI. Differential diagnosis is important with exclusion of potential underlying causes of seizure including metabolic abnormalities (ruled out with evaluation of routine laboratory chemistries), traumatic head injury (determined by history), and presence of underlying structural abnormalities such as tumor (ruled out through brain imaging studies).

Signs and Symptoms

The clinical presentation of epilepsy is dependent on the classification of seizure type.

- Partial seizures result in asymmetrical alterations in motor function and in sensory or somatosensory symptoms, and may or may not involve a loss of consciousness. Nervous ticks, aberrations of normal behavior, and memory loss are also possible.
- Generalized seizures have symptoms that indicate involvement of both hemispheres of the brain. Motor symptoms are bilateral and there may be a loss of consciousness.
  - Absence seizures manifest as sudden interruption of ongoing activities, a blank stare, or an upward rotation of the eyes.
  - Tonic-clonic seizures consist of sharp tonic muscle contractions, rigidity, and clonic movement that are accompanied by a loss of consciousness and may be preceded by an aura.

Guidelines

Efficacy and tolerability of the new antiepileptic drugs I: treatment of new onset epilepsy: report of the Therapeutics and Technology Assessment Subcommittee and Quality Standards Subcommittee of the American Academy of Neurology and the American Epilepsy Society. *Neurology*, no. 62 (8) (2004): 1252–60. http://www.guideline.gov/summary/summary.aspx?ss=15&doc_id=5183&nbr=3565.

Guidelines Summary

- Goals of treatment include a lack of seizure activity, minimal medication side effects of treatment, and improved quality of life.
- Treatment with antiepileptic drugs (AEDs) is warranted for patients that experience multiple seizures or have significantly affected quality of life. AED choice is based on the specific seizure type, the patient's age, comorbidities, ability to adhere to the regimen, and insurance coverage.
- AED monotherapy is preferred, but some patients do require combination therapy.

- First-line AEDs for partial seizures include carbamazepine, phenytoin, lamotrigine, valproic acid, and oxcarbazepine.
- First-line AEDs for generalized absence seizures include valproic acid and ethosuximide.
- First-line AEDs for tonic-clonic seizures include phenytoin, carbamazepine, and valproic acid.
- Alternative AEDs include gabapentin, topiramate, levetiracetam, zonisamide, tiagabine, primidone, felbamate, lamotrigine, phenobarbital, lacosamide, vigabatrin, and perampanel.
- In 2008, the FDA issued an alert regarding the relationship between the use of antiepileptic agents and suicidality (including suicidal behavior or ideation). Pooled analyses completed by the FDA indicated a significant increase of suicidality for patients treated with antiepileptic agents when compared to those given placebo. All antiepileptic agents appear to increase the risk similarly. Manufacturers of these agents are now required to include a boxed warning in their prescribing information and to include a medication guide for patients in their product labeling.

Anti-Epileptic Drugs

Generic	Brand	Dose & Max mg (frequency)	Contra-indications	Primary Side Effects	Key Monitoring Parameters	Med Pearls	Top 200
Mechanism of action – Carbamazepine inhibits voltage-gated sodium channels, thereby depressing electrical transmission in the nucleus ventralis anterior of the thalamus							
Carbamazepine	• Tegretol • Tegretol XR • Carbatrol	200–1,600 mg daily (BID)	• Bone marrow suppression • Hypersensitivity • Concomitant use with MAOIs or MRTIs	• Dizziness, drowsiness, unsteadiness, nausea, vomiting, blurred vision • Rare: aplastic anemia, agranulocytosis	• CBC periodically • Suicidality • Serum drug concentrations (4–12 mcg/mL) • Serum sodium • Seizure frequency	• First-line for partial seizures and generalized tonic-clonic seizures • Therapeutic concentration: 4–12 mcg/mL	Yes
Mechanism of action – valproic acid: not fully understood, thought to increase gamma amino butyric acid (GABA) concentrations in the brain							
Valproic acid (divalproex sodium)	• Depakote • Depakote ER • Depakene • Depacon	10–60 mg/kg/day	• Hepatic dysfunction • Hypersensitivity • Urea cycle disorders	• Hepatic impairment • Thrombocytopenia • Hyperammonemia • Weight gain • Pancreatitis • Headache • Somnolence • Dizziness • Alopecia	• Serum drug concentrations (50–100 mcg/mL) • Liver function tests (LFTs), at baseline and periodically • Periodic CBC and serum ammonia levels • Suicidality • Seizure frequency	• First-line for partial, generalized, tonic-clonic, and absence seizures • Highly teratogenic • Available in oral capsules, tablets, extended-release tablets, sprinkle caps, oral syrup, and IV solution • Therapeutic concentration: 50–100 mcg/mL	Yes
Mechanism of action – Phenytoin: promotes neuronal sodium efflux, thereby stabilizing the threshold against hyperexcitability							
Phenytoin	Dilantin	300–600 mg daily (divided TID)	Hypersensitivity	• Nystagmus, ataxia, slurred speech, dizziness, insomnia, headache, tremor, gingival hyperplasia • Rare: Stevens-Johnson rash	• Serum drug concentrations (10–20 mcg/mL) corrected for serum albumin <4 g/dL • Suicidality • Seizure frequency	• First-line option for partial and generalized tonic-clonic seizures • Abrupt discontinuation should be avoided; this may precipitate status epilepticus • Takes 7–10 days to reach steady state • Therapeutic concentration must be corrected for hypoalbuminemia (corrected phenytoin concentration = measured total concentration/ [0.2*albumin] + 0.1)	Yes

Anti-Epileptic Drugs *(cont'd)*

Generic	Brand	Dose & Max mg (frequency)	Contra-indications	Primary Side Effects	Key Monitoring Parameters	Med Pearls	Top 200
Mechanism of action – depresses motor cortex and elevates the threshold of the CNS to convulsive stimuli							
Ethosuximide	Zarontin	250–1,500 mg daily	Hypersensitivity	• Ataxia • Drowsiness • GI upset • Blood dyscrasias • Rash (Stevens-Johnson possible)	• Periodic CBC • Seizure frequency • Presence of adverse effects • Suicidality • Serum drug concentration (40–100 mcg/mL)	Available as capsules or syrup; used *only* for absence seizure	No
Mechanism of action – blocks voltage-sensitive sodium channels, resulting in stabilization of hyperexcitable neuronal membranes							
Oxcarbazepine	Trileptal tablets and oral suspension	600–2,400 mg daily (BID)	Hypersensitivity	• Sedation • Dizziness • Ataxia • Nausea • Rash (Stevens-Johnson possible) • Hyponatremia	• Periodic Na, renal function • Suicidality • Seizure frequency	CrCl <30 mL/min requires half of initial dose	Yes
Felbamate	Felbatol	1,200–3,600 mg daily (TID-QID)	• Hypersensitivity • Blood dyscrasias • Liver dysfunction	• Aplastic anemia • Acute lever failure • Anorexia • Nausea, vomiting • Insomnia • Headache	• Frequent CBC • Frequent liver transaminases • Suicidality • Seizure frequency • Presence of adverse effects	• AST or ALT >2 × ULN requires discontinuation • Not a first-line agent; reserved for refractory cases	No
Lamotrigine	• Lamictal • Oral tablets, chewable tablets	25–700 mg daily (once to BID)	Hypersensitivity, history of Stevens-Johnson rash	• Stevens-Johnson rash • Other rash • Diplopia • Dizziness • Headache	• Presence of side effects • Suicidality • Seizure frequency	• Risk of rash increased when combined with VPA • First-line option for partial seizures • Slow dose titration necessary	Yes

Anti-Epileptic Drugs *(cont'd)*

Generic	Brand	Dose & Max mg (frequency)	Contra-indications	Primary Side Effects	Key Monitoring Parameters	Med Pearls	Top 200
Lacosamide	Vimpat	• 50 mg PO BID; may be increased at weekly intervals by 100 mg/day • Maintenance dose: 200–400 mg/day BID • IV formulation available (equivalent dose)	None known	• Nausea/vomiting • Ataxia • Dizziness • Headache • Fatigue • Diplopia • Tremor	• Suicidality • Seizure frequency • ECG in patients with conduction abnormalities or CVD at baseline and at steady state	• Adjunctive therapy for partial-onset seizures • Only for adults (>17y) • Should not be abruptly discontinued	No
Mechanism of action – although structurally similar to GABA, pharmacological effects in epilepsy are not fully understood							
Gabapentin	• Neurontin • Tablets, capsules, oral solution	900–3,600 mg daily (TID)	Hypersensitivity	• Dizziness • Fatigue • Somnolence • Ataxia • Weight gain	• Presence of adverse effects • Suicidality • Seizure frequency	• No known drug interactions • Renal dose adjustment necessary when CrCl <60 mL/min	Yes
Mechanism of action – blocks voltage-dependent sodium channels, augments GABA activity, antagonizes glutamate receptors							
Topiramate	• Topamax • Tablets and sprinkle caps	25–400 mg daily (BID)	Hypersensitivity	• Difficulty concentrating • Psychomotor slowing • Speech problems • Somnolence • Fatigue • Dizziness • Headache • Weight loss • Kidney stones	• Presence of side effects • Suicidality • Seizure frequency	• Adjunctive therapy in patients with partial seizures • Slow titration necessary to avoid adverse effects	Yes
Mechanism of action – not well understood							
Levetiracetam	• Keppra • Tablets, oral solution, parenteral solution	1,000–3,000 mg daily (BID)	Hypersensitivity	• Dizziness • Asthenia • Behavioral disturbances (hostility, nervousness) • Somnolence • Infection	• Presence of side effects • Renal function • Suicidality • Seizure frequency	• No known drug interactions • Dose adjustment required in renal impairment (CrCl <60 mL/min) • Adjunctive therapy for partial seizures and for generalized tonic-clonic seizures	Yes

Anti-Epileptic Drugs *(cont'd)*

Generic	Brand	Dose & Max mg (frequency)	Contra-indications	Primary Side Effects	Key Monitoring Parameters	Med Pearls	Top 200
Mechanism of action – elevates seizure threshold by decreasing postsynaptic excitability through stimulation of postsynaptic GABA inhibitory responses							
Phenobarbital	• Solfoton • Tablets, capsules, elixir • Luminal IV injection	60–600 mg daily	Severe liver impairment, hypersensitivity, porphyria	• Sedation • Nystagmus • Ataxia • Hyperactivity • Headache • Nausea • Blood dyscrasias (agranulocytosis, granulocytopenia)	• Serum concentrations 20–40 mcg/mL • Periodic CBC • Periodic LFTs • Suicidality • Seizure frequency	• Drug of choice for neonatal seizures; otherwise, adjunctive therapy for partial and generalized (other than absence) seizures • Frequency of side effects limits use • Titrate dose slowly to minimize adverse effects • Avoid abrupt discontinuation • Takes 3–4 wks to reach steady-state	Yes
Primidone	Mysoline	125–2,000 mg daily (TID–QID)		• Rash • Behavior changes • Intellectual blunting • Mood change	• Serum concentrations 5–12 mcg/mL • Periodic CBC • Periodic LFTs • Suicidality	• Metabolized to phenobarbital • Avoid abrupt discontinuation	No
Mechanism of action – potent and specific inhibitor of GABA uptake into neuronal elements, thereby enhances GABA activity by decreasing its removal from the neuronal space							
Tiagabine	Gabitril	4–56 mg daily (BID–QID)	Hypersensitivity	• Dizziness • Fatigue • Difficulty concentrating • Nervousness • Tremor • Blurred vision • Depression • Weakness	• Presence of adverse effects • Suicidality • Seizure frequency	• Adjunctive therapy in partial seizures • Do not abruptly discontinue; taper dose	No
Mechanism of action – irreversible inhibition of gamma-aminobutyric acid transaminase (GABA-T), thereby increasing the levels of GABA within the brain							
Vigabatrin	Sabril	• 500 mg 2 × daily initially, increase daily dose by 500 mg at weekly intervals • Recommended dose: 3 g/day	None	• Permanent vision loss • Fatigue • Somnolence • Tremor • Nystagmus • Blurred vision • Memory impairment • Weight gain • Arthralgia • Confusion	• Ophthalmologic exam • Observe patient for excessive sedation • Suicidality • Seizure frequency	• Used as adjunctive therapy for refractory complex-partial seizures • Should not be abruptly discontinued • Renal dose adjustment required • Boxed warning due to ocular effects • Available only through special, restricted distribution program (SHARE)	No

Anti-Epileptic Drugs *(cont'd)*

Generic	Brand	Dose & Max mg (frequency)	Contra-indications	Primary Side Effects	Key Monitoring Parameters	Med Pearls	Top 200
Mechanism of action – blocks voltage-dependent sodium and calcium channels, thereby reducing repetitive neuronal firing							
Zonisamide	Zonegran	100–600 mg daily	Hypersensitivity to zonisamide or sulfonamides	• Sedation • Dizziness • Cognitive impairment • Nausea • Rash (Stevens-Johnson possible) • Anorexia	• Seizure frequency • Suicidality • BUN/SCr • Serum bicarb	• Adjunctive therapy in partial seizures • Takes up to 2 wks to achieve steady-state	Yes
Mechanism of action – antagonistic effects of ionotropic alpha-amino-3-hydroxy-5-methyl-4-isoxazolepropionic acid (AMPA) glutamate receptor							
Perampanel	Fycompa	2–12 mg PO once daily at bedtime	None	• Dizziness • Headache • Somnolence • Fatigue • Irritability • Anxiety • Aggression • Depression • Weight gain • Nausea • Peripheral edema	• Seizure frequency • Suicidality • Weight	Adjunctive therapy for partial-onset seizures	No

AED Drug Interactions

AED	Interacting Medication	Effect
Carbamazepine	Felbamate	↓ Carbamazepine
	Phenobarbital	↓ Carbamazepine
	Phenytoin	↓ Carbamazepine
	Cimetidine	↑ Carbamazepine
	Erythromycin	↑ Carbamazepine
	Fluoxetine	↑ Carbamazepine
	Isoniazid	↑ Carbamazepine
	Propoxyphene	↑ Carbamazepine
	Oral contraceptives	↓ Contraceptives
	Doxycycline	↓ Doxycycline
	Theophylline	↓ Theophylline
	Warfarin	↓ Warfarin
	Perampanel	↓ Perampanel
VPA	Carbamazepine	↓ VPA
	Lamotrigine	↓ VPA
	Phenobarbital	↓ VPA
	Primidone	↓ VPA
	Phenytoin	↓ VPA
	Cimetidine	↑ VPA
	Salicylates	↑ VPA
	Oral contraceptives	↓ Contraceptives
Phenytoin	Carbamazepine	↓ Phenytoin
	Felbamate	↑ Phenytoin
	Phenobarbital	↑ or ↓ Phenytoin
	VPA	↓ Phenytoin
	Antacids	↓ Phenytoin
	Cimetidine	↑ Phenytoin
	Chloramphenicol	↑ Phenytoin
	Disulfiram	↑ Phenytoin
	Ethanol (acute)	↑ Phenytoin
	Ethanol (chronic)	↑ Phenytoin
	Warfarin	↑ Phenytoin
	Propoxyphene	↑ Phenytoin
	Fluconazole	↑ Phenytoin
	Isoniazid	↑ Phenytoin
	Oral contraceptives	↓ Contraceptives
	Folic acid	↓ Folic acid
	Quinidine	↓ Quinidine
	Perampanel	↓ Perampanel
Oxcarbazepine	Carbamazepine	↓ Oxcarbazepine
	Phenytoin	↓ Oxcarbazepine
	Phenobarbital	↓ Oxcarbazepine
	Oral contraceptives	↓ Contraceptives
	Perampanel	↓ Perampanel

AED Drug Interactions *(cont'd)*

AED	Interacting Medication	Effect
Felbamate	Carbamazepine	↓ Felbamate
	Phenytoin	↓ Felbamate
	Simeprevir	↓ Simeprevir
	VPA	↑ VPA
Perampanel	Alcohol	↑ CNS depressant effect
	Aripiprazole	↓ Aripiprazole
	Buprenorphine	↑ CNS depressant effect
	Carbamazepine	↓ Perampanel
	Progestins	↓ Progestin
	Phenytoin	↓ Perampanel
	Oxcarbazine	↓ Perampanel
	Simeprevir	↓ Simeprevir
	CNS depressants	↑ CNS depressant effect
Lacosamide	Carbamazepine	↓ Lacosamide
	Phenobarbital	↓ Lacosamide
	Phenytoin	↓ Lacosamide
Lamotrigine	Carbamazepine	↓ Lamotrigine
	Phenobarbital	↓ Lamotrigine
	Phenytoin	↓ Lamotrigine
	Primidone	↓ Lamotrigine
	VPA	↑ Lamotrigine
Topiramate	Alcohol	↑ CNS depressant effect
	Carbamazepine	↓ Topiramate
	Metformin	↑ Metformin adverse effects
	Phenytoin	↓ Topiramate
	Simeprevir	↓ Simeprevir
	VPA	↓ VPA
	Oral contraceptives	↓ Contraceptives
Phenobarbital	Apixaban	↓ Apixaban
	Dronaderone	↓ Dronaderone
	Felbamate	↑ Phenobarbital
	Phenytoin	↑ Phenobarbital
	Rivaroxaban	↓ Rivaroxaban
	Simeprevir	↓ Simeprevir
	VPA	↑ Phenobarbital
	Oral contraceptives	↓ Contraceptives

AED Drug Interactions *(cont'd)*

AED	Interacting Medication	Effect
Primidone	Carbamazepine	↓ Primidone, ↑ Phenobarbital
	Phenytoin	↓ Primidone, ↑ Phenobarbital
	VPA	↑ Primidone, ↓ Phenobarbital
	Corticosteroids	↓ Corticosteroids
Tiagabine	Carbamazepine	↓ Tiagabine
	Phenytoin	↓ Tiagabine
Vigabatrin	CNS depressants	↑ CNS depressant effect
	Phenytoin	↓ Phenytoin
	Ketorolac	↓ Vigabatrin
Zonisamide	Carbamazepine	↓ Zonisamide
	Phenytoin	↓ Zonisamide
	Phenobarbital	↓ Zonisamide

Storage and Administration Pearls

- Valproic acid: Extended-release divalproex sodium should be swallowed whole and should not be chewed, crushed, or split. Divalproex sodium sprinkle caps may be swallowed whole or may be opened and sprinkled on a small amount (~ teaspoon) of soft food, such as pudding or applesauce.
- Phenytoin: Available in chewable tablets, capsules, extended-release capsules, oral suspension and parenteral solution (IM or IV).
- Oxcarbazepine oral suspension should be shaken well before administration and should be used within 7 weeks of opening the bottle.

Patient Education Pearls

- Antiepileptic medication should not be abruptly discontinued, as this may result in increased and emergent seizure activity.
- Any skin rash that develops should be reported to a healthcare provider immediately.
- When taking any new medications, patients should consult with their pharmacist, as multiple drug interactions are possible.
- Antiepileptic medications have been associated with an increased risk of suicidal thoughts and behaviors. Please discuss this with your healthcare provider and report any of these symptoms immediately.

PARKINSON'S DISEASE

Definitions

Parkinson's disease (PD) is a syndrome characterized by tremor, rigidity, bradykinesia, and/or postural instability caused by a progressive depletion of dopamine neurons in the substantia nigra of the basal ganglia. Symptoms are a result of the dopamine deficiency and subsequent relative acetylcholine excess.

Diagnosis

Diagnosis of PD is based on careful clinical history and physical exam. There are no agreed-upon objective or definitive lab or imaging criteria for diagnosis. Generally, patients need two of the four main symptoms (tremor, bradykinesia, rigidity, postural instability) to be diagnosed with PD.

Signs and Symptoms

PD has an insidious onset and begins with nonspecific symptoms such as malaise and fatigue. Tremor is generally the first of the cardinal signs and is generally unilateral and occurring at rest rather than upon intention. Rigidity of the limbs manifests as resistance to passive movement of the joints, and bradykinesia as slow movements or difficulty moving. Symptoms generally begin unilaterally and progress asymmetrically.

Summary of Treatment Recommendations

- Initial therapy generally consists of either a dopamine agonist or carbidopa/levodopa.
  - Patients ≥65 years of age or those with significant disability due to their PD should receive carbidopa/levodopa as initial therapy.
  - Patients <65 years of age should receive a dopamine agonist as initial therapy.
  - Inadequate response to maximum tolerable doses of initial therapy with a dopamine agonist or levodopa should result in the addition of the alternate medication.
  - Subsequently, COMT inhibitors may be added to ongoing levodopa therapy, and adjunctive therapies such as amantadine or anticholinergics may be utilized.
  - Anticholinergic agents are primarily useful for the treatment of tremor-predominant PD but should be used with caution in elderly patients and avoided in patients with pre-existing cognitive impairment.
  - Because dopamine agonists and levodopa therapies are aimed at increasing the available dopamine in the CNS, side effects such as hallucinations and delusions are possible. Psychiatric side effects which occur at the lowest effective doses of these drugs may be treated with the antipsychotic medication quetiapine.

Drugs for Parkinson's Disease

Mechanism of action – antiviral that blocks the uncoating of influenza A virus, preventing penetration of virus into host

Mechanism of action – monoamine-oxidase (MAO) B inhibitors: inhibit the catabolism of dopamine by selectively inhibiting the monoamine oxidase B enzyme

Generic	Brand	Dose & Max	Contra-indications	Primary Side Effects	Key Monitoring Parameters	Pertinent Drug Interactions	Med Pearls	Top 200
Amantadine	Symmetrel	200–300 mg daily	Hypersensitivity	Confusion, nightmares, hallucinations, insomnia, nervousness, irritability	• Response to therapy • Presence of adverse effects	• Triamterene increases plasma amantadine concentrations • Concomitant agents that cause QTc prolongation	Renal dose adjustment necessary for CrCl <50 mL/min	No
Selegiline	• Eldepryl: tablets • Emsam: transdermal patch • Zelapar: disintegrating tablets	5–10 mg daily (once to BID) ODT: max = 2.5 mg daily	• Hypersensitivity • Use of meperidine, methadone, or tramadol • MAOIs	• Nausea, hallucinations, insomnia, depression, orthostasis, arrhythmia • Rare: hypertensive crisis (if high-tyramine foods are ingested)	• Response to therapy • Presence of adverse effects	• Avoid use with meperide, other opioid analgesics, or dextromethorphan; may result in fatal increased activity of analgesics • Co-administration with other serotonergic agents increases risk of serotonin syndrome	• Avoid tyramine-containing foods • Discontinue 14 days prior to surgery if possible; should not be taken with general anesthesia	No
Rasagiline	Azilect	0.5–1 mg daily	• Hypersensitivity • MAOIs • Meperidine, methadone, tramadol within 14 days • Cyclobenzaprine, dextromethorphan, and St. John's wort	• Flu-like syndrome • Arthralgia • Depression • Dyspepsia • Hypertension • Nausea • Orthostasis	• Response to therapy • Presence of side effects • Blood pressure	• Avoid use with meperidine, opioid analgesics, or dextromethorphan; may result in fatal reaction • Co-administration with other serotonergic agents increases risk of serotonin syndrome • Ciprofloxaxin (and other CYP1A2 inhibitors) increases rasagiline plasma levels	• Should not be abruptly discontinued • Avoid tyramine-containing foods	No

Drugs for Parkinson's Disease (cont'd)

Generic	Brand	Dose & Max	Contra-indications	Primary Side Effects	Key Monitoring Parameters	Pertinent Drug Interactions	Med Pearls	Top 200
Mechanism of action – levodopa is a direct precursor to dopamine and is converted to dopamine once it crosses the blood-brain barrier; carbidopa is a dopa decarboxylase inhibitor, and it is necessary to combine this with levodopa in order to prevent the peripheral degradation of levodopa prior to entry into the blood-brain barrier.								
Carbidopa/ levodopa	• Sinemet • Sinemet CR • Parcopa: orally disintegrating tablets	• Carbidopa 75–300 mg daily (75 mg required, side effects if >300 mg/ day) • Levodopa 100–2,000 mg daily (individualized)	• Hypersensitivity • Narrow-angle glaucoma • History of melanoma	Nausea, vomiting, orthostasis, confusion, hallucinations, wearing-off fluctuations, dyskinesias	• Response to therapy • Presence of side effects • BP • LFTs • BUN/SCr	• Nonselective MAO inhibitors should be avoided; may cause hypertensive crisis • Pyridoxine (vitamin B6) decreases effectiveness of levodopa	Immediate-release (IR) and controlled-release (CR) tabs often used simultaneously; IR tabs can treat wearing-off symptoms of CR tabs; CR is less bioavailable (~30% less) than IR	Yes
Mechanism of action – dopamine agonists: direct stimulation of striatal dopamine receptors								
Bromocriptine (Ergot-derivative)	• Parlodel • Cycloset	1.25–40 mg daily (divided TID) (max = 100 mg/ day)	• Uncontrolled hypertension • Sensitivity to ergot alkaloids • Pregnancy • Postpartum fundus with CAD	• Cardiac valve fibrosis • Nausea, hallucinations, dizziness, drowsiness	• Response to therapy • Presence of adverse effects	Decrease levodopa dose by 20–30% when initiating	Cardiac side effects decrease clinical use; nonergot derivatives used much more commonly	No
Pramipexole (Nonergot derivative)	• Mirapex • Mirapex ER	• 1.5–4.5 mg daily • IR: TID • ER: once daily		Nausea, vomiting, constipation, orthostasis, hypersexuality, hallucinations, syncope, somnolence, impulse control disorders	• Response to therapy • Presence of adverse effects • BP • Weight	• Decrease levodopa dose by 20–30% when initiating • Metoclopramide and antipsychotics decrease efficacy	• Renal dose adjustment required when CrCl <50 mL/min • Titrate dose slowly and taper upon discontinuation	Yes

Drugs for Parkinson's Disease *(cont'd)*

Generic	Brand	Dose & Max	Contra-indications	Primary Side Effects	Key Monitoring Parameters	Pertinent Drug Interactions	Med Pearls	Top 200
Ropinirole (nonergot derivative)	• Requip • Requip XL	0.75–12 mg daily (divided TID) (max = 24 mg/day)	Hypersensitivity	• Syncope • Somnolence • Dizziness • N/V	• BP • Oversedation • Response to therapy			Yes
Rotigotine	Neupro transdermal delivery system	2–8 mg daily (apply 1 patch daily)	• Dementia • Hypersensitivity	• Application site reactions • N/V • Somnolence • Insomnia • Hallucinations • Abnormal dreams • Edema	• Response to therapy • Presence of adverse effects • BP • Skin checks	Decrease levodopa dose by 20–30% when initiating; metoclopramide and phenothiazines decrease efficacy	• Transdermal patch • Taper dose upon discontinuation	No

Mechanism of action – COMT inhibitors: inhibit the degradation of dopamine through inhibition of the catechol-0-methyltransferase enzyme

Generic	Brand	Dose & Max	Contra-indications	Primary Side Effects	Key Monitoring Parameters	Pertinent Drug Interactions	Med Pearls	Top 200
Tolcapone	Tasmar	300–600 mg daily (divided TID)	• AST or ALT >2 × ULN • Known liver disease • History or nontraumatic rhabdomyolysis	• Liver failure • Dyskinesias • N/V • Hallucinations	• Frequent LFT monitoring • Response to therapy • Presence of adverse effects • BP	• MOAIs • Increased activity of drugs known to be metabolized by COMT (dopamine, dobutamine, isoproterenol, methyldopa)	• Reserved for third-line therapy in patients that do not respond adequately to levodopa and dopamine agonists • Only used as adjunct therapy with levodopa	No
Entacapone	Comtan	200–1,600 mg daily (divided up to 8 × daily; administered with carbidopa/levodopa tablets)	Hypersensitivity	Dyskinesias, nausea, vomiting, hallucinations, urine discoloration	• Response to therapy • Presence of adverse effects, periodic LFTs	Increased activity of drugs known to be metabolized by COMT (dopamine, dobutamine, isoproterenol, methyldopa)	• Reserved for third-line therapy in patients that do not respond adequately to levodopa and dopamine agonists • Preferred over tolcapone, as no fatal liver injury has been reported with this agent	No

Drugs for Parkinson's Disease *(cont'd)*

Mechanism of action – anticholinergics: through diminished activity of acetylcholine, help to decrease the relative increase in activity compared to dopamine, thereby decreasing tremor

Generic	Brand	Dose & Max	Contra-indications	Primary Side Effects	Key Monitoring Parameters	Pertinent Drug Interactions	Med Pearls	Top 200
Benztropine	Cogentin	0.5–6 mg daily (BID)	Hypersensitivity	• Dry mouth • Blurred vision • Constipation • Urinary retention • Confusion • Memory impairment • Hallucinations	• Response to therapy • Presence of adverse effects	Additive anticholinergic side effects when co-administered with other anticholinergic medications	Caution use in elderly patients who are at risk for mental status changes with anticholinergic medications; primarily used for tremor and/or drooling	Yes
Trihexyphenidyl	Artane	1–15 mg daily (BID–TID)	None	• Dry mouth • Blurred vision • Constipation • Urinary retention • Confusion • Memory impairment • Hallucinations	• Response to therapy • Presence of adverse effects	Additive anticholinergic side effects when co-administered with other anticholinergic agents	Caution use in elderly patients; primarily used for tremor and drooling	Yes

KAPLAN) MEDICAL

Storage and Administration Pearls

- Selegiline is available as a tablet, capsule, transdermal patch, and oral disintegrating tablet. Oral disintegrating tablets should be taken in the morning before any food or water. Tablets dissolve on the tongue, and food/drink should be avoided for 5 minutes after dose.

- Carbidopa/levodopa extended-release tablets can be taken as whole tablets or half tablets but should not be chewed or crushed. Extended-release tablets are less bio-available than immediate-release tablets and patients may require up to a 30% dose increase to attain similar efficacy.

- Rotigotine patch should be worn continuously for 24 hours. Heat may increase absorption.

Patient Education Pearls

- Avoid concomitant alcohol with any antiparkinsonian agent.

- Rotigotine patch should be worn continuously for 24 hours. Heat may increase absorption. Patients should not take a hot bath or sauna or apply a heated pad while wearing patch.

- Hallucinations, delusions, or strange dreams should be immediately reported to a physician.

MIGRAINE HEADACHE

Definitions

Migraine headaches are defined as recurring headaches of moderate to severe intensity and are associated with gastrointestinal, neurological, and autonomic symptoms. Migraine headaches may or may not be preceded by an aura.

Diagnosis

Diagnostic criteria are established by the International Headache Society (IHS) and consist of distinct criteria for migraine with aura and migraine without aura.

Migraine with aura

- At least two attacks
- Aura symptoms that do not last more than 60 minutes
- Organic disorder ruled out or headaches do not relate temporally to organic disorder

Migraine without aura

- At least five attacks
- Headache lasts 4–72 hours

- Unilateral, pulsating, moderate/severe intensity, or aggravated by physical activity
- Nausea/vomiting, photophobia, or phonophobia
- Organic disorder ruled out or headaches do not relate temporally to organic disorder

Signs and Symptoms

Pain is the primary symptom of migraine headache. The pain is generally gradual in onset, peaks in intensity over minutes to hours, and lasts 4–72 hours if untreated. Intensity is often described as moderate to severe and generally stated as a 5 or greater on a 0–10 pain scale. Most commonly, pain occurs in the frontotemporal region and is most often unilateral and pulsating. Other symptoms that may accompany the pain include gastrointestinal symptoms of nausea/vomiting and neurological symptoms of photo- or phonophobia.

Guidelines

Evidence-based guideline update: Pharmacologic treatment for episodic migraine prevention in adults. Report of the Quality Standards Subcommittee of the American Academy of Neurology and the American Headache Society. *Neurology* 78(2012): 1337–1345.

Summary of Treatment Recommendations

- Migraine treatment is divided into abortive treatment, rescue treatment, and prophylactic treatment. The majority of patients will respond to abortive treatment and can be controlled without the addition of rescue or prophylactic therapy.
- Abortive treatment options include analgesics (over-the-counter and prescription), NSAIDs (detailed in bone and joint chapter), ergotamine and dihydroergotamine, serotonin agonists, and butorphanol. Over-the-counter analgesics, prescription non-opioid analgesics, and NSAIDs are reserved for patients with mild symptoms.
- The serotonin agonists are the mainstay of abortive therapy options for patients with moderate to severe symptoms. Various dosage forms are available and there is only slight variability between the efficacy and safety of available agents. Patients may respond to one agent in this class and not to another; therefore, trial and error is often the approach taken.
- For patients who have >2 headaches/week or >8 headaches/month, or who do not have an adequate response to abortive therapy, prophylactic therapy may be warranted.
- Available prophylactic agents include antihypertensive medications such as propranolol, atenolol, and metoprolol (detailed in cardiovascular chapter); antidepressant medications such as amitriptyline, paroxetine, fluoxetine, and sertraline (detailed in psychiatric disorders chapter); and anticonvulsant medications such valproic acid, gabapentin, tiagabine, and topiramate (detailed earlier in this chapter). In general, migraine prophylactic doses are low compared to normal doses of these medications.

Drugs for Migraine

Generic	Brand	Dose & Max	Contra-indications	Primary Side Effects	Key Monitoring Parameters	Pertinent Drug Interactions	Med Pearls	Top 200
Analgesics								
Acetaminophen, aspirin, caffeine	• Excedrin Migraine • Anacin	2 tablets PO at onset, then q6 hrs PRN	• Hypersensitivity to any component • Pregnancy	Minimal	• Response to therapy • Presence of adverse effects	Other acetaminophen-containing meds	Available OTC	No
Aspirin or acetaminophen with butalbital and caffeine	• Fiorinal • Fioricet	1–2 tabs PO q4–6 hrs PRN (max = 6 doses/day)	• Hypersensitivity to any component • Pregnancy	• Tachycardia • Dizziness • Drowsiness or insomnia • Orthostatic hypotension	• Response to therapy • Presence of adverse effects	• Alcohol • Additive CNS depression with butalbital	• Limit to 4 tablets/day and use max of 2 days/week • Dependence may develop with continued use	Yes
Isometheptene/dichloral-phenazone/APAP	Nodolor	2 caps PO at onset, 1 cap q hour PRN (max = 6 capsules/24 hr)	• Glaucoma • Severe renal disease • Hypertension • CVD • CVA • MAOI use	• Dizziness • Skin rash	• Response to therapy • Presence of adverse effects	MAOIs: potential for hypertensive crisis	Max 6 caps/day; 20 caps/month	No
Mechanism of action — ergotamine tartrate: exerts serotonergic agonist activity, resulting in vasoconstriction								
Ergotamine tartrate	Ergomar sublingual tablet	• 1 tab at onset and 1 tab q30 min PRN • Not to exceed 3 tabs/day	Peripheral arterial disease, heart disease, hypertension, impaired hepatic or renal function, hypersensitivity	• Chest pain • Hypertension • Tachycardia • Nausea • Edema	• Response to therapy • Presence of adverse effects	Other meds with potential to increase blood pressure	Potential for dependence with long-term use	No
Mechanism of action — dihydroergotamine: serotonin agonistic activity, results in cerebral vasoconstriction								
Dihydroergotamine	DHE 45 SC, IM, or IV injection 1 mg/mL	1 mg at onset, repeated at 1-hr intervals (max = 2 mg/day IV or 3 mg/day SC or IM)	• Ischemic heart disease • Uncontrolled hypertension • Peripheral arterial disease • History of MI • Angina • Within 24 hr of triptans	• Hypertension • Vasospasm • Myocardial infarction • Tachycardia • Fibrosis	• BP • HR • Response to therapy • Presence of side effects	Potent inhibitors of CYP3A4, including protease inhibitors and macrolide antibiotics	Use significantly limited by adverse effects	No
	Migranal nasal spray	1 spray (0.5 mg) in each nostril followed by repeat spray in each nostril >15 minutes (max = 3 mg/day)						

Drugs for Migraine (cont'd)

Mechanism of action – serotonin agonists (triptans): serotonin 5HT receptor agonists, resulting in vasoconstriction in the cerebral vasculature

Generic	Brand	Dose & Max	Contra-indications	Primary Side Effects	Key Monitoring Parameters	Pertinent Drug Interactions	Med Pearls	Top 200
Sumatriptan	Imitrex oral tablets	25–100 mg PO at onset, may redose at >2 hrs up to 200 mg/day	• Ischemic cardiac disease • Peripheral vascular disease • Cerebrovascular disease • Uncontrolled TITN • Within 24 hrs of an ergot product • Within 2 wks of an MAOI	• Fatigue • Dizziness • Flushing • Neck/throat pressure • Unpleasant taste	• Response to therapy • Presence of side effects • BP	MAO – A inhibitors – increased triptan levels can lead to serotonin syndrome and cardiac side effects; sibutramine and SSRI coadministration – increased risk of serotonin syndrome	• First approved serotonin agonist for migraine • Also available in combination with naproxen (Treximet) • Subcutaneous dosage form has fastest onset of action	Yes
	Imitrex SC injection	4–6 mg SC; may repeat in 1 hour (max = 2 doses/day)						
	Imitrex nasal spray	10–20 mg spray intranasally at onset; may repeat after 2 hrs (max = 40 mg/day)						
	• Sumavel Dosepro • Needle-free, SC injection	6 mg SC; may repeat in 1 hr						
Zolmitriptan	• Zomig • Oral tabs; rapid disintegrating tabs; nasal spray	1–5 mg at onset, redose >2 hrs if needed (max = 10 mg/day)						No
Naratriptan	Amerge oral tablets	1–2.5 mg at onset; may redose >4 hrs if needed (max = 5 mg/day)						No

Drugs for Migraine *(cont'd)*

Generic	Brand	Dose & Max	Contra-indications	Primary Side Effects	Key Monitoring Parameters	Pertinent Drug Interactions	Med Pearls	Top 200
Rizatriptan	• Maxalt • Maxalt MLT	5–10 mg PO at onset; redose >2 hrs (max = 30 mg/day)	• Ischemic cardiac disease • Peripheral vascular disease	• Fatigue • Dizziness • Flushing • Neck/throat pressure	• Response to therapy • Presence of side effects	MAO – A inhibitors – increased triptan levels can lead to serotonin syndrome and cardiac side effects; sibutramine and SSRI coadministration – increased risk of serotonin syndrome		Yes
Almotriptan	Axert	6.25–12.5 mg PO at onset; redose >2 hrs if needed (max = 25 mg/day)	• Cerebrovascular disease • Uncontrolled HTN • Within 24 hrs of an ergot product					No
Eletriptan	Relpax	20–40 mg PO at onset; redose >2 hrs if needed (max = 80 mg/day)	• Within 1 wk of an MAOI				• Metabolized by CYP3A4	No
Frovatriptan	Frova	2.5 mg PO at onset; redose >2 hrs if needed (max = 7.5 mg/day)						No

Mechanism of action – butorphanol: mixed opioid agonist/antagonist with opioid analgesic properties

Generic	Brand	Dose & Max	Contra-indications	Primary Side Effects	Key Monitoring Parameters	Pertinent Drug Interactions	Med Pearls	Top 200
Butorphanol	Stadol nasal spray	1 mg (1 spray) intranasally at onset; may repeat after 1 hour and then q3–4 hrs PRN	• Hypersensitivity, CrCl <30 mL/min • Patients with a history of narcotic dependence	• Somnolence • Dizziness • Nausea • Nasal congestion • Insomnia	• Response to therapy • Presence of adverse effects	Concurrent use of other CNS depressants will have additive adverse effects and should be avoided	• Not routinely used for migraine • High addiction potential; controlled substance	No

Storage and Administration Pearls

- Store all preparations between 2–30°C (36–86°F). Protect from light.
- Place rapid disintegrating tablets directly on tongue and allow them to dissolve.
- Sumatriptan and zolmitran nasal sprays are sprayed into one nostril only.
- Sumatriptan injection is self-administered subcutaneously using prefilled syringes and an autoinjector.

Patient Education Pearls

- Rapid disintegrating tablets should be placed directly on the tongue and allowed to dissolve.
- Follow dosing recommendations carefully to decrease risk of adverse effects or dependence.

Learning Points

- Disease-modifying drugs are the agents of choice in treating MS.
- First-line choice of antiepileptic drug is based on seizure classification. Options include carbamazepine, phenytoin, lamotrigine, valproic acid, and oxcarbazepine.
- Antiepileptic drugs have a significant number of drug-drug interactions due to their impact on and metabolism by the cytochrome P450 enzyme system.
- Carbidopa/levodopa is the mainstay of therapy for PD and is available in numerous dosage forms. Controlled-and immediate-release tablets are often prescribed simultaneously.
- Anticholinergic agents should be avoided in elderly patients.
- Agents affecting dopamine, including dopamine agonists and carbidopa/levodopa, may elicit psychiatric side effects.
- Serotonin agonists are the mainstay of treatment for migraine headache and are available in numerous dosage forms.

ALZHEIMER'S DISEASE

Definition

Alzheimer's disease (AD) is a dementia of progressive nature that affects, in the early stages, primarily cognition and in later stages behavior and functional status. The pathophysiology is not fully understood but is known to involve destruction of neurons and synapses and cortical atrophy.

Diagnosis

The *Diagnostic and Statistical Manual of Mental Disorders, Fifth Edition* (DSM 5) criteria describe an insidious onset of memory impairment plus one additional cognitive defect. The diagnosis is based upon evidence of progressive cognitive decline from baseline that has reached the point of impacting social or occupational functioning along with the ruling out of reversible causes such as thyroid abnormalities, vitamin deficiencies, medication side effects, and infections.

Signs & Symptoms

Problems with memory, difficulty performing familiar tasks, forgetting information that was recently acquired, poor judgment, difficulty with abstract concepts, mood changes, and loss of interest in usual activities include some of the most common elements of the clinical presentation. The Folstein Mini-Mental State Examination (MMSE) is often used to provide staging and clinical guidance. MMSE scores of 20 or greater are considered mild AD, scores of 10–19 indicated moderate disease, and scores less than 10 indicate severe cases.

Guidelines

American College of Physicians/American Academy of Family Physicians (ACP/AAFP). Current pharmacologic treatment of dementia: a clinical practice guideline from the American College of Physicians and the American Academy of Family Physicians. *Ann Intern Med* 2008 Mar 4;148(5):370–8.

Guidelines Summary:

- Goals of treatment include preservation of function and symptomatic slowing of cognitive decline. A commonly used benchmark is the change in MMSE within one year. Without therapy, MMSE would be expected to decrease approximately 2 to 4 points per year. Therapeutic efficacy is often determined if MMSE decreases by two or fewer points per year. None of the available therapies has an impact on halting disease progression or reversing pathophysiology.
- Cholinesterase inhibitors are the treatment of choice in mild to moderate AD. Although slight differences exist in the mechanisms of these agents, there is no evidence to indicate greater efficacy with one agent over another. Agent selection is typically made based upon patient preference, cost, and potential for drug interactions. There is insufficient evidence to support a dose-response relationship within this class. It is currently recommended that patients be started on the lowest dose and titrated slowly to the typical maintenance dose.

- Memantine is the only currently available NMDA receptor agonist and has been studied and approved in moderate to severe AD as either monotherapy or an adjunct to a cholinesterase inhibitor.
- The most widely accepted approach to treatment is to initiate a low-dose cholinesterase inhibitor at the time of diagnosis with slow titration to typical maintenance dose. After 6 months to one year, efficacy is assessed. If this therapy is not efficacious, the patient can be switched to an alternate cholinesterase inhibitor or memantine can be added (in moderate to severe disease).

Storage and Administration Pearls

- Donepezil: Should be taken in evening prior to bed with or without food. Oral disintegrating tablets should be allowed to dissolve on tongue and then followed with glass of water.
- Galantamine: Ensure adequate fluid intake while on therapy, and take with food. Do not crush, break, or chew extended-release capsules.
- Rivastigmine: Apply patch to a dry, hairless area of skin (preferably upper back) and rotate site of application daily.

Patient Education Pearls

- The most common side effects are nausea, vomiting, diarrhea, and dizziness.
- Abrupt discontinuation of therapy may cause worsening of symptoms.
- The expected outcome is that the medications will slow progression. Significant improvement is not likely to be observed.

Cholinesterase Inhibitors

Mechanism of action – inhibits the activity of cholinesterase enzyme, thereby allowing greater acetylcholine activity

Generic	Brand	Dose & Max	Contraindications	Primary Side Effects	Key Monitoring Parameters	Pertinent Drug Interactions	Med Pearls	Top 200
Donepezil	• Aricept • Tablets and orally disintegrating tablets	5 mg daily, titrated to 10 mg daily after 4–6 weeks (max = 23 mg daily in moderate–severe AD)	Hypersensitivity	• Nausea • Vomiting • Diarrhea • Urinary incontinence • Dizziness • Headache • Syncope • Salivation • Sweating • Bradycardia • Hypertension	• Presence of side effects • Heart rate, blood pressure, MMSE at 6–12 month intervals	• Succinylcholine: prolonged neuromuscular blockade (AVOID) • Oxybutynin/tolterodine: decrease efficacy of donepezil • Ramelteon, ketoconazole, bethanechol, quinidine	• Slow titration can increase tolerability • Donepezil and galantamine available as generic	Yes
Galantamine	• Razadyne: oral solution, tablet • Razadyne ER: extended release capsule	• 4–12 mg PO BID • 8–24 mg PO once daily				• Oxybutynin/tolterodine: decrease efficacy of galantamine • Quinidine, ketoconazole, paroxetine, fluoxetine, fluvoxamine: increased galantamine concentrations		No
Rivastigmine	• Exelon • Capsules, oral solution, transdermal patch	• 1.5–6 mg PO BID • 4.6–9.5 mg/24 hrs (transdermal)				• Metoclopramide: increased risk of EPS (contraindicated) • Oxybutynin/tolterodine: decrease efficacy of rivastigmine		No

NMDA Receptor Antagonists

Generic	Brand	Dose & Max	Contraindications	Primary Side Effects	Key Monitoring Parameters	Pertinent Drug Interactions	Med Pearls	Top 200
Mechanism of action – NMDA receptor antagonist								
Memantine	• Namenda • Namenda XR	• 5–10 mg PO BID • 7–28 mg PO daily	Hypersensitivity	• Confusion • Constipation • Dizziness • Headache • D/V • Hypertension	• Presence of side effects • BP • MMSE at 6–12 month intervals	• Carbonic anhydrase inhibitors • Nicotine polacrilex • Quinidine • Ranitidine • Sodium bicarbonate • Cimetidine • Hydrochlorothiazide	Indicated for moderate–severe AD as monotherapy or in combination with cholinesterase inhibitor	Yes

PRACTICE QUESTIONS

1. What is recommended first-line for newly diagnosed multiple sclerosis?

    (A) Oral prednisone 50 mg PO daily for 1 week, then slowly tapered over 1 month
    (B) Betaseron
    (C) Methylprednisolone 100–500 mg/day for 3–10 days
    (D) Natalizumab
    (E) Rebif + mitoxantrone

2. What patient counseling should be provided when dispensing an interferon injectable prescription for multiple sclerosis?

    (A) If the medication cannot be used within 1 month, freeze the syringe to allow beyond-date use.
    (B) Apply heat to the injection site before and after the injection.
    (C) Try to use the same injection site each time.
    (D) If the medication reaches room temperature, it is no longer usable and must be discarded.
    (E) NSAIDs may decrease the flu-like symptoms.

3. Which of the following is associated with the use of divalproex?

    (A) Hepatotoxicity
    (B) Hirsutism
    (C) Hypoglycemia
    (D) Renal dysfunction
    (E) Thrombocytosis

4. Which of the following medications is a contraindication to using sumatriptan?

    (A) Ibuprofen
    (B) Lisinopril
    (C) Phenelzine
    (D) Sertraline
    (E) Zolpidem

5. Which of the following is a contraindication to the use of rizatriptan?

    (A) Uncontrolled HTN
    (B) History of a stroke
    (C) Peripheral arterial disease
    (D) Concomitant use of phenelzine
    (E) All of the above

ANSWERS

1. **B**

Interferon agents (such as Betaseron, Avonex, and Rebif) and glatiramer acetate (Copax-one) are considered first-line disease-modifying drugs (DMDs) for the treatment of MS. Therefore, (B) is correct. Natalizumab (D) is reserved for patients who do not respond to traditional therapy. Treatment is usually initiated one agent at a time and, as the disease progresses, treatment with DMD + mitoxantrone pulse therapy (E) may be used. Corti-costeroids (A and C) are the cornerstone of acute exacerbations but will play no role in treating the disease itself.

2. **E**

Acetaminophen or NSAIDs can reduce the flu-like symptoms associated with the inter-feron injections. The injectables for multiple sclerosis should never be frozen (A) and should always be protected from light. To ease the discomfort of the injections, ice—not heat (B)—can be applied to the injection site prior to the injection, and the injection site should be rotated each time (making choice C incorrect). It is perfectly fine and recom-mended to allow the injectable to reach room temperature prior to the injection (D), but it should otherwise be stored in the refrigerator.

3. **A**

Divalproex is associated with elevations in AST and ALT with potential hepatotoxicity. Hirsutism (B) is not correct as divalproex is associated with alopecia. Divalproex is not associated with hypoglycemia (C) and may be associated with hyperglycemia in rare instances. Divalproex does not cause renal dysfunction (D), and thrombocytosis (E) is not correct as divalproex is associated with thrombocytopenia.

4. **C**

The triptans are contraindicated if a patient has taken an MAOI within 2 weeks of using the triptan, as there is a risk of serotonin syndrome. NSAIDs may be taken with trip-tans; therefore, ibuprofen (A) is not a contraindication. Patients with uncontrolled HTN may not take triptans, but antihypertensive medications such as lisinopril (B) can be used. Sertraline (D) and zolpidem (E) may be used with triptans, but sertraline should be used with caution as there is a risk of serotonin syndrome with concomitant use.

5. **E**

Triptans cause vasoconstriction and cannot be used with ischemic heart or cerebrovas-cular disease. Patients with uncontrolled HTN (A), history of a CVA or TIA (B), PAD (C), or vasospastic condition should avoid the use of any triptan. Triptans also may cause serotonin syndrome if used within 2 weeks on an MAOI, so the combination should be avoided.

Gastrointestinal Disorders

6

This chapter covers the following diseases:

- **Gastroesophageal reflux disease/peptic ulcer disease**
- **Inflammatory bowel disease**

 Suggested Study Time: **45 minutes**

GASTROESOPHAGEAL REFLUX DISEASE/ PEPTIC ULCER DISEASE

Definitions

Gastroesophageal reflux disease (GERD) is a condition in which patients have symptoms or mucosal damage resulting from the abnormal reflux of stomach contents into the esophagus. If the esophagus is chronically exposed to these contents, inflammation of the esophagus can develop which is termed reflux esophagitis, and/or the esophageal mucosa can become ulcerated, leading to erosive esophagitis. Often, GERD results because of reduced lower esophageal sphincter (LES) pressures; however, this condition may also arise because of a delay in gastric emptying, use of certain medications or foods, or a hiatal hernia. Various medications may precipitate GERD symptoms either by decreasing LES pressure (e.g., anticholinergics, benzodiazepines, β-agonists, calcium channel blockers, dopamine agonists, estrogen, opioid narcotics, nicotine, nitrates, progesterone, theophylline) or by irritating the esophageal mucosa (e.g., nonsteroidal anti-inflammatory drugs [NSAIDs], bisphosphonates, salicylates, iron, potassium chloride).

Peptic ulcer disease (PUD) refers to the development of duodenal or gastric ulcers. The majority of PUD cases are caused by either *Helicobacter pylori* (*H. pylori*) infection or the use of NSAIDs, but can also be induced by stress. A number of risk factors exist that may predispose patients to NSAID-induced ulcers, including a prior gastrointestinal (GI) ulcer or hemorrhage; age >65 years; concurrent use of corticosteroids, antiplatelets, or anticoagulants; and chronic debilitating disorders, especially cardiovascular (CV) disease.

Patients taking NSAIDs can be categorized as being at high risk, moderate risk, or low risk for GI injury:

- High risk
  - History of previously complicated ulcer (especially recent)
  - Multiple (>2 risk factors) (see above)
- Moderate risk (1–2 risk factors)
  - Age >65 years
  - High-dose NSAID therapy
  - Previous history of uncomplicated ulcer
  - Concurrent use of aspirin (including low dose), corticosteroids, or anticoagulants
- Low risk
  - No risk factors

Diagnosis

Gastroesophageal Reflux Disease

- Diagnosis for uncomplicated cases is based primarily on description of symptoms and potential risk factors. Response to treatment can also be used as a diagnostic strategy.
- Endoscopy is recommended for the following patients:
  - Age >45 years
  - Presenting with atypical or alarm symptoms (see below)
  - Refractory to initial treatment
- Ambulatory pH testing can also be used if patients continue to have symptoms despite either normal endoscopic findings or appropriate therapy.

Peptic Ulcer Disease

- Clinical history (including symptoms and history of medication use) can be helpful in arriving at a preliminary diagnosis (not important to differentiate between duodenal and gastric ulcers).
- All patients with a suspected diagnosis of PUD should be tested for *H. pylori*.
  - Invasive tests (endoscopy): rapid urease tests (80–95% sensitive, 95–100% specific; false negatives can occur if patients previously on proton pump inhibitor

[PPIs], H_2 receptor antagonist, or bismuth therapy; patient needs to be off these drugs for at least 1 week before performing this test)

- Noninvasive tests:
  - » Serological: 85% sensitive, 79% specific; not influenced by prior acid-suppressive therapy; can be used to confirm diagnosis but will not be helpful in determining eradication of infection
  - » Urea breath test: 97% sensitive, 95% specific; influenced by prior acid-suppressive and antibiotic therapy ($\uparrow$ risk of false negative); can be used to confirm diagnosis and eradication
  - » Stool antigen test: 88–92% sensitive, 87% specific; influenced by prior acid-suppressive therapy; can be used to confirm diagnosis and eradication

Signs and Symptoms

Gastroesophageal Reflux Disease

- Typical symptoms: Heartburn (pyrosis), regurgitation, belching, water brash ($\uparrow$ salivation)
- Atypical symptoms: Noncardiac chest pain, hoarseness, nausea, asthma-like symptoms, chronic cough, sore throat, dental erosions
- Alarm symptoms (indicate need for immediate evaluation): Dysphagia (difficulty swallowing), odynophagia (painful swallowing), bleeding, weight loss
- Long-term complications: Esophageal strictures, Barrett's esophagus, esophageal cancer

Peptic Ulcer Disease

- Abdominal pain (usually epigastric): The most common symptom
  - Can be described as burning, discomfort, or fullness
  - Duodenal ulcer: Pain often occurs 1–3 hours after a meal and is relieved with food
  - Gastric ulcer: Pain brought on by food
- Other symptoms: Heartburn, belching, bloating, nausea, anorexia
- Long-term complications: Upper GI bleeding, perforation

Guidelines

Gastroesophageal Reflux Disease

Katz PO, Gerson LB, Vela MF. Guidelines for the diagnosis and management of gastroesophageal reflux disease. *Am J Gastroenterol* 2013;108:308–28.

Peptic Ulcer Disease

Chey WD, Wong BC; Practice Parameters Committee of the American College of Gastroenterology. American College of Gastroenterology guideline on the management of *Helicobacter pylori* infection. *Am J Gastroenterol* 2007;102:1808–25.

Lanza FL, Chan FK, Quigley EM; Practice Parameters Committee of the American College of Gastroenterology. Guidelines for prevention of NSAID-related ulcer complications. *Am J Gastroenterol* 2009;104:728–38.

Lanza FL; Parameters of the American College of Gastroenterology. A guideline for the treatment and prevention of NSAID-induced ulcers. Members of the Ad Hoc Committee on Practice. *Am J Gastroenterol* 1998;93:2037–46.

Guidelines Summary

Gastroesophageal Reflux Disease

The goals of therapy are to relieve symptoms, promote healing of esophageal mucosa, prevent recurrence, and prevent complications.

- **Lifestyle modifications**
  - Unlikely to control symptoms, when used alone, in most patients
  - Dietary changes: Avoid foods that can worsen symptoms (alcohol, caffeine, chocolate, citrus juices, peppermint/spearmint, coffee, spicy foods, tomatoes, high-fatty meals, garlic, onions); avoid eating before bedtime; remain upright after meals
  - Weight loss
  - Smoking cessation
  - Head elevated off the bed by 6–8 inches
  - No tight-fitting clothes
  - No medications that can worsen symptoms
- **Pharmacological therapy**
  - Step 1: Antacids and over-the-counter (OTC) acid suppressants (H_2 receptor antagonists, omeprazole, lansoprazole) can be used initially on an as-needed basis for intermittent or mild symptoms. If symptoms persist after 2 weeks, proceed to Step 2.
  - Step 2: PPI or H_2 receptor antagonist (can be used at higher prescription doses).
    - » PPIs are considered more effective than H_2 receptor antagonists.
  - A promotility agent (e.g., metoclopramide) can be used as adjunctive therapy, if needed.

Peptic Ulcer Disease

The goals of therapy are to relieve symptoms, promote healing of the ulcer, eradicate *H. pylori* (if present), prevent recurrence, and prevent complications.

- **Lifestyle modifications:** Reduce stress, smoking cessation, discontinue NSAID use, avoid foods that can worsen symptoms
- **Pharmacological therapy**
  - *H. pylori*-associated ulcers: PPI + two antibiotics (usually clarithromycin and amoxicillin); duration = 10–14 days. If this therapy fails, four-drug therapy should be used (PPI + bismuth + metronidazole + tetracycline); duration = 14 days.
  - NSAID-induced ulcers
    - » Treatment:
      - First-line therapy: PPI (duration of therapy = 6–8 weeks; may be longer if recurrent symptoms, heavy smoker, or continued NSAID use)
      - Second-line therapies: Misoprostol or H_2 receptor antagonist
    - » Primary prevention:
      - Recommendations based on whether patient is at low, moderate, or high risk for NSAID GI toxicity (see Definitions) and the patient's risk for CV disease; high CV risk is defined by the patient's need for low-dose aspirin to prevent future CV events

	Low GI Risk	Moderate GI Risk	High GI Risk
Low CV Risk	NSAID alone	NSAID + PPI/misoprostol	Alternative therapy, if possible; or, cyclooxygenase-2 inhibitor + PPI/misoprostol
High CV Risk	Naproxen + PPI/misoprostol	Naproxen + PPI/misoprostol	Avoid NSAIDS or cyclooxygenase-2 inhibitors; use alternative therapy

Antacids

Mechanism of action – neutralize stomach acid and ↑ gastric pH

Generic	Brand	Dose	Contra-indications	Primary Side Effects	Key Monitoring	Pertinent Drug Interactions	Med Pearl	Top 200
Magnesium hydroxide/ aluminum hydroxide	Alamag	15 mL with meals and at bedtime	None	• Diarrhea (from magnesium [Mg^{2+}]) • Constipation (from aluminum [Al^{3+}] or calcium [Ca^{2+}])	S/S GERD	• May bind to numerous drugs (separate from other drugs by at least 2 hrs) • May ↓ absorption of drugs whose absorption is pH-dependent (e.g., itraconazole, ketoconazole, iron, atazanavir)	Use Mg^{2+}- and Al^{3+}- containing products with caution in patients with renal dysfunction	No
Calcium carbonate	• Tums • Maalox Chewables	1–2 tabs q2h as needed						No

H₂ Receptor Antagonists

Mechanism of action – reversibly inhibit histamine (H_2) receptors in the gastric parietal cells, which inhibits secretion of gastric acid

Generic	Brand	Dose	Dosage Forms	Primary Side Effects	Key Monitoring	Pertinent Drug Interactions	Med Pearl	Top 200
Cimetidine	Tagamet	200–1,600 mg/day	• Rx: Tabs, solution • OTC: Tabs	• Headache • Fatigue • Dizziness • Confusion • Gynecomastia (cimetidine)	S/S GERD/PUD	• Cimetidine inhibits CYP enzymes to greater extent than the other drugs (inhibits CYP1A2, CYP2C19, CYP2D6, and CYP3A4) • May ↓ absorption of drugs whose absorption is pH-dependent (e.g., itraconazole, ketoconazole, iron, atazanavir)	• Adjust dose of all drugs in renal dysfunction • Pepcid Complete also contains calcium carbonate + magnesium hydroxide	No
Famotidine	Pepcid	20–80 mg/day	• Rx: Tabs, suspension, injection • OTC: Tabs					Yes
Nizatidine	Axid	150–300 mg/day	• Rx: Caps, solution • OTC: Tabs					No
Ranitidine	Zantac	75–300 mg/day	• Rx: Tabs, syrup, injection • OTC: Tabs					Yes

Proton Pump Inhibitors

Generic	Brand	Dose	Dosage Forms	Primary Side Effects	Key Monitoring	Pertinent Drug Interactions	Med Pearl	Top 200
Mechanism of action – irreversibly inhibit H+/K+-ATPase in gastric parietal cells, which inhibits secretion of gastric acid								
Dexlansoprazole	Dexilant	30–60 mg/day	Caps	• Diarrhea • Headache	S/S GERD/PUD	• May ↓ absorption of drugs whose absorption is pH-dependent (e.g., itraconazole, ketoconazole, iron, atazanavir) • May ↓ antiplatelet effects of clopidogrel	• Zegerid is omeprazole + sodium bicarbonate (available as caps or suspension) • Vimovo is esomeprazole + naproxen • May be associated with: • Osteoporosis-related fractures • ↓ Mg^{2+} • ↑ risk of *Clostridium difficile*	Yes
Esomeprazole	Nexium	20–40 mg/day	Caps, granules for suspension, injection					Yes
Lansoprazole	Prevacid	15–30 mg/day	Caps, orally disintegrating tabs, suspension OTC: Caps					Yes
Omeprazole	Prilosec	20 mg/day	Rx: Caps, granules for suspension, suspension OTC: Tabs					Yes
Pantoprazole	Protonix	20–40 mg/day	Tabs, granules for suspension, injection					Yes
Rabeprazole	Aciphex	20 mg/day	Tabs, capsule sprinkle					Yes

Promotility Drug

Generic	Brand	Dose	Contra-indications	Primary Side Effects	Key Monitoring	Pertinent Drug Interactions	Med Pearl	Top 200
Mechanism of action – dopamine antagonist; ↑ LES pressure and accelerates gastric emptying								
Metoclopramide	• Reglan • Metozolv ODT	40–60 mg/day	Seizures	• Dizziness • Sedation • Diarrhea • Extrapyramidal symptoms (EPS)	• S/S GERD • EPS	Use with antipsychotic agents may ↑ risk of EPS	• Can also be used for diabetic gastroparesis; erythromycin is an alternative • ↓ dose in renal dysfuction	Yes

Mucosal Protectant Drug

Generic	Brand	Dose	Contra-indications	Primary Side Effects	Key Monitoring	Pertinent Drug Interactions	Med Pearl	Top 200
Mechanism of action – nonabsorbable aluminum salt that forms bonds with damaged and normal GI tissue; complex forms protective cover over ulcerated area								
Sucralfate	Carafate	4 g/day	None	Constipation	S/S PUD	May bind to numerous drugs (separate from other drugs by at least 2 hrs)	• Use cautiously in patients with chronic kidney disease (↑ risk of Al³⁺ toxicity) • Limited value in treatment of GERD; more useful in treatment of PUD	Yes

Prostaglandin Analog

Generic	Brand	Dose	Contraindications	Primary Side Effects	Key Monitoring	Pertinent Drug Interactions	Med Pearl	Top 200
Mechanism of action – prostaglandin E1 analog; replaces protective prostaglandins inhibited by NSAID therapy								
Misoprostol	Cytotec	400–800 mcg/day	Pregnancy (abortifacient) (Pregnancy Category X)	Diarrhea	S/S PUD	None	• Women of childbearing age should have pregnancy test before initiating therapy; educate regarding appropriate use of contraception • Can also be used for medical termination of pregnancy	No

Chapter 6: Gastrointestinal Disorders

Helicobacter pylori Treatment Regimens (for PUD)

Proton Pump Inhibitor	Drug #2	Drug #3	Drug #4	Comments
Three-Drug Regimen (PPI + two antibiotics; duration of therapy = 10–14 days; 14 days preferred)				
Esomeprazole 40 mg daily OR lansoprazole 30 mg 2 × daily OR omeprazole 20 mg 2 × daily OR pantoprazole 40 mg 2 × daily OR rabeprazole 20 mg 2 × daily	Amoxicillin 1,000 mg 2 × daily	Clarithromycin 500 mg 2 × daily		• Metronidazole (500 mg 2 × daily) can be used instead of amoxicillin or clarithromycin in patients with penicillin or macrolide allergy, respectively • Rabeprazole regimen should be given for 7 days • Prevpac is a compliance package that contains individual units of lansoprazole, amoxicillin, and clarithromycin • Omeclamox-Pak is a compliance package that contains individual units of omeprazole, amoxicillin, and clarithromycin
Four-Drug Regimen (PPI + bismuth subsalicylate + metronidazole + tetracycline; duration of therapy = 14 days)				
Esomeprazole 40 mg daily OR lansoprazole 30 mg 2 × daily OR omeprazole 20 mg 2 × daily OR pantoprazole 40 mg 2 × daily OR rabeprazole 20 mg 2 × daily	Bismuth subsalicylate 525 mg 4 × daily	Metronidazole 250 mg 4 × daily	Tetracycline 500 mg 4 × daily	• Pylera contains bismuth, metronidazole, and tetracycline in each capsule • Can alternatively use H_2 antagonist instead of PPI (4-drug regimen given for 2 weeks and then H_2 antagonist alone continued for additional 2 weeks)

KAPLAN) MEDICAL   201

Storage and Administration Pearls

- Esomeprazole
  - May be administered via nasogastric (NG) or orogastric (OG) tube
    - » Capsules: Open the capsule and mix with water
    - » Granules for oral suspension: Dilute granules in water
  - Capsules can be opened and mixed with applesauce (eat immediately)
  - Mix granules for oral suspension in water
- Lansoprazole
  - May be administered via NG or OG tube
    - » Capsules: Open the capsule and mix with apple juice
    - » Orally disintegrating tablets: Dilute tablet in water
  - Capsules can be opened and mixed with applesauce, Ensure pudding, cottage cheese, or yogurt (swallow immediately); can also mix in orange, apple, or tomato juice (swallow immediately)
- Dexlansoprazole
  - May be administered via NG tube: Open the capsule and mix with water
  - Capsules can be opened and mixed with applesauce (eat immediately); can also mix in water to be given via oral syringe
- Omeprazole
  - May be administered via NG or OG tube
    - » Granules for oral suspension: Dilute granules in water
  - Capsules can be opened and mixed with applesauce (eat immediately); **cannot be given via NG or OG tube**
  - **Tablets should not be crushed**
- Pantoprazole
  - May be administered via NG or OG tube
    - » Granules for oral suspension: Dilute in apple juice
  - Tablets: Should **not** be crushed; **cannot** be given via NG or OG tube
  - Granules for oral suspension can be mixed in apple juice or sprinkled on applesauce
- Rabeprazole
  - Tablets should **not** be crushed; **cannot** be given via NG or OG tube
  - Sprinkle capsules can be opened and sprinkled on apple sauce, baby food (fruit or vegetable-based), or yogurt or mixed in apple juice, infant formula, or pediatric electrolyte solution; **cannot** be given via NG or OG tube
- Misoprostol should be administered with meals
- Sucralfate should be administered 1 hour before meals

Patient Education Pearls

- Lifestyle changes should be continued throughout the course of therapy
- Patient should separate the administration of antacids from other medications by at least 2 hours
- PPIs should be taken 15–30 minutes before breakfast; if patient is taking two daily doses, final dose should be taken before dinner (not at bedtime).
- A patient who is being treated for *H. pylori* should complete the entire course of therapy to facilitate eradication of the infection.

INFLAMMATORY BOWEL DISEASE

Definitions

Inflammatory bowel disease (IBD) is a broad term used to describe two conditions: ulcerative colitis (UC) and Crohn's disease (CD). UC is a chronic inflammatory disease that consists of superficial mucosal lesions localized to the colon and rectum. CD is also a chronic inflammatory disease, but is characterized by transmural lesions that can occur anywhere along the GI tract. The etiology of both of these disorders is thought to be due to immunologic or infectious causes; however, environmental, psychological, or genetic factors may also contribute to the development of these diseases.

Diagnosis

Diagnosis is suspected on the basis of clinical presentation, but is confirmed through various studies, including sigmoidoscopy, colonoscopy, barium enema, and stool examination. A biopsy of the lesions is usually performed during the sigmoidoscopy or colonoscopy.

Signs and Symptoms

The following symptoms can occur with both UC and CD: fever, diarrhea, weight loss, rectal bleeding, and abdominal pain.

Clinical Findings Associated with Ulcerative Colitis or Crohn's Disease

Clinical Finding	Ulcerative Colitis	Crohn's Disease
Abdominal mass	No	Yes
Fistulas/strictures	No	Yes
Bowel involvement	Rectum/colon	Can affect anywhere from mouth to anus (often affects ileum)
Systemic complications (i.e., extraintestinal involvement)	Yes	Yes
Toxic megacolon	Yes	No
At risk for colorectal cancer	Yes	Rare
Pattern of inflammation	Continuous	Segmented ("cobblestone" appearance)

Severity of Disease: Ulcerative Colitis

- Mild: >4 stools/day (with or without blood), no systemic signs of toxicity, and normal erythrocyte sedimentation rate (ESR)
- Moderate: >4 stools/day and minimal signs of toxicity
- Severe: >6 stools/day (with blood) and evidence of toxicity (e.g., fever, tachycardia, anemia, or elevated ESR)

Severity of Disease: Crohn's Disease

- Mild-moderate: Ambulatory and able to tolerate oral intake without evidence of dehydration, systemic toxicity, abdominal tenderness, painful mass, intestinal obstruction, or >10% weight loss
- Moderate-severe: Fail to respond to treatment for mild-moderate disease or have fever, significant weight loss (>10%), abdominal mass/tenderness, intermittent nausea/vomiting (without findings of obstruction), or significant anemia
- Severe/fulminant: Persistent symptoms despite the initiation of treatment with corticosteroids or biologic agents as outpatients or presenting with high fevers, persistent vomiting, evidence of intestinal obstruction, significant peritoneal signs (e.g., rebound tenderness, cachexia, or evidence of abscess)

Guidelines

Kornbluth A, Sachar DB; Practice Parameters Committee of the American College of Gastroenterology. Ulcerative colitis practice guidelines in adults: American College of Gastroenterology, Practice Parameters Committee. *Am J Gastroenterol* 2010;105:501–23.

Lichtenstein GR, Hanauer SB, Sandborn WJ; Practice Parameters Committee of American College of Gastroenterology. Management of Crohn's disease in adults. *Am J Gastroenterol* 2009;104:465–83.

Guidelines Summary

The goals of therapy are to induce and maintain remission, to prevent and resolve complications and systemic symptoms, and to maintain quality of life. There is no pharmacologic cure for these diseases; therefore, treatment focuses on management of symptoms.

- **Nonpharmacologic therapy**
  - Lifestyle changes/diet: Avoid foods that may worsen disease symptoms
  - Possible surgery when complications (e.g., fistulas, strictures, perforation) develop or to manage refractory disease

- **Pharmacologic therapy**
  - Adjunctive therapies: antidiarrheals (e.g., loperamide), antispasmodics (e.g., dicyclomine, propantheline, hyoscyamine)
  - Ulcerative colitis:
    » Treatment based upon whether inflammation is distal (below the splenic flexure; topical therapy appropriate) or extensive (proximal to the splenic flexure; requires systemic therapy)
    » Mild/moderate distal disease:
      - Active disease: Topical mesalamine (enema or suppository preferred), oral aminosalicylate, topical corticosteroid
      - Maintenance of remission: Topical mesalamine or oral aminosalicylate
    » Mild/moderate extensive disease:
      - Active disease: Oral aminosalicylate (first-line), oral corticosteroids, azathioprine, 6-mercaptopurine, infliximab
      - Maintenance of remission: Oral aminosalicylate (first-line), azathioprine, 6-mercaptopurine, infliximab, adalimumab, or golimumab
    » Severe disease:
      - Infliximab (if urgent hospitalization not needed), intravenous (IV) corticosteroids (if urgent hospitalization needed), IV cyclosporine
  - Crohn's disease:
    » Mild/moderate active disease:
      - First-line: Oral aminosalicylate, budesonide (disease localized to ileum and/or right colon)
      - Second-line: Metronidazole, ciprofloxacin
    » Moderate/severe disease:
      - First-line: Prednisone
      - Second-line: Infliximab, adalimumab, certolizumab pegol, natalizumab, methotrexate (intramuscularly [IM] or subcutaneously [SC])
    » Severe/fulminant disease:
      - First-line: IV corticosteroids
      - Second-line: IV cyclosporine or IV tacrolimus
    » Maintenance therapy:
      - First line: Azathioprine, 6-mercaptopurine, methotrexate, infliximab, adalimumab, certolizumab pegol, or natalizumab

Aminosalicylates

Mechanism of action – ↓ inflammation in GI tract by inhibiting prostaglandin synthesis and subsequent production of various immune mediators; sulfasalazine is cleaved in colon to mesalamine (responsible for therapeutic effect) + sulfapyridine (causes side effects); olsalazine and balsalazide also contain mesalamine

Generic	Brand	Dose	Dosage Forms	Contra-indications	Primary Side Effects	Key Monitoring	Med Pearl	Top 200
Sulfasalazine	• Azulfidine • Azulfidine EN • Sulfazine	• Induction: 3–4 g/day • Maintenance: 2 g/day	Tabs, delayed-release (enteric-coated) tabs	• Aspirin allergy • Sulfa allergy • G6PD deficiency • Pregnancy (near term)	• Stevens-Johnson syndrome • Photosensitivity • Nausea/vomiting (N/V) • Headache • Folate deficiency • Hemolytic anemia • Agranulocytosis • Hepatitis	• S/S IBD • Liver function tests (LFTs) (with sulfasalazine) • Complete blood count (CBC) (with sulfasalazine)	• Mesalamine, olsalazine, and balsalazide are not sulfa derivatives; are poorly absorbed from GI tract (better tolerated than sulfasalazine) • Folic acid should be given to patients on sulfasalazine • Sulfasalazine may ↑ effects of warfarin and oral hypoglycemics • All may ↓ absorption of digoxin	No
Mesalamine	• Apriso • Asacol HD • Canasa • Delzicol • Lialda • Pentasa • Rowasa	• Oral: *Induction* 2.4–4.8 g/day; *Maintenance,* 1.5–4 g/day • Rectal enema (Rowasa): 4 g at bedtime • Rectal suppository (Canasa): 1 g at bedtime	Extended-release caps, delayed-release tabs, rectal enema, rectal suppository	• Aspirin allergy • G6PD deficiency	• Nausea • Diarrhea • Headache • Malaise			No
Olsalazine	Dipentum	1–3 g/day	Caps					No
Balsalazide	Colazal, Giazo	1.5–6.75 g/day	Caps, tabs					No

Corticosteroids

Generic	Brand	Dose	Dosage Forms	Contra-indications	Primary Side Effects	Key Monitoring	Med Pearl	Top 200
Mechanism of action – quickly ↓ inflammation during acute exacerbations of IBD								
Budesonide	• Entocort EC • Uceris	• Initial: 9 mg 1 × daily for up to 2 mo • Maintenance: 6 mg 1 × daily for up to 3 mo	Extended-release caps, extended release tabs	None	• Hyperglycemia • ↑ appetite • Insomnia • Hypertension • Edema • Adrenal suppression • Osteoporosis • Cataracts • Delayed wound healing	• S/S IBD • Blood glucose • Blood pressure (BP) • Electrolytes	• Should only be used to treat acute exacerbation (4–8 wks) and then tapered • IV therapy given for severe exacerbations for 7–10 days, then switched to oral therapy • Budesonide has localized effect; has minimal systemic side effects • Entocort EC indicated for CD • Uceris indicated for UC	No
Methylprednisolone	Solu-Medrol	10–100 mg/day	Injection, tabs					Yes
Prednisone	Sterapred	20–60 mg/day	Tabs					Yes

Immunosuppressants

Mechanism of action – ↓ production of inflammatory mediators (e.g., interleukins) through various mechanisms

Generic	Brand	Dose	Contra-indications	Primary Side Effects	Key Monitoring	Pertinent Drug Interactions	Med Pearl	Top 200
Azathioprine	Imuran	75–150 mg/day	• Pregnancy • Bone marrow suppression • Liver dysfunction	• Pancreatitis • Arthralgias • Nausea • Diarrhea • Rash • Bone marrow suppression • Hepatotoxicity	• Amylase/lipase (if symptoms) • CBC with differential • LFTs	• Allopurinol and febuxostat may ↑ risk of side effects (↓ azathioprine dose by 75% when used with allopurinol; avoid concomitant use with febuxostat) • Aminosalicylates may ↑ risk of side effects • May ↓ effects of warfarin	• 6-mercaptopurine is active metabolite of azathioprine • Adjust dose in patients with renal dysfunction	No
6-Mercaptopurine	Purinethol	50–100 mg/day						No
Cyclosporine	Sandimmune	4–8 mg/kg/day IV	Renal failure	• Hypertension • Nephrotoxicity • Hypomagnesemia • Infection • Anaphylaxis	• BP • Blood urea nitrogen (BUN)/serum creatinine (SCr) • Electrolytes • S/S infection • Cyclosporine levels	• Cyclosporine is a CYP3A4 substrate and inhibitor • CYP3A4 inhibitors may ↑ levels/toxicity • CYP3A4 inducers may ↓ effects • May ↑ effects of other CYP3A4 substrates	• Used only for severe disease that has not responded to corticosteroids • Used only for 7–10 days	No
Methotrexate	Rheumatrex	15–25 mg/wk IM or SC	• Pregnancy • Bone marrow suppression • Severe renal or hepatic dysfunction	• Hepatotoxicity • Bone marrow suppression • Pneumonitis • Rash • N/V • Diarrhea	• LFTs • CBC with differential • Chest x-ray (if symptoms)	• NSAIDs and salicylates ↑ risk of toxicity • Penicillins, sulfonamides, and tetracyclines may ↑ risk of toxicity	• Only effective for CD (useful for steroid-dependent and steroid-refractory CD) • Adjust dose in patients with renal dysfunction	Yes

Biological Agents

Mechanism of action — inhibit tumor necrosis factor (TNF)

Generic	Brand	Dose	Contraindications	Primary Side Effects	Key Monitoring	Pertinent Drug Interactions	Med Pearl	Top 200
Adalimumab	Humira	160 mg SC on day 1 or over 2 days, then 80 mg 2 wk later (day 15), then 40 mg every other wk beginning day 29	None	• Headache • Rash • Injection site reactions • Hypertension • Infection (especially tuberculosis or fungal infections) • Lymphoma • Heart failure exacerbation • Bone marrow suppression • Lupus-like syndrome	• S/S infection • S/S heart failure • CBC with differential	Do not administer live vaccines	• PPD should be done before initiating treatment • Approved for moderately to severely active CD or UC in patients who have not responded despite adequate therapy with a corticosteroid or immunosuppressant	No
Certolizumab pegol	Cimzia	400 mg SC at 0, 2, and 4 wks; then 400 mg every 4 wks	None	• Headache • Nausea • Hypersensitivity reactions • Hypertension • Infection (especially tuberculosis or fungal infections) • Lymphoma • Heart failure exacerbation • Bone marrow suppression • Lupus-like syndrome			• PPD should be done before initiating treatment • Only approved for moderately to severely active CD in patients who have not responded despite adequate therapy with a corticosteroid or immunosuppressant	No
Golimumab	Simponi	200 mg SC at wk 0, then 100 mg at wk 2, then 100 mg every 4 wk	None	• Hypersensitivity reactions • Hypertension • Infection (especially tuberculosis or fungal infections) • Lymphoma • Heart failure exacerbation • Bone marrow suppression	• S/S of infection • S/S of heart failure • CBC with differential	Do not administer live vaccines	• PPD should be done before initiating treatment • Only approved for moderately to severely active UC in patients who have not responded despite adequate therapy with a corticosteroid or immunosuppressant	No

Biological Agents (cont'd)

Generic	Brand	Dose	Contra-indications	Primary Side Effects	Key Monitoring	Pertinent Drug Interactions	Med Pearl	Top 200
Infliximab	Remicade	5 mg/kg IV at 0, 2, and 6 wks; then every 8 wks	• NYHA class III or IV heart failure (for doses >5 mg/kg) • Active infection	• Infusion reactions (hypotension, fever, chills, urticaria, pruritus) • Delayed hypersensitivity (fever, rash, myalgia, headache, sore throat) • Infection (especially tuberculosis or fungal infections) • Heart failure exacerbation • Bone marrow suppression • Lymphoma • Hepatitis	• BP • LFTs • S/S infection • S/S heart failure • CBC with differential	Do not administer live vaccines	• Delayed hypersensitivity reaction may occur 3–10 days after administration • PPD should be done before initiating treatment • Approved for moderately to severely active CD or UC in patients who have not responded despite adequate therapy with a corticosteroid or immunosuppressant	No

Mechanism of action – ↓ inflammation by binding to α4-subunit of integrins

Generic	Brand	Dose	Contra-indications	Primary Side Effects	Key Monitoring	Pertinent Drug Interactions	Med Pearl	Top 200
Natalizumab	Tysabri	300 mg IV every 4 wks; discontinue if no response by week 12	Progressive multifocal leukoencephalopathy (PML); concurrent use of tumor necrosis factor inhibitors or immunosuppressants	• Headache • Fatigue • Depression • Rash • Nausea • Arthralgia • Infusion reactions • PML (may be fatal) • Infection • Hepatotoxicity	• S/S PML • Brain MRI (at baseline) • S/S infection • LFTs	Do not administer live vaccines	• Patients need to be enrolled in CD-TOUCH program • Must be administered as monotherapy • Only approved for moderate to severely active CD in patients who are refractory to or unable to tolerate conventional therapies and TNF inhibitors	No

Mechanism of action – integrin receptor antagonist; monoclonal antibody

Generic	Brand	Dose	Contra-indications	Primary Side Effects	Key Monitoring	Pertinent Drug Interactions	Med Pearl	Top 200
Vedolizumab	Entyvio	300 mg IV at 0, 2, and 6 wks; then every 8 wks	None	• Hypersensitivity reactions • Infusion reactions (especially tuberculosis) • Infection • PML • Hepatotoxicity	• S/S of infection • S/S of PML • LFTs	Do not administer live vaccines	• Consider performing PPD before treatment • Approved for moderately to severely active CD or UC in patients who are refractory to or unable to tolerate TNF blocker or corticosteroid therapy	No

Storage and Administration Pearls

- Patients receiving infliximab should be pretreated with antihistamines (H_1 and H_2 blockers), acetaminophen, and/or corticosteroid to prevent infusion-related reaction.
- Infliximab should be administered as an IV infusion over 2 hours.
- Natalizumab should be administered as an IV infusion over 1 hour.
- If switching from prednisone to budesonide, prednisone should be tapered over a period of 2 weeks.

Patient Education Pearls

- Adherence to medication is very important as disease exacerbations can have a significant impact on quality of life.
- Mesalamine enemas and suppositories should be administered at bedtime to allow for direct contact of the drug with the rectal mucosa for at least 8 hours.
- Live vaccines should not be administered if a patient is receiving biological agents.
- Patients receiving azathioprine, 6-mercaptopurine, methotrexate, infliximab, adalimumab, certolizumab pegol, golimumab, or natalizumab are at increased risk for infection. They should wash their hands frequently and avoid crowds or other persons who are sick.
- Patients taking sulfasalazine should wear sunscreen and protective clothing. Sulfasalazine should be taken with meals to minimize GI effects. Patients taking sulfasalazine should take folic acid (1 mg/day) to prevent folate deficiency. Sulfasalazine may cause an orange discoloration of body fluids (urine, tears), which may stain clothing and contact lenses.
- Women receiving azathioprine, 6-mercaptopurine, or methotrexate should be counseled on using appropriate contraceptive methods.
- NSAIDs and high-dose salicylates (not the doses of aspirin used for prevention of CV diseases) may increase the risk of methotrexate toxicity and should be avoided if the patient is receiving this immunosuppressant.

Learning Points

- **GERD/PUD**
    - Antacids should be separated from other medications by at least 2 hours because of the risk for binding and $\downarrow$ the absorption of these drugs.
    - The majority of PUD cases are caused by either *H. pylori* infection or NSAIDs.
    - Three-drug regimen (PPI + two antibiotics [usually clarithromycin and amoxicillin]) is recommended for treatment of *H. pylori* infection.

- The dosage of all H_2 antagonists needs to be adjusted in patients with renal insufficiency.
- Of all the H_2 antagonists, cimetidine is the most likely to be involved with drug interactions involving the CYP450 system.
- Of all the PPIs, only esomeprazole and pantoprazole are available as IV injection; also be familiar with the various dosage forms of the PPIs.

- **IBD**
  - Sulfasalazine should not be used in patients with sulfa allergies. The other aminosalicylates—mesalamine, olsalazine, and balsalazide—can be used in these patients.
  - Folic acid should be administered to patients receiving sulfasalazine to prevent folate deficiency.
  - Know the various dosage forms of the aminosalicylates.
  - Be familiar with the side effects of systemic corticosteroids.
  - Methotrexate is only effective for CD.
  - PPD should be performed prior to starting adalimumab, certolizumab pegol, golimumab, or infliximab.
  - Infliximab is associated with infusion reactions; patients need to be pretreated with antihistamine, acetaminophen, and/or corticosteroid.
  - Natalizumab is associated with PML.

PRACTICE QUESTIONS

1. Remicade is the brand name for which of the following drugs?

    (A) Azathioprine
    (B) Budesonide
    (C) Cyclosporine
    (D) Infliximab
    (E) Balsalazide

2. Which of the following is a contraindication for the use of metoclopramide?

    (A) Hyperkalemia
    (B) Myasthenia gravis
    (C) Porphyria
    (D) Seizure disorder
    (E) Sulfa allergy

3. A patient using NSAIDs for chronic pain develops a bleeding ulcer. Which of the following drugs would be MOST appropriate to treat his condition?

    (A) Aluminum hydroxide
    (B) Bismuth subsalicylate
    (C) Calcium carbonate
    (D) Metoclopramide
    (E) Misoprostol

4. A patient who is taking warfarin for chronic atrial fibrillation develops GERD. Which of the following drugs would be MOST likely to interact with the warfarin and increase this patient's risk for bleeding?

    (A) Cimetidine
    (B) Pantoprazole
    (C) Magnesium hydroxide
    (D) Misoprostol
    (E) Sucralfate

5. Which of the following reasons MOST likely explains why the plasma levels of ketoconazole are decreased in patients who are taking lansoprazole?

    (A) Lansoprazole induces the CYP450 enzymes that metabolize ketoconazole.
    (B) Ketoconazole requires an acidic environment for its oral absorption.
    (C) Lansoprazole binds acidic drugs in the GI tract.
    (D) Lansoprazole has prokinetic effects, which increase GI transit time.
    (E) There is a competition for transport mechanisms in the GI tract.

6. Which of the following medications needs to be dose-adjusted in patients with renal dysfunction?

    I. Esomeprazole
    II. Metoclopramide
    III. Ranitidine

(A) I only
(B) III only
(C) I and II only
(D) II and III only
(E) I, II, and III

7. A patient with ulcerative colitis (UC) has a history of anaphylaxis when taking trimethoprim/sulfamethoxazole. Which of the following drugs would be safe to use for the treatment of UC in this patient?

    I. Azulfidine
    II. Dipentum
    III. Asacol HD

(A) I only
(B) III only
(C) I and II only
(D) II and III only
(E) I, II, and III

8. Which of the following characteristics is more likely to occur with UC than Crohn's disease (CD)?

(A) Confinement of the disease to the colon and rectum
(B) Fistula formation
(C) Cobblestone pattern of inflammation
(D) Transmural lesion in the GI tract
(E) Systemic complications

9. Which of the following supplements may be needed in a patient taking chronic sulfasalazine therapy for IBD?

(A) Calcium carbonate
(B) Folic acid
(C) Iron
(D) Vitamin B_{12}
(E) Vitamin C

10. Which of the following baseline tests should be performed before a patient begins certolizumab pegol therapy for CD?

    (A) Brain MRI
    (B) LFTs
    (C) PPD
    (D) Serum creatinine
    (E) Uric acid

ANSWERS

1. **D**

Remicade is the brand name for infliximab. Imuran is the brand name for azathioprine (A). Entocort EC is the brand name for oral budesonide (B). Sandimmune, Gengraf, and Neoral are brand names for cyclosporine (C). Colazal is the brand name for balsalazide (E).

2. **D**

Seizure disorder is a contraindication for the use of metoclopramide; therefore, choice (D) is correct.

3. **E**

The first-line therapy for an NSAID-induced ulcer is a PPI. However, no PPIs are listed as answer choices. Appropriate second-line therapies for an NSAID-induced ulcer are either misoprostol or an H_2 receptor antagonist. Misoprostol is a prostaglandin E1 analog that acts to replace protective prostaglandins that have been inhibited by NSAID therapy. Aluminum hydroxide (A), bismuth subsalicylate (B), calcium carbonate (C), and metoclopramide (D) would not be appropriate treatments for a NSAID-induced ulcer.

4. **A**

Cimetidine is a strong inhibitor of CYP3A4 and a moderate inhibitor of CYP1A2. It is also a weak inhibitor of CYP2C9. (R)-warfarin is a substrate of CYP3A4 and CYP1A2, while (S)-warfarin is a substrate of CYP2C9. Therefore, cimetidine has the potential to inhibit the metabolism of both the (S)- and (R)-enantiomers of warfarin, which could lead to an increased risk of bleeding. Pantoprazole (B), magnesium hydroxide (C), misoprostol (D), and sucralfate (E) do not inhibit CYP450 system and therefore should not increase the risk of bleeding with warfarin.

5. **B**

The absorption of ketoconazole is pH-dependent; this antifungal drug requires an acidic environment to be adequately absorbed; therefore, the bioavailability of this drug decreases as gastric pH increases. By increasing gastric pH, lansoprazole may reduce the absorption of ketoconazole, which would lead to decreased plasma concentrations. Lansoprazole is not known to be an inducer of CYP450 isoenzymes (A). If anything, it may be a weak inhibitor of CYP2C19; however, this inhibition would not have any effect on ketoconazole plasma concentrations. Lansoprazole does not bind to acidic drugs in the GI tract (C). Lansoprazole also does not have prokinetic effects in the GI tract (D); metoclopramide has these properties. Lansoprazole does not compete with ketoconazole for transport mechanisms in the GI tract (E).

6. **D**

Both metoclopramide (II) and ranitidine (III) are primarily excreted in the urine as unchanged drug. Therefore, the doses of these drugs need to be adjusted in patients with renal dysfunction. In fact, the dose of all H2 receptor antagonists needs to be adjusted in this patient population. None of the PPIs (I) needs to be dose adjusted in patients with renal dysfunction.

7. **D**

Sulfasalazine (Azulfidine) (I) is a sulfa derivative and should be avoided in patients with a history of anaphylaxis to sulfa products (e.g., trimethoprim/sulfamethoxazole). Olsalazine (Dipentum) (II), mesalamine (Asacol HD) (III), and balsalazide are not sulfa derivatives and could be safely used in this patient with UC.

8. **A**

UC is more likely to be confined to the colon and rectum, whereas CD can affect anywhere in the GI tract from the mouth to the anus. Fistulas (B) are more likely to develop in patients with CD as opposed to those with UC. The inflammation in CD occurs in a segmented or cobblestone pattern (C), while it occurs in a more continuous fashion in UC. The mucosal lesions in UC are more superficial than those in CD, which are more transmural (D). Systemic complications can occur with either UC or CD (E).

9. **B**

Sulfasalazine can impair folate absorption. Therefore, patients taking chronic sulfasalazine therapy are at risk for developing folate deficiency and should supplement folic acid to prevent this adverse effect. Sulfasalazine does not impair the absorption of calcium (A), iron (C), vitamin B_{12} (D), or vitamin C (E). Therefore, routine supplementation of these vitamins/minerals during sulfasalazine is not necessary.

10. **C**

Before starting therapy with certolizumab pegol, patients should be evaluated for tuberculosis risk factors and latent tuberculosis infection with a PPD. Cases of reactivation of tuberculosis or new tuberculosis infections have been reported in patients receiving therapy with TNF-inhibitors, including certolizumab pegol; patients who are receiving these drugs are at increased risk for developing serious infections. Certolizumab pegol has not been associated with PML (life-threatening), so there is no need to perform a brain MRI (A) before starting therapy with this drug; baseline brain MRI is taken prior to initiating therapy with natalizumab. The drug is not associated with hepatotoxicity or nephrotoxicity, so there is no need to monitor baseline LFTs (B) or SCr (D). Finally, certolizumab pegol does not affect uric acid levels, so this parameter does not need to be monitored at baseline.

Renal Disorders

This chapter covers the following disorder:

- **Renal disorders**

 Suggested Study Time: **20 minutes**

RENAL DISORDERS

Definition

Chronic kidney disease (CKD) is defined as either kidney damage (albuminuria ≥30 mcg:mg creatinine) and/or decreased glomerular filtration rate (GFR) (<60 mL/min) for ≥3 months.

Diagnosis

Among individuals meeting the criteria for CKD just listed, staging is based upon GFR, with higher stages indicating worsening renal function (lower GFR).

Stage	GFR (mL/min/1.73m^2)
1	>90 (+ kidney damage)
2	60–89 (+ kidney damage)
3	30–59
4	15–29
5	<15 (or dialysis)

Signs and Symptoms

The earliest detectable sign of kidney damage is microalbuminuria. The majority of signs and symptoms do not become apparent until later in the course of disease. Symptoms may include sequelae of hypervolemia including edema, weight gain, and fatigue. Signs may include anemia, hyperkalemia, vitamin D deficiency, hyperparathyroidism, hypercalcemia, and hyperphosphatemia.

Albuminuria is a helpful measure of disease progression. It is classified as listed in the following table:

Collection	Normal	Microalbuminuria	Macroalbuminuria
Spot collection albumin:creatinine ratio	<30 mcg/mg Cr	30–300 mcg/mg Cr	>300 mcg/mg Cr
24-hr collection (mg of albumin/24hrs)	<30 mg/24hrs	30–300 mg/24 hrs	>300 mg/24 hrs
Timed collection (mcg of protein/min)	<20 mcg/min	20–200 mcg/min	>200 mcg/min

Guidelines

National Kidney Foundation. K/DOQI clinical practice guidelines for chronic kidney disease: evaluation, classification, and stratification. *Am J Kidney Dis* 2002;39(2 Suppl 1): S1–266.

Guidelines Summary

- Goals of therapy:
  - Slow the progression of the disease, reduce proteinuria, prevent complications, correct and manage reversible risk factors
  - Blood pressure (BP) <130/80 mmHg for CKD + any degree of proteinuria
  - BP <140/90 mmHg for CKD with no proteinuria (<30 mcg/mg) (patient with diabetes mellitus [DM], use DM-specific goal)
- Pharmacologic therapy for CKD
  - CKD and hypertension
    » Patient with any degree of proteinuria should be initiated on an angiotensin-converting enzyme inhibitor (ACEI) or an angiotensin II receptor blocker (ARB).
    » Patient with no degree of proteinuria (<30 mcg/mg) should be initiated on diuretic therapy (thiazide if creatinine clearance [CrCl] >30 mL/min or loop if <30 mL/min).

» Patients with BP that is elevated >20/10 mmHg above goal should be initiated on ACEI + diuretic.

- CKD without hypertension

    » Patient with macroalbuminuria should be initiated on ACEI or ARB.

    » Patient with microalbuminuria and diabetes should be initiated on ACEI or ARB.

    » Patient with microalbuminuria without diabetes should not be initiated on pharmacologic therapy.

- With initiation of ACEI or ARB, up to 30% increase in serum creatinine is acceptable/expected.

■ Pharmacologic therapy for complications of CKD

- Edema: loop diuretics

    » Hyperkalemia: loop diuretics, sodium polystyrene sulfonate, calcium, insulin, dialysis

    » Anemia

    – When Hgb falls below 10 g/dL, erythropoietin stimulating agents (ESAs) are indicated. Iron indices should also be monitored and appropriated supplemented.

    » Renal osteodystrophy

    – Hyperphosphatemia (phosphate goals: 2.7–4.6 mg/dL for stages 3 and 4; 3.5–5.5 mg/dL for stage 5)

        ○ Calcium-containing phosphate binders are the treatment of choice as long as corrected calcium <10.2 mg/dL and calcium phosphate product <55 mg^2/dL^2.

        ○ Non–calcium containing phosphate binders such as sevelamer and lanthanum are appropriate for patients with corrected calcium >10.2 or calcium phosphate product >55 mg^2/dL^2.

        ○ Aluminum-containing phosphate binders are only indicated in severe hyperphosphatemia (serum phosphate >7 mg/dL) because they have a high side effect profile.

    – Secondary hyperparathyroidism (intact parathyroid hormone [PTH] goals: 35–70 pg/mL for stage 3; 70–110 pg/mL for stage 4; and 150–300 pg/mL for stage 5)

        ○ Phosphate should be at goal before treating elevated PTH.

        ○ Activated vitamin D analogs are paricalcitol, calcitriol, doxercalciferol.

    – Vitamin D insufficiency/deficiency (goal 25(OH) vitamin D >30 ng/mL)

        ○ Insufficiency 16–30 ng/mL

        ○ Deficiency ≤15

- ○ Treatment: loading dose (ergocalciferol) followed by maintenance dose
- ○ Treatment timeframe determined by severity of deficiency

Dosing Considerations in Patients with Renal Disease

Estimating Renal Clearance

As serum creatinine increases, this indicates declining renal function. The Cockcroft-Gault equation is the most commonly used method of estimating creatinine clearance (CrCl). The CrCl serves as an approximation of the GFR when considering the renal clearance of medications.

$$\text{Creatinine clearance (female) (mL/min)} = \frac{(140 - age) \times IBW \times 0.85}{72 \times serum\ creatinine}$$

$$\text{Creatinine clearance (male) (mL/min)} = \frac{(140 - age) \times IBW}{72 \times serum\ creatinine}$$

This formula is not ideal for use in the very elderly, very young, or in end stage renal disease (ESRD). IBW is ideal body weight.

Medications Requiring Dose Adjustment in Renal Disease

Medications that are primarily eliminated via renal excretion often require dose and/or interval adjustment in advanced stages of renal disease. Reducing medication doses results in reduced peak concentrations while trough concentrations are maintained. Extending dosing intervals results in reduced trough concentrations while peak concentrations are maintained. Certain renally eliminated medications should be avoided in the setting of advanced renal disease due to the risk of serious side effects related to accumulation. Examples of commonly used medications that should be avoided and that require renal dose adjustment are provided in this list.

Commonly used medications requiring dose/interval adjustment in renal disease

• Acyclovir	• Gabapentin
• Allopurinol	• Ganciclovir
• Amphotericin	• Lamivudine
• Aminoglycosides	• Metoclopramide
• Aztreonam	• Penicillins
• Beta-lactam antibiotics	• Pregabalin
• Colchicine	• Quinolones
• Clarithromycin	• Sulfamethoxazole/trimethoprim
• Dabigatran	• Tramadol
• Didanosine	• Valacyclovir
• Digoxin	• Vancomycin
• Enoxaparin	• Venlafaxine
• Ethambutol	• Zidovudine
• Famotidine	• Zoledronic acid

Commonly used medications that should be avoided or discontinued in advanced renal disease

• Alendronate	• Lithium
• Chlorpropamide	• Meperidine
• Cidofovir	• Metformin
• Dabigatran	• Nitrofurantoin
• Dofetilide	• NSAIDs
• Duloxetine	• Rivaroxaban
• Eplerenone	• Sotalol
• Fondaparinux	• Spironolactone
• Foscarnet	• Tadalafil
• Glyburide	• Tenofovir

Dosing Considerations in Dialysis

Patients with ESRD who require dialysis also require careful consideration of medication regimens to determine if medications are removed during dialysis and if replacement dosing is necessary post-dialysis. Some factors affecting removal of a drug via dialysis include the drug's volume of distribution, molecular size, and degree of protein binding as well as the type of dialysis membrane. Drugs with larger volume of distribution, larger molecular size, and higher degree of protein binding will be less effectively cleared via dialysis. High-flux dialysis membranes remove more medication than low- or medium-flux membranes.

Generic	Brand	Dose & Max	Contraindications	Primary Side Effects	Key Monitoring	Pertinent Drug Interactions	Med Pearl	Top 200
Vitamin D analog								
Ergocalciferol	• Calcidiol • Calciferol • Drisdol	50,000 units 2 × /wk for 8–12 wks	• Hypercalcemia • Malabsorption syndrome	• Constipation • N/V • Hypercalcemia	Serum calcium and phosphorous every 2 weeks	• Cimetidine, phenytoin, phenobarbital, and carbamazepine result in decreased levels • Thiazide diuretics may increase hypercalcemic effects	Dosing may differ depending on level of vitamin D deficiency	No
Calcium-containing phosphate binders								
Calcium carbonate	• Rolaids • Tums	1,000 mg of elemental calcium/day (max should not exceed 2,000 mg/day)	Hypercalcemia	• Constipation • Flatulence • Swollen abdomen • Hypercalcemia • Milk-alkali syndrome	Serum calcium and phosphate levels	• Antacids decrease concentration; separate 2 hrs before or 4 hrs after phenytoin, ketoconazole, levothyroxine, tetracycline antibiotics • If taken with digoxin, can cause an arrhythmia	• For females ≥51 yrs old, dose is changed to 1200 mg of elemental calcium/day • Take with meals • Take in doses of <500 mg (elemental calcium) at a time for greatest absorption	No
Calcium acetate	• Calphron • PhosLo • Eliphos	Initial: 1,334 mg with each meal, can be increased every 2–3 weeks to usual dose: 2,001–2,668 mg calcium acetate with each meal	• Hypercalcemia • Renal calculi	• Hypercalcemia • N/V/D	• Serum calcium • Phosphorus • PTH	• Antacids decrease concentration; separate 2 hrs before or 4 hrs after phenytoin, ketoconazole, levothyroxine, tetracycline antibiotics • If taken with digoxin can cause an arrhythmia	Do not give additional calcium supplements	Yes
Non–calcium containing phosphate binders								
Sevelamer hydrochloride	• Renvela • Renagel	800–1,600 mg 3 × /day with meals; the initial dose may be based on serum phosphorus levels	Bowel obstruction	• N/V/D • Dyspepsia • Abdominal pain • Constipation	Serum phosphate (want ≤5.5 mg/dL), serum bicarbonate and chloride	Ciprofloxacin, mycophenolate, and levothyroxine all have decreased concentrations when taken with Sevelamer	Initial dose may be based on serum phosphorous	No

Generic	Brand	Dose & Max	Contraindications	Primary Side Effects	Key Monitoring	Pertinent Drug Interactions	Med Pearl	Top 200
Lanthanum carbonate	Fosrenol	Initial dose of 500 mg TID with meals, can increase up to 750 mg/day every 2–3 weeks for a max dose of 3,000 mg	• Bowel obstruction • Fecal impaction • Ileus	• N/V • Abdominal pain • Constipation	Serum phosphate and calcium	Quinolone antibiotics, mycophenolate, and levothyroxine all have decreased concentrations when taken with Lanthanum	• Take with meals and do not swallow intact tablets • Only available as a chewable tablet	No
Aluminum-containing phosphate binders								
Aluminum carbonate		400–500 mg PO TID with meals	Hypersensitivity	• Hypomagnesemia • Hypophosphatemia	• Phosphate, calcium • Magnesium	• Antacids decrease concentration; separate 2 hrs before or 4 hrs after phenytoin, ketoconazole, levothyroxine, tetracycline antibiotics • Allopurinol: antacids decrease absorption		No
Aluminum hydroxide		300–600 mg PO TID with meals		• Constipation • Anemia • Neurotoxicity				No
Active vitamin D analog								
Paricalcitol	Zemplar	• Stages 3 and 4: 1 mcg PO daily or 2 mcg PO 3 ×/wk • Stage 5: 2.5–5 mcg IV 3 ×/wk	• Hypersensitivity • Hypercalcemia • Vitamin D toxicity	• Hypercalcemia • Calciphylaxis • N/D • Edema	• Calcium, phosphorus • Vitamin D • PTH	• CYP 3A4 substrate • Strong CYP3A4 inducers/inhibitors	Paricalcitol and doxercalciferol are synthetic forms of vitamin D that have less effect on calcium and phosphate	No
Calcitriol	Rocaltrol	• Stages 3 and 4: 0.25 mcg PO daily • Stage 5: 0.5–1.5 mcg PO/IV 3 ×/wk				• Aluminum hydroxide: increase aluminum concentration • Bile acid sequestrants: decrease serum concentration of vitamin D analogs • Sucralfate: vitamin D analogs increase concentration		Yes
Doxercalciferol	Hectorol	• Stages 3 and 4: 1 mcg PO daily or 2.5 mcg PO 3 ×/wk • Stage 5: 5 mcg PO or 2 mcg IV 3 ×/wk						No
Erythropoietin stimulating agents								
Epoetin alfa	Procrit	50–100 U/kg 3 ×/wk	Hypersensitivity	• Hypertension • Stroke • Fever • Thromboembolism	• Hemoglobin • Ferritin • Transferrin • BP		• Boxed warning: increase risk of death, MI, stroke, thrombosis, and tumor progression or recurrence	No
Darbepoetin alfa	Aranesp	• 0.45 mcg/kg 1 ×/wk • 0.75 mcg/kg 1 × every 2 wk		• Nausea • Headache			• Hemoglobin <10 g/dL before starting treatment	No
Peginesatide	Omontys	0.04 mg/kg 1 ×/month	• Hypersensitivity • Uncontrolled hypertension				• Indicated only for patients receiving dialysis	No

Storage and Administration Pearls

- Preferred route of administration for erythropoietin-stimulating agents (ESAs) is subcutaneous, except when administered to patients undergoing hemodialysis, for whom intravenous administration is preferred.
- ESAs should be protected from light, should be stored in the refrigerator from 2°C to 8°C (36°–46°F), and should not be frozen or shaken.
- Phosphate binders should be administered with meals.

Patient Education Pearls

- Patients should report experience injection-site reactions with ESAs to their health care professional. Patients should seek emergency medical care for shortness of breath, wheezing, or swelling of the tongue.
- Phosphate binders should be administered with meals.

PRACTICE QUESTIONS

1. A 66-year-old female (5′2″, 80 kg) has a stable serum creatinine of 1.5 mg/dL. Which is an accurate assessment of her renal function?

   (A) Stage 1 CKD
   (B) Stage 2 CKD
   (C) Stage 3 CKD
   (D) Stage 4 CKD

2. A 58-year-old man (5′10″, 92 kg) presents for routine follow-up. He has a medical history of hypertension. At last visit 4 months ago, BP was 148/96 mmHg, serum creatinine was 1.6 mg/dL, and urine albumin:creatinine was 10 mcg:mg. Data today includes BP 146/94 mmHg, HR 84 bpm, serum potassium 4.5 mEq/L, serum creatinine 1.5 mg/dL, and urine albumin:creatinine 10 mcg:mg. Which of the following is the best recommendation?

   (A) Initiate chlorthalidone
   (B) Initiate lisinopril
   (C) Initiate amlodipine
   (D) Non-pharmacological therapy only

3. A female patient with stage 3 CKD and hypertension presents for follow-up after a BP reading at last visit of 138/88 mmHg. She began non-pharmacological therapy for BP at that time. Vital signs today include BP 136/84 mmHg and HR 88 bpm. Serum labs include potassium 4.2 mEq/L, sCr 1.4 mg/dL, and urine albumin:creatinine ratio 100 mg:g. Which is the best recommendation?

   (A) Initiate chlorthalidone
   (B) Initiate lisinopril
   (C) Initiate amlodipine
   (D) Non-pharmacological therapy only

4. Which is the most appropriate therapy in a patient with stage 4 CKD and edema?

   (A) Indapamide
   (B) Spironolactone
   (C) Bumetanide
   (D) Chlorthalidone

5. A patient with stage 3 CKD presents for a routine follow-up and has the following serum lab results: 25(OH) vitamin D 40 ng/mL, PTH 115 pg/mL, phosphate 5.3 mg/dL, calcium 9.9 mg/dL, albumin 3 mg/dL. Which is the most appropriate therapy to recommend at this time?

   (A) Sevelamer
   (B) Calcitriol
   (C) Calcium carbonate
   (D) Ergocalciferol

6. A patient with stage 4 CKD presents for routine follow up with the following serum lab results: 25(OH) vitamin D 35 ng/mL, PTH 105 pg/mL, phosphate 5.3 mg/dL, calcium 9.2 mg/dL, albumin 3.8 mg/dL. Which is the most appropriate therapy to recommend?

   (A) Sevelamer
   (B) Calcitriol
   (C) Calcium carbonate
   (D) Ergocalciferol

ANSWERS

1. **D**

$$Creatinine\ clearance\ (female) = \frac{(140 - age) \times IBW \times 0.85}{72 \times serum\ creatinine}$$

(mL/min)

$$= \frac{(140 - 66) \times 50.1 \times 0.85}{72 \times 1.5} = 29\ mL/min$$

This patient has an estimated creatinine clearance of 29 mL/min calculated via the Cockcroft-Gault equation. Stage 4 CKD includes estimated GFR (calculated CrCl) of 15–29 mL/min.

2. **A**

This patient's estimated GFR (calculated CrCl) is 52 mL/min placing him into stage 3 CKD (30–59 mL/min). His urine protein assessment is below the range considered positive for microalbuminuria (<30 mcg:mg). Patient's with non-proteinuric CKD have a BP goal of <140/90 mmHg and, therefore, pharmacotherapy is indicated making (D) incorrect. First line therapy per NKF is thiazide-type diuretic such as chlorthalidone (A). Lisinopril (B), an ACEI, would be an appropriate second line choice or would be appropriate first line option for him if he had proteinuria. Calcium channel blockers are appropriate for add on therapy for hypertension.

3. **B**

Because this patient has CKD with proteinuria, her evidence-based BP goal is <130/80 mmHg and her BP readings require treatment. Therefore, option (D) is incorrect. First line therapy for hypertension in patients with CKD and proteinuria is an ACEI such as lisinopril (B) or an ARB per National Kidney Foundation (NKF) guidelines. Thiazide diuretics such as chlorthalidone (A) are appropriate first line therapy in a patient with non-proteinuric CKD or as second line therapy in a patient with proteinuric CKD per the NKF. Calcium channel blockers such as amlodipine (C) are appropriate add-on agents for BP reduction but are not first line treatment.

4. **C**

Patients with stage 4 CKD have an estimated glomerular filtration rate (GFR) of <30 mL/min. In this setting, loop diuretics (e.g., [C] bumetanide) maintain efficacy, whereas thiazide diuretics such as (A) indapamide and (D) chlorthalidone do not. Additionally, loop diuretics are more effective in treating edema as compared to aldosterone antagonists (B) spironolactone and thiazide diuretics.

5. **A**

This patient has complications of CKD including hyperphosphatemia and secondary hyperparathyroidism. Before treating hyperparathyroidism, the phosphate should be brought into the goal range. Both sevelamer (A) and calcium carbonate (C) are phosphate binders. The calcium-containing phosphate binder, calcium carbonate, should be avoided because the patient's corrected calcium is >10.2 mg/dL and the calcium × phosphate product is >55 mg^2/dL^2. Ergocalciferol (D) is incorrect because patient's 25(OH) vitamin D level is at goal of >30 ng/mL.

6. **C**

This patient has hyperphosphatemia as a complication of CKD. Because the patient's corrected calcium is <10.2 mg/dL (9.4 mg/dL) and calcium × phosphate product is <55 mg^2/dL^2, a calcium-containing phosphate binder such as calcium carbonate (C) is the best recommendation. Sevelamer (A) is reserved for hyperphosphatemia in the setting of elevated corrected calcium (>10.2 mg/dL) or elevated calcium × phosphate product (>55 mg^2/dL^2). Calcitriol (B) would not be indicated as the patient's intact PTH is within the stage 4 CKD range of 70–110 pg/mL. Ergocalciferol (D) is not indicated because 25(OH) vitamin D level is at goal of >30 ng/mL.

Oncology

8

This chapter covers the following topics:

- **Lymphoma**
- **Leukemia**
- **Lung cancer**
- **Colorectal cancer**
- **Breast cancer**
- **Prostate cancer**
- **Ovarian cancer**
- **Supportive care**

 Suggested Study Time: **2 hours**

Since many of the drugs used in chemotherapy are indicated for multiple types of cancer, the background information for all of the hematologic malignancies and solid tumors will be discussed first, with the drug therapies described in charts at the end of the section. Because cancer therapy is generally protocol-driven, your focus should be mostly on toxicities and on certain cases where a specific drug is indicated on the basis of cell-surface markers such as CD20 or HER-2 overexpression. Supportive care (pain management, antinauseant and antiemetic agents, and colony-stimulating factors) is covered at the end of this chapter.

LYMPHOMA

Definitions

Lymphomas are tumors of the lymphoid cells. Hodgkin's lymphoma (or Hodgkin's disease, HD) is less common than other types of lymphoma and is marked by the presence of Reed-Steinberg cells. HD may have a genetic component and, while HD is not contagious, certain infections (particularly Epstein-Barr and human immunodeficiency virus [HIV]) may increase the risk of acquiring the disease. HD is more common in young adults (15–35 years) and those over 55.

Non-Hodgkin's lymphomas (NHLs) are a group of related cancers including follicular, diffuse large B-cell, and Burkitt's lymphoma. NHL is the eighth leading cause of cancer in the United States, and the incidence increases with age (median age of diagnosis is 50 years). Immunodeficiency and infections are risk factors for NHL, as is prior chemotherapy. The various types of NHL are typified by proliferation of malignant B or T lymphocytes. The cancer may be classified as either aggressive (fast-growing) or indolent (slow-growing).

Diagnosis

HD

- Lymph node biopsy → Presence of Reed-Sternberg cells
- Computed tomography (CT) scan, magnetic resonance imaging (MRI), position emission tomography (PET) scan, or bone marrow biopsy to determine staging

NHL

- Lab values:
  - Elevated white blood cells (WBCs)
  - Lactate dehydrogenase levels may be high
- Lymph node or tissue biopsy
- Flow cytometry — cell surface marker analysis

Staging is the same for HD and NHL. Each stage is subdivided into A and B; B denotes the presence of systemic symptoms, specifically night sweats, weight loss, and fever:

- Stage 1: present in one lymph node or one part of tissue or organ
- Stage 2: present in ≥2 lymph nodes on the same side of the diaphragm
- Stage 3: present in lymph nodes above and below the diaphragm
- Stage 4: present in several parts of ≥1 tissues, or in an organ and distant lymph nodes
- Recurrent: disease returns after remission

Signs and Symptoms

HD

- Painless enlargement of lymph nodes, especially in the neck
- Fever, night sweats, and/or weight loss
- Malaise
- Possible bone pain

NHL

- Swollen lymph nodes on neck, underarms, and groin
- Fever, weight loss, and night sweats
- Fatigue
- Weakness

LEUKEMIA

Definitions

The leukemias are a group of blood malignancies characterized by unregulated growth of blood-forming cells in the bone marrow. These immature white cells crowd out normal cells in the bone marrow, leading to low red cell, white cell, and platelet counts. Four major types of leukemia exist: Acute lymphocytic (ALL), acute myeloid (AML), chronic lymphocytic (CLL), and chronic myeloid (CML) leukemias. Acute leukemias worsen rapidly; chronic leukemias worsen slowly. Exposure to radiation and chemicals (particularly benzene and formaldehyde) can increase leukemia risk.

Although the overall incidence of acute leukemias is low, they are the most common cancers in children, and ALL is the leading cause of cancer-related death in those under 35 years. AML occurs with increasing frequency in the elderly.

Virtually all patients with CML have a specific chromosomal abnormality (Philadelphia chromosome).

Diagnosis

- Bone marrow biopsy → Send for morphologic examination
- AML diagnosis requires 20% blasts

Signs and Symptoms

- Weight loss, fatigue, malaise
- Palpitations and dyspnea on exertion
- Fever and chills; night sweats
- Bruising
- Bone pain

LUNG CANCER

Definitions

Lung cancer is the leading cause of cancer death in men and women. Most lung cancers are non-small cell (NSCLC); while this type of cancer is slow-growing, it does not respond well to chemotherapy and only about 14% of patients can be cured. Small-cell lung cancer (SCLC) is very aggressive and, though it is chemotherapy-sensitive, most patients die within 2 years of diagnosis. Smoking is the primary risk factor for lung cancer; over 80% of patients have a history of smoking. Occupational exposure to asbestos, radon, and other agents may also increase risk, as can certain genetic abnormalities and family history of the disease.

Diagnosis

- Chest x-ray, CT scans, and PET scan to detect lesions and determine extent of disease
- Pathological confirmation by sputum cytology or tumor biopsy

Signs and Symptoms

- Cough—most common
- Other lung-related symptoms (sputum production, dyspnea, wheezing); often misattributed to concomitant pulmonary conditions
- Weight loss, fever, bone pain
- Paraneoplastic syndromes:
  - Occur in 10% of cases; may be first sign or symptom
  - Inappropriate secretion of antidiuretic hormone (SIADH)
  - Hypercalcemia
  - Eaton-Lambert myasthenic syndrome: muscle weakness and autonomic dysfunction

COLORECTAL CANCER

Definitions

Colorectal cancer is the fourth leading cause of cancer death in the United States. Incidence is highest in industrialized countries and may be linked to a higher-fat, lower-fiber diet in such locations. Genetic predisposition also plays a role in 5–10% of cases. Primary prevention strategies involve dietary change (increase calcium, fiber, and antioxidants and decrease fat).

Diagnosis

- Fecal occult blood testing (FOBT) may decrease cancer mortality by one-third, but has a high false-negative rate as many early stage tumors do not bleed.
- FOBT plus immunochemical assays lead to improved specificity and sensitivity.
- Flexible sigmoidoscopy can detect lesions in distal and sigmoid colon; early detection and excision can decrease mortality by 60%.
- Colonoscopy is preferred screening method as it shows entire colon, but it requires more bowel preparation.
- Double-contrast barium enema plus flexible sigmoidoscopy may be used instead of colonoscopy.

Signs and Symptoms

- Change in bowel habits (diarrhea, constipation, stools narrower than usual)
- Rectal bleeding/blood in the stool
- Nausea, vomiting, and abdominal discomfort (gas pains or cramps, bloating)
- Fatigue (generally related to anemia)
- Weight loss
- Leg edema (result of lymph node involvement)
- Hepatomegaly and jaundice

BREAST CANCER

Definitions

Breast cancer is the most common cancer in women and is second only to lung cancer as a cause of cancer death in women. Family history plays a large role in the development of breast cancer, with mutations in the *BRCA1/BRCA2* tumor suppressor genes leading to high risk. Long-term progestin use and other endocrine factors (early menarche, late menopause, advanced age at first pregnancy) and lifestyle factors (high fat intake, alcohol consumption, obesity) also increase risk of developing breast cancer. Prognosis is poor in younger (<35 years) and premenopausal patients, African Americans, and those with *HER2/neu* overexpression.

Diagnosis

- Palpable mass on physical examination
- Breast imaging techniques: mammography and/or ultrasound
- Biopsy if mass or cluster of calcifications is detected

Signs and Symptoms

- May be asymptomatic
- Painless lump: Initial sign in 90% of patients
- Stabbing or aching pain is initial sign in remaining 10%
- Nipple discharge, retraction, dimpling
- Scaly, red, or swollen skin of breast or nipple
- Advanced disease: Bone pain, difficulty breathing, jaundice, abdominal enlargement, mental status changes

PROSTATE CANCER

Definitions

Prostate cancer is the most common cancer in men, and the second most common cause of cancer death in men. One-third to one-half of men present with advanced disease, for which there is no cure. High-fat diet and hormonal factors are two of the primary risk factors; as prostate cancer is androgen-dependent, high levels of testosterone can fuel tumor growth. This may explain the increased incidence in African-American men, who generally have testosterone levels 15% higher than Caucasian men.

Diagnosis

- Transrectal ultrasound or cystoscopy
- Biopsy: Only sure method of diagnosis

Signs and Symptoms

- Elevated prostate-specific antigen (PSA)
- Nodule on digital rectal exam of the prostate
- Localized disease: Generally asymptomatic; symptoms of prostatic enlargement may indicate cancer, benign prostatic hyperplasia, or infection; further investigation warranted
  - Urinary difficulty
  - Difficulty in having an erection
  - Blood in the urine or semen

- Advanced disease:
  - Bone pain
  - Anemia and fatigue
  - Weight loss
  - Back pain
  - Edema of the legs

OVARIAN CANCER

Definitions

Ovarian cancer typically occurs postmenopause. Risk factors include family history of ovarian or breast cancer, personal history of other types of cancer, nulliparity, and long-term estrogen therapy (without progesterone). Genetics also play a role; breast cancer and ovarian cancer are linked to mutation in *BRCA1/BRCA2*, along with other genetic alterations.

Diagnosis

- Ovarian size/contour on pelvic exam
- Elevation of CA-125 (antigen common to most ovarian cancers)
- Pelvic ultrasound
- Biopsy

Signs and Symptoms

Symptoms may be vague and nonspecific, but may include:

- Fatigue
- Back pain
- Bloating, constipation, abdominal pain
- Palpable abdominal mass, abdominal distention
- Hepatic and renal function abnormalities

Alkylating Agents

Mechanism of action – alkylate DNA, making it more prone to breakage; most effective against rapidly dividing cells

Generic	Brand/Route of Administration	Contraindications	Primary Side Effects	Key Monitoring	Pertinent Drug Interactions	Med Pearl	Top 200
Cyclophosphamide	Only available generically (IV and PO)	Hypersensitivity to any alkylating agent	• Alopecia • Hemorrhagic cystitis • Infertility • Nausea, vomiting (N/V), mucositis, stomatitis • Bone marrow suppression	• Complete blood count (CBC) with differential • Blood urea nitrogen (BUN)/serum creatinine (SCr) • Uric acid (UA)	CYP3A4 inducers may ↑ levels of active metabolite (acrolein)	• Maintain adequate hydration to avoid hemorrhagic cystitis; can also use mesna • High emetogenic potential • Tablets should be taken with food	No
Chlorambucil	Leukeran (PO)		• Bone marrow suppression • Infertility • Secondary leukemias • Seizures • Stevens-Johnson syndrome • Hepatotoxicity	• CBC with differential • LFTs	None	• Take on empty stomach • Avoid alcohol	No
Carmustine	• BiCNU (IV) • Gliadel (intracranial implant)		• Bone marrow suppression • Pulmonary fibrosis • Severe N/V • Hypotension (IV) • Secondary leukemias (with long-term use) • Reversible elevation of liver function tests (LFTs)	• CBC with differential • Pulmonary function tests • LFTs • Blood pressure (BP) (during IV administration)	IV solution contains ethanol; do not give aldehyde-dehydrogenase inhibitors	Very high emetogenic potential	No

Platinum-Based Agents

Generic	Brand/Route of Administration	Contraindications	Primary Side Effects	Key Monitoring	Pertinent Drug Interactions	Med Pearl	Top 200
Mechanism of action – crosslink DNA, causing it to break							
Cisplatin	Only available generically (IV)	• Hypersensitivity to any platinum-containing compounds • Renal insufficiency • Pre-existing hearing impairment (cisplatin)	• Anaphylaxis • Dose-related myelosuppression • N/V • Ototoxicity (cisplatin) • Nephrotoxicity with cumulative doses (esp. cisplatin) • Peripheral neuropathy	• BUN/SCr • Electrolytes • Neurologic exam • CBC with differential • Urine output	• Administration with taxane derivatives may ↑ myelosuppression and ↓ efficacy of platinum agents • May ↓ digoxin levels (oxaliplatin)	• Do not administer doses exceeding 100 mg/m^2 every 3 wks • High emetogenic potential	No
Carboplatin	Only available generically (IV)					Moderate emetogenic potential	No
Oxaliplatin	Eloxatin (IV)					• Moderate emetogenic potential • Warn patients to wear a scarf if being treated during cold weather to prevent laryngeal spasms	No

Enzyme Inhibitors

Generic	Brand/Route of Administration	Contraindications	Primary Side Effects	Key Monitoring	Pertinent Drug Interactions	Med Pearl	Top 200
Mechanism of action – target enzymes responsible for DNA replication and repair							
Irinotecan	Camptosar (IV)	Concurrent therapy with ketoconazole or St. John's wort	• Bone marrow suppression • Severe, life-threatening diarrhea	• CBC with differential • Electrolytes (esp. if diarrhea)	CYP3A4 substrate	• Diarrhea may be early or late onset • High emetogenic potential	No
Etoposide	Only available generically (IV and PO)	None	• Bone marrow suppression • Hepatotoxicity	• CBC with differential • LFTs	CYP3A4 substrate	• Do NOT give IV push (may cause hypotension) • Do NOT give IM (necrosis)	No

Antimitotic Agents

Mechanism of action – spindle poisons; interfere with mitotic spindle; prevent chromosome segregation and lead to cell death

Generic	Brand/Route of Administration	Contraindications	Primary Side Effects	Key Monitoring	Pertinent Drug Interactions	Med Pearl	Top 200
Vincristine	Vincasar PFS (IV)	None	• Peripheral neuropathy (dose-limiting) • Paralytic ileus (secondary to neurologic toxicity) • Hepatotoxicity	• Neurologic exam • LFTs • Change in frequency of bowel movements	None	• Do NOT give intrathecally (IT) (fatal) • All patients should be on a prophylactic bowel management regimen • Avoid extravasation (vesicant) • Should NOT exceed 2 mg/dose	No
Vinblastine	Only available generically (IV)	None	• Peripheral neuropathy • Bone marrow suppression (dose-limiting)	• CBC with differential • Neurologic exam	None	• Do not give IT (fatal) • Avoid extravasation (vesicant)	No
Paclitaxel	Taxol (IV)	• Hypersensitivity to Cremophor • Absolute neutrophil count (ANC) <1,500/mm^3 (ovarian, lung, or breast cancer) • ANC ≤1,000/mm^3 (Kaposi's sarcoma)	• Bone marrow suppression (dose-limiting) • Peripheral neuropathy • Cardiac rhythm abnormalities • Hepatotoxicity • Mucositis, stomatitis (severe)	• CBC with differential • Electrocardiogram (ECG) • LFTs • Neurologic exam	• CYP2C8 and CYP3A4 substrate • Administer prior to platinum derivatives to limit myelosuppression and enhance efficacy	Pretreat with dexamethasone, diphenhydramine, and H$_2$-receptor antagonist	No
Paclitaxel protein-bound particles	Abraxane (IV)	Baseline neutrophils <1,500/mm^3				No need for pretreatment	No
Docetaxel	Taxotere, Docefrez (IV)	• Hypersensitivity to polysorbate 80 • Baseline neutrophils <1,500/mm^3 • Severe hepatic impairment	• Significant, dose-dependent fluid retention • Bone marrow suppression • Hypersensitivity reactions	• CBC with differential • LFTs • Weight, signs of edema	• CYP3A4 substrate • Administer prior to platinum derivatives to limit myelosuppression and enhance efficacy	• Avoid doses >100 mg/m^2 • Pretreat with corticosteroids for 1–5 days to prevent fluid retention and hypersensitivity reactions	No

Antimetabolites

Generic	Brand/Route of Administration	Contraindications	Primary Side Effects	Key Monitoring	Pertinent Drug Interactions	Med Pearl	Top 200
Mechanism of action – nucleoside analogs							
Cytarabine	Cytosar-U (IV)	None	• Severe bone marrow suppression • Cytarabine syndrome: myalgia, bone pain, rash, conjunctivitis, and fever	CBC with differential	May ↓ levels of digoxin	• Pretreat with corticosteroid; may prevent cytarabine syndrome • May also be administered IT or subcutaneously (SC) • Moderate emetogenic potential	No
Cytarabine liposomal	DepoCyt (IT)	Active meningeal infection	• Chemical arachnoiditis (N/V, headache, and fever) • Neurotoxicity	Monitor closely for signs of immediate reactions and neurotoxicity	None reported; limited systemic exposure	• Co-administer dexamethasone to lessen chemical arachnoiditis • Moderate emetogenic potential	No
5-Fluorouracil	Adrucil (IV)	Dihydropyrimidine dehydrogenase (DPD) deficiency	• Hand-and-foot syndrome • N/V/D • Mucositis • Stomatitis • Bone marrow suppression	CBC with differential	May ↑ effects of warfarin	• Leucovorin ↑ effectiveness and toxicity; dose of fluorouracil may need to be ↓	No
Mechanism of action – folic acid antagonist							
Methotrexate	Trexall (PO) Only available generically (IV, IM, IT)	None	• Nephrotoxicity • Bone marrow suppression • Stevens-Johnson syndrome • Severe diarrhea and ulcerative stomatitis • Neurotoxicity • Hepatotoxicity	• CBC with differential • SCr • LFTs	NSAIDs may ↑ risk of toxicity	• Give leucovorin rescue 24 hrs after dosing to limit toxicity; do not administer concurrently • Can be given IT for leukemias • Also used SC as DMARD for rheumatoid arthritis	Yes

Anthracyclines

Mechanism of action – intercalate DNA and generate reactive oxygen species

Generic	Brand/Route of Administration	Contraindications	Primary Side Effects	Key Monitoring	Pertinent Drug Interactions	Med Pearl	Top 200
Daunorubicin	Cerubidine (IV)	Pre-existing severe myocardial insufficiency or arrhythmia	• Dose-related cardiotoxicity • Severe bone marrow suppression • Red coloration of body fluids	• CBC with differential • ECG • Left ventricular ejection fraction (LVEF)	↑ risk of cardiotoxicity with trastuzumab, cyclophosphamide, and taxane derivatives	• Greatest risk of irreversible myocardial damage at cumulative dose >550 mg/m^2 • Moderately emetogenic	No
Doxorubicin	Adriamycin (IV)		• Dose-related cardiotoxicity • Severe bone marrow suppression • Secondary leukemias • Red coloration of body fluids				No

Hormonal Agents

Mechanism of action — treat cancers in which growth is accelerated by hormones

Generic	Brand/Route of Administration	Contraindications	Primary Side Effects	Key Monitoring	Pertinent Drug Interactions	Med Pearl	Top 200
Leuprolide	Only available generically (SC)	• Spinal cord compression • Undiagnosed abnormal vaginal bleeding	• Abnormal menses • Exacerbation of endometriosis • Hot flashes/sweats • ↓ bone mineral density (if used >6 mo) • Spinal cord compression and urinary tract obstruction in prostate cancer • Tumor flare • Depression, mood disturbances	• Leutinizing hormone (LH) and follicle-stimulating hormone (FSH) levels • Serum testosterone (males), estradiol (females) • Bone mineral density	None	• Administered daily • Rotate injection sites	No
	Lupron depot (IM)					• Administered every 1–6 mo, depending on dosage • Rotate injection sites	
	Eligard (SC depot formulation)						
Tamoxifen	Soltamox (PO)	• Concurrent warfarin therapy • History of deep vein thrombosis (DVT) or pulmonary embolism	• Thromboembolic events • ↑ risk of endometrial cancer • Hot flashes • Altered menses • Mood disturbances, depression • ↓ bone mineral density	Annual gynecologic exams	• CYP3A4 substrate • May ↑ effects of warfarin	• Bone pain may indicate a good therapeutic response; manage with mild analgesic • Used in premenopausal women with breast cancer • Should not exceed 5 years of therapy	Yes
Anastrozole	Arimidex (PO)	None	• ↓ bone mineral density • Hyperlipidemia • Mood disturbances	• Bone mineral density • Low-density lipoprotein (LDL) and total cholesterol	None	Used in postmenopausal women with breast cancer	Yes
Letrozole	Femara (PO)	None	• ↓ bone mineral density • Hyperlipidemia • Hot flashes	• Bone mineral density • LDL and total cholesterol	None	Used in postmenopausal women with breast cancer	No

Chemotherapy Agents: Common Adverse Effects

- Cardiotoxicity
  - Doxorubicin
  - Daunorubicin
  - Idarubicin
  - Mitoxantrone
  - Trastuzumab
- N/V
  - Cisplatin
  - Carboplatin
  - Cytarabine
  - Doxorubicin
  - Cyclophosphamide
- Mucositis
  - Cytarabine
  - Cyclophosphamide
  - 5-Fluorouracil
  - Methotrexate
- Neuropathy
  - Vincristine
  - Vinblastine
  - Oxaliplatin
  - Paclitaxel
- Renal dysfunction
  - Cisplatin
  - Cyclophosphamide
  - Ifosfamide
- Pulmonary fibrosis
  - Bleomycin
  - Busulfan
- Infusion reactions
  - Monoclonal antibodies
  - Paclitaxel

Targeted and Biologic Agents

Monoclonal Antibodies

- Ibritumomab tiuxetan (Zevalin) (IV)
  - Used for CD20-positive, B-cell NHL (including rituximab-resistant)
  - Linked to a radioisotope that targets B cells, including malignant ones
  - Used in combination with rituximab as part of a two-step process using indium-111 (step 1) and yttrium-90 (step 2) ibritumomab tiuxetan
  - Major toxicities: Infusion-related reactions, myelosuppression (prolonged), secondary leukemia, myelodysplastic sydrome, Stevens-Johnson syndrome, toxic epidermal nectolysis, exfoliative dermatitis
  - Premedicate with diphenhydramine and acetaminophen
- Obinutuzumab (Gazyva) (IV)
  - Used for CLL (targeted against CD20 antigen)
  - Major toxicities: Infusion-related reactions, tumor lysis syndrome, myelosuppression (prolonged), progressive multifocal leukoencephalopathy (PML)
  - Premedicate with diphenhydramine, acetaminophen, and glucocorticoid
- Ofatumumab (Arzerra) (IV)
  - Used for CLL (targeted against CD20 antigen)
  - Major toxicities: Infusion-related reactions, tumor lysis syndrome, myelosuppression (prolonged), PML
  - Premedicate with diphenhydramine, acetaminophen, and glucocorticoid
- Rituximab (Rituxan) (IV)
  - Used for CD20-positive, B-cell NHL and CD20-positive CLL
  - Also used for rheumatoid arthritis
  - Major toxicities: Infusion-related reactions, tumor lysis syndrome, Stevens-Johnson syndrome, toxic epidermal necrolysis, PML, cardiotoxicity
  - Premedicate with diphenhydramine and acetaminophen

Epidermal Growth Factor Receptor (EGFR) Inhibitors

- Afatinib (Gilotrif) (PO)
  - Used for metastatic NSCLC
  - Major toxicities: Diarrhea, rash (can be severe), interstitial lung disease, hepatotoxicity
- Cetuximab (Erbitux) (IV)
  - Used for squamous cell cancer of head and neck and colorectal cancer (EGFR positive)
  - Major toxicities: Infusion-related reactions, rash (can be severe), interstitial lung disease
  - Premedicate with diphenhydramine

- Erlotinib (Tarceva) (PO)
  - Used for locally advanced/metastatic NSCLC or locally advanced, surgically unresectable, or metastatic pancreatic cancer
  - Major toxicities: Rash (can be severe), diarrhea, interstitial lung disease
  - CYP3A4 substrate
- Lapatinib (Tykerb) (PO)
  - Used for metastatic breast cancer with tumor overexpression of HER2
  - Major toxicities: Diarrhea, hepatotoxicity, rash (can be severe), QT interval prolongation, interstitial lung disease
  - CYP3A4 substrate
- Panitumumab (Vectibix) (IV)
  - Used for metastatic colorectal cancer
  - Major toxicities: Rash (can be severe), infusion-related reactions, interstitial lung disease
- Pertuzumab (Perjeta) (IV)
  - Used for HER2-positive metastatic breast cancer (used with trastuzumab and docetaxel)
  - Major toxicities: Cardiotoxicity, infusion-related reactions, myelosuppression
  - Should not be used with anthracyclines (↑ risk for cardiotoxicity)
- Trastuzumab (Herceptin) (IV)
  - Used for HER2-positive metastatic breast cancer and metastatic gastric cancer
  - Major toxicities: Cardiotoxicity, infusion-related reactions (can be treated with diphenhydramine, acetaminophen, and meperidine), myelosuppression, interstitial lung disease
  - Should not be used with anthracyclines (↑ risk for cardiotoxicity)
- Ado-trastuzumab emtansine (Kadcyla) (IV)
  - Used for HER-2 positive metastatic breast cancer
  - Major toxicities: Hepatotoxicity, cardiotoxicity, infusion-related reactions (treatment same as trastuzumab), interstitial lung disease, neutropenia, thrombocytopenia, peripheral neuropathy
  - CYP3A4 substrate (avoid medications with inducing or inhibiting properties)

Vascular Endothelial Growth Factor (VEGF) Inhibitors

- Axitinib (Inlyta) (PO)
  - Used for metastatic renal cell carcinoma
  - Major toxicities: Thromboembolic events, hypertension, bleeding, heart failure, reversible posterior leukoencephalopathy syndrome (RPLS)
  - CYP3A4 substrate

- Bevacizumab (Avastin) (IV)
  - Used for metastatic colorectal cancer, locally advanced, recurrent or metastatic nonsquamous NSCLC, glioblastoma, metastatic renal cell carcinoma, and persistent, recurrent, or metastatic cervical cancer
  - Major toxicities: Thromboembolic events, hypertension, bleeding, RPLS
- Ramucirumab (Cyramza) (IV)
  - Used for advanced or metastatic gastric cancer
  - Major toxicities: Thromboembolic events, hypertension, bleeding, infusion-related reactions, RPLS
  - Premedicate with diphenhydramine
- Sunitinib (Sutent) (PO)
  - Used for gastrointestinal stromal tumor (GIST), renal cell carcinoma, and pancreatic neuroendocrine tumors
  - Major toxicities: Diarrhea, rash, hypertension, heart failure, RPLS
  - CYP3A4 substrate
- Sorafenib (Nexavar) (PO)
  - Used for advanced renal cell carcinoma and unresectable hepatocellular carcinoma, and locally recurrent or metastatic, progressive differentiated thyroid cancer
  - Major toxicities: Diarrhea, rash, hypertension, hand-foot syndrome
  - CYP3A4 substrate

Tyrosine Kinase Inhibitors

- Dasatinib (Sprycel) (PO)
  - Used for Philadelphia-positive (Ph+) CML and Ph+ ALL
  - Major toxicities: Myelosuppression, fluid retention, QT interval prolongation
  - CYP3A4 substrate
- Imatinib (Gleevec) (PO)
  - Used for Ph+ CML, Kit (CD117)-positive GIST, Ph+ ALL, and a variety of other disorders
  - Major toxicities: Fluid retention, Stevens-Johnson syndrome, myelosuppression, heart failure, hepatotoxicity
  - CYP3A4 substrate and inhibitor; CYP2D6 inhibitor
- Nilotinib (Tasigna) (PO)
  - Used for Ph+ CML
  - Major toxicities: Myelosuppression, QT interval prolongation, pancreatitis, hepatotoxicity
  - CYP3A4 substrate and inhibitor; CYP2C9 and CYP2D6 inhibitor; CYP2C9 inducer

Anaplastic Lymphoma Kinase (ALK) Inhibitors

- Ceritinib (Zykadia) (PO)
  - Used for ALK-positive, metastatic NSCLC
  - Major toxicities: Diarrhea, hepatotoxicity, interstitial lung disease, QT interval prolongation, hyperglycemia, bradycardia
  - CYP3A4 substrate
- Crizotinib (Xalkori) (PO)
  - Used for ALK-positive, metastatic NSCLC
  - Major toxicities: Diarrhea, hepatotoxicity, interstitial lung disease, QT interval prolongation, bradycardia, visual disturbances
  - CYP3A4 substrate

Storage and Administration Pearls

- Do not administer live vaccines during chemotherapy cycles.

Patient Education Pearls

- Patient should not breastfeed or attempt to become pregnant while taking chemotherapy.
- Because Zevalin contains radioactive isotopes, patients should be instructed on proper handwashing, special disposal of bodily waste, and other ways to limit exposure to family members postdischarge.

SUPPORTIVE CARE

Nausea and Vomiting

About 55% of cancer patients experience nausea and vomiting during the first week of chemotherapy. 5HT3 antagonists are useful in most cases, but should be used only for prevention of nausea and vomiting. Corticosteroids should be given unless contraindicated, as they are synergistic with the 5HT3 antagonists; other drug therapies depend on the type of nausea and vomiting experienced.

- Benzodiazepines: Treatment of choice for anticipatory nausea and vomiting (caused by the sights and smells of the chemotherapy environment)
- Aprepitant: Useful for delayed nausea and vomiting caused by drugs with high emetic potential (cisplatin, cyclophosphamide, doxorubicin)
- Prochlorperazine or metoclopramide: May be used in less severe cases

Pain Management

Pain is one of the most common symptoms associated with cancer and occurs in up to 75% of advanced cases, greatly affecting quality of life. Cancer pain frequently requires much higher analgesic doses than pain from other causes. As a result, cancer pain is often undertreated.

For uncontrolled pain, drug choice depends on prior opioid use and severity of pain. If opioids have not been used:

- Severe pain: Rapid titration with short-acting opioids
- Moderate pain: Slower titration with short-acting opioids
- Mild pain: NSAID, acetaminophen, or slow titration with short-acting opioids

Morphine, codeine, oxycodone, oxymorphone, hydromorphone, and fentanyl are the most commonly used opioids for cancer pain; all are short-acting agents unless given in a controlled-release dosage form. Controlled-release formulations are recommended only for non–opioid naïve patients, as they cannot be easily titrated. Methadone is occasionally used in cancer pain, and has a longer half-life and duration of action. Patients taking controlled-release formulations should also receive a prescription for a short-acting, fast-onset analgesic for breakthrough pain. Likewise, patient-controlled analgesia devices should have on-demand bolus doses available for acute pain, with a lockout setting to reduce the risk of overdose.

Management of Neutropenia and Anemia

Neutropenia and its major complication, neutropenic fever, are major concerns in many types of cancer. The nadir, or lowest, concentration of WBCs in the peripheral blood usually occurs 1–2 weeks following the administration of chemotherapy and is typically proportional to the dose. Subsequent chemotherapy is delayed until the ANC recovers, which explains the 3- to 4-week cycle length of most chemotherapy regimens. Classification of ANC is:

- Normal: 3,000–7,000 neutrophils/mm^3
- Mild neutropenia: 500–1,000/mm^3
- Moderate neutropenia: 100–500/mm^3
- Severe neutropenia: <100/mm^3

Colony-stimulating factors (CSF) such as filgrastim have been shown to shorten the duration of neutropenia, but they have little effect on mortality and are very expensive. CSFs do decrease hospitalizations, however, and clinical judgment should be used to determine which patients are most likely to benefit. Because infection leads to death in a large percentage of neutropenic patients (possibly up to 30%), anti-infective therapy is frequently needed. Broad-spectrum bactericidal antibiotics are generally used (third- and fourth-generation cephalosporins, carbapenems, or fluoroquinolones with or without aminoglycosides or β-lactams), with antipseudomonal activity being particularly important. If antifungal therapy is needed, amphotericin B is the drug of choice.

Anemia is also common in cancer patients. Treatment of anemia is currently the subject of much controversy; use of erythropoiesis-stimulating agents, including erythropoietin and darbepoetin, is no longer supported in myeloid malignancies (these agents have been associated with increase in mortality compared to patients not receiving erythropoietin). The hypothesis is that the drug may be stimulating cancer growth. These drugs should NOT be used in patients with myeloid malignancies who are receiving chemotherapy when the anticipated outcome is a cure. This finding may not apply to solid tumors; more information is needed.

Antiemetic Drugs

Generic	Brand	Dose	Contraindications	Primary Side Effects	Key Monitoring	Pertinent Drug Interactions	Med Pearl	Top 200
Mechanism of action – 5HT3 antagonists; prevent release of serotonin in GI mucosa								
Ondansetron	• Zofran • Zuplenz	16–24 mg PO or 8–12 mg IV	Current nausea and vomiting (useful only for prevention)	• Headache • Constipation or diarrhea • Fatigue • Dry mouth • Transient ↑ LFTs • QT interval prolongation	None	• CYP3A4 substrate • Use with serotonergic agents may ↑ risk of serotonin syndrome	• Single dose prior to chemotherapy; repeat doses do not ↑ effect • Palonosetron effective in preventing delayed N/V • Ondansetron also available as orally-disintegrating tabs (ODT), oral solution, and oral films (Zuplenz) • Granisetron also available as oral solution, transdermal patch (Sancuso)	Yes
Granisetron	Sancuso	2 mg PO or 1 mg IV						No
Dolasetron	Anzemet	100 mg IV/PO						No
Palonosetron	Aloxi	0.25 mg IV						No
Mechanism of action – neurokinin-1 (NK-1) antagonist; blocks substance P from NK-1 receptor								
Aprepitant	Emend	PO: 125 mg on day 1, then 80 mg daily on days 2 and 3 IV: 150 mg on day 1	None	• Asthenia • Fatigue • Diarrhea • Hiccups • Dizziness • Dehydration	Monitor levels of chemotherapy agents metabolized by CYP3A4	• CYP3A4 substrate • Inhibits CYP3A4 • Induces CYP2C9	• Use in combination with 5HT3 antagonist and dexamethasone • Prevents delayed N/V	No
Mechanism of action – corticosteroids; potentiate antiemetic properties of 5HT3 antagonists								
Dexamethasone	Decadron	8–40 mg daily PO/IV	Systemic fungal infections	• Hyperglycemia • Immunosuppression • Adrenal suppression • Insomnia • Mood changes, anxiety • GI irritation • Weight gain	• Hemoglobin/hematocrit • Serum potassium • Glucose	CYP3A4 substrate	• Synergistic with 5HT3 antagonists • Can use as single agents for mild chemotherapy-induced N/V	No
Methylprednisolone	Solu-Medrol	40–125 mg daily PO/IV						Yes
Mechanism of action – dopamine-2 antagonists								
Metoclopramide	Reglan	10–20 mg PO/IV q4–6h PRN	Seizures	• Dizziness • Sedation • Diarrhea • Extrapyramidal symptoms (EPS)	EPS	Antipsychotic agents may ↑ risk of EPS	Should not drive or operate heavy machinery while taking this drug	Yes

Cancer Pain Drugs

Mechanism of action: narcotic opioid analgesics; stimulate the mu(μ) opioid receptor, inhibiting pain pathways

Generic	Brand	Dose	Contraindications	Primary Side Effects	Key Monitoring	Pertinent Drug Interactions	Med Pearl	Top 200
Codeine	Generic (tabs, injection)	15–60 mg q4–6h	• ↑ intracranial pressure • Severe respiratory depression • Severe or acute asthma • Paralytic ileus	• Drowsiness • Dizziness • Hypotension • N/V • Constipation • Xerostomia • Respiratory depression	• Pain relief • Respiratory status • Mental status • BP	• Central nervous system (CNS) depression with alcohol or sedative/hypnotics • Mixed agonist/antagonist analgesics (could precipitate withdrawal) • Use of monoamine oxidase inhibitors (MAOIs) within 14 days may ↑ risk of severe reactions (↓ morphine dose by 25%)	• Often used in combination with aspirin, acetaminophen, or NSAIDs • Poor metabolizers of CYP2D6 cannot convert to morphine and receive no pain relief; start immediately on another drug	Yes (combination products)
Morphine	Roxanol (liquid) Generic (injection immediate-release [IR] tabs, rectal suppository) Extended release (ER) tabs/caps: • MS Contin • Avinza • Kadian	2.5–5 mg IV/IM q3–4hr 0.8–10 mg/hr continous infusion • 5–30 mg PO q4h • 10–20 mg rectally q4h Varies widely in opioid-tolerant patients; no max dose in chronic pain					• Drug of choice for severe pain • Use IR products to titrate and to control breakthrough pain • Do not crush ER products; Kadian and Avinza may be opened • Do not give Kadian through nasogastric (NG) tube	Yes
Hydromorphone	• Dilaudid (tabs, liquid, injection, rectal suppository) • Exalgo (ER tabs)	2.5–10 mg (PO) q3–6h (IR) 1–2 mg SC or IM q4–6h 8–64 mg PO q24h (ER)	• ↑ intracranial pressure • Severe respiratory depression • Severe or acute asthma • Paralytic ileus	• Drowsiness • Dizziness • Hypotension • N/V • Constipation • Xerostomia • Respiratory depression	• Pain relief • Respiratory status • Mental status • BP	• CNS depression with alcohol or sedative/hypnotics • Mixed agonist/antagonist analgesics (could precipitate withdrawal) • Cimetidine may ↑ effects • Use of MAOIs within 14 days may ↑ risk of severe reactions	• More potent than morphine • Short half-life; requires frequent dosing • Do not crush ER tabs	Yes

Cancer Pain Drugs *(cont'd)*

Generic	Brand	Dose	Contraindications	Primary Side Effects	Key Monitoring	Pertinent Drug Interactions	Med Pearl	Top 200
Oxycodone	• Generic (IR tabs, caps, liquid) • OxyContin (ER tabs) • Percocet (with acetaminophen)	• 10–30 mg q4h (IR) • 10 mg q12h (ER); titrate dosage upward as needed					Do not crush ER tabs	Yes
Fentanyl	Actiq (transmucosal lozenge)	200 mcg per episode (limit to ≤4 units/day)					• Actiq, Fentora, Lazanda, Abstral, Subsys, and Onsolis should be used for breakthrough pain only; they are not interchangeable • Duragesic should be used only for chronic pain in patients who are opioid-tolerant • Also available as injection	No
	Fentora (buccal tab)	100–200 mcg per episode (limit to ≤4 applications/day)						
	Duragesic (transdermal)	25–100 mcg/hr						
	Onsolis (buccal film)	200 mcg per episode (limit to ≤4 applications/day)						
	Lazanda (nasal spray)	100–200 mcg per episode (limit to ≤4 episodes/day)						
	Abstral (sublingual tab)	100 mcg per episode (limit to ≤4 episodes/day)						
	Subsys (sublingual spray)	100 mcg per episode (limit to ≤4 episodes/day)						
Hydrocodone (available only in combination products)	With acetaminophen: only available generically With ibuprofen: • Ibudone • Vicoprofen • Reprexain	• 1 tab (5–10 mg) q4–6h • Maximum of 5 tabs/24 hrs					• Combination with other drugs (i.e. ibuprofen, acetaminophen) limit ability to titrate upward • Formulations limited to ≤325 mg of acetaminophen/unit	Yes

Colony-Stimulating Factors

Generic	Brand	Dose	Contra-indications	Primary Side Effects	Key Monitoring	Pertinent Drug Interactions	Med Pearl	Top 200
Mechanism of action – stimulate production of WBCs								
Filgrastim	Neupogen	300–480 mcg SC daily	Hypersensitivity to *E. coli*	• Bone pain • Hypertension • Swelling • Redness • Hypersensitivity reactions	CBC with differential	Use lithium with caution, as it can potentiate neutrophil release	• Requires daily administration • Neutrophil-specific	No
PEG-Filgrastim	Neulasta	6 mg SC with each chemo-therapy cycle					• PEG unit increases half-life; can give 1x per chemotherapy cycle • Neutrophil-specific	No
Sargramostim	Leukine	250–500 mcg/m² /day SC	• Hypersensitivity to yeast • Excessive leukemic myeloid blasts in bone marrow	• Fever, chills • Bone pain • Myalgia • Hypertension • Hypersensitivity reactions			• Requires daily administration • Stimulates formation of all WBCs except lymphocytes	No

Storage and Administration Pearls

- Dolasetron injection may be diluted in apple or apple-grape juice and taken orally; stable for 2 hours.
- Zofran ODT contains phenylalanine.

Patient Education Pearls

- Kadian and Avinza may be opened and sprinkled on applesauce; do not chew, crush, or let dissolve or too much drug will be absorbed too quickly.
- Patient should take morphine with food if it causes stomach upset.
- Patient should not take echinacea if taking corticosteroids.

Learning Points

- Chemotherapy protocols vary tremendously; do NOT spend your time memorizing drugs of choice for the various cancers (pharmacists usually do not play a role in selecting drug therapies as treatment is usually protocol driven).
    - Focus more on the toxicity profile of the most commonly used drugs and less on dosing and specific drug combinations.
- Because of the increasing importance of pharmacogenomics, you should know which drugs target specific receptors (e.g., Trastuzumab, HER2 receptor; Cetuximab, EGFR; Rituximab, CD20 cell surface protein, etc.).
- Leucovorin is used as a rescue agent in patients receiving methotrexate but enhances the effect of 5-fluorouracil.
- To treat N/V, most patients should receive a corticosteroid, a 5HT3 antagonist, and possibly a benzodiazepine. For severe cases, aprepitant should be added.
- Short-acting opioids are the pain management drugs of choice for cancer pain. As severity increases, titration should be performed more quickly.

PRACTICE QUESTIONS

1. Which of the following chemotherapeutic agents may cause left ventricular systolic dysfunction as a toxicity?

    > I.   Doxorubicin
    > II. Trastuzumab
    > III. Cisplatin

    (A) I only
    (B) III only
    (C) I and II only
    (D) II and III only
    (E) I, II, and III

2. Which of the following chemotherapeutic agents is associated with profound acute- and late-onset diarrhea?

    (A) Irinotecan
    (B) Doxorubicin
    (C) Daunorubicin
    (D) Trastuzumab
    (E) Methotrexate

3. The mechanism of action of Emend is

    (A) 5HT3 receptor antagonist.
    (B) neurokinin-1 receptor antagonist.
    (C) D2 receptor antagonist.
    (D) benzodiazepine receptor agonist.
    (E) histamine receptor antagonist.

4. A patient with NHL is to be started on cyclophosphamide, doxorubicin, vincristine, and prednisone. Which of the following drugs is MOST likely to be protective against the toxicity of doxorubicin?

    (A) Amifostine
    (B) Dexrazoxane
    (C) Folic acid
    (D) Leucovorin
    (E) Mesna

5. A patient receiving cancer chemotherapy presents to the emergency room complaining of an increase in urinary frequency and dysuria. No apparent findings are apparent on physical examination. This patient's urinalysis reveals (–) WBC, (+) blood, (–) bacteria, (–) casts. If the symptoms experienced by the patient are related to the cancer chemotherapy, what drug is MOST likely the cause?

    (A) Cyclophosphamide
    (B) Irinotecan
    (C) Methotrexate
    (D) Paclitaxel
    (E) Tamoxifen

6. Which of the following BEST describes the mechanism of action of Zofran?

    (A) It competes for the binding sites of serotonin receptors.
    (B) It inhibits the substance P/neurokinin-1 receptor.
    (C) It inhibits histamine H_1 receptors.
    (D) It stimulates dopamine-2 receptors.
    (E) It stimulates cannabinoid receptors.

7. Etoposide should not be administered IV push because of the increased risk of which of the following adverse effects?

    (A) Diarrhea
    (B) Hepatotoxicity
    (C) Hypotension
    (D) Pulmonary fibrosis
    (E) Seizure

8. Pulmonary fibrosis is MOST likely to be occur as a toxicity of which of the following chemotherapy drugs?

    (A) Bleomycin
    (B) Cisplatin
    (C) Daunorubicin
    (D) Trastuzumab
    (E) Vincristine

9. Which of the following antiemetic drugs is available as a transdermal patch?

    (A) Aprepitant
    (B) Dexamethasone
    (C) Granisetron
    (D) Metoclopramide
    (E) Prochlorperazine

10. Which of the following drugs is/are considered VEGF inhibitors?

    I. Bevacizumab
    II. Rituximab
    III. Trastuzumab

(A) I only
(B) III only
(C) I and II only
(D) II and III only
(E) I, II, and III

11. Fentanyl is available in which of the following formulations?

    I. Injection
    II. Transmucosal lozenge
    III. Transdermal patch

(A) I only
(B) III only
(C) I and II only
(D) II and III only
(E) I, II, and III

ANSWERS

1. C

Cardiotoxicity is a major adverse effect associated with both doxorubicin (I) and trastuzumab (II). Cisplatin (III) does not cause cardiotoxicity. Instead, this chemotherapeutic agent is associated with nephrotoxicity.

2. A

Of the drugs listed, only irinotecan exhibits major GI adverse effects. The other drugs are more likely to lead to cardiomyopathy (trastuzumab, doxorubicin, and daunorubicin) or neuro-, nephro-, and hepatotoxicity (methotrexate).

3. B

Emend (aprepitant) is a highly selective emetogenic agent that works against the neurokinin-1 receptor. It has little to no affinity for the other receptor targets of chemotherapy-induced or postoperative nausea and vomiting.

4. B

Dexrazoxane can be used to reduce the incidence and severity of cardiomyopathy associated with doxorubicin administration (cumulative doses >300 mg/m^2). Amifostine (A) is used to reduce the cumulative renal toxicity associated with repeated administration of cisplatin. The use of methotrexate can lead to folate deficiency; folic acid (C) can be administered to patients receiving methotrexate to prevent side effects. Leucovorin (D) can be given after administration of methotrexate to limit its toxicity. Mesna (E) is used to prevent hemorrhagic cystitis associated with cyclophosphamide or ifosfamide.

5. A

This patient is most likely exhibiting signs of chemotherapy-induced hemorrhagic cystitis. This adverse effect is most commonly associated with cyclophosphamide and ifosfamide. The major toxicity associated with irinotecan (B) is diarrhea. Methotrexate (C) can cause numerous organ toxicities, including nephrotoxicity (acute renal failure), neurotoxicity, and hepatotoxicity. Paclitaxel (D) can be associated with peripheral neuropathy. The major adverse effect associated with tamoxifen (E) is thromboembolic events.

6. A

The antiemetic Zofran (ondansetron) is a selective serotonin (5HT$_3$) receptor antagonist. Another antiemetic, aprepitant (Emend), inhibits the substance P/neurokinin-1 receptor (B). By inhibiting dopamine (DA2) receptors—not stimulating them (D)—metoclopramide (Reglan) also acts as an antiemetic.

7. **C**

Administering etoposide via IV push may lead to hypotension. Etoposide should be administered over 30–60 minutes to minimize the risk of this adverse effect.

8. **A**

Pulmonary fibrosis is a significant adverse effects associated with bleomycin and busulfan. The major toxicity associated with cisplatin (B) is nephrotoxicity. Daunorubicin (C) and trastuzumab (D) are associated with cardiotoxicity. Vincristine (E) is associated with dose-limiting peripheral neuropathy.

9. **C**

Of the listed antiemetic drugs, only granisetron, a 5HT3 antagonist, is available as a transdermal patch (Sancuso). Aprepitant (A) is available as a capsule and an IV injection. Dexamethasone (B) is available as a tablet, oral solution, and IV injection. Metoclopramide (D) is available as a tablet, orally disintegrating tablet, oral solution, and IV injection. Prochlorperazine (E) is available as a tablet, rectal suppository, and IV injection.

10. **A**

Only bevacizumab (I) is considered a VEGF inhibitor. Rituximab (II) is a monoclonal antibody directed against the CD20 antigen on B-lymphocytes. Trastuzumab (III) is a monoclonal antibody targeted against the HER2 receptor.

11. **E**

Fentanyl is available as an IV injection (I), transmucosal lozenge (II) (Actiq), and transdermal patch (III) (Duragesic). Fentanyl is also available as a buccal tablet, buccal film, nasal spray, sublingual tablet, and sublingual spray.

Psychiatric Disorders

This chapter covers the following disease states:

- **Depression**
- **Anxiety**
- **Bipolar disorder**
- **Schizophrenia**
- **Insomnia**
- **ADHD**

 Suggested Study Time: **60 minutes**

DEPRESSION

Definition

Depression, or major depressive disorder, is a complex mood disorder that has many subtypes and is due to multiple etiologies. Depression can be classified as single-episode, recurrent, or chronic and as depression with or without psychotic features, with typical or atypical symptoms, etc.

Diagnosis

The diagnosis of depression is based on the *Diagnostic and Statistical Manual of Mental Disorders*, 5th Edition (DSM V). Criteria for diagnosis are based primarily on symptoms. Five or more of the following symptoms must have been present during the same 2-week period and must represent a change from previous functioning; at least one of the symptoms is either (*1*) depressed mood or (*2*) loss of interest or pleasure.

- Depressed mood most of the day, nearly every day
- Markedly diminished interest or pleasure in all, or almost all, activities

- Significant weight loss when not dieting, or weight gain
- Insomnia or hypersomnia nearly every day
- Psychomotor agitation or retardation nearly every day
- Fatigue or loss of energy nearly every day
- Feelings of worthlessness or of excessive or inappropriate guilt
- Diminished ability to think or concentrate, or indecisiveness
- Recurrent thoughts of death (not just fear of dying), recurrent suicidal ideation without a specific plan, or a suicide attempt or a specific plan for committing suicide

Signs and Symptoms

Signs and symptoms are detailed in the diagnostic criteria.

Guidelines

American Psychiatric Association practice guideline for the treatment of patients with major depressive disorder, 3rd ed. www.psychiatryonline.org/guidelines/aspx.

Guidelines Summary

- The primary goal of therapy is remission of symptoms.
- There are various antidepressant medications available. Clinical evidence indicates that, in general, efficacy is similar between classes.
- Initial choice of pharmacotherapy agent is based on anticipated side effects, tolerability of these side effects for an individual patient, patient preference, quantity and quality of clinical evidence, and cost.
- First-line options for most patients include selective serotonin reuptake inhibitors (SSRIs), desipramine, nortriptyline, bupropion, and venlafaxine. Because of the potential for serious side effects and drug interactions, monoamine oxidase inhibitors (MAOIs) should be reserved for patients who do not respond to other therapies.
- An adequate therapy trial requires at least 6–8 weeks. Dose adjustments or treatment changes are made at 6- to 8-week intervals at the earliest.
- There is significant interpatient variability in response to antidepressants. Patients may respond to classes/agents that have been effective in the past or that have been effective for family members. Bupropion has a lower incidence of sexual side effects and may be preferred in patients presenting with this complaint related to therapy.
- In 2005, the FDA required that all product labeling for antidepressants include a boxed warning regarding the potential for increased risk of clinical worsening and suicidality in children, adolescents, and young adults taking these agents.

Antidepressants

Mechanism of action – SSRIs: inhibit reuptake of serotonin, allowing more serotonin availability in synapses

Generic	Brand	Dose & Max mg (frequency)	Contra-indications	Primary Side Effects	Key Monitoring Parameters	Pertinent Drug Interactions	Med Pearls	Top 200
Citalopram	Celexa	10–60 mg daily	• MAOI • Pimozide • Hypersensitivity	• Lightheadedness • Syncope • Sweating • Diarrhea • Nausea • Xerostomia • Confusion • Dizziness • Somnolence • Tremor • Hallucinations • Disorder of ejaculation • Impotence • Rhinitis • Fatigue • Female sexual disorder	• Reduction or resolution of symptoms • Withdrawal symptoms from abrupt discontinuation • Abnormal bleeding • Worsening of depression, suicidality, or unusual behavior at initiation of therapy or when changing dose	• Other serotonergic medications, such as MAOI, SSRI, triptans, linezolid, St. John's wort, tramadol	Racemic mixture R and S isomer	Yes
Escitalopram	Lexapro	10–20 mg daily	• Hypersensitivity				Only contains the S isomer of citalopram	Yes
Fluoxetine	• Prozac • Prozac Wkly • Sarafem • Rapiflux	20–60 mg daily or 80 mg wkly				• Other serotonergic medications such as MAOI, SSRI, triptans, linezolid, St. John's wort, tramadol, phenytoin • Drugs metabolized by cytochrome P450	• Allow 5 wks washout prior to MAOI due to long half-life • Does not require taper due to long half-life	Yes
Fluvoxamine	Luvox	50–300 mg daily	• MAOI • Pimozide • Thioridazine • Alosetron • Astemizole • Terfenadine • Tizanidine • Hypersensitivity					No
Paroxetine	Paxil	20–60 mg daily	• MAOI • Pimozide • Thioridazine • Hypersensitivity			Other serotonergic medications such as MAOI, SSRI, triptans, linezolid, St. John's wort, tramadol		Yes
Sertraline	Zoloft	50–200 mg daily	• MAOI • Pimozide • Disulfiram-like compounds (oral concentrate) • Linezolid • Hypersensitivity				Oral concentrate contains alcohol	Yes
Vortioxetine	Brintellix	5–20 mg daily	• MAOI (within 21 days) • Linezolid • Hypersensitivity • Methylene blue			• Major substrate of CYP3A4 and 2D6 • Strong CYP3A4 inducers/inhibitors • Other serotonergic medications such as MAOIs, SSRIs, triptans, linezolid, St. John's wort, tramadol		No

Antidepressants *(cont'd)*

Mechanism of action – selective serotonin reuptake inhibitor, partial 5HT1A receptor agonist

Generic	Brand	Dose & Max mg (frequency)	Contra-indications	Primary Side Effects	Key Monitoring Parameters	Pertinent Drug Interactions	Med Pearls	Top 200
Vilazodone	Viibryd	10–40 mg PO once daily	MAOI	• Diarrhea • Nausea • Xerostomia • Dizziness • Insomnia	• Reduction or resolution of symptoms • Worsening of depression/suicidality	• Other serotonergic medications such as MAOI, SSRI, triptans, linezolid, St. John's wort, tramadol • Warfarin, NSAIDs, antiplatelet agents—increased risk of bleeding	• Should be taken with food • Avoid abrupt discontinuation • Risk of bleeding is unique among antidepressants	No

Mechanism of action – tricyclic antidepressants (TCAs): increased synaptic concentration of norepinephrine and serotonin

Generic	Brand	Dose & Max mg (frequency)	Contra-indications	Primary Side Effects	Key Monitoring Parameters	Pertinent Drug Interactions	Med Pearls	Top 200
Amitriptyline	• Elavil • Vanatrip	50–300 mg daily (q day–TID)	• MAOI • Post-myocardial infarction (MI) acute recovery • Hypersensitivity	• Anticholinergic symptoms • Weight gain • Bloating • Blurred vision • Xerostomia • Constipation • Asthenia • Dizziness • Somnolence • Headache • Fatigue	• Reduction or resolution of symptoms • Withdrawal symptoms from abrupt discontinuation • Worsening of depression, suicidality, or unusual behavior at initiation of therapy or when changing dose • Blood pressure (BP) • Electrocardiogram (ECG) in patients with cardiac disease or hyperthyroidism	Other serotonergic medications such as MAOI, SSRI, triptans, linezolid, St. John's wort, tramadol	• Dangerous in overdose situations • Avoid in patients with high suicidality • Avoid dispensing large quantities • Also used for sleep disorders	Yes
Amoxapine	Ascendin	50–600 mg daily (BID–TID)						No
Clomipramine	Anafranil	75–250 mg daily (divided TID)						No
Desipramine	Norpramin	100–300 mg daily (q day or divided doses)						No
Doxepin	• Sinequan • Prudoxin • Zonalon	25–300 mg daily (q day–TID)						Yes
Imipramine	Tofranil	100–300 mg daily (q day–divided)						Yes
Nortriptyline	• Pamelor • Aventyl	25 mg TID–QID (max = 150 mg daily)						Yes
Protriptyline	Vivactil	15–60 mg daily (TID–QID)						No
Trimipramine	Surmontil	75–300 mg daily (q day–TID)						No

Antidepressants (cont'd)

Mechanism of action – serotonin and norepinephrine reuptake inhibitors (SNRI): inhibit the reuptake of serotonin and norepinephrine to allow higher available synaptic concentrations

Generic	Brand	Dose & Max mg (frequency)	Contra-indications	Primary Side Effects	Key Monitoring Parameters	Pertinent Drug Interactions	Med Pearls	Top 200
Duloxetine	Cymbalta	30–120 mg daily (q day)	• MAOI • Hypersensitivity • Uncontrolled narrow-angle glaucoma	• Palpitations • Diaphoresis • Constipation • Decreased appetite • D/N • Xerostomia • Asthenia • Dizziness • Insomnia • Somnolence • Vertigo • Blurred vision • Polyuria • Reduced libido • Cough • Nasopharyngitis • Fatigue	• Reduction or resolution of symptoms • Withdrawal symptoms from abrupt discontinuation • Worsening of depression	Other serotonergic medications such as MAOI, SSRI, Triptans, Linezolid, St. John's wart, Tramadol;	Doses >60 mg did not provide additional benefit in generalized anxiety disorder	Yes
Venlafaxine	• Effexor • Effexor XR	37.5–375 mg daily (q day–TID)	• MAOI • Hypersensitivity	• Hypertension • Sweating • Weight loss • Constipation • Loss of appetite • Nausea • Xerostomia • Insomnia or somnolence • Erectile dysfunction	• Reduction or resolution of symptoms • Withdrawal symptoms from abrupt discontinuation • Worsening of depression • BP			Yes

Antidepressants *(cont'd)*

Generic	Brand	Dose & Max mg (frequency)	Contra-indications	Primary Side Effects	Key Monitoring Parameters	Pertinent Drug Interactions	Med Pearls	Top 200
Levomilnacipran	Fetzima	20–120 mg daily	• MAOI (within 21 days) • Linezolid • Hypersensitivity • Methylene blue • Uncontrolled narrow angle glaucoma			• Major substrate of CYP3A4 • Strong CYP3A4 inducers/inhibitors • Other serotonergic medications such as MAOIs, SSRIs, triptans, linezolid, St. John's wort, tramadol • Enhanced bleeding risk with anticoagulants, thrombolytics	Renal dosing CrCl <60 mL/min	No
Desvenlafaxine	Pristiq	50–400 mg PO daily	• Hypersensitivity • MAOI therapy	• Orthostatic hypotension (elderly) • Nausea • Dizziness • Insomnia • Hyperhidrosis • Constipation • Somnolence • Decreased appetite • Anxiety • Male sexual dysfunction	• Renal function • Response to therapy • BP • Worsening of depressive symptoms • Suicidality	• MAOI, serotonergic agents increase risk of serotonin syndrome • Increased risk of bleeding when used in combination with anticoagulants, thrombolytics	• Renal dose adjustment required • Should not be abruptly discontinued	Yes
Desvenlafaxine ER	Khedezla							
Nefazodone	Serzone	200–600 mg daily (BID)	• Previous nefazodone-induced hepatic damage • Hypersensitivity • Astemizole • Carbamazepine • Cisapride • Triazolam • Terfenadine • Pimozide	• Lightheadedness • Constipation • Indigestion • Nausea • Xerostomia • Asthenia • Confusion • Dizziness • Headache • Insomnia • Memory impairment • Somnolence	• Reduction or resolution of symptoms • Withdrawal symptoms from abrupt discontinuation • Worsening of depression			No

Antidepressants *(cont'd)*

Mechanism of action – MAOIs: increase epinephrine, norepinephrine, dopamine, and serotonin

Generic	Brand	Dose & Max mg (frequency)	Contra-indications	Primary Side Effects	Key Monitoring Parameters	Pertinent Drug Interactions	Med Pearls	Top 200
Isocarboxazid	Marplan	20–60 mg daily (BID–QID)	• Cardiovascular disorder • Hypertension • Cerebrovascular disorder • Concurrent administration of interacting medications • General anesthesia • History of headache • Hypersensitivity • Pheochromocytoma • Severe renal function impairment	• Weight gain • Constipation • Xerostomia • Dizziness • Headache • Insomnia • Somnolence • Blurred vision • Anxiety • Mania	• Reduced depression and associated symptoms • BP • Liver function • Worsening of depression, suicidality, or unusual changes in behavior	• Other serotonergic medications such as SSRI, triptans, linezolid, St. John's wort, tramadol • Concurrent administration of antihistaminic, sedative, or anesthetic substances • Bupropion • Buspirone • Narcotics • Barbiturates • Ethanol • Dextromethorphan • Excessive caffeine • Foods containing high concentrations of tyramine • Meperidine • SSRI • Sympathomimetic drugs • MAOI • Tricyclic antidepressants (TRAs) • Maprotiline • Carbamazepine • Cyclobenzaprine	Used very infrequently due to poor side effect profile and frequency of drug interactions	No
Phenelzine	Nardil	45–90 mg daily (TID–QID)	• Cardiovascular disorder • Hypertension • Cerebrovascular disorder • Concurrent administration of interacting medications • General anesthesia • History of headache • Hypersensitivity • Pheochromocytoma • Severe renal function impairment					No
Tranylcypromine	Parnate	30–60 mg daily (divided doses)						No

Antidepressants *(cont'd)*

Generic	Brand	Dose & Max mg (frequency)	Contra-indications	Primary Side Effects	Key Monitoring Parameters	Pertinent Drug Interactions	Med Pearls	Top 200
Selegiline	Emsam	6 mg daily transdermal patch (q day)	• Cardiovascular disorder • Hypertension • Cerebrovascular disorder • Concurrent administration of interacting medications • General anesthesia • History of headache • Hypersensitivity • Pheochromocytoma • Severe renal function impairment			• Other serotonergic medications such as SSRI, triptans, linezolid, St. John's wort, tramadol • Concurrent administration of antihistaminic, sedative, or anesthetic substances • Bupropion • Buspirone • Narcotics • Barbiturates • Ethanol • Dextromethorphan • Excessive caffeine • Foods containing high concentrations of tyramine • Meperidine • SSRI • Sympathomimetic drugs • MAOI • TCA • Maprotiline • Carbamazepine • Cyclobenzaprine	Used primarily for Parkinson's disease and less frequently for depression	No

Antidepressants (cont'd)

Generic	Brand	Dose & Max mg (frequency)	Contra-indications	Primary Side Effects	Key Monitoring Parameters	Pertinent Drug Interactions	Med Pearls	Top 200
Mechanism of action – aminoketone: weak inhibitor of dopamine and norepinephrine reuptake								
Bupropion	• Wellbutrin • Wellbutrin SR • Wellbutrin XL • Zyban	100–450 mg daily (q day–QID)	• MAOI • Bulimia or anorexia • Patients in withdrawal from alcohol • Seizure disorders	• Taste disturbance • Agitation • Increased seizure activity	• Reduction or resolution of symptoms • Withdrawal symptoms from abrupt discontinuation • Worsening of depression • Seizure activity	MAOI	• Also used for smoking cessation • Mostly dopamine reuptake activity	Yes
Mechanism of action – tetracyclic antidepressants: increase available synaptic concentrations of norepinephrine, serotonin, or both								
Maprotiline	Ludiomil	75–225 mg daily (BID–TID)	• MAOI • Hypersensitivity • Seizure disorder • Post-MI acute recovery period	• Hypotension • Tachyarrhythmia • Rash • Weight gain • Constipation • Nausea • Pancreatitis • Reduced salivation • Vomiting • Xerostomia	• Reduction or resolution of symptoms • Withdrawal symptoms from abrupt discontinuation • Worsening of depression	MAOI		No
Mirtazapine	• Remeron • Solutab	15–45 mg daily (q HS)		• Increased appetite • Hyperlipidemia • Weight gain • Constipation • Elevated transaminases		• MAOI • Clonidine • Tramadol • Fluoxetine • Fluvoxamine • Linezolid • Olanzapine • Venlafaxine	• Dosed at bedtime due to somnolence • Off-label use for appetite stimulation	Yes

Storage and Administration Pearls

- Store at room temperature in a dry place that is protected from light.

Patient Education Pearls

- It may take several weeks for medication to demonstrate maximal efficacy. Allow adequate trial before determining if medication is ineffective.
- Patients should not abruptly discontinue their medication. They should consult with a healthcare professional to determine appropriate tapering procedures.
- Patients on MAOIs should avoid excessive caffeine intake, chocolate, and foods containing high levels of tyramine, including red wine, aged cheeses, avocado, eggplant, figs, and soy-based foods.

ANXIETY

Definition

Anxiety disorders consist of a number of disorders, including generalized anxiety disorder (GAD) and panic disorder. This chapter focuses on these two most common subtypes of anxiety disorders. The pathophysiology of anxiety is poorly understood but is theoretically linked to abnormal function of several neurotransmitters, including GABA, serotonin, and norepinephrine.

Diagnosis

GAD diagnosis is based on the presence of anxiety or excessive worry (1) that has been present on most days over at least 6 months, and (2) over which the patient feels a lack of control. Three or more subjective symptoms must be present in order to make the diagnosis.

Panic disorder is a complex disorder characterized by panic attacks. During a panic attack, at least four psychic and somatic symptoms will be present. In order to be diagnosed with panic disorder, a patient must have a history of recurrent panic attacks

Signs and Symptoms

- Subjective symptoms of GAD include restlessness, feeling easily fatigued, difficulty concentrating, irritability, muscle tension, and sleep difficulties.
- Psychic symptoms of panic disorder include depersonalization, fear of dying, derealization, fear of losing control, and fear of going "crazy."
- Somatic symptoms of panic disorder include sweating, trembling, shaking, choking, chest pain, nausea, abdominal pain, palpitations, tachycardia, shortness of breath, dizziness, light-headedness, chills, and hot flashes.

Summary of Treatment Recommendations

- Goals of therapy include improvement in overall functionality and quality of life through reduction of symptom frequency and intensity. Complete remission of illness is the long-term treatment goal.
- Treatment options are detailed in the medication charts and no consensus exists as to the preferred initial therapy or order of options thereafter.
- Many clinicians prefer the SSRIs as initial therapy due to their favorable side-effect profile as compared to other therapies. Subsequently, other antidepressants such as venlafaxine or tricyclics can be utilized. Benzodiazepines are commonly used, especially in acute situations. Although efficacious, these agents lend themselves to issues related to dependence, increased fall risk in the elderly, and potential for negative cognitive effects in general. Buspirone is a unique treatment option that is effective but requires 2 to 3 weeks to reach efficacy; thus, it is not useful in acute situations.
- Benzodiazepine selection should take into account varying pharmacokinetic profiles of agents. In elderly patients, preference is given to those agents that are shorter-acting (less accumulation) and those metabolized by glucoronidation (e.g., lorazepam, oxazepam) versus oxidation (e.g., alprazolam, diazepam). Agents with a rapid onset have a greater potential for dependence.

Anxiolytics

Mechanism of action – benzodiazepines bind to GABA receptors, causing an influx of chloride which results in hyperpolarization and a less excitable state; metabolized by CYP450, benzodiazepines have a potential interaction with all CYP450 inhibitors and inducers

Generic	Brand	Dose & Max mg (frequency)	Contra-indications	Primary Side Effects	Key Monitoring Parameters	Pertinent Drug Interactions	Med Pearls	Top 200
Alprazolam	• Xanax • Xanax XR • Nirazax ODT • Alprazolam • Intensol	• Immediate release (IR) 0.25–2 mg (q day–TID) • Extended release (ER) 0.5–3 mg (q day) (max = 4 mg/day)	• Hypersensitive • Narrow-angle glaucoma	• Somnolence • Ataxia • Dizziness • Changes in appetite • Decreased libido • Confusion • Constipation • Blurred vision	• Orthostasis • Excessive sedation • Signs of withdrawal • Periodic basic metabolic panel (BMP) • Liver function tests (LFTs) and complete blood count (CBC) in chronic therapy	• Ketoconazole • Itraconazole • Alcohol • Central nervous system (CNS) depressants • Digoxin • Fluoxetine • Propoxyphene • Nefazodone	• Schedule C-IV • Pregnancy category D • Smoking decreases concentration up to 50% • Pediatric dosing • Rapid onset, short-acting	Yes
Chlordiazepoxide	Librium	5–25 mg (TID–QID)				• Alcohol • CNS depressants • Ketoconazole	• CrCl <10% give 50% of recommended dose • IV injection available • Avoid in elderly • Schedule C-IV • Pregnancy category D • Slower-onset, long-acting	No
Clonazepam	• Klonopin • Klonopin Wafers	• 0.5–2 mg (BID) • Orally disintegrating tablet (ODT) 0.125–2 mg (BID)					• Decrease dose by 50% in elderly and hepatic disease • Pregnancy category D • Schedule C-IV • Rapid-onset, long-acting	Yes
Clorazepate	• Gen-XENE • Tranxene T-Tab • Tranxene-SD • Tranxene	• IR: 3.75–15 mg (BID–QID) • ER: 11.25–22.5 mg (q day)					• Avoid in elderly • Schedule C-IV • Pregnancy category D • Rapid-onset, long-acting	No
Diazepam	• Valium • Diazepam Intensol	2–10 mg (BID–QID)					• IV and liquid dosage forms available • Schedule C-IV • Pregnancy category D • Rapid-onset, long-acting	Yes

Anxiolytics *(cont'd)*

Generic	Brand	Dose & Max mg (frequency)	Contra-indications	Primary Side Effects	Key Monitoring Parameters	Pertinent Drug Interactions	Med Pearls	Top 200
Lorazepam	• Ativan • Lorazepam • Intensol	0.5–2 mg (BID–TID) (max = 10 mg/day)					• Available in IV and liquid form • Schedule C-IV • Pregnancy category D • Medium-onset, short-acting	Yes
Oxazepam	• Alepam • Medopam • Murelax • Noripam • Oxpam • Purata • Serax • Serepax	10–30 mg (TID–QID)					• Schedule C-IV • Pregnancy category D • Medium-onset, short-acting	No

Mechanism of action — SSRIs: selectively inhibit the reuptake of serotonin by presynaptic neuronal membranes with little to no effect on norepinephrine or dopamine reuptake

Generic	Brand	Dose & Max mg (frequency)	Contra-indications	Primary Side Effects	Key Monitoring Parameters	Pertinent Drug Interactions	Med Pearls	Top 200
Citalopram	Celexa	Details above in antidepressants table			Unlabeled use for panic disorder, GAD, posttraumatic stress disorder (PTSD), and obsessive-compulsive disorder (OCD)			Yes
Escitalopram	Lexapro				Indicated for GAD			Yes
Fluoxetine	• Prozac • Sarafem				Indicated for OCD, panic disorder			Yes
Paroxetine	• Paxil • Paxil CR				Indicated for panic disorder, PTSD, GAD, OCD, social anxiety disorder (SAD)			Yes
Sertraline	Zoloft				Indicated for OCD, panic disorder, SAD, PTSD			Yes
Fluvoxamine	Luvox				Indicated for OCD			No

Anxiolytics *(cont'd)*

Generic	Brand	Dose & Max mg (frequency)	Contra-indications	Primary Side Effects	Key Monitoring Parameters	Pertinent Drug Interactions	Med Pearls	Top 200
Mechanism of action – nonselective beta-adrenergic blocker which competitively blocks response to beta1- and beta2-adrenergic stimulation in the heart muscle, vascular smooth muscle, and bronchial muscles								
Propranolol (nonselective BB)	• Inderal, Inderal LA • InnoPran XL • Propranolol • Intensol	10–80 mg 1 hr prior to anxiogenic event	• Hypersensitivity • Severe bradycardia • Heart block • Uncompensated congestive heart failure (CHF) • Severe chronic obstructive pulmonary disease (COPD) or asthma	• Dizziness • Fatigue • Gastrointesinal (GI) upset • Hypotension	• Heart rate • BP	• Inhibitors/inducers of CYP450 (major CYP1A2) • Non-dihydropyridine calcium channel blockers (CCBs)	Unlabeled for situational anxiety, acute panic	Yes
Mechanism of action – exact mechanism is unknown; high affinity for 5-HT$_{1A}$ and 5-HT$_2$ receptors, mild affinity for dopamine D$_2$ receptors								
Buspirone	BuSpar	5–30 mg (BID–TID) (max = 60 mg/day)		• Headache • Dizziness • Nausea • Hostility • Confusion • Drowsiness	• Mental status • Symptoms of anxiety • Pseudo-parkinsonism	• MAOIs • Nondihydropyridine CCBs • Inhibitors/inducers of CYP450 • Macrolides • SSRIs	• Pregnancy category B • Avoid use in renal and hepatic impairment • Pediatric dosing for 6 yrs and older • Takes 2–3 wks to reach efficacy	Yes
Mechanism of action – serotonin norepinephrine reuptake inhibitor (SNRI): inhibits reuptake of neuronal serotonin and norepinephrine; may have weak inhibitory effect on reuptake of dopamine								
Venlafaxine	• Effexor • Effexor XR	• 25–100 mg (q day) • ER: 37.5–150 mg (q day) (max = 225 mg/day)	• Hypersensitivity • Concurrent use of MAOI	• Drowsiness • Dizziness • Insomnia • Xerostomia • Weakness (generalized) • Changes in appetite	• BP • Mental status • Symptoms/ signs of serotonin syndrome	• Alcohol • CNS depressants— SSRIs • TCAs • MAOIs • Buspirone • Tramadol • Lithium • Haloperidol • Clozapine • Nefazodone • Trazodone	• Labeled for GAD, panic disorder, SAD • Pregnancy category C • Use with caution in renal impairment	Yes

Anxiolytics *(cont'd)*

Mechanism of action – competes with histamine for H$_1$-receptor sites on effector cells in GI, blood vessels, and respiratory tract

Generic	Brand	Dose & Max mg (frequency)	Contra-indications	Primary Side Effects	Key Monitoring Parameters	Pertinent Drug Interactions	Med Pearls	Top 200
Hydroxyzine	Vistaril	10–100 mg (QID)	• Hypersensitivity • Early pregnancy	• Dizziness • Drowsiness • Fatigue • Xerostomia • Blurry vision • Urinary retention	• BP • Mental status • Blood urea nitrogen (BUN) serum creatinine (SCr) with chronic use	• Antihistamines • MAOIs • CNS depressants	• Use with caution in benign prostatic hyperplasia (BPH), respiratory disease, glaucoma • Pregnancy category C • Avoid in elderly • Avoid in renal impairment	Yes

Mechanism of action – appears to affect the thalamus and limbic system; also appears to inhibit multineuronal spinal reflexes

Generic	Brand	Dose & Max mg (frequency)	Contra-indications	Primary Side Effects	Key Monitoring Parameters	Pertinent Drug Interactions	Med Pearls	Top 200
Meprobamate	Miltown	200–400 mg (TID–QID) (max = 2,400 mg/day)	• Hypersensitivity to carbamates • Porphyria	• Drowsiness • Ataxia • N/V/D • Anorexia • Hypotension	• S/S of withdrawal • Mental status • LFTs with chronic use	• Alcohol • CNS depressants	• Schedule C-IV • Pregnancy category D • Dose adjustment in hepatic and renal insufficiency	No

Storage and Administration Pearls

- Tablets and capsules should all be stored at room temperature, in dry area out of direct sunlight.
- Keep liquid preparations from freezing or overheating. Do not expose to temperatures >77°F (25°C).

Patient Education Pearls

- Take as directed by physician.
- Patients should *not* abruptly discontinue any anxiety medication.
- SSRIs, SNRIs, MAOIs may take up to several weeks (2–4 weeks) to see effect
- Patients should avoid alcohol when taking any of these medications.
- Patients should avoid driving or operating heavy machinery while taking benzodiazepines until they know how they respond to the medication.

Bipolar Disorder

Definition

Bipolar disorder is an episodic, lifelong illness with symptoms of depression alternating with symptoms of mania or hypomania. Bipolar disorder is classified on the basis of the frequency of alternating symptoms and the subtype of manic symptoms demonstrated. Bipolar I disorder is defined as one or more manic episodes plus one or more major depressive episodes. Bipolar II disorder is defined as one or more episodes of major depression and one or more hypomanic episodes with no history of a full manic or mixed episode.

Diagnosis

The diagnosis of bipolar disorder is based on the DSM V criteria for each of the subtype mood disorders (mania, hypomania, depression, mixed episode). Bipolar disorder diagnosis requires that a patient exhibits diagnosed episodes of both major depression plus manic, hypomanic, or mixed episodes. Acute manic symptoms are hallmarks of the disorder and consist of elevated, expansive, or irritable mood lasting for at least 1 week or requiring hospitalization. Hypomania is defined as symptoms of mania that do not meet the criteria for manic episode and last for at least 4 days. Mixed episode is one that meets criteria for major depression and a manic episode for at least 1 week.

Signs and Symptoms

Acute mania requires that three of the following symptoms must be present: flight of ideas or racing thoughts, decreased need for sleep, inflated self-esteem or grandiosity, more talkative than usual or pressured speech, distractibility, psychomotor agitation, and excessive involvement in pleasurable activities with high potential for negative consequences.

Major depressive symptoms are detailed in the depression section of this chapter.

Guidelines

Texas Implementation of Medication Algorithms: update to the algorithms for the treatment of bipolar disorder. *J Clin Psychiatry*, no. 66 (2005): 870–86.

Guidelines Summary

- First-line treatment options for patient with acute manic episodes include lithium, valproate, aripiprazole, quetiapine, risperidone, ziprasidone, olanzapine, or carbamazepine. Antipsychotic medications are detailed in medication charts later in this chapter.
- First-line treatment options for acute depressive episodes include lamotrigine monotherapy or lamotrigine in combination with antimania therapy.
- Maintenance therapy generally consists of continuation of therapy used in acute phases. Lithium and valproate have long history of clinical success in maintenance therapy.

Mood Stabilizers

Generic	Brand	Dose & Max mg (frequency)	Contra-indications	Primary Side Effects	Key Monitoring Parameters	Med Pearls	Top 200
Mechanism of action – lithium: altered sodium transport leads to a shift toward intraneuronal metabolism of catecholamines; the specific mechanism in mania is not fully understood							
Lithium	• Tablets • Lithobid extended-release tablets	• 300–1,200 mg daily (TID) • 300–1,200 mg daily (BID)	• Significant renal or cardiovascular disease • Dehydration	• D/V • Drowsiness • Muscle weakness • Lack of coordination • Ataxia • Blurred vision • Tinnitus	Serum drug concentration 0.6–1.5 mEq/L	Significant drug interactions with angiotensin converting enzyme (ACE) inhibitors and diuretics which decrease lithium clearance and increase toxicity	Yes
Mechanism of action – valproic acid: not fully understood; thought to increase gamma amino butyric acid (GABA) concentrations in the brain							
Valproic acid (divalproex sodium)	• Depakote • Depakote ER • Depakene • Depacon	10–60 mg/kg/day	• Hepatic dysfunction • Hypersensitivity • Urea cycle disorders	• Hepatic impairment • Thrombocytopenia • Hyperammonemia • Weight gain • Pancreatitis	• Serum drug concentrations (50–100 mcg/mL) • LFTs at baseline and periodically • Periodic CBC and serum ammonia levels	• Highly teratogenic • Available in oral capsules, tablets, ER tablets, sprinkle caps, oral syrup, and IV solution • Drug interactions detailed in neurological disorders chapter	Yes
Mechanism of action – oxcarbazepine: blocks voltage-sensitive sodium channels, resulting in stabilization of hyperexcitable neuronal membranes							
Oxcarbazepine	Trileptal tablets and oral suspension	600–2,400 mg daily (BID)	Hypersensitivity	• Sedation • Dizziness • Ataxia • Nausea • Rash (Stevens-Johnson possible) • Hyponatremia	Periodic Na, renal function; serum concentrations 12–30 mcg/mL	• CrCl <30 mL/min requires half of initial dose • Drug interactions detailed in neurological disorders chapter	Yes
Mechanism of action – lamotrigine: affects sodium channels stabilizing neuronal membranes; the exact mechanism in bipolar disorder is unknown							
Lamotrigine	Lamictal oral tablets, chewable tablets	25–700 mg daily (once to BID)	• Hypersensitivity • History of Stevens-Johnson rash	• Stevens-Johnson rash • Other rash • Diplopia • Dizziness • Headache	• Response to therapy • Presence of side effects	• Risk of rash increased when combined with valproate • Slow dose titration necessary • Drug interactions detailed in neurological disorders chapter	Yes

Storage and Administration Pearls

- All medications should be stored at room temperature in a dry area away from direct sunlight.
- Patient may take medications with food if GI upset occurs.

Patient Education Pearls

- It is important that medications be continued once the symptoms have resolved.
- Patients should discuss any new medications with a healthcare professional prior to use due to risk of drug interactions.

SCHIZOPHRENIA

Definition

Schizophrenia is a psychiatric disorder that manifests as symptoms including hallucinations or delusions, and has a dramatic impact on the affected individual's functionality and quality of life. The pathophysiology is not fully understood, but theories suggest an excessive firing of dopamine and potential activity of additional neurotransmitters such as norepinephrine, serotonin, and glutamate.

Diagnosis

Persistent disturbances in social, occupational, and self-care functioning must be present for at least 6 months, with 1 month of symptoms including at least two of the following: hallucinations, delusions, disorganized speech, disorganized behavior, or negative symptoms.

Signs and Symptoms

There are multiple subtypes of schizophrenia and symptoms vary widely between them, ranging from catalepsy or stupor to disorganized speech. Potential symptoms include auditory or visual hallucinations, delusions, disorganized speech or behavior, flat or inappropriate affect, and catatonic behavior.

Guidelines

American Psychiatric Association. *Practice Guideline for the Treatment of Patients with Schizophrenia*, 2nd ed. Arlington, VA: American Psychiatric Association; 2004: 1–114.

Guideline Watch. Practice guideline for the treatment of patients with schizophrenia (2009): *http://psychiatryonline.org/content.aspx?bookid=28&sectionid=1682213.*

Guidelines Summary

For many years, atypical antipsychotics were considered the obvious first-line choice because of significantly reduced incidence of extrapyramidal side effects. Recently, considerable controversy has surfaced, because of the ability of these medications to increase the risk of the metabolic syndrome. At this time, choice of either class is appropriate as first-line therapy. It should be considered, however, that atypical agents have better efficacy in treating negative symptoms.

- Goals of therapy include: Reduce or eliminate symptoms, minimize adverse effects of pharmacological treatment, and prevent relapse.
- Atypical and typical antipsychotics have similar efficacy profiles. Decision on first-line therapy is based on consideration of side-effect profiles, adherence issues, history of response, and cost.

Typical Antipsychotics

Mechanism of action – phenothiazines: block postsynaptic mesolimbic dopaminergic receptors in the brain

Generic	Brand	Dose & Max mg (frequency)	Contra-indications	Primary Side Effects	Key Monitoring Parameters	Pertinent Drug Interactions	Med Pearls	Top 200
Chlorpromazine	Thorazine	10–200 mg (BID–QID) (max = 2,000 mg/day)	• Hypersensitivity • Severe CNS depression • Coma	• Orthostatic hypotension • Drowsiness • Xerostomia • Constipation • Nausea	• Vital signs • Mental status • Lipid profile • Fasting blood glucose • Severity of EPS	• Alcohol • CNS depressants • Lithium • Warfarin • Other phenothiazine	• Available in IV • May produce false-positive phenylketonuria (PKU) test results and pregnancy • Pregnancy category C	No
Fluphenazine	Prolixin	1–10 mg (TID–QID) (max = 40 mg/day)	• Hypersensitivity • Severe CNS depression	• Urinary retention • Blurred vision • Photosensitivity	• LFTs • Involuntary movement	• Propranolol • Pindolol • Valproic acid	• Available as elixir and injection • Pregnancy category C	No
Perphenazine	Trilafon (only generic available)	2–16 mg (BID–QID) (max = 64 mg/day)	• Coma • Subcortical brain damage • Blood dyscrasias • Hepatic disease	• Extrapyramidal symptoms (EPS)	• Neuroleptic malignant syndrome (NMS) • CBCs	• Phenytoin • Atropine	Pregnancy category C	No
Trifluoperazine	Stelazine (only generic available)	1–10 mg (q day–BID) (max = 40 mg/day)					• Pregnancy category C • False-positives on PKU and pregnancy tests	No
Prochlorperazine	• Compazine • Compro (suppository)	• 5–15 mg (TID–QID) • 2.5–25 mg (BID) (max = 150 mg/day)					False-positives on PKU and pregnancy tests	Yes
Thioridazine	Mellaril (only generic available)	10–200 mg (BID–QID) (max = 800 mg/day)				• Alcohol • CNS depressants • Propranolol • Pindolol • Drugs that prolong QT interval	• Pregnancy category C • Black box warning for altered cardiac conduction • Use with caution in respiratory disease and hepatic disease	No

Typical Antipsychotics *(cont'd)*

Mechanism of action – haloperidol: not well established; thought to block postsynaptic mesolimbic dopaminergic D_2 receptors in the brain

Generic	Brand	Dose & Max mg (frequency)	Contra-indications	Primary Side Effects	Key Monitoring Parameters	Pertinent Drug Interactions	Med Pearls	Top 200
Haloperidol	• Haldol • Haldol Deconade (Injection)	• 0.5–20 mg (BID–TID) • 50–100 mg/mL (q day) (max = 100 mg/day)	• Hypersensitivity • Parkinson's disease • Severe CNS depression • Bone marrow suppression • Severe cardiac or hepatic disease • Coma	• Xerostomia • Drowsiness • Constipation • Nausea • Urinary retention • Blurred vision • EPS • Dyspepsia • Priapism • QT prolongation	• Vital signs • CBCs • Mental status • ECG at baseline • EPS • Involuntary movement	• Alcohol • CNS depressants • Antiparkinson medication • Lithium • Inhibitors/inducers of CYP450	• Available in IV and liquid dosage form • Pregnancy category C • IV form uses sesame oil	Yes

Mechanism of action – pimozide: a potent, centrally acting dopamine–receptor antagonist

Generic	Brand	Dose & Max mg (frequency)	Contra-indications	Primary Side Effects	Key Monitoring Parameters	Pertinent Drug Interactions	Med Pearls	Top 200
Pimozide	Orap	• 1–2 mg (q day) (max = 0.2 mg/kg or 10 mg, whichever is less)	• Severe CNS depression • Coma • History of dysrhythmia • Prolonged QT syndrome • Hypokalemia, hypomagnesemia • Drugs that are inhibitors of CYP3A4 (azole antifungals, fluvoxamine, macrolide antibiotics)	• Somnolence • Drowsiness • Rash • Xerostomia • Constipation • Diarrhea • Increased appetite • Taste disturbance • Impotence • Weakness • Visual disturbance • Speech disorder • Hypotension	• Vital signs • CBCs • Mental status • ECG at baseline • EPS • Involuntary movement	• Alcohol • CNS depressants • Anticonvulsants • Propranolol macrolide antibiotics • Lithium • Sertraline • TCAs • CYP3A4 inhibitors	• FDA-labeled for Tourette's disorder • Pregnancy category C	No

Typical Antipsychotics *(cont'd)*

Generic	Brand	Dose & Max mg (frequency)	Contra-indications	Primary Side Effects	Key Monitoring Parameters	Pertinent Drug Interactions	Med Pearls	Top 200
Mechanism of action – loxapine: blocks postsynaptic mesolimbic D_1 and D_2 receptors in the brain, and also possesses serotonin 5-HT_2 blocking activity								
Loxapine	• Loxitane • Adasure inhalation	5–50 mg (BID–QID) (max = 250 mg/day)	• Hypersensitivity • Severe CNS depression • Coma	• Hypotension • Nausea • Constipation • Vomiting • Xerostomia • Weakness • Sexual disturbance • Dizziness	• Vital signs • Mental status • EPS • CBCs • Thyroid function tests • Involuntary movement	• Lorazepam • Alcohol • CNS depressants • TCAs • Anticonvulsants • Lithium	• Use with extreme caution in patients with thyroid disease • False-positive PKU test • Pregnancy category C	No
Mechanism of action – molindone: exerts effect on the ascending reticular activating system								
Molindone	Moban	5–50 mg (TID–QID) (max = 225 mg/day)	• Severe cardiovascular disorders • Hypersensitivity	• Drowsiness • Xerostomia • Constipation • Hypotension • Tachycardia	• Vital signs • Mental status • EPS • CBCs	• Phenytoin • Tetracycline • Alcohol • CNS depressants	Pregnancy category C	No
Mechanism of action – thiothixene: blocks postsynaptic dopamine receptors, resulting in inhibition of dopamine-mediated effects; also has alpha-adrenergic blocking activity.								
Thiothixene	Navane	1–20 mg (TID) (max = 60 mg/day)	• Hypersensitivity • Severe CNS depression • Circulatory collapse • Blood dyscrasias • Coma	• Hypotension • Dizziness • GI upset • Constipation • Libido changes • Tachycardia • Insomnia	• Vital signs • CBCs • Thyroid function tests • EPS	• Alcohol • CNS depressants	May cause false-positive pregnancy tests	No

Typical Antipsychotics

Generic	Brand	Dose & Max mg (frequency)	Contra-indications	Primary Side Effects	Key Monitoring Parameters	Pertinent Drug Interactions	Med Pearls	Top 200
Mechanism of action – mixed and varied (per agent) D_2/5-HT_2 antagonist activity								
Aripiprazole	• Abilify • Abilify Discmelt • Oral tablet, disintegrating tablet, solution, immediate IM injection	• 10–30 mg PO daily (q day) • 9.75 IM (q 2 hrs up to 30 mg/day)	Hypersensitivity	• Weight gain • Constipation • N/V/D • Akathisia • Hyperglycemia • Hyperlipidemia • Anxiety • Restlessness • Sedation • Prolonged QT interval • Hyperprolactinemia (rare) • EPS (rare) • Tardive dyskinesia (rare) • Tachycardia	• Blood sugar • Fasting lipid panel, BP, and HR • Weight/body mass index • Symptoms of psychosis or EPS • ECG	• Ranolazine • Carbamazepine • Quinidine • Ketoconazole • Medications that prolong QT interval • Metodopramide	Among the lowest risk of metabolic syndrome	Yes
Aripiprazole ER injectable	Abilify Maintena	300–400 mg IM 1 ×/mo						
Olanzapine	Zyprexa oral tablets; oral disintegrating tablets; immediate IM injection	• 10–20 mg IM daily (q day) • 10–30 mg IM daily					Higher degree of weight gain than some other atypicals	Yes
Paliperidone	Invega	• 6–12 mg daily (q day)					• Major active metabolite of risperidone • Newest med in this class, least clinical evidence	Yes
Quetiapine	Seroquel oral tablets, ER tablets	• IR: 50–750 mg daily (BID–TID) • ER: 300–800 mg daily (q day)					Dosed at bed time due to somnolence	Yes
Iloperidone	Fanapt	Initial: 1 mg BID recommended dosage range: 6–12 mg BID (max = 24 mg/day) Recommended titration schedule: increase in 2 mg increments every 24 hrs on days 2–7					Lower risk of weight gain than many atypical, low risk of somnolence; may improve cognitive function	No
Asenapine	Saphris	• Schizophrenia: 5 mg BID • Bipolar disorder: 10 mg BID					Very low incidence of EPS	No

Atypical Antipsychotics *(cont'd)*

Generic	Brand	Dose & Max mg (frequency)	Contra-indications	Primary Side Effects	Key Monitoring Parameters	Pertinent Drug Interactions	Med Pearls	Top 200
Risperidone	• Risperdal • Risperdal Consta • Risperdal M–Tab • Tablet, liquid, disintegrating tablet, long-acting injection	• 2–16 mg PO daily (q day–BID) • 25–50 mg IM q 2 wks	(same as above)	(same as above)	(same as above)	(same as above)	Sedation often leads to bed time dosing	Yes
Ziprasidone	Geodon	40–160 mg daily (BID)	• History of cardiac arrhythmias • Uncompensated heart failure • Hypersensitivity • Acute or recent MI • QT prolongation history • Drugs that cause QT prolongation				Lower risk of metabolic syndrome when compared to other atypicals	Yes
Lurasidone	Latuda	40–80 mg PO once daily	Hypersensitivity; concomitant use with CYP3A4 inhibitors or inducers			• Potent inducers (rifampin) and inhibitors (ketoconazole) of CYP3A4, diltiazem • Metoclopramide (increased risk of EPS)	Metabolized by CYP3A4	No

Atypical Antipsychotics *(cont'd)*

Generic	Brand	Dose & Max mg (frequency)	Contra-indications	Primary Side Effects	Key Monitoring Parameters	Pertinent Drug Interactions	Med Pearls	Top 200
Clozapine	• Clozaril • FazaClo	12.5–900 mg daily (q day–TID)	• History of clozapine-induced agranulocytosis or severe granulocytopenia • Myelo-proliferative disorder • Paralytic ileus • CNS depression or comatose states • Other agents that cause agranulocytosis	• Hypotension • Tachyarrhythmia • Rash • Weight gain • Agranulocytosis • Neuroleptic malignant syndrome (rare)	• WBC and absolute neutrophil count (ANC) wkly for 6 mo, q 2 wks for 6 mo, and then q 4 wks • S/S of psychotic behavior • Blood sugar, fasting lipid panel • Symptoms of neuroleptic malignant syndrome • BP and HR • Orthostatic hypotension • ECG	• Droperidol • Buspirone • Carbamazepine • Lithium • Tramadol • Zotepine	• Used less frequently than other atypicals due to requirement for frequent monitoring • Effective in treatment of refractory cases and in patients at high risk for suicide	Yes
	Versacloz suspension	125–900 mg daily (once–TID)						

Storage and Administration Pearls

- All medications should be stored at room temperature in a dry area away from direct sunlight.
- Patient may take medications with food if GI upset occurs.

Patient Education Pearls

- Grapefruit juice should be avoided when taking these medications.
- Alcohol should be avoided due to excessive CNS depression.
- Driving or operating heavy machinery should be avoided until patients know how they respond to medication.
- All medications can take up to several weeks (2–4 weeks) to see full effect.
- Medications should *not* be abruptly discontinued.
- Patients should not self-adjust dose.
- Patients should report to a physician any side effects that disrupt their daily life (i.e., EPS).

Learning Points

- The most commonly used antidepressants are the SSRIs. These agents may take several weeks to reach maximal efficacy.
- Bupropion is the antidepressant of choice in patients with sexual side effects resulting from other classes of antidepressants.
- The treatment of anxiety and panic disorder may include acute therapies such as benzodiazepines but may also include chronic prophylactic therapies with antidepressants.
- Mood stabilizer therapy is the mainstay of treatment for bipolar disorder. Lithium has a narrow therapeutic window and requires therapeutic serum monitoring.
- While atypical antipsychotic medications exhibit fewer extrapyramidal side effects than typical agents, they do carry a greater risk of metabolic side effects such as weight gain, hyperglycemia, and hyperlipidemia. Atypical antipsychotics are more effective in treating the negative symptoms of schizophrenia.

INSOMNIA

Definition

According to the American Academy of Sleep Medicine insomnia is the subjective perception of difficulty with sleep initiation, duration, consolidation, or quality that occurs despite adequate opportunity for sleep that results in some form of daytime impairment.

Diagnosis

The diagnosis of insomnia is made primarily based upon patient history with assessment of complaints, pre-sleep conditions, sleep-wake patterns, other symptoms, and daytime consequences. Some instruments that may aid in diagnosis include patient questionnaires, sleep diaries, polysomnography, symptom checklists, and psychological assessments. Diagnostic criteria include:

- Complaint of difficulty initiating sleep, maintaining sleep, waking too early, or sleep that is of nonrestorative/poor quality. This difficulty occurs despite adequate opportunity and circumstances for sleep.
- At least one form of daytime impairment is reported: fatigue, impairment in concentration/attention/memory, social/vocational impairment, poor school performance, mood disturbance/irritability, daytime sleepiness, decreased motivation/energy/initiation, proneness for errors/accidents, tension, headaches, or gastrointestinal symptoms in response to sleep loss, concerns, or worries about sleep.

Signs and Symptoms

Detailed in the diagnostic description, most patients complain of difficulty with falling asleep, staying asleep, or with chronically nonrestorative/quality sleep. These common complaints may also be accompanied by other nocturnal symptoms including snoring, coughing, kicking, restlessness, walking/movement, vocalization, pain, or anxiety.

Guidelines

Schutte-Rodin S, Broch L, Buysse D, Dorsey C, Sateia M. Clinical guideline for the evaluation and management of chronic insomnia in adults. *J Clin Sleep Med.* 2008;4:487–504.

Guideline Summary

- Goals of therapy: Improve quality and quantity of sleep and improve daytime sleep-related impairment.

- All patients should be educated about good sleep hygiene. Nonpharmacological measures are the preferred initial treatment.

- Pharmacological therapy should be combined with behavioral therapy to achieve the best results.

- Medication selection is based upon the following patient-specific elements: (*1*) symptom pattern, (*2*) patient preference, (*3*) availability, (*4*) cost, (*5*) prior response, (*6*) comorbid conditions, (*7*) contraindications, (*8*) concurrent medications, (*9*) side effect profile, and (*10*) treatment goals.

- Pharmacological classes for insomnia include benzodiazepines, benzodiazepine receptor agonists (BzRA), melatonin receptor agonists, and sedating antidepressants.

- Short-intermediate acting benzodiazepine receptor agonist (BzRAs), benzodiazepines (BZDs), or the melatonin receptor agonist are first-line therapy options for most patients. BzRAs and BZDs ideally should be limited to short-term use (7–10 days), but there is limited evidence to support use extended to 6–12 months.

- Inadequate response after initial trial can be followed with a trial on a second agent from within these therapeutic class options.

- Third-line options include sedating antidepressants or off-label combination therapy or self-care therapies such as antihistamines.

Treatment Algorithm

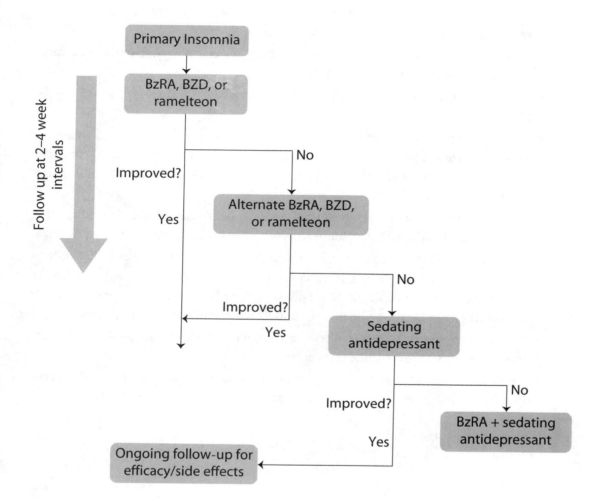

Drugs for Insomnia

Nonbenzodiazepine benzodiazepine receptor antagonists (schedule IV controlled substances)

Generic	Brand	Dose & Max	Contra-indications	Primary Side Effects	Key Monitoring	Pertinent Drug Interactions	Med Pearl	Top 200
Eszopiclone	Lunesta	1–3 mg PO QHS	Hypersensitivity	• Headache • Taste disturbance • Xerostomia • Dizziness • Nausea • Somnolence • CNS depression • Sleep-related activities: hazardous activities such as sleep-driving and cooking have been reported (rare), incidence increased with alcohol use or above max doses. • Behavior changes such as decreased inhibition, aggression, agitation, hallucinations, and depersonalization (rare)	• Improvement in sleep quality/quantity • Presence of side effects	Avoid combination with: • CNS depressants due to additive CNS depression • Strong CYP 3A4 inhibitors due to resultant increased sedative serum concentration	• CYP 3A4 substrate • High fat/heavy meal will delay absorption, best efficacy when administered on empty stomach. • Re-evaluate need every 6 months	Yes
Zolpidem immediate release	Ambien, Zolpimist	• 5 mg PO HS (females) • 5–10 mg PO HS (males)					• CYP 3A4 substrate • Take immediately before bedtime • Heavy/high fat meal will delay absorption	Yes
Zolpidem sublingual	Edluar	• 5 mg SL HS (females) • 5–10 mg SL HS (males)					• CYP 3A4 substrate • Placed under the tongue and allowed to disintegrate; do not chew or swallow • Intermezzo helpful for nighttime awakenings	No
	Intermezzo	• 1.75 mg SL/night (females) • 3.5 mg SL/night (males)						
Zolpidem controlled release	Ambien CR	• 6.25 mg PO HS (females) • 6.25–12.5 mg PO HS (males)					• CYP 3A4 substrate • Heavy/high fat meal will delay absorption. • Do not crush or chew	No
Zaleplon	Sonata	5–20 mg PO HS	Hypersensitivity				• CYP 3A4 substrate • Heavy/high fat meal will delay absorption. • Headache incidence 30%–40%	No

Drugs for Insomnia (cont'd)

Generic	Brand	Dose & Max	Contra-indications	Primary Side Effects	Key Monitoring	Pertinent Drug Interactions	Med Pearl	Top 200
Benzodiazepines (schedule IV controlled substances)								
Estazolam	Estazolam generics	1–2 mg PO HS	• Pregnancy • Narrow-angle glaucoma • Concurrent use with itra- or ketoconazole	• Somnolence • Dizziness • Hypokinesia • Hangover effect • Abnormal coordination	• Improvement in sleep quality/quantity • Presence of side effects	CYP 3A4 substrate: • Avoid use with ketoconazole or itraconazole. • Avoid use with CNS depressants due to risk of additive CNS depression.	Time to peak 0.5–6 hrs, T½ 10–24 hrs	No
Temazepam	Restoril	7.5–30 mg PO HS	Pregnancy, narrow-angle glaucoma	• Confusion • Xerostomia • Constipation		Avoid use with CNS depressants due to risk of additive CNS depression.	Time to peak 1.2–1.6 hrs, T½ 3.5–18 hrs	Yes
Triazolam	Halcion	0.125–0.5 mg PO HS	• Pregnancy • Narrow-angle glaucoma • Concurrent use with itra- or ketoconazole or nefazodone			CYP 3A4 substrate: • Avoid use with potent inhibitors such as itra- or ketoconazole or nefazodone due to potential for increased triazolam serum concentration/effect. • Avoid use with CNS depressants due to risk of additive CNS depression.	Time to peak 1–2 hrs, T½ 1.5–5.5 hrs	No
Flurazepam	Flurazepam generics	15–30 mg PO HS	Pregnancy, narrow-angle glaucoma			CYP 3A4 substrate: • Avoid use with potent inhibitors such as itra- or ketoconazole or nefazodone due to potential for increased flurazepam serum concentration/effect. • Avoid use with CNS depressants due to risk of additive CNS depression.	Time to peak 3–6 hrs, T½ 2.5 hrs (active metabolite ~70 hrs)	No
Melatonin Receptor Agonist								
Ramelteon	Rozerem	8 mg within 30 min of bedtime	Angioedema with prior use, concomitant fluvoxamine	• Dizziness • Fatigue • Depression • Nausea • Myalgia	• Improvement in sleep quality/quantity • Presence of side effects	Fluvoxamine • Increases ramelteon serum concentration. Avoid this combination. • Avoid concomitant CNS depressants due to risk of additive CNS depression.	• CYP 1A2 substrate • Not scheduled/controlled	No

Storage and Administration Pearls

- Intermezzo should be taken in bed if patient wakes in the middle of the night (i.e., if ≥4 hours left before desired wake time) and has difficulty returning to sleep.

- Ambien CR tablets should be swallowed whole; do not divide, crush, or chew.

- Zolpidem sublingual tablets should be placed under the tongue and allowed to disintegrate; do not swallow or administer with water.

- Zolpimist oral spray should be sprayed directly into the mouth over the tongue. Prior to initial use, pump should be primed by spraying 5 times. If pump is not used for at least 14 days, reprime pump with 1 spray.

Patient Education Pearls

- Proper sleep hygiene is essential for effective insomnia management.
  - Avoid daytime naps.
  - Keep the bedroom dark, comfortable, free from noise/distractions.
  - Stay on a routine sleep schedule.
  - Avoid heavy meals and exercise prior to bedtime.
  - Avoid caffeine in the evening.
  - Limit liquid consumption in the evening.

- Benzodiazepines and benzodiazepine receptor agonists should be reserved for short-term use in most instances. Some patients may require use for longer periods but need should be re-evaluated every 6 months.

- BZDs and BzRAs should not be abruptly discontinued following long-term use due to the potential for withdrawal. Work with your health care provider to determine an appropriate dosage taper.

- BzRAs should not be taken with heavy/high-fat meal due to the potential for delayed absorption.

ATTENTION DEFICIT HYPRACTIVITY DISORDER (ADHD)

Definition

ADHD is a chronic illness that often initially presents in childhood and may persist into adulthood. Patients affected exhibit core symptoms include inattention, hyperactivity and/or impulsivity.

Diagnosis

The diagnosis of ADHD is based upon the *Diagnostic and Statistical Manual of Mental Disorders,* 5th Edition (DSM-V). Criteria provide examples of inattention and hyperactivity/impulsivity and require a persistent pattern of at least six symptoms of either inattention or hyperactivity/impulsivity that have been present for at least 6 months and that interfere with functioning or development. Criteria further specify that several symptoms were present prior to age 12 and in two or more settings.

Signs and Symptoms

- Inattention:
  - Failure to pay attention
  - Trouble holding attention
  - Lack of follow through on instructions
  - Failure to finish schoolwork
  - Difficulty organizing tasks
  - Avoidance/dislike of tasks requiring mental effort
  - Loss of things/demonstrates forgetfulness
  - Easy distractibility
- Hyperactivity/impulsivity:
  - Fidgets/squirms
  - Leaves seat unexpectedly
  - Inability to play quietly
  - Excessive talking
  - Trouble waiting
  - Interrupts/intrudes
  - Blurts out answer/responses
  - Runs around when not appropriate
  - Inability to keep still

Guidelines

Subcommittee on Attention-Deficit/Hyperactivity Disorder; Steering Committee on Quality Improvement and Management. Wolraich M, Brown L, Brown RT, et al. ADHD: clinical practice guideline for the diagnosis, evaluation, and treatment of attention-deficit/hyperactivity disorder in children and adolescents. *Pediatrics* 2011;128:1007–22.

Guideline Summary

- First-line pharmacologic therapy for ADHD includes stimulant medications. Approved options included methylphenidate, dexmethylphenidate, dextroamphetamine, dextroamphetamine + amphetamine, and lisdexamfetamine.

- Nonstimulant options approved for ADHD and are generally reserved for one of the following: concerns related to abuse/diversion, strong family/patient preference for nonstimulant medications, or as adjunctive therapy to stimulants. Options include atomoxetine, guanfacine, and clonidine. Of these options, atomoxetine monotherapy is preferred to guanfacine and clonidine, which are generally reserved for adjunctive therapy.

- When selecting a stimulant, patient-specific factors such as ability to swallow tablets/capsules, affordability, number of daily doses required, and presence of a tic disorder are considerations.

- Interpatient variability in efficacy is recognized and alternate stimulant agents are recommended as second- and third-line options after appropriate titration to maximal effective/tolerated dose of initial stimulant selected.

Drugs for Attention Deficit Hyperactivity Disorder

Generic	Brand	Dose & Max	Contraindications	Primary Side Effects	Key Monitoring	Pertinent Drug Interactions	Med Pearl	Top 200
Stimulants								
Methylphenidate IR	• Ritalin • Methylin chewable, oral suspension	2.5–20 mg BID-TID	• Anxiety • Tension • Agitation • Glaucoma • Recent MAOI use (within 14 days) • Family history of Tourette's syndrome or tics • Metadate CD and ER: Uncontrolled, severe hypertension, heart failure, arrhythmias, hyperthyroidism, recent myocardial infarction, angina • Ritalin products: pheochromocytoma	General: • Anorexia • Nausea • Insomnia • Dizziness • Light-headedness • Irritability • Blurred vision • Priapism (rare) Cardiovascular: • Increased BP • Tachycardia Psychiatric: • May exacerbate anxiety, mania, aggression, hostility, depression • Use with caution in patients with pre-existing psychiatric diagnoses	• Efficacy: Resolution of symptoms • BP • HR • Weight • ECG at baseline and if chest pain or syncope • Signs of misuse/abuse	MAOIs require 14 day washout period prior to stimulant initiation	• Black box: Potential for dependency • CI: Prescriptions issued 1 mo at a time • Generally taken QAM to avoid insomnia • Remove patch after 9 hrs of wear, alternate application site (hips) • Withdrawal potential, titrate slowly and taper upon discontinuation	Yes
Methylphenidate LA	Ritalin LA	10–40 mg						
Methylphenidate SR	Ritalin SR	20 mg						
Methylphenidate ER	• Methylin ER • Metadate ER • Wuilivant XR suspension							
Methylphenidate IR-ext-release	Concerta	18–54 mg QAM						
Methylphenidate IR-extended release	Metadate CD	10–60 mg daily						
Methylphenidate transdermal patch	Daytrana	1.1–3.3 mg/hr						
Dexmethylphenidate IR	Focalin	2.5–10 mg BID						No
Dexmethylphenidate ER	Focalin XR	5–20 mg QAM						
Dextroamphetamine and amphetamine IR	Adderall	5–30 mg QAM or BID					• Black box: Potential for dependency • CI: Prescriptions issued one month at a time • Generally taken QAM to avoid insomnia • First dose given QAM, second dose (when applicable) 4–6 hrs later • With or without food • Withdrawal potential; titrate slowly and taper upon discontinuation	
Dextroamphetamine and amphetamine ER	Adderall XR	5–30 mg QAM						Yes
Dextroamphetamine IR	• Dexedrine • Dextrostat	5–10 mg QAM or BID						No
Dextroamphetamine SR and IR	• Dexedrine Spansules • ProCentra	5–15 mg QAM						
Lisdexamfetamine	Vyvanse	20–70 mg QAM					• Pro-drug of dextroamphetamine; rapid effect muted if injected or snorted (designed to decrease abuse potential) • Contents can be mixed with water—drink immediately	Yes

Drugs for Attention Deficit Hyperactivity Disorder *(cont'd)*

Generic	Brand	Dose & Max	Contraindications	Primary Side Effects	Key Monitoring	Pertinent Drug Interactions	Med Pearl	Top 200
Nonstimulant								
Atomoxetine	Strattera	40–100 mg daily or divided BID (max = 80 mg/day)	• Glaucoma, pheochromocytoma • Use with caution if pre-existing cardiovascular conditions	• Headache • Insomnia • Nausea • Anorexia • Somnolence • Xerostomia • Menstrual changes • Orthostasis • Can exacerbate pre-existing psychiatric illness including hallucinations/mania • Priapism (rare) • Liver injury (rare)	• Efficacy: Resolution of symptoms • Safety: Symptoms of liver injury (fatigue, abdominal pain, yellowed skin, darkened urine), period liver enzymes	• Metabolized by CYP2D6, decrease dose if on strong inhibitor (paroxetine, fluoxetine, quinidine) • MAOIs – 14 day washout required	• Risk of suicidal ideation observed in children • Risk of severe liver injury • Capsules cannot be opened	Yes
Guanfacine	Intuniv	1–4 mg daily		• Dizziness • Fatigue • Somnolence • Xerostomia • Constipation • Bradycardia • Headache • Hypotension • Syncope • Skin rash (rare; discontinue if develops)	• Efficacy: Resolution of symptoms • Safety: BP, HR at each office visit	• Metabolized by CYP3A4: Limit daily dose to 2 mg if used in combination with 3A4 inhibitors • Additive CNS depressant effects with other depressants • Additive BP lowering with other antihypertensives	• High fat meals increase medication absorption • Can be used as monotherapy or as adjunctive to stimulant therapy • Also used for treatment of hypertension—formulations not interchangeable • Cannot be crushed	Yes
Clonidine	Kapvay	0.1–0.4 mg daily		• Headache • Somnolence • Bradycardia • Hypotension • Rebound • Hypertension, if abrupt discontinuation	• Efficacy: Resolution of symptoms • Safety: BP, HR at each visit	• Additive sedation with other CNS depressants • Additive BP lowering with other antihypertensives	• Do not crush • Do not stop abruptly	Yes

Storage and Administration Pearls

- Store stimulants where they cannot be accessed by others or stolen.
- Some of the formulations including Focalin XR, Ritalin LA, Metadate CD, and Adderall XR can be mixed with room temperature or cool applesauce and eaten right away if patient has difficulty swallowing capsules.
- Vyvanse can be mixed with water but must be taken immediately once mixed.
- Daytrana patches are applied to the hip approximately 2 hours prior to desire effect and rotated to alternate hip every morning. Remove after 9 hours of wear. Patient can bathe/swim while wearing the patch. Dispose of used patches in a place that is not accessible to small children or pets.
- Do not crush guanfacine or clonidine tablets.
- Extended-release formulations can be used to avoid the need for doses delivered during school day.

Patient Education Pearls

- Most side effects to stimulant medications are minor and many subside with continued use. Lack of appetite or trouble sleeping may occur initially or with increases in dose but often resolve with continued use. If these side effects persist, discuss with your prescriber.
- Report any significant chest pain, shortness of breath, or fainting to a health care professional immediately.
- Report any hallucinations or changes in personality to a health care professional immediately.
- Store stimulant medications where they cannot be accessed by others or stolen.
- Stimulant medications should not be abruptly discontinued due to the potential for withdrawal.
- Clonidine should not be abruptly discontinued due to the potential for rebound hypertension.

PRACTICE QUESTIONS

1. Which of the following is first-line in the treatment of acute depressive episode in a patient with bipolar disorder?

   (A) Lithium
   (B) Valproic acid
   (C) Oxcarbazepine
   (D) Lamictal
   (E) Carbamazepine

2. A 48-year-old woman is newly diagnosed with depression. She has a medical history significant for type 2 diabetes and hypertension. Current medications include metformin 1,000 mg PO BID and lisinopril 40 mg PO daily. Her blood pressure remains elevated at today's visit. Which antidepressant has the greatest potential to worsen this patient's hypertension?

   (A) Citalopram
   (B) Desipramine
   (C) Venlafaxine
   (D) Vilazodone

3. To avoid withdrawal symptoms, most antidepressants require tapering upon discontinuation. Which SSRI does not require a taper upon discontinuation due to its long elimination half-life?

   (A) Escitalopram
   (B) Fluoxetine
   (C) Paroxetine
   (D) Sertraline

4. Antidepressants with serotonergic activity should be avoided in combination with which of the following antibiotics due to the clinically significant risk of serotonin syndrome?

   (A) Cefazolin
   (B) Meropenem
   (C) Vancomycin
   (D) Linezolid

5. A 36-year-old woman with bipolar disorder is on lithium 300 mg PO TID with a serum drug concentration of 0.9 mEq/L. She is diagnosed with hypertension and her physician is considering therapy initiation. Which of the following medications would result in a significant drug interaction with the patient's lithium, increasing the risk for lithium toxicity? (Select **ALL** that apply.)

   (A) Chlorthalidone
   (B) Metoprolol
   (C) Lisinopril
   (D) Amlodipine

6. Which of the following antipsychotics would have the greatest risk of extrapyramidal side effects?

   (A) Olanzapine
   (B) Risperidone
   (C) Clozapine
   (D) Asenapine

7. Coadministration with a high-fat meal would result in delayed absorption of which of the following medications?

   (A) Eszopiclone
   (B) Triazolam
   (C) Ramelteon
   (D) Melatonin

8. An 11-year-old male adolescent is diagnosed with attention deficit hyperactivity disorder (ADHD). He has an older brother (18 years) with ADHD and opioid dependence. The patient's want to avoid pharmacological treatment options with potential for dependency. Which of the following would be the most appropriate first-line pharmacological therapy for this patient's ADHD?

   (A) Methylphenidate
   (B) Atomoxetine
   (C) Guanfacine
   (D) Clonidine

ANSWERS

1. **D**

According to the guidelines, first-line treatment options for acute depression episodes include lamotrigine as monotherapy or in combination with antimania agents. Lithium (A) and valproic acid (B) are used as first-line treatment options for acute manic episodes. Oxcarbazepine (C) and carbamazepine (E) would also be used as first-line treatment options of acute manic episodes. Maintenance therapy may consist of a combination of medications for both depression and manic episodes.

2. **C**

Serotonin, norepinephrine reuptake inhibitors, specifically venlafaxine, can increase blood pressure due the impact on norepinephrine. SSRIs such as citalopram (A) and vilazodone (D) are not associated with increasing blood pressure. Tricyclic antidepressants such as desipramine (B) can result in orthostatic hypotension due to anticholinergic side effects.

3. **B**

Fluoxetine's terminal half-life is measured in days (4–16) rather than hours; this pharmacokinetic principle allows the medication to slowly eliminate thereby diminishing the need for tapering upon discontinuation. The other drugs' half-lives are: escitalopram (A) about 28 hours, paroxetine (C) 21 hours, and sertraline (D) 26 hours.

4. **D**

Linezolid is a reversible, nonselective inhibitor of monoamine oxidase, and coadministration with serotonergic agents such as SSRIs should be avoided due to the significant risk of serotonin syndrome.

5. **A and C**

Both thiazide diuretics such as chlorthalidone (A) and ACEIs such as lisinopril (C) decrease the clearance of lithium and increase the risk of lithium toxicity. Although these medications may be used in combination with lithium, the concomitant administration should be monitored very closely. Beta blockers such as metoprolol (B) and calcium channel blockers such as amlodipine (D) do not interact with lithium.

6. **B**

Risperidone has a relatively low risk of EPS among the first generation (typical) antipsychotics. Its risk is greater, however, compared with the atypical antipsychotics such as olanzapine (A), asenapine (C), and clozapine (D).

7. **A**

BzRAs such as eszopiclone have demonstrated delayed absorption when co-administered with high-fat/heavy meals. The same precaution does not apply to benzodiazepines such as triazolam (B), melatonin receptor agonists such as ramelteon (C), or melatonin (D).

8. **B**

Atomoxetine is a nonstimulant option that is not a scheduled/controlled substance. Methylphenidate (A) is a stimulant option and would not address the family's concerns related to dependence. For patients/families with concerns regarding dependence, atomoxetine is considered the first-line option, while other nonstimulants such as guanfacine (C) and clonidine (D) are reserved for second-line/adjunctive therapy.

Bone and Joint Disorders

10

This chapter covers the following disease states:

- **Osteoarthritis**
- **Rheumatoid arthritis**
- **Osteoporosis**
- **Gout**

 Suggested Study Time: **45 minutes**

OSTEOARTHRITIS

Definition

Osteoarthritis (OA) is a disease of the cartilage resulting from an imbalance between cartilage destruction and formation with subsequent bony proliferation within the joint, which results in pain, potentially decreased range of motion, and local inflammation.

Diagnosis

The diagnosis of OA is based on history, physical exam, and radiographs. History and physical exam will reveal symptoms and signs consistent with OA (detailed below) and should be used to rule out other potential conditions such as rheumatoid arthritis. Radiologic changes may include joint space narrowing, osteophytes, or subchondral bone sclerosis.

Signs and Symptoms

- Osteoarthritis signs: Physical exam may reveal tenderness, crepitus, and/or enlargement of the affected joints. Radiologic evaluation is necessary to identify presence of OA and disease progression. Radiographic changes may not be easily identifiable in early, mild disease but with disease progression may include narrowing of the joint spaces, presence of osteophytes, subchondral bony sclerosis, and eventual subluxation and deformity.

- Osteoarthritis symptoms: Patients with OA present with pain, stiffness, and instability of joints that can be unilateral or bilateral. The pain is often worsened with weight-bearing activity and is described as deep and aching. Stiffness may resolve with motion but may limit physical activity. Commonly affected joints include the hands, knees, and hips.

Guidelines

Hochberg MC, Altman RD, April KT, et al. American College of Rheumatology 2012 recommendations for the use of nonpharmacologic and pharmacologic therapies in osteoarthritis of the hand, hip, and knee. *Arthritis Care Res* 2012;64:465–74.

Guidelines Summary

The goals of therapy are to decrease pain and stiffness, maintain/improve joint mobility and limit functional impairment, and increase the quality of life.

- Osteoarthritis of the hand:
  - First-line options: Topical capsaicin, topical NSAIDs, oral NSAIDs, tramadol
  - Topical NSAIDs preferred over oral NSAIDs in patients ≥75 years of age

- Osteoarthritis of the knee or hip:
  - First-line option: Acetaminophen (scheduled, up to maximum of 4 g/day)
  - Second-line options: Topical or oral NSAIDs (topical preferred in patients ≥75 years of age) or intra-articular corticosteroid injections
  - Third-line options: Duloxetine, tramadol, or intra-articular hyaluronan injections

Treatment Algorithm

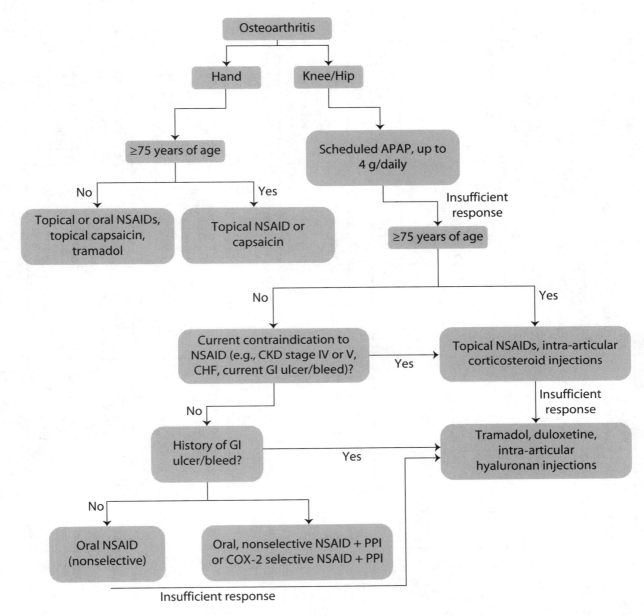

Drugs for Osteoarthritis

Generic	Brand	Dose & Max mg (frequency)	Contraindications	Primary Side Effects	Key Monitoring Parameters	Pertinent Drug Interactions	Med Pearls	Top 200
Mechanism of action – decreases pain through inhibition of central cyclo-oxygenase, which in turn inhibits prostaglandin synthesis								
Acetaminophen	Tylenol	• 325–1,000 • TID–QID (max dose = 4 g/day)	• Hepatic disease • Alcoholism	Very few	Pain relief	Alcohol	• Over-the-counter (OTC) • Best if taken on scheduled basis vs. as needed (PRN)	No, OTC
Tramadol	• Ultram • Ultram ER	• Immediate release (IR) 25–400 daily (q 4–6 hrs) • Extended release (ER) 100–300 daily	Hypersensitivity	Confusion, sedation, rash, stomach upset, orthostatic hypotension	• Pain relief • Renal and hepatic function periodically	• Alcohol • Opioids • Selective serotonin reuptake inhibitors (SSRIs) • Monamine oxidase inhibitors (MAOIs) • Warfarin	Renal dose adjustment for CrCl <30 mL/min	Yes
Mechanism of action – induces the release of substance P, the principle chemomediator of pain impulses from the periphery								
Capsaicin cream	Various	0.025–0.1% applied 3–4 × daily	Do not apply to wounds or damaged skin	Localized stinging	Pain relief	None	• OTC • Must be used regularly for 2 wks or more for maximal efficacy	No
Mechanism of action – nonsteroidal anti-inflammatory drugs (NSAIDs): decrease pain and inflammation by inhibition of prostaglandin synthesis through inhibition of cyclooxygenase enzymes								
Aspirin	Various	• IR 325–3,600 daily (q 4–6 hrs) • XR product 650–1,300 TID	• Allergy • Fever in children • Active bleeding	• Gastrointestinal (GI) (upset stomach, bleeding) • Rash	• Pain relief • GI symptoms	• Warfarin • Other NSAIDs • Angiotensin-converting enzyme (ACE) inhibitors • Antiplatelets	• OTC • Anti-inflammatory only at high doses (>3 g/day)	No, OTC
Nonacetylated salicylates								
Salsalate	Various	500–3,000 daily (BID–TID)	Hypersensitivity	• GI (upset stomach, bleeding) • Rash • Diminished renal function • Edema	• Pain relief • GI symptoms	• Other salicylates • Warfarin • ACE inhibitors	• Monitor serum salicylate levels with chronic use or very high doses • Desired range 10–30 mg/100 mL	No
Diflunisal	None	500–1,500 daily (BID)					Administer with food	No

Drugs for Osteoarthritis *(cont'd)*

Generic	Brand	Dose & Max mg (frequency)	Contraindications	Primary Side Effects	Key Monitoring Parameters	Pertinent Drug Interactions	Med Pearls	Top 200
Acetic acids								
Etodolac	None	200–1,200 daily (Q 6–8 hrs)	Hypersensitivity	• GI (upset stomach, bleeding) • Rash • Diminished renal function • ↑ Blood pressure (BP) • Edema	• Pain relief • GI symptoms • Renal function • Blood pressure	• Other salicylates • Warfarin • Lithium • ACE inhibitors	Administer with food	No
Diclofenac	• Cataflam • Voltaren	50–150 daily (BID–TID)						Yes
Indomethacin	• Indocin • Indocin SR	• IR 25–200 daily (BID–TID) • Sustained release (SR) 75–150 1× daily		• GI (upset stomach, bleeding) • Rash • Diminished renal function • ↑ BP • Edema • Central nervous system (CNS) disturbances			• Most commonly used for treatment of gout • Fat-soluble, crosses blood brain barrier • Administer with food	Yes
Ketorolac	Toradol	30 mg IM or 15 mg IV initial; 10 mg PO q 4–6 hrs up to 40 mg daily	• Active peptic ulcer disease (PUD) or bleeding • History of GI bleeding • Severe renal impairment • Labor and delivery	• GI (upset stomach, bleeding) • Rash • Diminished renal function • ↑ BP • Edema			• Only approved for moderate-severe pain for ≤5 days duration • Available IM and IV as well	No
Nabumetone	Relafen	500–2,000 daily (q day–BID)	Hypersensitivity				Administer with food	Yes

Drugs for Osteoarthritis *(cont'd)*

Generic	Brand	Dose & Max mg (frequency)	Contraindications	Primary Side Effects	Key Monitoring Parameters	Pertinent Drug Interactions	Med Pearls	Top 200
Propionic acids								
Fenoprofen	Nalfon	200–3,200 daily (TID–QID)	Hypersensitivity	• GI (upset stomach, bleeding) • Rash • Diminished renal function • Increase BP • Edema	• Pain relief • GI symptoms • Renal function • BP	• Other salicylates • Warfarin • ACEIs • Lithium	Administer with food	No
Flurbiprofen	Ansaid	50–300 daily (BID–QID)						No
Ibuprofen	• Motrin • Advil	200–3,200 daily (TID–QID)					• Available OTC and Rx (400–800 mg tabs) • Administer with food • Available in pediatric preparations	Yes
Ketoprofen	• Orudis • Oruvail • Rhodis • Apo-Keto-E	• IR: 50–300 daily (TID–QID) • SR: 75–200 daily					• Administer with food	No
Naproxen	• Naprosyn • Naprosyn • Naprelan	• IR: 250–1,500 daily (BID) • EC: 375–1,500 daily (BID) • Controlled release (CR): 375–1,500 daily (BID)					• Available OTC and Rx • Administer with food	Yes
Naproxen sodium	Anaprox	275–1,650 daily (BID)						
Oxaprozin	Daypro	600–1800 daily (1 × daily)					Administer with food	No

Drugs for Osteoarthritis *(cont'd)*

Generic	Brand	Dose & Max mg (frequency)	Contraindications	Primary Side Effects	Key Monitoring Parameters	Pertinent Drug Interactions	Med Pearls	Top 200
Fenamates								
Meclofenamate	None available	50–400 mg daily (q 4–6 hrs)	Hypersensitivity	• GI (upset stomach, bleeding) • Rash • Diminished renal function • ↑ BP • Edema	• Pain relief • GI symptoms • Renal function • BP	• Other salicylates • Warfarin • ACEIs • Lithium	Administer with food	No
Oxicams								
Piroxicam	Feldene	10–20 mg daily (1 × daily)	Hypersensitivity	• GI (upset stomach, bleeding) • Rash • Diminished renal function • ↑ BP • Edema	• Pain relief • GI symptoms • Renal function • BP	• Other salicylates • Warfarin • ACEIs • Lithium	More COX-2 selectivity than traditional NSAIDs; slightly less GI symptoms	Yes
Meloxicam	Mobic	7.5–15 mg daily (1 × daily)						Yes
Selective COX-2 inhibitors								
Celecoxib	Celebrex	50–200 mg daily (q day–BID)	Hypersensitivity	• GI (upset stomach, bleeding— less than other NSAIDs) • Rash • Diminished renal function • ↑ BP • Edema	• Pain relief • GI symptoms • Renal function • BP	• Other salicylates (including aspirin) • Warfarin • ACEIs • Lithium	• Lower incidence of GI toxicity than with nonselective NSAIDs • Concern about cardiovascular adverse effects prompted withdrawal of similar drug from market (rofecoxib)	Yes
Adjunctive therapies/nutritional supplements								
Glucosamine sulfate	Various	500–1,500 daily (q day–BID)	Unknown	• Itching • GI upset	• Pain relief • Presence of side effects	Unknown	• Nutritional supplement • Available OTC • Conflicting clinical trial data	No

Drugs for Osteoarthritis *(cont'd)*

Generic	Brand	Dose & Max mg (frequency)	Contraindications	Primary Side Effects	Key Monitoring Parameters	Pertinent Drug Interactions	Med Pearls	Top 200
Intra-articular injections								
Mechanism of action – serves as a lubricant for joint tissue								
Hyaluronate and derivates	• Synvisc • Synvisc-One	• Inject 16 mg (2 mL) once weekly for 3 wks (total of 3 injections) • Inject 48 mg (6 mL) once per knee	Hypersensitivity	• Injection site reaction • Bruising • Erythema • Lumps • Pain • Swelling • Pruritus • Skin discoloration • Arthralgia • Infection	• Intraocular pressure • S/S of inflammation or infection	No known significant drug interactions	None	No

Storage and Administration Pearls

- NSAIDs should be administered with food to decrease the risk of gastrointestinal side effects.
- Capsaicin cream may take several weeks for maximal efficacy to be demonstrated. Regular daily use, 2–4 times daily for 4 weeks, is considered an adequate trial.

Patient Education Pearls

- Take NSAIDs with food to avoid stomach upset.
- Avoid alcohol when taking acetaminophen or narcotic analgesics due to the risk of liver damage.
- Avoid driving or operating heavy machinery while taking narcotics.
- Capsaicin cream may take 2–4 weeks to become effective. Allow an adequate trial before determining efficacy.
- Wash your hands very thoroughly after capsaicin application.

RHEUMATOID ARTHRITIS

Definition

Rheumatoid arthritis (RA) is an autoimmune disease characterized by chronic inflammation of the synovial tissue lining the joint capsule. The erosive synovitis is generally symmetrical and extra-articular involvement may also occur, including rheumatoid nodules, cardiopulmonary disease, lymphadenopathy, splenomegaly, and neurological dysfunction.

Diagnosis

RA diagnosis is based on history and physical, laboratory evidence, and radiographic evaluation. History and physical will reveal consistent signs and symptoms of RA. Laboratory evidence will demonstrate rheumatoid factor (RF) presence in 60–70% of affected patients, elevated erythrocyte sedimentation rate and c-reactive protein, and radiographic evidence of joint space narrowing or erosions. Level of disease activity and presence of poor prognostic features guide treatment decisions.

- Disease activity: Categorized as low, moderate, or high based upon validated scales based upon clinical assessment.
- Poor prognostic features: Functional limitation, extra-articular disease (e.g., rheumatoid nodules, vasculitis), bony erosions by radiograph, or positive RF or anti-cyclic citrullinated peptide antibodies.

Signs and Symptoms

- Symmetrical symptoms of joint pain and stiffness (especially in the morning) for more than 6 weeks' duration
- Joint tenderness, erythema, swelling, and, potentially, rheumatoid nodules

Guidelines

American College of Rheumatology 2008 recommendations for the use of nonbiologic and biologic disease-modifying antirheumatic drugs in rheumatoid arthritis. At: http://www.rheumatology.org/practice/clinical/guidelines/recommendations.pdf.

Singh JA et al. 2012 update of the 2008 American College of Rheumatology recommendations for the use of disease-modifying antirheumatic drugs and biological agents in the treatment of rheumatoid arthritis. *Arthritis Care & Research* 64(May 2012):5, 625–639.

Guidelines Summary

- Goals of therapy include achieving low disease activity or remission.
- Disease-modifying antirheumatic drug (DMARD) should be initiated within 3 months of diagnosis to retard disease progression.
- Leflunomide, sulfasalazine, hydroxychloroquine, and methotrexate are first-line DMARD options.
- In patients with moderate to severe disease activity or those with features of poor prognosis (functional limitation, extra-articular disease, rheumatoid factor positivity, bony erosions) at the time of diagnosis, combination therapy may be considered initially.
- NSAIDs are useful for symptomatic relief during onset of DMARD and PRN otherwise. NSAIDs do not alter disease progression in RA.
- Corticosteroids are used as adjunctive therapy in patient with refractory symptoms.
- Biologic agents are used generally when initial DMARD has been demonstrated to be ineffective as monotherapy. Additional DMARDs may be tried prior to use of biologics.
- Biologic therapies increase the risk of serious infections and should not be initiated in a patient with an active infection or in combination with live vaccines.

Treatment Algorithm

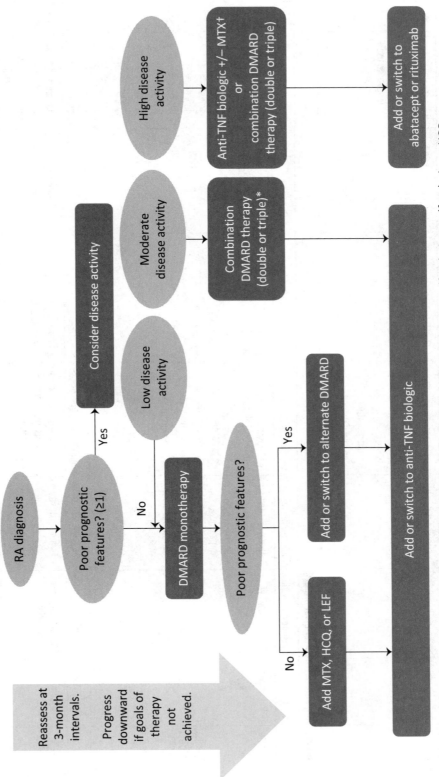

Drugs for Rheumatoid Arthritis

Mechanism of action – corticosteroids: exert anti-inflammatory and immunosuppressive effects by inhibiting prostaglandins and leukotrienes, which results in decreased inflammation, decreased pain, and a potential decrease in joint destruction

Generic	Brand	Dose & Max mg (frequency)	Contraindications	Primary Side Effects	Key Monitoring Parameters	Pertinent Drug Interactions	Med Pearls	Top 200
Prednisone	Various	5–60 mg daily initially; individualized	• Systemic fungal infection • Hypersensitivity	• High blood sugar • High BP • Reduced bone mineral density • Fluid retention • Impaired wound healing	• Blood sugar • BP • Bone mineral density • Presence of edema/weight	Warfarin	Side effects generally present with chronic and/or long-term use	Yes

Disease-modifying antirheumatic drugs (DMARDs)

Mechanism of action – inhibits cytokine production, inhibits purine biosynthesis, thereby decreasing inflammation in affected joints

Generic	Brand	Dose & Max mg (frequency)	Contraindications	Primary Side Effects	Key Monitoring Parameters	Pertinent Drug Interactions	Med Pearls	Top 200
Methotrexate (MTX)	• Rheumatrex • Trexall	7.5 mg 1 × wkly	• Hypersensitivity • Alcoholism • Severe hepatic impairment • Immuno-deficiency • Significant blood dyscrasias/anemias • Pregnancy • CrCl <40 mL/min	• GI upset (nausea, diarrhea, abdominal pain) • Stomatitis • Thrombocytopenia • Leukopenia • ↑ liver enzymes • Malaise • Fatigue • Fever/chills • Infections	• Pain relief • Liver function tests (LFTs) • Periodic complete blood count (CBC) • Folate	• Salicylates • Sulfonamides • Phenytoin	• May supplement folic acid to decrease adverse effects and prevent folate deficiency • Myelosuppression is biggest concern • Should be taken with food	Yes

Mechanism of action – not fully understood; thought to be related to immunosuppressant properties

Generic	Brand	Dose & Max mg (frequency)	Contraindications	Primary Side Effects	Key Monitoring Parameters	Pertinent Drug Interactions	Med Pearls	Top 200
Hydroxy-chloroquine	Plaquenil	200–600 mg daily (1 × daily)	• Hypersensitivity • Retinal changes with agent in past	Macular damage, corneal deposits; retinopathy; rash; nausea, diarrhea	• Ocular exams q 3 mo • Periodic CBC	• Cyclosporine • Digoxin	Older drug without risk of myelosuppression but ocular risk	Yes

Drugs for Rheumatoid Arthritis (cont'd)

Mechanism of action – leflunomide: inhibits pyrimidine synthesis, thereby decreasing lymphocyte proliferation and inflammation

Generic	Brand	Dose & Max mg (frequency)	Contraindications	Primary Side Effects	Key Monitoring Parameters	Pertinent Drug Interactions	Med Pearls	Top 200
Leflunomide (LEF)	Arava	Load 100 mg daily for 3 days; 20 mg daily maintenance	• Hepatic disease • Pregnancy • Immuno-deficiency	• Diarrhea • Elevated liver enzymes • Alopecia • Rash	Alanine transaminase (ALT) monthly × 6 mo, then periodically	• Cholestyramine • Rifampin	• Oral DMARD with low risk of bone marrow toxicity • Appropriate contraception should be used • Highly teratogenic	No

Mechanism of action – not fully understood; related to anti-inflammatory properties

Sulfasalazine	Azulfidine	250–2,000 mg daily (BID)	Hypersensitivity to any sulfa-containing drug	• Frequent diarrhea, nausea, vomiting • Rash • Urticaria • Photosensitivity • Leukopenia • Alopecia • Stomatitis • Elevated liver enzymes	• Response to therapy • Presence of adverse effects • CBC • Liver enzymes	• Warfarin • Methotrexate • Cyclosporine • Digoxin • Thiopurines	• Warfarin interaction very clinically significant • Monitor international normalized ratio (INR) closely	No

Biologics

Anti-TNF Biologic Agents

Mechanism of action – binds to and inhibits the cytokine tumor necrosis factor (TNF), thereby inhibiting the subsequent inflammatory cascade

Etanercept	Enbrel	50 mg SC 1 × wk	• Sepsis • Active infection • Hypersensitivity	• Local injection site reactions • Infections	Response to therapy	• Anakinra • Cyclophosphamide • Live vaccines	• Refrigerate prior to use • Discontinue temporarily if infection occurs • Can be self-administered • Can be used alone or in combination with methotrexate (MTX)	No

Drugs for Rheumatoid Arthritis (cont'd)

Generic	Brand	Dose & Max mg (frequency)	Contraindications	Primary Side Effects	Key Monitoring Parameters	Pertinent Drug Interactions	Med Pearls	Top 200
Mechanism of action – monoclonal antibody that binds to TNF and prevents interaction with TNF receptors on inflammatory cells								
Infliximab	Remicade	3–10 mg/kg IV infusion at initiation; wks 2 and 6 and q8 wks thereafter	• Active infection • Hypersensitivity	• Infections (upper respiratory common) • Acute infusion reactions (fever, chills, rash)	Response to therapy	• Anakinra • Live vaccines	• *Always* used in combination with MTX • Dose limited to ≤5 mg/kg in patients with heart failure	No
Mechanism of action – TNFα inhibitor								
Golimumab	Simponi	50 mg SC once per month	None	• Infection • Nasopharyngitis • Injection site reaction • Elevated AST/ALT	• Latent TB screening prior to initiation and during therapy • S/S of infection and heart failure • CBC • Hepatitis B virus (HBV) screening	• May diminish the therapeutic effect of immunosuppresants • Not to be given with live vaccines	• Once monthly SC injection may increase use due to convenience • Indicated for use in combination with MTX • Caution use in patients with heart failure • Discontinue use if serious infection • Refrigerated (not frozen)	No
Mechanism of action – monoclonal antibody that binds to TNF, blocking its interaction with cell surface receptors and decreasing inflammation								
Adalimumab	Humira	40 mg subcutaneously (SC) q other wk to wkly	• Active infection • Untreated latent tuberculosis (TB)	• Injection-site reactions • Infections	• Ongoing monitoring for response to therapy and presence of infection • Response to therapy • Latent tuberculosis (TB) screening prior to initiation	• Anakinra • Live vaccines	• Caution use in patients with heart failure • Discontinue during serious infections • Used as monotherapy or in combination with MTX or other DMARDs	No

Drugs for Rheumatoid Arthritis *(cont'd)*

Generic	Brand	Dose & Max mg (frequency)	Contraindications	Primary Side Effects	Key Monitoring Parameters	Pertinent Drug Interactions	Med Pearls	Top 200
Certolizumab pegol	Cimzia	400 mg SC at wks 0, 2, and 4 then 200 mg SC q other week	• Active, severe infection • Use with caution in NYHA class III or IV HF	• Infections • Injection site reactions • Worsening heart failure symptoms	• Latent TB and HBV screening prior to and during treatment • Response to therapy • CBC periodically • Signs and symptoms of infection	• May diminish the therapeutic effect of immunosuppressants • Not to be given with live vaccines	• Not to be given with live vaccines • Caution use in HF • Discontinue use during serious infection	No

Mechanism of action – binds to interleukin-1 (IL-1) receptors on target cells, thereby preventing release of chemotactic factors and adhesion molecules and subsequently decreasing inflammation and connective tissue damage

Generic	Brand	Dose & Max mg (frequency)	Contraindications	Primary Side Effects	Key Monitoring Parameters	Pertinent Drug Interactions	Med Pearls	Top 200
Anakinra	Kineret	100 mg SC daily	• Hypersensitivity • Active infections	Injection-site reactions (inflammation, ecchymosis); infections; neutropenia	• CBC periodically • Response to therapy • Presence of adverse effects	• Etanercept, infliximab, adalimumab • Live vaccines	Used alone or in combination with DMARDs (other than TNF blockers)	No

Mechanism of action – interleukin-6 (IL-6) receptor antagonist

Generic	Brand	Dose & Max mg (frequency)	Contraindications	Primary Side Effects	Key Monitoring Parameters	Pertinent Drug Interactions	Med Pearls	Top 200
Tocilizumab	Actemra	IV: Initial: 4 mg/kg every 4 wks; may be increased to 8 mg/kg based on clinical response (max = 800 mg per infusion)	None	• Serious: potentially fatal infections, TB • Common: upper respiratory tract infection, nasopharyngitis, elevated aspartate aminotransferase (AST)/ alanine aminotransferase (ALT)	• Signs and symptoms of infection • Latent TB screening prior to initiation and during therapy • CBC, lipid panel, and AST/ ALT prior and every 4–8 weeks during therapy • Signs and symptoms of CNS demyelinating disorders	• May diminish the therapeutic effect of immunosuppressants • Not to be used with live vaccines	• Discontinue use if serious infection • Do not use with live vaccines • Monotherapy or in addition to MTX • Indicated for patients that have failed one or more TNF agents	No

Drugs for Rheumatoid Arthritis *(cont'd)*

Mechanism of action – selective co-stimulation modulator; inhibits T-cell activation

Generic	Brand	Dose & Max mg (frequency)	Contraindications	Primary Side Effects	Key Monitoring Parameters	Pertinent Drug Interactions	Med Pearls	Top 200
Abatacept	Orencia	IV according to body weight; repeat dose at 2 wks, 4 wks, and every 4 wks thereafter • <60 kg: 500 mg • 60–100 kg: 750 mg • >100 kg: 1,000 mg	Hypersensitivity	• Headache • Nausea • Nasopharyngitis • Upper respiratory tract infection • Antibody formation	• Latent TB and HBV screening prior to initiation • S/S of infection and infusion reaction	• May diminish the therapeutic effect of immunosuppresants • Should not be given with live vaccines • Increased risk of infection with TNF antagonists	• Not to be given with TNF antagonists or live vaccines • Discontinue use if serious infection • Infections more likely in patients with chronic obstructive pulmonary disease (COPD) • Can be used as monotherapy or in combination with MTX	No

Mechanism of action – inhibits Janus kinase thereby reducing cytokine signaling

Generic	Brand	Dose & Max mg (frequency)	Contraindications	Primary Side Effects	Key Monitoring Parameters	Pertinent Drug Interactions	Med Pearls	Top 200
Tofacitinib	Xeljanz	5 mg PO (1 × –2 × daily)	None	• Infections • Latent infection reactivation • Elevated AST/ALT • Elevated lipids (total cholesterol, LDL) • Elevated serum creatinine • Diarrhea	• Latent TB screening prior to initiation • S/S of infection • HBV screening • Liver enzymes and lipid panel periodically	• Metabolized by CYP3A4, concentrations effected by potent inducers or inhibitors • Should not be given with live vaccines	• Indicated as monotherapy or in conjunction with other nonbiologic DMARDs • Oral therapy offers advantage over many available biologics	No

Storage and Administration Pearls

- NSAIDs should be administered with food to decrease risk of gastrointestinal side effects.
- Oral methotrexate should be administered with food to avoid stomach upset.
- The following medications should be refrigerated to 2–8°C (36–46°F): MTX injectable, etanercept, infliximab, adalimumab, anakinra, golimumab, and certolizumab pegol. These medications should *not* be frozen and should be protected from light.
- The following medications are administered through SC injection: etanercept, adalimumab, anakinra, golimumab, and certolizumab pegol.
- Methotrexate is administered orally or through intramuscular (IM) injection.
- Infliximab, tocilizumab, and abatacept cannot be self-administered and are delivered through IV infusion.
- The following medications are available in prefilled syringes and/or pen devices: etanercept, adalimumab, anakinra, golimumab, and certolizumab pegol.

Patient Education Pearls

- Promptly report any signs of infection to your physician. A temporary withdrawal of medication may be necessary during this time.
- Do not receive live vaccines while you are on biologic therapies.
- Appropriate administration of injectable therapies is as follows:
  - Visually inspect the products for particulate matter or discoloration. Do not use if either is present.
  - MTX is injected IM.
  - All other self-injectables are SC administration.
  - Rotate injection site.
  - Do not inject into tender, bruised, hard, or ulcerated skin.
  - Do not reuse needles or syringes.
  - Properly dispose of needles in a puncture-proof container.

OSTEOPOROSIS

Definition

Osteoporosis is a condition of low bone mass, which results in increased fragility of bone and subsequent increased risk of fracture. Potential etiologies of the characteristic decreased bone mass include age-related physiologic changes, disorders of estrogen or testosterone levels, or use of medications associated with drug-induced osteoporosis. Although more common in women, osteoporosis also occurs in men.

Normal bone physiology includes constant bone remodeling, which consists of bone formation via osteoblasts and bone resorption via osteoclasts. Bone mineral density (BMD) reflects the balance between resorption and formation. Osteoporosis occurs when there is an imbalance between formation and resorption resulting in a decreased BMD.

Diagnosis

The diagnosis of osteoporosis is most commonly based on the results of BMD measurement with dual energy x-ray absorptiometry (DXA) at the hip and spine. Results of the DXA are reported as the T score. The T score represents the number of standard deviations away from the mean BMD for a young, healthy individual. Normal BMD would be considered any T score greater than –1, while osteopenia would be a T score –1 to –2.5; a T score of less than –2.5 would be diagnostic for osteoporosis. Osteoporosis can also be diagnosed based on the occurrence of a nontraumatic fracture.

Signs and Symptoms

Typical signs of osteoporosis include kyphosis, shortened stature, and nontraumatic fractures of the vertebrae, hip, or forearm. Some patients may have symptoms of bone pain, and often vertebral fractures go undiagnosed as patients complain of chronic back pain. In a patient with risk factors for osteoporosis, radiographic investigation of back pain is warranted. Pain and physical changes associated with osteoporosis may lead to depression and lowered self-esteem. The FRAX® tool can be used to estimate 10-year fracture risk and guide treatment strategy.

Guidelines

National Osteoporosis Foundation. *Clinician's Guide to Prevention and Treatment of Osteoporosis*. Washington, DC: National Osteoporosis Foundation; 2013. www.nof.org /hcp/clinicians-guide.

Guidelines Summary

- Dietary and supplemental calcium and vitamin D are important prerequisites to pharmacological therapy. Without adequate calcium and vitamin D available, other therapies will be limited in their ability to improve bone architecture.

- Bisphosphonates are the first-line therapy for the prevention and treatment of osteoporosis in patients without contraindications.

- Oral bisphosphonates are approved for prevention and treatment of osteoporosis (including glucocorticoid-induced osteoporosis) in men and women.

- Efficacy of bisphosphonates beyond five years is limited, with rare but serious side effects such as osteonecrosis of the jaw and atypical femur fractures. It is reasonable to reassess fracture risk and consider therapy discontinuation after three to five years.

- Raloxifene is recommended as an alternative choice for the treatment of osteoporosis in patients with contraindications to bisphosphonates or in patients who are unable to comply with the appropriate bisphosphonate administration instructions.

- Calcitonin is reserved for third-line therapy because of a lack of compelling evidence indicating fracture reductions and lack of long-term data. Calcitonin is approved for the treatment of acute pain secondary to vertebral fractures and is well tolerated, so may have specific role in certain situations.

- Teriparatide is approved for treatment of osteoporosis and is indicated in patients with a history of fracture secondary to osteoporosis and in those with multiple risk factors for fracture who have not responded or are intolerant to bisphosphonate therapy, as well as for patients with glucocorticoid-induced osteoporosis.

- Denosumab is reserved for second-line therapy for the treatment of osteoporosis in postmenopausal females at high risk for fracture (previous osteoporotic fractures, multiple fracture risk factors, failed other therapies).

- Estrogens and tissue-selective estrogen complex (conjugated estrogens/bazedoxifene) are approved for the prevention of osteoporosis in postmenopausal women. Use should consider potential risks (cardiovascular, breast cancer, venous thromboembolism) and should be at the lowest effective dose for the shortest duration.

Drugs for Osteoporosis

Mechanism of action – bisphosphonates: adsorb to bone apatite and inhibit osteoclast activity

Generic	Brand	Dose & Max	Contra-indications	Primary Side Effects	Key Monitoring Parameters	Pertinent Drug Interactions	Med Pearls	Top 200
Alendronate	• Fosamax • Binosto effervescent	• 10 mg daily or 70 mg 1 × wk (treatment) • 5 mg daily or 35 mg 1 × wk (prevention)	• Esophageal stricture • Hypersensitivity • Inability to sit upright or stand for 30 minutes	• Nausea • Dyspepsia • Esophageal irritation	BMD	NSAIDs/aspirin increase risk of GI symptoms	• Must be taken with at least 8 oz of water ≥30 minutes prior to other medications/food • Patient should remain upright for 30 min or more	Yes
Risedronate	Actonel	5 mg daily or 35 mg 1 × wk	• CrCl <35 mL/min; hypocalcemia	• Ulceration • Muscle pain				Yes
Ibandronate	Boniva	150 mg PO 1 × month or 3 mg IV q3mo						Yes
Zoledronic acid	Reclast	5 mg IV infusion 1 × year	• Hypersensitivity • CrCl <35 mL/min	• Hypotension • Agitation • Confusion • Fever • Nausea • Constipation • Hypocalcemia • Muscle pain	BMD	Aminoglycosides	Annual IV infusion	No

Mechanism of action – selective estrogen receptor modulators: through selective binding to estrogen receptors, decreases bone resorption and reduces biochemical markers of bone turnover

Generic	Brand	Dose & Max	Contra-indications	Primary Side Effects	Key Monitoring Parameters	Pertinent Drug Interactions	Med Pearls	Top 200
Raloxifene	Evista	60 mg 1 × daily	• Hypersensitivity • History of pulmonary embolism or deep vein thrombosis • Pregnancy/lactation	• Hot flushes • Leg cramps • Thromboembolism	• BMD • Presence of adverse effects	• Cholestyramine • Warfarin	• Monitor international normalized ratio (INR) closely for patients on warfarin (expect INR increase) • Lipid effects include decreased LDL with no effect on HDL/triglycerides	Yes

Drugs for Osteoporosis *(cont'd)*

Miscellaneous agents

Mechanism of action – inhibits bone resorption through inhibition of osteoclast activity, to a small decrease stimulates bone formation through stimulation of osteoblast activity

Generic	Brand	Dose & Max	Contra-indications	Primary Side Effects	Key Monitoring Parameters	Pertinent Drug Interactions	Med Pearls	Top 200
Calcitonin	• Miacalcin Nasal Spray • Injection	• 200 units (1 spray) daily intranasally • 100 units q other day (SC or IM)	Hypersensitivity	• Nasal irritation and dryness • Rhinitis	BMD	None	• Refrigerate • Keep nasal spray at room temp while in use (<86°F/30°C) • Discard unused nasal spray after 30 days	No

Mechanism of action – acts as a parathyroid hormone (PTH) agonist; thereby increases bone formation by the stimulation of osteoblast activity and increases renal reabsorption of calcium

Generic	Brand	Dose & Max	Contra-indications	Primary Side Effects	Key Monitoring Parameters	Pertinent Drug Interactions	Med Pearls	Top 200
Teriparatide (PTH)	Forteo	20 mcg 1 × daily SC	• Hypersensitivity • Primary hyperparathyroidism • Hypercalcemia • Paget's disease	• Orthostatic hypotension • Dizziness • Nausea • Hypercalcemia	BMD	Digoxin (may predispose to digoxin toxicity)	Reduces risk of vertebral and nonvertebral fractures	No

Mechanism of action – monoclonal antibody, bone-modifying agent

Generic	Brand	Dose & Max	Contra-indications	Primary Side Effects	Key Monitoring Parameters	Pertinent Drug Interactions	Med Pearls	Top 200
Denosumab	Prolia	60 mg SC q6 months	Hypocalcemia	• Fatigue • Diarrhea • Nausea • Hyperlipidemia • Hypophosphatemia	• BMD • Serum phosphorous • Calcium • Magnesium	None	• Refrigerate • Should be clear and colorless	No

Storage and Administration Pearls

- Oral bisphosphonates should be taken on an empty stomach first thing in the morning with at least 8 oz of water. At least 30 to 60 minutes should pass prior to ingestion of any medication or food. Patient should remain upright for 30 to 60 minutes after taking dosage.

- Zoledronic acid solution for injection should be refrigerated prior to use. IV infusion administered only by healthcare professional.

- Calcitonin injection and nasal spray should be refrigerated at 2–8°C (36–46°F). Nasal spray can be kept at room temperature up 30°C to (86°F) during use.

- Nasal spray should be primed prior to use. Discard unused portion after 30 days.

- Calcitonin injection can be administered SC or IM.

- Teriparatide injection is available in a prefilled pen device and should be refrigerated at 2–8°C (36–46°F). The product should not be frozen, and any unused portion should be discarded after 28 days of use.

- Denosumab injection is available in a prefilled pen device and should be refrigerated at 2–8°C (36–46°F). The product should be brought to room temperature prior to injection (15–30 minutes) and injected by a health care professional. Once at room temperature it should be used within 14 days.

Patient Education Pearls

- Take oral bisphosphonates on an empty stomach first thing in the morning with at least 8 oz of plain water. You should then remain upright for 30–60 minutes and avoid lying down. Avoid ingestion of food, beverages (other than water), and other medications for 30–60 minutes after taking this medication.

- Calcitonin nasal spray should be primed prior to use and any unused portion should be discarded after 30 days.

- Teriparatide injection should be refrigerated at all times and should be discarded after 28 days of use.

- Denosumab injection should be refrigerated prior to use and brought to room temperature in its original container prior to injection into the upper arm, thigh, or abdomen. Once at room temperature, the prefilled syringe should be used within 14 days. Injection is typically administered by a health care professional.

- Oral bisphosphonate therapy has been associated with a low potential risk for osteonecrosis of the jaw. Use of bisphosphonate therapy should be shared with your dental health professional.

GOUT

Definition

Gout is a syndrome of acute or chronic recurrent arthritis characterized by deposits of monosodium urate crystals in synovial fluid and/or tissues and is most often associated with hyperuricemia. Hyperuricemia can result from either an overproduction or underexcretion of uric acid. Overproduction of uric acid is most common in myeloproliferative and lymphoproliferative disorders. A decrease in the renal excretion of uric acid can be the result of renal dysfunction, certain drugs, or a number of predisposing conditions, including obesity and hypothyroidism. Acute gouty attacks may be precipitated by a number of conditions including stress, trauma, and alcohol ingestion.

Diagnosis

The diagnosis of gout is based on clinical presentation along with the presence of uric acid crystals detected on joint aspiration of the synovial fluid of affected joints. Evaluation of a 24-hour urinary uric acid will allow classification of the patient as a uric acid overproducer (urinary uric acid excretion ≥600 mg) or a uric acid underexcretor (urinary uric acid >600 mg), which will assist in pharmacotherapeutic decisions.

Signs and Symptoms

Patients presenting with acute gouty arthritis complain of a quick onset of excruciating pain, inflammation, and swelling that most commonly affects the first metatarsophalangeal (MTP) joint and can also affect the feet, ankles, heels, knees, wrists, fingers, and elbows. Severe cases of gout can result in uric acid nephrolithiasis, nephropathy, or urate deposits (tophi) in affected joints.

Guidelines

Khanna D, Fitzgerald JD, Khanna PP, Bae S, Singh MK, Neogi T, et al; American College of Rheumatology. 2012 American College of Rheumatology Guidelines for Management of Gout. Part 1: Systematic nonpharmacologic and pharmacologic therapeutic approaches to hyperuricemia. *Arthritis Care Res (Hoboken).* 2012;64(10):1431–46.

Treatment of Acute Gouty Arthropathy

- Asymptomatic hyperuricemia does not require therapy.
- First-line treatment for gout includes the use of an NSAID. The majority of acute gout attacks will respond to an NSAID within 72 hours of therapy. Indomethacin is the most common NSAID used in the treatment of gout, but other NSAIDs are also

appropriate. Please see the medication chart in the osteoarthritis section of this chapter for more specific NSAID information.

- If patients have a contraindication to the use of an NSAID, evaluation of the time course of symptoms is necessary.
  - If gout symptoms have been present for less than 48 hours, colchicine is recommended for acute treatment.
  - If gout symptoms have been present for more than 48 hours, use of a corticosteroid is recommended.
- If the patient demonstrates an inadequate response to either NSAIDs or colchicine, corticosteroids should be considered.
- The use of oral (preferred) or parenteral corticosteroids is recommended for multijoint involvement, while an intraarticular corticosteroid can be used to target one specific symptomatic joint.
- Allopurinol or febuxostat should never be used in the treatment of acute gout. These agents are reserved for chronic prophylactic therapy in patients with multiple gout exacerbations each year. If these agents are used in the treatment of an acute gout exacerbation, the symptoms may be worsened due to the mobilization of uric acid stores.

Prophylaxis of Gout

- Colchicine maintenance therapy is indicated for prophylaxis in patients with only slightly elevated serum uric acid levels.
- Allopurinol is indicated for prophylaxis of gout exacerbations in patients with a moderately elevated serum uric acid level and a history of nephrolithiasis, tophi, serum creatinine >2.0 g/dL, or urinary uric acid excretion indicative of overproduction.
- Uricosuric drugs are indicated for prophylaxis of gout exacerbations in patients who are not candidates for allopurinol or febuxostat therapy and have a urinary uric acid excretion indicative of underexcretion.
- When initiating prophylactic therapy in a patient with gout, colchicine should be initiated with allopurinol, febuxostat, or a uricosuric and continued for the first 3–6 months of therapy to avoid causing an exacerbation.
- Pegloticase is indicated for refractory chronic gout in patients that do not respond to or have contraindications to traditional therapy.

Drugs for Gout

Generic	Brand	Dose & Max	Contra-indications	Primary Side Effects	Key Monitoring Parameters	Pertinent Drug Interactions	Med Pearls	Top 200
Mechanism of action – colchicine: inhibits lactic acid production, decreases uric acid deposition, reduces phagocytosis, and decreases inflammation								
Colchicine	Colcrys	1.2 mg then 0.6 mg 1 hr later (max = 1.8 mg)	Hypersensitivity; serious GI, renal, hepatic or cardiac disorders	• D/N/V • Rare: bone marrow suppression, aplastic anemia, thrombocytopenia	• Response to therapy • Serum uric acid • GI symptoms • Periodic CBC	None significant	• Patients may be provided with a prescription to be filled on a PRN basis and used during an exacerbation • Used for treatment and prophylaxis	No
Mechanism of action – xanthine oxidase inhibitor: by inhibition of xanthine oxidase, impairs the conversion of xanthine to uric acid, thereby decreasing the production of uric acid								
Allopurinol	Zyloprim	100–800 mg daily (renal dose adjustment necessary)	Hypersensitivity	• Skin rash • Leukopenia • GI upset	• Response to therapy • Serum uric acid • Renal function	• Mercaptopurine • Azathioprine	Renal dose adjustment	Yes
Febuxostat	Uloric	40–80 mg PO daily	Concurrent use with azathioprine, mercaptopurine, or theophylline	• Rash • Liver abnormalities • Arthralgia	• LFTs 2 and 4 months after initiation and periodically thereafter • Serum uric acid levels	• Azathioprine • Mercaptopurine • Theophylline • Didanosine	• No renal dose adjustment necessary • Not to be used during acute gout flares	No
Mechanism of action – uricosuric agents: increase the renal clearance of uric acid by inhibiting tubular reabsorption								
Sulfinpyrazone	Anturane	50–800 mg daily (BID)	• Hypersensitivity • CrCl <50 mL/min • History of renal calculi • Overproducers of uric acid • PUD	• GI upset • Rash • Stone formation	• Response to treatment • Serum uric acid • Renal function	• Warfarin (↑ INR) • Salicylates	May precipitate acute gouty attacks; avoid use during acute gouty arthritis	No
Probenecid	None	250–2,000 mg daily (BID)	• Hypersensitivity • CrCl <50 mL/min • History of renal calculi • Overproducers of uric acid • PUD	• GI upset • Rash • Stone formation	• Response to treatment • Serum uric acid • Renal function	• Methotrexate (↓ MTX levels) • Salicylates • Penicillins	May precipitate acute gouty attacks; avoid use during acute gouty arthritis	No

Drugs for Gout *(cont'd)*

Mechanism of action — catalyzes oxidation of uric acid to allantoin, thereby decreasing serum uric acid

Generic	Brand	Dose & Max	Contra-indications	Primary Side Effects	Key Monitoring Parameters	Pertinent Drug Interactions	Med Pearls	Top 200
Pegloticase	Krystexxa	8 mg IV infusion (over 2 or more hours) q2 weeks	• Glucose-6-phosphate-dehydrogenase deficiency • Risk of hemolysis • Methemoglobinemia	Acute gout exacerbation, infusion reactions	• Serum uric acid • S/S of anaphylaxis/infusion reactions 1 hr after infusion • Symptoms of congestive heart failure after infusion	None	• Indicated only for refractory cases • Patient should receive pre-treatment with antihistamines and corticosteroids • Gout flare prophylaxis with colchicine or NSAID one week prior to administration is recommended	No

Storage and Administration Pearls

- Medications should be stored in a dry place and protected from light.

Patient Education Pearls

- Patient should drink plenty of water (6–8 eight-oz glasses) while taking sulfinpyrazone or probenecid to avoid formation of kidney stones.

Learning Points

- First-line therapy for mild to moderate osteoarthritis is acetaminophen.
- NSAIDs and other pain medication should be administered with food to minimize stomach upset.
- Biologic therapies for RA suppress immunity and therefore cannot be initiated during infection and may be temporarily withdrawn during active infection.
- Biologic therapy for RA requires parenteral administration.
- First-line therapy for osteoporosis is the bisphosphonate class. Frequency of administration varies greatly from once daily to once annually. Oral formulations require very specific adherence to administration instructions to avoid esophageal side effects.
- Allopurinol and febuxostat are used for gout prophylaxis only and should be avoided during acute attacks because of their ability to exacerbate acute gout arthropathy by mobilizing uric acid stores.

PRACTICE QUESTIONS

1. Which of the following is NOT correctly matched with its trade name?

    (A) Methotrexate – Rheumatrex
    (B) Hydroxychloroquine – Azulfidine
    (C) Leflunomide – Arava
    (D) Etanercept – Enbrel
    (E) Infliximab – Remicade

2. A 60-year-old woman on etanercept 50 mg subcutaneously once weekly is requesting that her immunizations be updated. Which immunization would be contraindicated?

    (A) Varicella zoster
    (B) Seasonal influenza vaccine (intramuscular)
    (C) 23-valent pneumococcal vaccine
    (D) Tetanus, diphtheria, pertussis (Tdap)

3. A 64-year-old man with a medical history significant for hypertension and obesity takes bisoprolol 5 mg daily. His serum uric acid concentration is 7.3 mg/dL on routine laboratory examination. Which is the most appropriate therapeutic strategy?

    (A) Start allopurinol 100 mg/day.
    (B) Start febuxostat 40 mg/day.
    (C) Start probenecid 500 mg twice daily.
    (D) Therapy is not indicated because the patient has not yet experienced a gout attack.

4. A 52-year-old man with a medical history of hypertension, obesity, and gout (one episode, 6 months ago) takes enalapril 40 mg daily, amlodipine 10 mg daily, and aspirin 81 mg daily. He presents with symptoms, starting this morning, of gout in his left first metatarsophalangeal joint and left ankle. The metatarsophalangeal joint is swollen, inflamed, erythematous, and sensitive to light touch. Which is the best approach to therapy?

    (A) Colchicine 1.2 mg by mouth, then 0.6 mg 1 hour later
    (B) Colchicine 1.2 mg by mouth, then 0.6 mg 1 hour later; start allopurinol 300 mg once daily
    (C) Colchicine 1.2 mg by mouth, then 0.6 mg every hour as tolerated
    (D) Colchicine 1.2 mg by mouth, then 0.6 mg every hour as tolerated; start allopurinol 300 mg once daily

5. An 80-year-old woman is diagnosed with osteoarthritis of the right hand. Her medical history is significant for of peptic ulcer disease (PUD), hypertension, and hyperlipidemia. Which is the most appropriate therapy recommendation?

    (A) Glucosamine sulfate 500 mg by mouth three times daily
    (B) Naproxen 500 mg by mouth twice daily
    (C) Diclofenac 1% gel topically four times daily
    (D) Duloxetine 60 mg by mouth once daily

6. A 62-year-old man with hyperlipidemia, allergic rhinitis, and a history of PUD with an upper gastrointestinal bleed 2 years ago is diagnosed with osteoarthritis of the knee. He has tried maximum-dose, scheduled acetaminophen with insufficient pain relief. Current medications include atorvastatin and loratadine. Which is the best recommendation for the management of this patient's osteoarthritis of the knee?

    (A) Naproxen
    (B) Naproxen plus esomeprazole
    (C) Intraarticular corticosteroid
    (D) Diclofenac topical gel

7. A 44-year-old woman is newly diagnosed with rheumatoid arthritis (determined to be moderate–high disease activity with poor prognostic features) following more than 3 months of bilateral symptoms involving her metacarpophalangeal (MCP) and wrist joints. Laboratory results include AST 33 IU/L, ALT 36 IU/L, SCr 1.0 mg/dL, Hgb 13 g/dL, Hct 39%, (+) RF. Which is the most appropriate therapy selection?

    (A) Hydroxychloroquine
    (B) Methotrexate
    (C) Leflunomide
    (D) Adalimumab

8. A 56-year-old woman with rheumatoid arthritis complains of worsening joint pain in wrists and elbows over the past month. Upon physical exam, new rheumatoid nodules are noted on both elbows. Current medications include adalimumab, methotrexate, and folic acid. Prior medications include hydroxychloroquine (in combination with methotrexate), leflunomide, and etanercept. Which is the most appropriate therapy recommendation?

    (A) Replace adalimumab with abatacept
    (B) Replace methotrexate with sulfasalazine
    (C) Add sulfasalazine
    (D) Add minocycline

9. A 72-year-old woman with osteoporosis and a history of multiple vertebral fractures presents with intolerance to both alendronate and risedronate due to dyspepsia and esophageal irritation. She has followed administration instructions closely but continues to complain of bothersome side effects and indicates that she will no longer consider taking the medications. Her medical history is significant for chronic heart failure and history of venous thromboembolism (×2). Current medications include calcium, vitamin D, lisinopril, digoxin, furosemide, and rivaroxaban. Which of the following is the most appropriate therapy for her osteoporosis?

   (A) Ibandronate
   (B) Raloxifene
   (C) Denosumab
   (D) Teriparitide

ANSWERS

1. **B**

Hydroxychloroquine is generic for Plaquenil. Azulfidine is the brand name for sulfasalazine. The other answer choices are correctly matched with their trade names. Methotrexate (A) is generic for Rheumatrex or Trexall.

2. **A**

Patients with RA receiving biologic DMARDs should not be administered live vaccines such as varicella zoster. Trivalent seasonal influenza vaccine (B) and 23-valent pneumococcal vaccine (C) are acceptable to give to all patients, according to the schedule recommended by the Centers for Disease Control and Prevention (CDC) and Advisory Committee on Immunization Practices (ACIP). The Tdap vaccine (D) may also be safely administered to patients who are considered (non-HIV) immune compromised or receiving immune system–compromising agents.

3. **D**

Patients should not receive for asymptomatic hyperuricemia until they have experienced their first gouty attack. One to 2 weeks after the first attack, patients may begin uric acid–lowering therapy, and they should be treated to a serum uric acid concentration of <6 mg/dL.

4. **A**

Because this patient is suffering from an acute gouty attack, the use of allopurinol (B and D) is not appropriate. Allopurinol should be initiated only after the episode of acute gout has resolved. With respect to the colchicine dose, current recommendations support the lower cumulative dose due to equal efficacy and superior tolerability (fewer GI adverse events). The "as-tolerated" instructions for choices (C) and (D) put the patient at risk of overdosing and could potentially cause the patient GI adverse effects and even life-threatening hematologic effects.

5. **C**

First-line options for osteoarthritis of the hand include topical and oral NSAIDs, topical capsaicin, and tramadol. The ACR 2012 guidelines do not recommend glucosamine (A) for the treatment of OA of the hand. For patients over age 75, topical NSAIDs are preferred over oral NSAIDs, making choice (B) incorrect. Although duloxetine (D) is a second-line option in osteoarthritis of the knee and hip, this agent is not recommended prior to topical NSAIDs and is not preferred in OA of the hand.

6. **B**

Patients with a history of a GI bleed >1 year ago should receive an NSAID plus a proton pump inhibitor (B) or a COX2 selective NSAID. According to the ACR 2012 guidelines, oral NSAIDs such as naproxen (A) are the first-line option following inadequate response to maximum dose acetaminophen in patients with OA of the knee. Duloxetine, tramadol, and intraarticular injections (C) are reserved for patients with NSAID nonresponse or NSAID contraindications. Diclofenac topical gel (D) is also reserved for patients with NSAID contraindication or over the age of 75.

7. **D**

According to the 2012 ACR recommendations, patients with moderate–high disease activity and poor prognostic features should receive combination DMARD therapy or ant-TNF biologic DMARD with or without methotrexate. Therefore, the only appropriate monotherapy option in this patient would be an anti-TNF agent such as adalimumab.

8. **A**

Based upon the 2012 ACR recommendations for rheumatoid arthritis treatment in patients with established disease, health care providers should replace adalimumab in patients with high disease activity (persistently worsening symptoms on escalating therapy) and poor prognosis (development of new rheumatoid nodules); the options include an alternate anti-TNF agent, rituximab, or abatacept. Using an alternate nonbiologic DMARD such as sulfasalazine in place of (B) or in addition to methotrexate (C) would not likely alter the disease progression or symptoms at this stage. Minocycline (D) is reserved for patients with low disease activity and good prognostic features.

9. **C**

Denosumab is an appropriate agent for the treatment of osteoporosis in postmenopausal female patients at high risk of fracture (prior fractures) that have been intolerant to or failed alternate therapy options. Ibandronate (A) is a bisphosphonate; although this is the first-line class, the patient has not tolerated two agents in this class of medications. Raloxifene (B) is contraindicated due to the patient's history of venous thromboembolism. Teriparatide (D) would be an appropriate selection in a patient with osteoporosis and a history of fracture but would interact with this patient's digoxin, increasing the risk of digoxin toxicity.

Pain Management

11

This chapter covers the following drug classes:

- **Nonsteroidal anti-inflammatory drugs (NSAIDs)**
- **Nonopioid pain management**
- **Opioid pain management**

The text also provides an overview of basic treatment and management of pain.

 Suggested Study Time: **30 minutes**

PAIN MANAGEMENT

Definitions

Pain management can be a very complicated and a very involved condition because pain is subjective and therapy must be individualized. Such objective measures as tachycardia are not reliable. There are five main types of pain: Acute, chronic, chronic cancer, breakthrough, and neuropathic pain. Pain can also be classified as somatic, visceral, nociceptive, neuropathic, psychologically based pain syndromes, and mixed or undetermined pathophysiology. Acute pain usually requires only temporary therapy for less than 30 days but may last up to 3 months. Chronic pain is persistent and adversely affects the function or well-being of the patient for longer than 3 months. Somatic and visceral pain are most likely to be treated like acute pain but may persist and become chronic in nature. Nociceptive, neuropathic, psychologically based pain syndromes, and mixed or undetermined pathophysiologic pain, however, are chronic pain types. Nonnarcotic preparations should be used when possible. However, chronic pain will intensify, requiring more complex regimens and combination therapy with narcotics and nonnarcotics. Chronic cancer pain occurs in 60–90% of patients with cancer. It is similar to chronic nonmalignant pain. Breakthrough pain is intermittent and occurs at a greater intensity over baseline chronic pain. Neuropathic pain is characterized by a burning or tingling feeling, and can often be treated using anticonvulsants and antidepressants (also known as co-analgesics) with great success.

Diagnosis

Because pain is identified principally through self-reports and is very much subjective, it is challenging for a clinician to accurately assess and is virtually impossible to diagnose.

- Pain is always subjective.
- No neurophysiological or laboratory test can measure pain.
- The clinician should conduct a thorough history to fully understand the patient's pain.

Signs and Symptoms

- Objective observations such as grimacing, limping, or tachycardia may be helpful in assessing patients, but theses signs are often absent in patients with chronic pain.
- Pain intensity scales help patients communicate the signs and symptoms and pain intensity. This assessment can help guide treatments.
- Most adults and children above the age of 7 can score their pain intensity on a verbal numerical rating scale: 0 = no pain; 10 = the worst pain imaginable.

Guidelines

- Chou R, Fanciullo GJ, Fine PG, Adler JA, Ballantyne JC, Davies P, et al; American Pain Society-American Academy of Pain Medicine Opioids Guidelines Panel. Clinical guidelines for the use of chronic opioid therapy in chronic noncancer pain. *J Pain* 2009;10:113–30.
- NCCN Clinical Practice Guidelines in Oncology Adult Cancer Pain. Version 2.2014. National Comprehensive Cancer Network, Inc. 2014.

Guidelines Summary

- Drug therapy is the mainstay of management for acute pain. The drugs discussed in this review are classified into three categories: Nonopioid analgesics, including acetaminophen and nonsteroidal anti-inflammatory drugs (NSAIDs); opioid pain management; and co-analgesics. The drug classes can be used in monotherapy and combination for pain.
- As the pain increases, so does the dose of medications, the migration to stronger medications, and the use of combinations of medications with different mechanisms of actions.

- Acetaminophen and NSAIDs are useful for acute and chronic pain arising from a variety of causes, including surgery, trauma, arthritis, and cancer.
- NSAIDs are indicated for pain involving inflammation because acetaminophen lacks clinically effective anti-inflammatory properties.
- NSAIDs differ from opioid analgesic by the following mechanisms:
  - NSAIDs are both analgesics and inflammatory in nature.
  - There is a dose ceiling of effect in relationship with adverse effects.
  - NSAIDs do not produce physical or psychological dependence.
  - NSAIDs are antipyretic.
- Initiation of opioid analgesics should be based on a pain-directed history and physical that includes repeated pain assessment.
  - Opioid analgesics should be added to nonopioids to manage acute pain and cancer-related pain that does not respond to nonopioids alone.
  - There is enormous variability in doses of opioids required to provide pain relief, even among opioid-naïve patients.
  - It is important to give each analgesic an adequate trial. As a result, a clinician will increase the opioid dose until unacceptable side effects appear before changing to another opioid.
  - It is recommended to administer analgesics on a regular schedule if pain is present most of the day. This allows the patient to stay ahead of the pain.
    - » For chronic pain, consider having a scheduled long-acting agent on board and a short-acting agent for times of breakthrough pain.
- Patient-controlled intravenous opioid administration (PCA) for acute pain is a commonly used technique for pain control.
  - PCA is used with a microprocessor-controlled infusion pump.
  - PCA is most often used for the intravenous (IV) administration of opioids for acute pain.
  - PCA allows patients considerable control over the experience of pain.
  - PCA is not recommended in situations in which oral opioids could readily manage pain.

Nonnarcotic Oral and Nonsteroidal Anti-inflammatory Drugs (NSAIDs)

Generic	Brand	Dose & Max mg (frequency)	Contraindications	Primary Side Effects	Key Monitoring Parameters	Pertinent Drug Interactions	Med Pearls	Top 200
Mechanism of action – decreases pain through inhibition of central cyclooxygenase, which in turn inhibits prostaglandin synthesis								
Acetaminophen	Tylenol	325–1,000 mg TID–QID (max = 3,000 mg)	• Hepatic disease • Alcoholism	Very few	Pain relief	Alcohol	• Over-the-counter (OTC) • Best if taken on scheduled basis vs. as needed (PRN)	No
Mechanism of action – NSAIDs: decrease pain and inflammation by inhibition of prostaglandin synthesis through inhibition of cyclooxygenase enzymes								
Aspirin	Various	• Immediate release (IR): 325–3,600 mg daily (q4–6 hrs) • Extended release (ER) product: 650–1,300 mg TID (max = 5.4 g/day)	• Allergy to aspirin • Active bleeding • Age <16 years	• Gastrointestinal (GI) (dyspepsia, GI ulceration) • Bleeding	• Pain relief • GI symptoms	• Warfarin • Other NSAIDs • Angiotensin-converting enzyme inhibitors (ACEIs) • Anticoagulants	• OTC • Anti-inflammatory only at high doses (>3 g/day)	No
Nonacetylated salicylates								
Salsalate	None	500–3,000 mg daily (BID–TID) (max = 3 g/day)	• Hypersensitivity • Allergy to aspirin or NSAIDs	• GI (upset stomach, bleeding) • Rash • Diminished renal function • Edema	• Pain relief • GI symptoms	• Other salicylates • Warfarin • ACEIs	• Monitor serum salicylate levels with chronic use or very high doses • Desired range 10–30 mg/100 mL	No
Diflunisal	None	500–1,500 mg daily (BID)	Hypersensitivity				Administer with food	No

Nonnarcotic Oral and Nonsteroidal Anti-inflammatory Drugs (NSAIDs) (cont'd)

Generic	Brand	Dose & Max mg (frequency)	Contraindications	Primary Side Effects	Key Monitoring Parameters	Pertinent Drug Interactions	Med Pearls	Top 200
Acetic acids								
Etodolac	None	200–1,200 mg daily (q6–8 hrs)	Hypersensitivity	• GI (upset stomach, bleeding) • Rash • Diminished renal function • ↑ blood pressure • Edema	• Pain relief • GI symptoms • Renal function • Blood pressure	• Other salicylates • Warfarin • Lithium • ACEIs	• Administer with food	No
Diclofenac	• Cataflam • Voltaren-XR	50–150 mg daily (BID–TID)	Hypersensitivity	• GI (upset stomach, bleeding) • Rash • Diminished renal function • ↑ blood pressure • Edema	• Pain relief • GI symptoms • Renal function • Blood pressure	• Other salicylates • Warfarin • Lithium • ACEIs	• Administer with food • Available as gel or patch	Yes
	• Zipsor	25 mg QID						
	• Flector	1.3% patch: apply 1 patch BID						
	• Pennsaid	1.5% or 2% solution: apply 2 sprays BID						
Indomethacin	Indocin	• IR: 25–200 mg daily (BID–TID) • Extended release 75–150 mg daily (BID) (max = 200 mg/day)	Hypersensitivity	• GI (upset stomach, bleeding) • Rash • Diminished renal function • ↑ blood pressure • Edema • Central nervous system (CNS) disturbances	• Pain relief • GI symptoms • Renal function • Blood pressure	• Other salicylates • Warfarin • Lithium • ACEIs	• Most commonly used for treatment of gout • Fat-soluble, crosses blood-brain barrier • Administer with food	Yes
Ketorolac	Toradol	• 10 mg PO q4–6 hrs up to 40 mg daily • IM or IV 30 mg 96 hrs up to 120 mg daily	• Active peptic ulcer disease (PUD) or bleeding • History of GI bleeding • Severe renal impairment • Labor and delivery	• GI (upset stomach, bleeding) • Rash • Diminished renal function • ↑ blood pressure	• Pain relief • GI symptoms • Renal function • Blood pressure	• Other salicylates • Warfarin • Lithium • ACEIs	Only approved for moderate-severe pain for ≤5 days' duration, due to risk of renal and GI dysfunction	No
Nabumetone	Relafen	500–2,000 mg daily (q day–BID)	Hypersensitivity				Administer with food	No

Nonnarcotic Oral and Nonsteroidal Anti-inflammatory Drugs (NSAIDs) *(cont'd)*

Generic	Brand	Dose & Max mg (frequency)	Contraindications	Primary Side Effects	Key Monitoring Parameters	Pertinent Drug Interactions	Med Pearls	Top 200
Propionic acids								
Fenoprofen	Nalfon	200–3,200 mg daily (TID–QID)	Hypersensitivity	• GI (upset stomach, bleeding) • Rash • Diminished renal function • ↑ blood pressure	• Pain relief • GI symptoms • Renal function • Blood pressure	• Other salicylates • Warfarin • Lithium • ACEIs	Administer with food	No
Flurbiprofen	Ansaid	50–300 mg daily (BID–QID)	Hypersensitivity				Administer with food	No
Ibuprofen	• Motrin • Advil • Caldolor	200–3,200 mg daily (TID–QID) (max = 3.2 g/day)	Hypersensitivity				• Available OTC and Rx (400–800 mg tabs) • Administer with food • Available in pediatric preparations	Yes
Ketoprofen	• Nexcede • Orudis Nexcede	• IR: 50–300 mg daily (TID–QID) • SR: 75–200 mg daily	Hypersensitivity				Administer with food	No
Naproxen	• Naprosyn • EC Naprosyn • Naprelan	• IR: 250–1,500 mg daily (BID) • Enteric coated (EC) 375–1,500 mg daily (BID) • Controlled release (CR) 375–1,500 mg daily (BID)	Hypersensitivity				• Available OTC and Rx • Administer with food	Yes
Naproxen sodium	• Anaprox • Aleve	275–1,650 mg daily (BID)	Hypersensitivity				• Available OTC and Rx • Administer with food	Yes
Oxaprozin	Daypro	600–1,200 mg daily (1 × daily)	Hypersensitivity				Administer with food	No

Nonnarcotic Oral and Nonsteroidal Anti-inflammatory Drugs (NSAIDs) *(cont'd)*

Generic	Brand	Dose & Max mg (frequency)	Contraindications	Primary Side Effects	Key Monitoring Parameters	Pertinent Drug Interactions	Med Pearls	Top 200
Fenamates								
Meclofenamate	Meclomen	50–400 mg daily (q 4–6 hrs)	Hypersensitivity	• GI (upset stomach, bleeding) • Rash • Diminished renal function • ↑ BP	• Pain relief • GI symptoms • Renal function • BP	• Other salicylates • Warfarin • Lithium • ACEIs	Administer with food	No
Oxicams								
Piroxicam	Feldene	10–20 mg daily (q day–BID)	Hypersensitivity	• GI (upset stomach, bleeding) • Rash • Diminished renal function • ↑ BP	• Pain relief • GI symptoms • Renal function • BP	• Other salicylates • Warfarin • Lithium • ACEIs	• More COX -2 selectivity than traditional NSAIDs • Slightly less GI symptoms	Yes
Meloxicam	Mobic	7.5–15 mg daily (1 × daily)	Hypersensitivity					Yes
Selective COX -2 inhibitors								
Celecoxib	Celebrex	50–200 mg daily (q day–BID)	• Hypersensitivity • Sulfa allergy	• GI (upset stomach, bleeding—less than other NSAIDs) • Rash • Diminished renal function • ↑ BP • Edema	• Pain relief • GI symptoms • Renal function • BP	• Other salicylates (including aspirin) • Warfarin • Lithium • ACEIs	• Lower incidence of GI toxicity than with NSAIDs • Concern about cardiovascular adverse effects prompted withdrawal of similar drug from market (rofecoxib)	Yes

Narcotic Analgesics

Narcotic analgesics: stimulate opioid receptors in the brain

Generic	Brand	Dose & Max mg (frequency)	Contraindications	Primary Side Effects	Key Monitoring Parameters	Pertinent Drug Interactions	Med Pearls	Top 200
Hydrocodone	Zohydro ER	• Initial: 10 mg PO q12 hrs • No max dose	• Hypersensitivity • Severe hepatic impairment • Alcoholism	• Constipation • CNS depression • Confusion • Sedation • Respiratory depression • Hypotension • Bradycardia	• Presence of side effects (constipation, confusion) • Pain relief • Respiratory rate • BP • HR	• Alcohol • Other CNS depressants • MAOIs	• May take with food if nausea occurs • Often need a laxative for constipation	No
Hydrocodone/APAP	• Lorcet • Vicodin	• Dose is limited by APAP component • Do not exceed 4 g per day					• High abuse potential • Schedule II controlled substance (hydrocodone content)	Yes
Codeine	None	15–60mg q4 hrs (max = 360 mg/day)					• Good antitussive properties	Yes
Codeine/APAP	• Tylenol 3 • Tylenol 4	15–60 mg codeine q4–6 hrs (max = 360 mg/day of codeine and 4 g/day of APAP)						
Morphine	• Astramorph • Kadian • MS Contin	• No max dose • Available in PO, IM, IV, IT formulations • Kadian administered q12 hrs or q24 hrs • MS Contin administered q8 hrs or q12 hrs	• Hypersensitivity to morphine or naltrexone • Respiratory depression • Acute or severe bronchial asthma • Hypercapnia • Paralytic ileus				• Available in PO, IM, IV, IT formulations • May take with food if nausea occurs • Often need a laxative for constipation • High abuse potential • Most often started on IR then switched to ER/CR	Yes
	Avinza	• 1,600 mg/day • Administered q24 hrs						
Morphine sulfate and naltrexone	Embeda	20 mg/0.8–100 mg/4 mg daily		• Constipation • Nausea • Somnolence				No

Narcotic Analgesics *(cont'd)*

Generic	Brand	Dose & Max mg (frequency)	Contraindications	Primary Side Effects	Key Monitoring Parameters	Pertinent Drug Interactions	Med Pearls	Top 200
Oxycodone	• OxyContin • Roxicodone	• No max dose • IR products dosed q4–6 hrs • OxyContin dosed q12 hrs		• Constipation • CNS depression • Confusion • Sedation • Respiratory depression • Hypotension • Bradycardia	• Presence of side effects (constipation, confusion) • Pain relief • Respiratory rate • BP • HR		• OxyContin has abuse deterrent formulation • May take with food if nausea occurs • Often need a laxative for constipation • High abuse potential	Yes
Oxycodone/APAP	• Percocet • Roxicet • Endocet	Dose is limited by APAP component, do not exceed 4 g per day						Yes

Narcotic Analgesics *(cont'd)*

Generic	Brand	Dose & Max mg (frequency)	Contraindications	Primary Side Effects	Key Monitoring Parameters	Pertinent Drug Interactions	Med Pearls	Top 200
Fentanyl	• Duragesic • Actiq • Fentora • Onsolis • Subsys • Abstral • Lazanda	• Infusion, injection, lozenge, tab, transdermal patch, buccal film, buccal tablet, nasal spray • No max • Dosages different for each delivery system				CYP3A4 inducers and inhibitors	• Patch takes 24 hrs to begin working • Fentanyl remains in patch at 72 hrs; fold in half to avoid diversion	Yes
Hydromorphone	• Dilaudid • Dilaudid – HP • Exalgo	• No max • Tablet, IV, IM, SC, rectal administration • Exalgo is dose q24 hrs	• Hypersensitivity • Asthma • Respiratory depression • CNS depression			None	• High potential for abuse • Dilaudid-HP is highly concentrated	Yes
Meperidine	Demerol	Injection, PCA pump, tablet 25–100 mg	Same as above		Same as above; add seizure due to potential metabolite-normeperidine		• Not recommended as an analgesic • Use less than 48 hrs and in doses <600 mg/day • Avoid in renal failure	No
Methadone	• Dolophine • Methadose	• Initial opioid naïve: 2.5–10 mg q8–12 hrs (no max)	Same as above and concurrent use of selegiline		• Pain relief • Mental status • BP • QTc interval	• Alcohol • Other CNS depressants • Other drugs that prolong the QTc interval	• Long half-life and difficult to titrate • Available in IV formulation	Yes
Tapentadol	• Nucynta • Nucynta ER	• 50–100 mg q4–6 hrs (max = 600 mg/day) • Nucynta ER: q12 hrs dosing (max = 500 mg/day)	Impaired pulmonary function, paralytic ileus, or use of MAOIs	• Nausea • Dizziness • Vomiting • Somnolence • Along with the other side effects of the drugs in this class	Pain relief and signs of abuse	• Alcohol • Other CNS depressants		No

Analgesic Adjuncts

Generic	Brand	Dose & Max mg (frequency)	Contraindications	Primary Side Effects	Key Monitoring Parameters	Pertinent Drug Interactions	Med Pearls	Top 200
Mechanism of action – increases synaptic concentration of norepinephrine, desensitization of adenyl cyclase, downregulation of serotonin receptors								
Desipramine	Norpramin	Initial: 10–25 mg/day (max = 150 mg)	Use of MAOI past 14 days; acute recovery phase following a myocardial infarction	• Orthostatic hypotension • Tachycardia • Anticholinergic effects • Arrythmias • Constipation	• Blood pressure • Suicidal ideation	CYP450 inhibits CYP1A2, CYP2C9, CYP2D6, CYP2E1	• Increased suicidal behavior in young adults age 18–24 yrs • Neuropathic pain is an unlabeled indication	No
Amitriptyline	Elavil	Initial: 25–50 mg/day (max = 150 mg)					• Taper off when medication is disontinued	Yes
Mechanism of action – induces the release of substance P, the principle chemomediator of pain impulses from the periphery								
Gabapentin	• Neurontin • Gralise	• Initial 300 mg TID (max = 3,600 mg) • Gralise (max = 1,800 mg/day q24 hrs)	None	• Somnolence • Dizziness • Peripheral edema • Viral infection	• Pain scale • Drowsiness	Sedative effects: CNS depressants, alcohol, opiates	• Chronic neuropathic pain is not a labeled indication for IR product • Gralise is labeled to treat post-herpetic neuralgia	Yes
Pregabalin	Lyrica	Initial: 75 mg BID (max = 450 mg/day)					• Controlled substance (C5) • Has official FDA indication for neuropathic pain associated with diabetes	Yes
Duloxetine	Cymbalta	40–60 mg/day; BID or daily (max = 60 mg/day)	• MAOI within 14 days • Concomitant linezolid therapy	• Headache • Somnolence • Nausea • Dry mouth • Dizziness • Insomnia	• Pain relief • BP	• MAOIs • Linezolid	Used to treat neuropathic pain and fibromyalgia	Yes

Analgesic Adjuncts *(cont'd)*

Generic	Brand	Dose & Max mg (frequency)	Contraindications	Primary Side Effects	Key Monitoring Parameters	Pertinent Drug Interactions	Med Pearls	Top 200
Mechanism of action – binds to μ-opiate receptors in the CNS, causing inhibition of ascending pain pathways								
Tramadol	• Ultram • Ultram ER	• IR: 25–400 daily (q4–6 hrs) • ER: 100–300 daily	• Hypersensitivity • Caution in patients with seizures	• Confusion • Sedation • Rash • Stomach upset • Orthostatic hypotension • Seizures	• Pain relief • Renal and hepatic function periodically	• Alcohol • Opioids • SSRIs • MAOIs • Warfarin	• Renal dose adjustment for CrCl <30 mL/min • Schedule IV controlled substance	Yes
Tramadol/APAP	Utracet	Max = 8 tablets/day						
Mechanism of action – induces the release of substance P, the principal chemomediator of pain impulses from the periphery								
Capsaicin Cream	• Salonpas • Zostrix	• Cream, gel, lotion: 0.025–0.1% applied 3–4 × daily • Patch: apply to affected area 3–4 × /day	Do not apply to wounds or damaged skin	Localized stinging	Pain relief	None	• OTC • Must be used regularly for 2 wks or more for maximal efficacy	No

Storage and Administration Pearls

- Do not freeze acetaminophen suppositories.
- Hydrolysis of aspirin occurs upon exposure to water or moist air, resulting in salicylate and acetate, which possess a vinegar-like odor. Do not use if a strong odor is present.
- Ibuprofen, indomethacin, ketoprofen, and ketoralac must be protected from light.
- Amitriptyline, oxycodone, fentanyl, hydromorphone, meperidine, and methadone all need to be protected from light.
- Wash hands after application of capsaicin products.

Patient Education Pearls

- The patient should always take exactly what is prescribed. Never increase the dose without discussing with the prescriber
- The narcotic medications may cause physical and psychological dependence.
- While using pain medications, it is recommended not to use alcohol or other prescription or OTC medications.

Learning Points

- NSAIDs are both analgesics and anti-inflammatory in nature.
- No NSAID is any more effective than any other in the general population.
- Symptoms of overdose for narcotic medications include: CNS depression, bradycardia, hypotension, respiratory depression, miosis, apnea, pulmonary edema, and convulsions.
- Onset of action of most pain medication occurs within 45 minutes, with peak drug effect in 1 to 2 hours after oral administration for most immediate-release medications.
- PCA provides the important advantage of medication that is rapidly administered when needed, delaying pain exacerbation.
- In chronic pain, continuous opioid administration is recommended with controlled release medication, transdermal patch, or infusion. Short-acting medications should be available for breakthrough pain.

PRACTICE QUESTIONS

1. Which of the following is a caution with the use of tramadol?

    (A) Bradycardia
    (B) GI bleed
    (C) HTN
    (D) Hyperglycemia
    (E) Seizures

2. Which of the following is true regarding meperidine?

    (A) May be used for long-term analgesia
    (B) Normeperidine may cause seizures
    (C) Only available in oral formulation
    (D) Preferred agent for use in renal failure
    (E) Recommended first line for analgesia

3. Which of the following should be avoided in PUD?

    I.   Aleve
    II. Toradol
    III. Diclofenac

    (A) I only
    (B) III only
    (C) I and II only
    (D) II and III only
    (E) I, II, and III

4. Which of the following can be used to treat neuropathic pain?

    (A) Acetaminophen
    (B) Capsaicin
    (C) Gabapentin
    (D) Ibuprofen
    (E) Ketorolac

5. Which of the following is associated with methadone use?

    (A) Diarrhea
    (B) GI bleeding
    (C) Hyperkalemia
    (D) Hypertension
    (E) QTc prolongation

ANSWERS

1. **E**

Tramadol is associated with a risk of seizures and should be used with caution in patients with epilepsy or a history of a seizure disorder. The risk of seizures is increased if given concomitantly with other agents that may lower the seizure threshold.

2. **B**

Normeperidine is a toxic metabolite of meperidine that is known to cause seizures. Meperidine should not be used for >48 hours (A) and should be avoided in renal failure to prevent the accumulation of normeperidine (D). Meperidine is available in oral and IV formulations (C). Meperidine should not be used as a first-line agent (E) due to the risk associated with the medication.

3. **E**

All of the agents are NSAIDs and should not be used if a patient has PUD or a history of a GI bleed. If an NSAID must be used in a patient with PUD or a GIB, a COX-2 selective inhibitor, celecoxib, would be preferred.

4. **C**

Gabapentin may be used to treat neuropathic pain. Neuropathic pain does not respond well to acetaminophen (A) or NSAIDs such as ibuprofen (D) or ketorolac (E).

5. **E**

Methadone is known to prolong the QTc interval and should not be used with other agents that prolong the QTc interval. Methadone is associated with constipation (not diarrhea, A), hypokalemia (not hyperkalemia, C), and hypotension (not hypertension, D). I is not known to cause GI bleeding (B).

Ophthalmologic and Otic Disorders

12

This chapter covers the following disorders:

- **Glaucoma**
- **Impacted cerumen, water-clogged ears, and otitis externa**

 Suggested Study Time: **25 minutes**

GLAUCOMA

Definitions

Glaucoma is a group of eye disorders caused by damage to an area of the optic nerve (optic disk), which results in loss of visual sensitivity and field. The two types of glaucoma include open-angle and closed-angle glaucoma. Open-angle glaucoma is the most common form of this disorder and can be due to either genetic causes (most prevalent is primary open-angle glaucoma [POAG]) or other factors such as trauma, surgery, or medications (secondary open-angle glaucoma). Although it was previously believed that increased intraocular pressure (IOP) was solely responsible for the damage to the optic disk, it appears that factors such as ischemia, changes in blood flow, and autoimmune factors may also play a role.

Given that up to 70% of all cases of glaucoma in the United States are characterized as POAG, the discussion in this chapter focuses only on this form of the ocular disorder.

Diagnosis

The diagnosis of POAG is based on the presence of characteristic changes to the optic disk and visual field loss with or without an increased IOP. An increased IOP does not need to be present to confirm the diagnosis of POAG. In general, an IOP greater than 21 mmHg is considered to be elevated.

Signs and Symptoms

Symptoms for glaucoma usually do not develop until significant damage to the optic disk and significant visual field loss has already occurred. Patients may complain of blind spots, reduced peripheral vision, and changes in color perception.

Guidelines

American Academy of Ophthalmology. http://one.aao.org/CE/PracticeGuidelines/default.aspx.

Overview of Treatment

Because the above guidelines do not specify which drugs should be used as first-line or second-line therapy, this section should not be considered as a "Guidelines Summary" but rather as a general overview of the pharmacologic treatment of glaucoma.

The initial goal is to achieve at least a 20% reduction in the IOP. Additional lowering may be necessary based upon the baseline IOP, the extent of damage to the optic disk, and the extent of visual field loss.

- β-blockers or prostaglandin analogs are considered first-line therapy for POAG. Prostaglandin analogs are often used as initial therapy. These agents can be used as monotherapy or in combination with each other.
  - If a patient does not tolerate or does not respond at all (no reduction in IOP) to an agent, an alternative drug should be used.
  - If a patient partially responds to an agent (some reduction in IOP, but not at goal), addition of another drug should be considered.
- α_2 agonists or topical carbonic anhydrase inhibitors can be considered if the patient does not respond to or tolerate one of the above first-line agents.
- Cholinergic agonist are usually considered as last-line drug therapies because of their increased risk of side effects.
- Laser or surgical procedures may also be considered during the course of therapy.

β-Blockers

Mechanism of action — ↓ IOP by ↓ production of aqueous humor

Generic	Brand	Dose	Contra-indications	Primary Side Effects	Key Monitoring	Pertinent Drug Interactions	Med Pearl	Top 200
Betaxolol (β₁-selective)	Betoptic-S	• Solution: 1–2 drops 2 × daily • Suspension: 1 drop 2 × daily	• Sinus bradycardia • ≥2nd-degree heart block (in absence of pacemaker) • Decompensated heart failure • Severe chronic obstructive pulmonary disease/asthma	Local effects • Burning • Stinging • Tearing • Blurred vision • Dry eyes; Systemic effects • Bradycardia • Heart block • Hypotension • Heart failure exacerbation • Bronchospasm • Fatigue	IOP every 2–4 wks until target achieved, then every 6 mo	• ↑ risk of systemic side effects with oral β-blockers • ↑ risk of bradycardia or heart block with digoxin, verapamil, diltiazem, or clonidine	• All have similar efficacy in ↓ IOP • Tachyphylaxis may occur with long-term use	No
Carteolol (nonselective, ISA properties)	Only available generically	1 drop 2 × daily					• Effect on IOP may be lessened in patients receiving oral β-blockers	No
Levobunolol (nonselective)	Betagan	1–2 drops 1–2 × daily						No
Metipranolol (nonselective)	OptiPranolol	1 drop 2 × daily						No
Timolol (nonselective)	• Solution: Timoptic, Betimol, Istalol • Gel-forming solution: Timoptic-XE	• Solution: 1 drop 1–2 × daily • Gel-forming solution: 1 drop 1 × daily						Yes

Prostaglandin Analogs

Mechanism of action — ↓ IOP by ↑ outflow of aqueous humor

Generic	Brand	Dose	Contraindications	Primary Side Effects	Key Monitoring	Pertinent Drug Interactions	Med Pearl	Top 200
Bimatoprost	Lumigan	1 drop 1× daily in evening	Hypersensitivity	• Change in iris, eyelash, and eyelid pigmentation (become darker) • Growth of eyelashes • Eyelid edema • Itching, redness, blurred vision, dry eyes	IOP every 2–4 wks until target achieved, then every 6 mo	No significant interactions	• Do not exceed 1x daily dosing (may worsen IOP) • Iris discoloration is not reversible (highest incidence with latanoprost) • Eyelid discoloration and eyelash changes may be reversible • Travatan Z does not contain benzalkonium chloride • Most effective in ↓ IOP • Bimatoprost also available as Latisse ⟶ to ↑ eyelash growth	Yes
Latanoprost	Xalatan	1 drop 1× daily in evening						Yes
Tafluprost	Zioptan	1 drop 1× daily in evening						No
Travoprost	Travatan Z	1 drop 1× daily in evening						Yes

α$_2$-Agonists

Mechanism of action — ↓ IOP by ↓ production of aqueous humor (brimonidine may also ↑ outflow of aqueous humor)

Generic	Brand	Dose	Contraindications	Primary Side Effects	Key Monitoring	Pertinent Drug Interactions	Med Pearl	Top 200
Apraclonidine	Iopidine	1 drop 3× daily	Concurrent or recent use (within 14 days) of monoamine oxidase inhibitors	Local effects • Eyelid edema • Itching, redness, burning Systemic effects • Dizziness • Fatigue • Dry mouth • Headache • Hypotension • Bradycardia	IOP every 2–4 wks until target achieved, then every 6 mo	↑ risk of systemic side effects with central nervous system depressants (e.g., alcohol, opiates, sedatives, barbiturates)	• Structurally similar to clonidine	No
Brimonidine	Alphagan P	1 drop 3× daily					• Apraclonidine primarily used to control postoperative ↑ IOP	Yes

Carbonic Anhydrase Inhibitors

Generic	Brand	Dose	Contra-indications	Primary Side Effects	Key Monitoring	Pertinent Drug Interactions	Med Pearl	Top 200
Mechanism of action – ↓ IOP by ↓ production of aqueous humor								
Brinzolamide	Azopt	1 drop 3 × daily	Sulfa allergy (risk of cross-sensitivity)	• Eyelid reactions • Burning, stinging, tearing, blurred vision • Bitter taste in mouth	IOP every 2–4 wks until target achieved, then every 6 mo	No significant interactions	• Topical therapy rarely associated with systemic side effects • Oral carbonic anhydrase inhibitor therapy (e.g., acetazolamide) may be used in patients refractory to maximal doses of topical therapy; associated with higher risk of side effects	No
Dorzolamide	Trusopt	1 drop 3 × daily						No

Cholinergic Agonists (Direct-Acting)

Generic	Brand	Dose	Contra-indications	Primary Side Effects	Key Monitoring	Pertinent Drug Interactions	Med Pearl	Top 200
Mechanism of action – ↓ IOP by ↑ outflow of aqueous humor								
Carbachol	Isopto Carbachol	1–2 drops 2–3 × daily	Ocular inflammatory condition (may worsen condition)	• Impaired night vision • Headache • Eyelid twitching • Stinging, burning, tearing	IOP every 2–4 wks until target achieved, then every 6 mo	No significant interactions	• Patients with darker eyes may require higher concentrations of pilocarpine to ↓ IOP • Pilocarpine PO (Salagen) used for Sjögren's syndrome	No
Pilocarpine	Solution: Isopto Carpine	1–2 drops 3–4 × daily						No

Combination Drugs

Generic	Brand
Brimonidine/brinzolamide	Simbrinza
Timolol/brimonidine	Combigan
Timolol/dorzolamide	Cosopt

Storage and Administration Pearls

- Most ophthalmic preparations (gels, solutions, suspensions) should be stored at room temperature.
  - Latanoprost should be refrigerated until opened; once opened, the bottle can be stored at room temperature.
- Ophthalmic suspensions should be shaken well prior to using.

Patient Education Pearls

- Patient should be educated on the appropriate administration of ophthalmic preparations:
  - Wash and dry hands.
  - If suspension is being used, shake the bottle well.
  - Contact lenses should be removed prior to administration.
  - Tilt head back and look at the ceiling.
  - Pull down the lower eyelid to form a pocket into which the medication will be instilled.
  - Place the dropper over the eye, look up, and then place a single drop in the eye.
  - To avoid contamination, the tip of the dropper should not touch any part of the eye.
  - Close the eyes for several minutes. Do not rub the eyes.
- If the patient is using more than one ophthalmic drug, administration of these drugs should be separated by at least 10 minutes to prevent loss of the initially administered drug.
- Patient should be educated on use of nasolacrimal occlusion when administering eye drops to minimize the development of systemic side effects and to enhance drug efficacy.
  - Once the eye drop is instilled, instruct patient to close eye and place index finger over nasolacrimal drainage system in the inner corner of the eye for 1–3 minutes.

OTIC DISORDERS

Definitions

Impacted cerumen, water-clogged ears, and swimmer's ear (otitis externa) are three common otic disorders that can be managed with various ear drop products. Cerumen normally helps to protect the ear by lubricating the external auditory canal, trapping foreign particles, and preventing organisms from penetrating into the ear. However, certain individuals, including those who have abnormally shaped external auditory canals, increased hair growth in their ears, or hearing aids, may be at increased risk for the cerumen to become impacted. Water-clogged ears are most likely to occur in patients who have abnormally shaped external auditory canals or excessive cerumen in their ears. Otitis externa occurs when inflammation or infection of the external auditory canal or outer ear develops.

Signs and Symptoms

- Impacted cerumen: Fullness/pressure in ear, hearing impairment, vertigo, tinnitus, otalgia
- Water-clogged ears: Fullness/pressure in ear, hearing impairment
- Otitis externa: Otalgia, otorrhea

Overview of Treatment

Drugs for Treatment of Impacted Cerumen

- Carbamide peroxide (Debrox)

Drugs for Treatment of Water-Clogged Ears

- 95% isopropyl alcohol in 5% anhydrous glycerin (Auro-Dri; Swim Ear)

Drugs for Treatment of Otitis Externa

- Acetic acid otic solution (VoSol) (also available with hydrocortisone [VoSol HC Otic])
- Neomycin with polymyxin B and hydrocortisone (Cortisporin Otic)
- Neomycin with colistin, hydrocortisone, and thonzonium (Coly-Mycin S)
- Ofloxacin (Floxin Otic)
- Ciprofloxacin (Cetraxal)
- Ciprofloxacin with hydrocortisone (Cipro HC Otic)
- Ciprofloxacin with dexamethasone (Ciprodex)

Storage and Administration Pearls

- Most otic preparations should be stored at room temperature
- Otic solutions/suspensions should be warmed to body temperature by holding containers in hand for a few minutes.
- Otic suspensions should be shaken well before using.

Patient Education Pearls

- Patient should be educated about the appropriate administration of otic preparations:
  - Wash and dry hands.
  - If a suspension is being used, shake the bottle well.
  - Warm the solution/suspension container in the hand for a few minutes.
  - Carefully wash and dry outside of the ear (being careful not to get water inside the ear canal).
  - Tilt head to the side or lie down with affected ear up.
  - Position the dropper tip near, but not inside, the opening of the ear canal. To avoid contamination, the tip of the dropper should not touch any part of the ear.
  - Pull the ear backward and upward to open the ear canal. If the patient is younger than 3 years, pull the ear backward and downward.
  - Instill the appropriate number of drops into the ear canal.
  - Gently press the small skin flap over the ear canal opening to push the ear drops down into the canal.
  - Remain in the same position for ≥1 minute to allow penetration of the medication.
  - Wash hands.

Learning Points

- Know examples of ophthalmic β-blockers, prostaglandin analogs, and α_2 agonists.
- β-blocker eye drops can cause systemic adverse effects. Use caution in patients also receiving oral β-blocker therapy.
- Prostaglandin analogs can cause pigmentation changes in the iris, eyelid, and eyelashes.
- Carbonic anhydrase inhibitors should not be used in patients with sulfa allergies.
- Know ophthalmic combination drug products.
- Know which otic products are used for impacted cerumen, water-clogged ears, and otitis externa.

PRACTICE QUESTIONS

1. Which of the following medications is likely to cause a darkening of the iris of the eye?

    (A) Apraclonidine
    (B) Carbachol
    (C) Dorzolamide
    (D) Latanoprost
    (E) Timolol

2. Lumigan belongs to which of the following classes of drugs?

    (A) α_2 agonist
    (B) Antihistamine
    (C) β-blocker
    (D) Cholinergic agonist
    (E) Prostaglandin analog

3. Which of the following products contains a carbonic anhydrase inhibitor?

    (A) Alphagan P
    (B) Azopt
    (C) Betoptic-S
    (D) Combigan
    (E) Lumigan

4. A patient with glaucoma has a history of anaphylaxis when taking trimethoprim/sulfamethoxazole. Which of the following drugs should be avoided in this patient?

    I. Travatan Z
    II. Simbrinza
    III. Trusopt

    (A) I only
    (B) III only
    (C) I and II only
    (D) II and III only
    (E) I, II, and III

5. Which of the following drugs reduce IOP by decreasing the production of aqueous humor?

      I. Bimatoprost
     II. Dorzolamide
   III. Timolol

(A) I only
(B) III only
(C) I and II only
(D) II and III only
(E) I, II, and III

ANSWERS

1. **D**

Latanoprost, an ophthalmic prostaglandin analog, is likely to cause darkening of the iris, so choice (D) is correct. This class of drugs may also cause increased pigmentation of the eyelid and eyelashes.

2. **E**

Lumigan, the brand name for bimatoprost, is a prostaglandin analog, so choice (E) is correct.

3. **B**

Azopt contains brinzolamide, which is a carbonic anhydrase inhibitor. Alphagan-P (A) contains brimonidine, an α_2-agonist. Betoptic-S (C) contains betaxolol, a β-blocker. Combigan (D) is a combination product that contains timolol (β-blocker) and brimonidine (α_2-agonist). Lumigan (E) contains bimatoprost, a prostaglandin analog.

4. **D**

The ophthalmic carbonic anhydrase inhibitors—brinzolamide and dorzolamide—are sulfa derivatives and should be avoided in patients with a history of anaphylaxis to sulfa products (e.g., trimethoprim/sulfamethoxazole). Both Simbrinza (II) (brimonidine/brinzolamide) and Trusopt (III) (dorzolamide) contain carbonic anhydrase inhibitors. Travatan Z (I) contains travoprost, a prostaglandin analog; this drug is not a sulfa derivative.

5. **D**

Ophthalmic β-blockers, α_2-agonists, and carbonic anhydrase inhibitors reduce IOP by decreasing the production of aqueous humor. Dorzolamide (II) is a carbonic anhydrase inhibitor, while timolol (III) is a β-blocker. Prostaglandin analogs such as bimatoprost (I) reduce IOP by increasing the outflow of the aqueous humor.

Hematologic Disorders

13

This chapter covers the following diseases:

- **Iron deficiency anemia**
- **Anemia of chronic kidney disease and dialysis**
- **Pernicious anemia**

 Suggested Study Time: **45 minutes**

IRON DEFICIENCY ANEMIA

Definitions

Iron deficiency anemia (IDA) is a common disorder worldwide. In the United States, most cases are caused by menstrual blood loss, GI blood loss, and increased iron requirements of pregnancy. Decreased iron absorption or increased iron requirements may also lead to iron deficiency.

Diagnosis

- Evidence of a source of blood loss should be sought.
- Iron deficiency anemia is classically described as a microcytic anemia (MCV <80).
- The differential diagnosis includes thalassemia, sideroblastic anemias, some types of anemia of chronic disease, and lead poisoning.
- Cells start out normochromic but become more hypochromic as the anemia progresses.
- Serum ferritin is the preferred initial diagnostic test. Total iron-binding capacity, transferrin saturation, serum iron, and serum transferrin receptor levels may be

helpful if the ferritin level is between 46 and 99 ng/mL (46 and 99 mcg/L); bone marrow biopsy may be necessary in these patients for a definitive diagnosis.

- Laboratory tests:
  - Low serum Fe
  - Low ferritin (main lab indicator)
  - Increased TIBC
  - Hgb and Hct decrease in later stages
  - Decreased MCV, MCH, MCHC
  - Decreased transferrin saturation

Signs and Symptoms

There are many symptoms of IDA. Different patients will experience different combinations of symptoms; and, if the anemia is mild, the symptoms may not be noticeable. Some of the symptoms are: Pale skin color, fatigue, irritability, dizziness, weakness, shortness of breath, sore tongue, brittle nails, decreased appetite (especially in children), and frontal headaches.

Guidelines

American Family Physicians. *Am Fam Physician* 2007;75:671–8. www.aafp.org/afp/20070301/671.pdf.

Guidelines Summary

Routine iron supplementation is recommended for high-risk infants 6 to 12 months of age. In children, adolescents, and women of reproductive age, a trial of iron is a reasonable approach if the review of symptoms, history, and physical examination are negative; however, the hemoglobin should be checked at 1 month. If there is not a 1–2 g/dL increase in the hemoglobin level in that time, possibilities include malabsorption of oral iron, lack of compliance, continued bleeding, or presence of an unknown lesion.

Transfusion should be considered for patients of any age with IDA who are complaining of symptoms such as fatigue or dyspnea on exertion. Transfusion should also be considered for asymptomatic cardiac patients with hemoglobin less than 10 g/dL (100 g/L). However, oral iron therapy is usually the first-line therapy for patients with IDA. As noted in the etiology section, iron absorption varies widely based on type of diet and other factors.

- Bone marrow response to iron is limited to 20 mg/day of elemental iron.
- An increase in the hemoglobin level of 1 g/dL (10 g/L) should occur every 2 to 4 weeks on iron therapy.

- It may take up to 4 months for the iron stores to return to normal after the hemoglobin has corrected. Iron sulfate in a dose of 300 mg provides 60 mg of elemental iron, whereas 325 mg of iron gluconate provides 36 mg of elemental iron.

- Sustained-release formulations of iron are not recommended as initial therapy because they reduce the amount of iron that is presented for absorption to the duodenal villi.

- Gastrointestinal (GI) absorption of elemental iron is enhanced in the presence of an acidic gastric environment, which can be accomplished through simultaneous intake of ascorbic acid (i.e., vitamin C).

- Patients should be counseled to take iron 2 hours before or 4 hours after antacids.

- Although iron absorption occurs more readily when taken on an empty stomach, this increases the likelihood of stomach upset because of iron therapy. Increased patient adherence should be weighed against the inferior absorption.

- Laxatives, stool softeners, and adequate intake of liquids can alleviate the constipating effects of oral iron therapy.

- Indications for the use of intravenous (IV) iron include:
  - Chronic uncorrectable bleeding
  - Intestinal malabsorption
  - Intolerance to oral iron: Often results in nonadherence by the patient
  - Hemoglobin levels less than 6 g/dL (60 g/L) with signs of poor perfusion

Drugs for Iron Deficiency Anemia

Generic	Brand	Dose	Contraindications	Primary Side Effects	Key Monitoring	Pertinent Drug Interactions	Med Pearl	Top 200
Mechanism of action – replaces iron found in hemoglobin, myoglobin; allows the transportation of oxygen via hemoglobin								
Ferrous sulfate, gluconate, fumarate	• Sulfate: Feosol, Fer-In-Sol, Fer-Iron, Slow-FE • Gluconate	• Sulfate treatment: 300 mg BID-QID • Gluconate/ fumarate: 60 mg BID-QID • Prophylaxis 1 dose/day	Hypersensitivity to iron salts, hemochromatosis (GI absorbs excess iron), hemolytic anemia	• GI irritation • Epigastric pain • Nausea • Dark stools • Vomiting • Stomach cramping • Constipation	• Serum iron • Total iron-binding capacity • Reticulocyte count • Hemoglobin	• ↓ Absorption of tetracyclines, fluoroquinolones, levodopa, methyldopa, penicillamine • Proton pump inhibitors (PPIs) and H$_2$ blockers can ↓ iron absorption	Administer with vitamin C (or orange juice) to ↑ absorption	No
Mechanism of action – release iron from the plasma; eventually replenishes the depleted iron stores in the bone marrow								
Iron dextran complex	• Dexferrum • Infed	Max = 100 mg/ day	Hypersensitivity to dextran	• Mild hypotension • Tightness in the chest • Wheezing	• Anaphylactoid reaction • Hemoglobin • Hematocrit • Serum ferritin		• Rifabutin often will be used with drug interaction to prevent the use of rifampin • Test dose is required	No
Sodium ferric gluconate	Ferrlecit	IV: 125 mg/10 mL infused approximately 8×	Hypersensitivity to components	• Angina, bradycardia • Hypotension • Agitation • Chills, dizziness, fatigue	• Serum iron • Vital signs	Decrease the absorption of oral iron	• A safer form of parenteral iron compared to dextran • No test dose is required	No
Ferumoxytol	Feraheme	IV: 510 mg followed by 510 mg 3–8 days later	Hypersensitivity	• Hypersensitivity reaction • Diarrhea • Constipation • Hypotension	Column will include points listed for joint boxes of iron dextran complex and sodium ferric gluconate		May interfere with MRI readings for ≤3 months after use	No
Mechanism of action – iron sucrose is dissociated by the reticuloendothelial system into iron and sucrose; increases serum iron levels								
Iron sucrose	Venofer	IV: 100 mg administered 1–3 ×/ wk during dialysis	• Evidence of iron overload • Anemia not caused by iron deficiency	• Hypotension • Peripheral edema • Headache and nausea	• Circulatory overload • Anaphylactoid reaction • Hemoglobin • Hematocrit • Electrolytes • Vital signs	Decrease the absorption of oral iron	Safety profiles are similar to sodium ferric gluconate	No

Storage and Administration Pearls

- Sodium ferric gluconate and iron sucrose should not be frozen.
- Iron is a leading cause of fatal poisoning in children. Store out of children's reach and in child-resistant containers.

Patient Education Pearls

Oral iron products can be taken with vitamin C or orange juice to increase absorption.

ANEMIA OF CHRONIC KIDNEY DISEASE AND DIALYSIS

Definitions

Anemia of chronic kidney disease is a hypoproliferative disorder associated with certain infectious or inflammatory processes, tissue injury, or conditions that release proin-flammatory cytokines. It is attributed primarily to decrease endogenous erythropoietin (EPO) production and may occur as the creatinine clearance declines below approximately 50 mL/min. Eventually, the patient may require dialysis to filtrate metabolic waste. There are several types of dialysis, including:

- Hemodialysis, which diffuses small molecular-weight solutes across a semipermeable membrane
- Peritoneal dialysis, which uses the peritoneum as a dialysis membrane
- Ultrafiltration and hemofiltration, which removes large volumes of fluid with minimal removal of metabolic wastes

Diagnosis

- There is currently no definitive test for anemia of chronic kidney disease. It is a diagnosis of exclusion.
- May coexist with iron deficiency and folate deficiency
- Low serum iron
- Normal or increased ferritin
- Decreased TIBC
- Normal MCV
- Normochromic red blood cells on peripheral smear

Signs and Symptoms

There are many symptoms of anemia of kidney disease. Different patients will experience different combinations of symptoms; and, if the anemia is mild, the symptoms may not be noticeable. Some of the symptoms are: Pale skin color, fatigue, irritability, dizziness, weakness, shortness of breath, sore tongue, brittle nails, decreased appetite (especially in children), and frontal headaches.

Guidelines

National Kidney Foundation. KDOQI Clinical Practice Guidelines and Clinical Practice Recommendations for Anemia in Chronic Kidney Disease. Am J Kidney Dis. 2006;47(5).

Guidelines Summary

- Treatment guidelines for stress treatment are based on hemoglobin (Hb).
- Hb should be between 11–12 mg/dL.
- Initial goal for ESA is to increase Hb levels 1–2 g/dL per month.
- Hb targets are not intended to apply to the treatment of iron deficiency in patients receiving iron therapy without the use of erythropoiesis-stimulating agents (ESAs).
- ESAs are the drug of choice.
- In dialysis and nondialysis patients with chronic kidney disease (CKD) receiving ESA therapy, the Hb target should not be greater than 13.0 g/dL.
  - Hb should not be greater than 13.0 g/dL due to the all-cause mortality and adverse cardiovascular event in patients with CKD and Hb greater than 13.0 g/dL.

Drugs for Anemia of Chronic Renal Disease and Dialysis

Mechanism of action – induces erythropoiesis by stimulating the division and differentiation of committed erythroid progenitor cells; induces the release of reticulocytes from the bone marrow into the bloodstream

Generic	Brand	Dose	Contraindications	Primary Side Effects	Key Monitoring	Pertinent Drug Interactions	Med Pearl
Epoetin alfa	• Procrit • Epogen	IV, subcutaneous (SC) initial: 50–100 units/kg 3 × wk	• Hb >12 g/dL • Hb increase >1 g/dL per 2-wk time period	• Hypertension • Peripheral edema • Headache • Nausea • Arthralgia	• Hb 1–2x wk until maintenance dose established and after dosage changes • Iron stores • Blood pressure	None	Not indicated for myelosuppressive anemia when the anticipated outcome of chemotherapy is curative
Darbepoetin alfa	Aranesp	IV, SC initial: 0.45 mcg/kg 1 × wkly	• Uncontrolled hypertension • Pure red cell aplasia				

Storage and Administration Pearls

- Refrigerate vial between 36–46°F.
- Do not freeze or shake.
- Multidose vials, with preservative, are stable for 1 week at room temperature.

Patient Education Pearls

- These medications can be administered only by infusion or injection.
- Frequent blood tests will be needed to determine appropriate dosages.
- Avoid alcohol and do not make significant changes in dietary iron without consulting prescriber.
- Check blood pressure frequently.

PERNICIOUS ANEMIA

Definitions

Pernicious anemia is a type of megaloblastic anemia. Pernicious anemia is a decrease in red blood cells that occurs when the body cannot properly absorb vitamin B12 (cyanocobalamin) from the GI tract or is deficient in folate. Vitamin B12 is necessary for the formation of RBCs. Megaloblastic anemia is a blood disorder characterized by RBCs that are larger than normal due to deficiency in folate or cyanocobalamin.

Diagnosis

- Detecting antibodies to intrinsic factor is specific for the diagnosis of pernicious anemia.
- A Schilling test may be used to detect antibodies to intrinsic factor.
- Serum vitamin B12-folate should be measured.
- B12 <200 pg/mL is diagnostic of B12 deficiency.
- Folate <2 ng/mL is diagnostic of folate deficiency.
- Serum methylmalonic acid and homocysteine are elevated in pernicious anemia.
- Increased MCV may be present.

Signs and Symptoms

- Symptoms similar to IDA
- May find glossitis, jaundice, and splenomegaly
- Ataxia, paresthesias, confusion, and dementia
- Folate acid deficiency: does not result in neurologic disease

Treatment Summary

- No major guidelines have been recently published on the treatment of pernicious anemia.
- Treatment is directed toward replacing the deficient factor.
- Blood transfusions are rarely required.
- Treatment is often initiated with intramuscular injections before moving to oral formulations.
- With therapy the reticulocytosis should begin within 1 week, followed by a rising Hb over 6–8 weeks.
- Coexisting iron deficiency is present in one-third of patients and is a common cause of incomplete response to therapy.

Drugs for Pernicious Anemia

Generic	Brand	Dose	Contraindications	Primary Side Effects	Key Monitoring	Pertinent Drug Interactions	Med Pearl	Top 200
Mechanism of action – coenzyme for various metabolic functions, cell replication, and hematopoiesis								
Cyanocobalamin (B12)	• Nascobal • Vitamin B12	• Initial: 1,000 mcg IM daily for 1 week, then 1,000 mcg IM monthly for 6 months • Maintenance: 1,000 mcg IM monthly • Oral: 1 mg/day • Intranasal: 500 mcg in 1 nostril weekly	Hypersensitivity to cobalt	• Anxiety • Itching • Diarrhea	• Vitamin B12 • Hb/HCT • Reticulocyte count • Folate • Iron	Long-term treatment with metformin may decrease the absorption of vitamin B12	Hydroxocobalamin is a longer-acting form of vitamin B12	No
Mechanism of action – coenzyme in many metabolic systems, particularly for purine and pyrimidine synthesis								
Folic acid (folate)	Apo-Folic	• Oral: 0.4–1 mg/day • Prevention of neural tube defects 0.4 – 0.8 mg/day	Hypersensitivity to folic acid	• Allergic reaction • Bronchospasm • Flushing • Malaise • Pruritus • Rash	• HCT • Reticulocyte count • Folate • Iron	Folic acid administration may decrease serum levels of phenytoin	• Phenytoin and other anticonvulsant may inhibit folic acid absorption • Products containing >0.8 mg of folic acid are Rx only	Yes

Storage and Administration Pearls

- Cyanocobalamin injection is clear pink-to-red solution, stable at room temperature.
- Cyanocobalamin must be protected from light.
- Intranasal spray must be stored in the refrigerator and not frozen.

Patient Education Pearls

- Pernicious anemia may require treatment for life.
- Report rashes on extremities or acute persistent diarrhea.

Learning Points

- Coexisting iron deficiency is present in many forms of anemia and should always be assessed.
- When treating with ESA, Hb should not be greater than 13.0 g/dL due to the all-cause mortality and adverse cardiovascular event in patients with CKD and Hb greater than 13.0 g/dL.
- Iron absorption is enhanced through simultaneous intake of ascorbic acid (i.e., vitamin C).
- Laxatives, stool softeners, and adequate intake of liquids should be regularly recommended to patients taking iron therapy, to alleviate the medication's constipating effects.
- Long-term metformin therapy can decrease the absorption of vitamin B12.

PRACTICE QUESTIONS

1. Which of the following can be administered with ferrous sulfate to increase absorption?

    (A) Calcium carbonate
    (B) Ascorbic acid
    (C) Omeprazole
    (D) Famotidine

2. Which of the following is an adverse effect associated with epoetin alfa?

    (A) Thrombocytopenia
    (B) Bradycardia
    (C) Constipation
    (D) Hypertension

3. Which of the following is true regarding cyanocobalamin?

    (A) Levels may be depleted by sulfonylureas.
    (B) It must be initiated with the nasal form.
    (C) Injection solution is red to pink in color.
    (D) It is used for the treatment of folate deficiency.

ANSWERS

1. **B**

Oral iron products need an acidic environment for absorption. Ascorbic acid (vitamin C) or a glass of orange juice can be administered with oral iron products to increase absorption. Calcium carbonate (A) is an antacid, omeprazole (C) is a proton pump inhibitor, and famotidine (D) is an H2 antagonist, all of which would decrease the acidification needed for iron absorption.

2. **D**

Hypertension is associated with the use of ESAs and should be monitored for while on therapy. If a patient has uncontrolled HTN before starting ESAs, it may preclude the use until the blood pressure is more optimally managed. Thrombocytopenia (A), bradycardia (A), and constipation (C) are not associated with ESAs.

3. **C**

The injection solution for cyanocobalamin is red to pink and is stable at room temperature. Levels of B12 may be depleted with metformin, not sulfonylureas (A). B12 therapy is often initiated with the IM formulation and is then transitioned to oral therapy; the nasal formulation (B) is rarely used. Cyanocobolamin is used to treat B12 deficiency, not folate deficiency (D).

Dermatologic Disorders

14

This chapter covers the following disease states:

- **Acne**
- **Psoriasis**

 Suggested Study Time: **15 minutes**

ACNE

Definitions

Acne vulgaris is an inflammatory skin disorder that results in comedones, papules, pustules, nodules, or cysts on the face, back, or chest. The disorder occurs most commonly in teenagers at or near puberty but can occur at any age.

Diagnosis

Although no strict diagnostic criteria exist, the presence of five or more lesions (of any type) is generally considered sufficient for diagnosis.

Signs and Symptoms

Acne vulgaris lesions appear most commonly on the face but also on the back and chest. The severity of acne vulgaris varies and is based on the types of lesions present. Type I acne is the mildest form and is associated with a mostly noninflammatory presentation of open and closed comedones. Type II acne is a more moderate form with multiple papules present. Type III acne is associated with a more severe form of acne consisting of an inflammatory condition with multiple pustules. Type IV is the most severe form, consisting of inflammatory nodules and cysts that lead to scarring.

Guidelines

Guidelines of care for acne vulgaris management. *J Am Acad Dermatol*, no. 56 (4) (April 2007): 651–63.

http://www.aad.org/File%20Library/Global%20navigation/Education%20and%20 quality%20care/Guidelines-Acne-Vulgaris.pdf

Guideline Summary

- Topical benzoyl peroxide is the first-line therapy recommendation for most mild to moderate forms of acne vulgaris (type I).
- Topical antibiotics and topical retinoids are considered first-line for moderate acne vulgaris (type II) and second-line for mild-moderate (type I).
- Topical antibiotics are most effective when used in combination with benzoyl peroxide or retinoid due to risk of antibiotic resistance when used as monotherapy.
- Moderate to severe, inflammatory acne (type III) should be treated with topical therapy (benzoyl peroxide, retinoids, or antibiotics) plus oral antibiotics.
- Severe, inflammatory acne (type IV) can be treated with the combination of oral antibiotics and topical therapy but often requires the use of oral isotretinoin therapy.
- Oral isotretinoin is an effective therapy option for the treatment of severe, inflammatory acne, or more moderate forms that have been refractory to other treatment options.
- All females of child-bearing age that have been prescribed isotretinoin must agree to use two forms of contraception during isotretinoin use. Because of the known teratogenic risk associated with isotretinoin therapy, all patients, pharmacies, physicians, and wholesalers must register with the iPLEDGE program. This is an FDA program designed to monitor and decrease the risk of fetal exposure to isotretinoin.

Drugs for Acne

Generic	Brand	Dose & Max	Contraindications	Primary Side Effects	Key Monitoring Parameters	Pertinent Drug Interactions	Med Pearls	Top 200
Topical								
Nonprescription								
Benzoyl peroxide	Many	2.5–10% cream, lotion, gel, wash	Hypersensitivity	Excessive drying, photo sensitivity, peeling, erythema	Presence of adverse effects, efficacy	Retinoids: combination causes significant irritation	Over-the-counter (OTC)	No
Sulfur	SAStid	3–8% soap				Other topical agents: additive drying		No
Salicylic acid	Many	0.5–2% wash						No
Antimicrobials								
Clindamycin	• Cleocin T • Clinda gel	1% gel, lotion, solution: apply BID	Hypersensitivity, ulcerative colitis	Burning, itching, dryness, irritation	Presence of adverse effects, efficacy	Neuromuscular blocking agents		No
Erythromycin	• Akne-Mycin • Ery-Tab • Erygel	2% gel, liquid, ointment, pads	Hypersensitivity			None		No
Retinoids								
Tretinoin	• Retin-A • Renova • Avita • Atralin • Refissa • Tretinx	0.015–0.1% gel, cream	Hypersensitivity	Photosensitivity, burning, dryness, erythema, irritation	Presence of adverse effects	Other topical drying agents – additive drying Other photosensitizing medications	Apply after freshly washed face is completely dry	No
Tazarotene	• Tazorac • Avage • Fabior	0.05–0.1% gel, cream, foam						No
Alitretinoin	Panretin	0.1% gel						No
Adapalene	• Differin • Differin XP	0.1% gel, cream, lotion; 0.3% gel					Does not require waiting until face is dry for application	No
Other								
Azelaic acid	• Azelex • Finacea	• 15% gel, 20% cream • Apply BID	Hypersensitivity	Burning, stinging, tingling, pruritus, photosensitivity	Presence of adverse effects	None		No

Drugs for Acne (cont'd)

Oral

Antimicrobials

Generic	Brand	Dose & Max	Contraindications	Primary Side Effects	Key Monitoring Parameters	Pertinent Drug Interactions	Med Pearls	Top 200
Tetracycline	• Achromycin • Sumycin	250–3,000 mg daily (divided BID–QID)	Hypersensitivity	Rash, photosensitivity, gastrointestinal (GI) upset	Presence of adverse effects	Antacids, penicillin, oral contraceptives, anticoagulants	Take 2 hrs before or after meals, avoid calcium containing foods (dairy)	No
Doxycycline	Many	50–200 mg daily (divided BID)						Yes
Minocycline	Minocin	50–200 mg daily (divided BID)				As above, and isotretinoin		Yes
Erythromycin	• E.E.S. • Erythrocin	250–3,000 mg daily (divided BID)	Hypersensitivity; use of terfenadine, astemizole, cisapride	GI upset, diarrhea, nausea, vomiting, abdominal pain	Presence of adverse effects	Terfenadine, astemizole, cisapride: combination of these agents with erythromycin increases the risk of fatal arrhythmia; anticoagulants, lovastatin, digoxin	Significant drug interactions and GI side effects limit use	No

Isotretinoin

Generic	Brand	Dose & Max	Contraindications	Primary Side Effects	Key Monitoring Parameters	Pertinent Drug Interactions	Med Pearls	Top 200
Isotretinoin	• Absorica • Amnesteem • Claravis • Myorisan • Zenatane	0.5–2 mg/kg/day (divided BID)	Pregnancy, hypersensitivity	Cheilitis, dry mouth, dry skin, pruritus, erythema, GI upset, headaches, hyperlipidemia, depression (rare)	Periodic lipid panel, presence of adverse effects	Isotretinoin increases concentrations of corticosteroids, phenytoin; and has additive toxicity with vitamin A	• Females must agree to at least 2 forms of contraception during therapy • Must register in iPLEDGE program • Highly teratogenic	No

Available combination products:

- Adapalene/benzoyl peroxide topical
- Benzoyl peroxide/hydrocortisone topical
- Clindamycin/benzoyl peroxide topical
- Clindamycin/tretinoin topical
- Erythromycin/benzoyl peroxide
- Sulfur/sulfacetamide

Storage and Administration Pearls

- Apply topical acne products only after washing the face and then waiting for the skin to dry completely (approximately 30 minutes).
- Protect tetracycline from light. Tetracycline, doxycycline, and minocycline should be taken 2 hours before or after a meal; they interact with calcium-containing products such as dairy items.

Patient Education Pearls

- Topical agents and antimicrobials increase risk of excessive burning from the sun. Apply sunscreen prior to sun exposure.

PSORIASIS

Definitions

Psoriasis is a chronic inflammatory skin disease associated with silvery scalelike lesions. There are two primary types of psoriasis identified: Type I is diagnosed early in life in patients with a family history, while type II develops later in life and generally has no family history present.

Diagnosis

Diagnosis is based on thorough history and physical and depends primarily on the observation of lesions.

Signs and Symptoms

Sharp, demarcated, erythematous papules and plaques covered with silvery scales is a sign. Affected areas may include the scalp, trunk, back, arms, legs, palms, soles, face, and/or genitalia. Psoriatic arthritis refers to secondary joint inflammation that occurs in patients with psoriasis. The most commonly affected joints are the elbows, wrists, ankles, and knees.

Guidelines

Guidelines of care for the management of psoriasis and psoriatic arthritis: Section 4. Guidelines of care for the management and treatment of psoriasis with traditional systemic agents. *J Am Acad Dermatol* 2009;61(3):451–85.

Summary of Treatment Recommendations

- The goal of therapy is complete resolution of lesions.
- There is significant interpatient variability in response to the available medications. Options for initial treatment include topical agents such as emollients and keratolytics (salicylic acid or sulfur), coal tar, anthralin, calcipotriene, or retinoids.
- Systemic treatment is considered as initial therapy in very severe cases or as second-line therapy in patients that do not respond to topical options. Systemic options include antimetabolite therapy (methotrexate, cyclosporine, tacrolimus), oral corticosteroids, psoralens, immunosuppressants, or retinoids.

Drugs for Psoriasis

Generic	Brand	Dose & Max	Contraindications	Primary Side Effects	Key Monitoring Parameters	Pertinent Drug Interactions	Med Pearls	Top 200
Coal Tar								
Coal tar	• Medotar • Fototar	1–25% ointment, cream, lotion apply 1–4 × daily	Hypersensitivity	Photosensitivity	Presence of adverse effects	Other photosensitizing agents	OTC	No
Retinoids								
Tretinoin	• Retin-A • Renova • Avita • Atralin • Refissa • Tretinx	0.015–0.1% gel, cream	See details above					No
Tazarotene	• Tazorac • Avage • Fabior	0.05–0.1% gel, cream, foam						No
Alitretinoin	Panretin	0.1% gel						No
Adapalene	• Differin • Differin XP	0.1% gel, cream, lotion; 0.3% gel					Does not require waiting until face is dry for application	No
Anthralin								
Dithranol	• Anthralin • Psoriatec	0.5–1% cream, apply 1 × daily	Hypersensitivity, inflamed eruptions	Discoloration of skin, hair, fabrics, irritation	Presence of adverse effects	Topical steroids	Staining of fabric can be permanent	No
Calcipotriene								
Calcipotriene	Dovonex	0.005% cream, ointment, solution; apply 1–2 × daily	Hypersensitivity, hypercalcemia	Burning, itching, skin irritation, drying	Presence of adverse effects	Other topical agents: additive drying		No

Drugs for Psoriasis *(cont'd)*

Generic	Brand	Dose & Max	Contraindications	Primary Side Effects	Key Monitoring Parameters	Pertinent Drug Interactions	Med Pearls	Top 200
Topical Vitamin D Analog								
Calcitriol	Vectical	Apply 2 × (max = 200 g/week)	Do not apply to face or eyes	Pruritis, erythema, blisters, skin discomfort, dermatitis, photosensitivity	Response to therapy	Concomitant use with vitamin D or calcium supplements, or calcium- or magnesium- containing antacids may increase likelihood of clinically significant increases in serum levels	Topical product unlikely to cause drug interactions or serum abnormalities due to limited systemic absorption	No
Systemic								
Antimetabolites								
Methotrexate (MTX)	None	7.5 mg PO 1 × wkly	• Hypersensitivity • Alcoholic liver disease • Pre-existing blood dyscrasias	• Leukopenia • Nausea • Fatigue • Chills • Fever • Hepatotoxicity • Photosensitivity	• Periodic complete blood count (CBC) • Liver enzymes	• NSAIDs • Salicylates • Probenecid • Phenytoin • Sulfonamides Increase MTX levels	Necessary to use contraception in female patients (pregnancy category X)	Yes
Immunosuppressants								
Etanercept	Enbrel	50 mg SC 2 × wkly	Hypersensitivity	• Injection site reactions • Infections • Headache • Rash • Nausea • Neutropenia	Periodic WBC	Risk of blood dyscrasias and infection when combined with anakinra or other immuno-suppressants	• Available in prefilled syringes • Pregnancy registry for pregnant females on medication	No

Drugs for Psoriasis *(cont'd)*

Generic	Brand	Dose & Max	Contraindications	Primary Side Effects	Key Monitoring Parameters	Pertinent Drug Interactions	Med Pearls	Top 200
Ustekinumab	Stelara	45–90 mg SC every 12 wks	Hypersensitivity	• Nasopharyngitis • Upper respiratory tract infection • Headache • Fatigue	• PPD prior to initiation of therapy • Response to therapy • Presence of infection	Not to be given with live vaccines or other immunosuppressants	Indicated for moderate to severe plaque	No
Golimumab	Simponi	50 mg SC 1 ×/month	None	• Infection • Nasopharyngitis • Injection site reactions • Elevated AST/ALT	• Latent TB and HBV screening prior to initiation and during therapy • S/S of infection and heart failure • CBC periodically	• May diminish the therapeutic effect of immuno-suppressants • Not to be given with live vaccines	• Once monthly injection • Discontinue/hold if serious infection • Caution use in patients with heart failure • Refrigerated (not frozen)	No

Retinoids

Generic	Brand	Dose & Max	Contraindications	Primary Side Effects	Key Monitoring Parameters	Pertinent Drug Interactions	Med Pearls	Top 200
Acitretin	Soriatane	25–50 mg PO daily	• Hypersensitivity • Impaired hepatic or renal function • Use with MTX	• Dry skin • Alopecia • Rash • Chelitis • Peeling • Pruritus	Presence of adverse effects	• MTX: increased risk of hepatitis • Tetracyclines: increased intra-cranial pressure	• Law requires medication guide be given to the patient each time acitretin is dispensed • Pregnancy category X	No

Storage and Administration Pearls

- Store out of reach of children.
- Avoid application of topical agents near the eyes.
- Alefacept and ustekinumab should be stored in a refrigerator between 2–8°C (36–46°F), protected from light, and retained in drug/diluent pack until time of use.
- Efalizumab (lyophilized powder) must be refrigerated at 2–8°C (36–46°F). Protect the vial from exposure to light. Store in original carton until time of use.
- Etanercept solution must be refrigerated at 2–8°C (36–46°F) and should not be frozen.

Patient Education Pearls

- Wash hands thoroughly after application of topical agents.
- Keep topical agents away from eyes.

Learning Points

- First-line therapy for mild to moderate acne vulgaris is topical benzoyl peroxide.
- Topical retinoids should not be combined with other topical acne agents due to risk of excessive drying and photosensitivity.
- Oral isotretinoin is reserved for refractory or severe cases of acne vulgaris. Patients, pharmacists, and physicians must register with the FDA iPLEDGE program to use this medication.
- Oral isotretinoin is associated with significant teratogenicity. Females on isotretinoin therapy must agree to use two forms of contraception during the course of therapy.
- Significant interpatient variability exists in the response to psoriasis treatments. Initial therapy generally consists of topic agents such as keratolytics, coal tar, or anthralin.
- Antimetabolite and immunosuppressant therapy carries significantly greater adverse effect risk and therefore should be reserved for severe or refractory cases.

PRACTICE QUESTIONS

1. Which of the following is appropriate initial treatment for type III acne?

    (A)   Topical antibiotics and topical retinoids
    (B)   Topical retinoids + oral antibiotics
    (C)   Topical benzoyl peroxide
    (D)   Oral antibiotics
    (E)   Isotretinoins

2. Which of the following topical products should be applied after the face is washed and completely dried in order to minimize the risk of excessive drying? (Select **ALL** that apply.)

    (A)   Clindamycin gel
    (B)   Tretinoin cream
    (C)   Alitretinoin gel
    (D)   Adapalene cream

3. A 22-year-old woman is diagnosed with moderate acne vulgaris (type II). She has no significant medical history and takes no medications. Which of the following is the best therapy recommendation?

    (A)   Benzoyl peroxide wash
    (B)   Adapalene gel
    (C)   Doxycycline oral
    (D)   Isotretinoin oral

4. Live vaccines should be avoided with which of the following medications for psoriasis? (Select **ALL** that apply.)

    (A)   Calcipotriene
    (B)   Dithranol
    (C)   Alefacept
    (D)   Efalizumab

ANSWERS

1. **B**

First-line therapy for type III acne is topical therapy (benzoyl peroxide, retinoids, or antibiotics) plus oral antibiotics. First-line therapy for type I acne is topical benzoyl peroxide (C). First-line therapy for type II acne is topical antibiotics and topical retinoids (A). Oral antibiotics are not used alone (D) without topical agents. Isotretinoins (E) are usually reserved for type IV or other types that are refractory to other treatment options.

2. **B** and **C**

Retinoids including tretinoin (B) and alitretinoin (C) should be applied only after the face is washed and completely dried in order to minimize risk of excessive drying. This precaution is not necessary with topical antibiotics such as clindamycin (A) or with adapalene (D), a retinoid.

3. **B**

Preferred treatment for moderate (type II) acne vulgaris is topical retinoid or topical antibiotic therapy. Topical benzoyl peroxide (A) is preferred for mild (type I) acne vulgaris. Oral antibiotics such as doxycycline (C) are recommended in combination with topical retinoids, benzoyl peroxide, or antibiotics for moderate–severe (type III) or type II that is unresponsive to topical monotherapy. Isotretinoin therapy (D) is reserved for severe (type IV) or treatment-resistance/refractory acne vulgaris.

4. **C** and **D**

Live vaccines should be avoided in combination with immunosuppressants. Alefacept (C) and efalizumab (D) are both immunosuppressants. Calcipotriene (A) and dithranol (B) are topical agents and do not interact with immunizations.

Antidotes

The following chapter addresses drugs that are used as antagonist drugs:

- **Antidotes**
- **General antidotes**

Suggested Study Time: **15 minutes**

ANTIDOTES

Definitions

The drugs included in this chapter act in a variety of ways to counter the toxic effects of exogenous and endogenous substances in the body. Therefore, they are used in the management of poisoning and overdosage. Many antidotes are used to protect against the toxicity of drugs such as antineoplastics, and in the management of metabolic disorders such as Wilson's disease, where toxic substances accumulate.

Accidental and deliberate drug overdosage is a common problem seen by ambulance staff and emergency workers. The majority of these episodes of poisoning are dealt with along similar lines with general supportive care, but some require more specific action.

Some antagonists, such as the opioid antagonist naloxone, compete with the poison for receptor sites. Other antagonists, such as atropine, block substances that mediate the effects of the toxin. This may reduce absorption of the toxin from the gastrointestinal tract, inactivate or reduce the activity of the toxin, or increase the toxin's elimination via drugs that affect the metabolism of the toxin.

Some antidotes, such as fomepizole in methyl alcohol poisoning, act by reducing the rate of metabolism to a toxic metabolite. Others, such as methionine and glutathione, promote the formation of inactive metabolites. Acetylcysteine also acts by bypassing the effect of the toxin. On the NAPLEX, antidotes questions can be an easy way to earn points if you learn the correct antidote for the toxicity.

ACUTE POISONING

In the management of suspected acute poisoning, it is often impossible to determine with any certainty the identity of the poison or the size of the dose received. As a result, a common procedure needs to be in place:

- First, call the poison control center: (800) 222–1222.
- Next, take a history of the event and drug, or substance, involved.
  - What mode of poisoning has occurred (i.e., ingestion or inhalation)?
  - When did it happen?
  - Has any treatment occurred yet (i.e., induced vomiting)?

Few poisons have specific antidotes or methods of elimination, and the mainstay of treatment for patients with suspected acute poisoning is therefore supportive and symptomatic therapy; in many cases, nothing further is required. Clinicians should assess the ABCDs: airway, breathing, circulation, dextrose, decontamination. Symptoms of acute poisoning are frequently nonspecific, particularly in the early stages. Maintenance of the airway and ventilation is the most important initial measure; other treatment—for example, for cardiovascular or neurological symptoms—may be added as appropriate.

Some centers also recommend the routine administration of dextrose to all unconscious patients since hypoglycemia may be a cause of unconsciousness, although blood glucose measurements should be obtained first where facilities are immediately available.

Specific antidotes are available for a number of poisons and are the primary treatment where there is a severe poisoning with a known toxin. These antidotes may be lifesaving in such cases but their use is not without hazard and, in many situations, they are not necessary. These agents are discussed in greater detail in the chart below.

Measures to reduce or prevent the absorption of the poison are widely advocated. For inhalational poisoning, the victim is removed from the source of poisoning. Some toxins, particularly pesticides, may be absorbed through the skin, and clothing should be removed and the skin thoroughly washed to avoid continued absorption. Caustic substances are removed from the skin or eyes with copious irrigation. However, for orally ingested poisons the best method of gastrointestinal (GI) decontamination remains controversial; this is addressed in the following sections.

GENERAL ANTIDOTES

Activated Charcoal

Activated charcoal absorbs a wide range of toxins and is often given to reduce absorption within the GI tract. A single dose is generally effective, particularly if it is given within 1 hour of ingestion. Delayed use, however, may be beneficial for modified-release preparations or for drugs that slow GI transit time, such as those with antimuscarinic properties. Charcoal is generally well tolerated, although vomiting is common, and there is a risk of aspiration if the airway is not adequately protected. Repeated doses may be useful in eliminating some substances even after systemic absorption has occurred.

Active removal of poisons from the stomach by induction of emesis or gastric lavage has been widely used, but there is little evidence to support its role. Emesis should not be induced if the poison is corrosive or petroleum-based, or if the poison is removable by treatment with activated charcoal.

Ipecac

When used appropriately, ipecac is a safe emetic. However, its efficacy in preventing deaths has never been proven, and the routine use of ipecac at home has been questioned.

A recent survey found that increased home use of ipecac was not associated with referral to an emergency department. Additionally, there was no difference in adverse outcome rate between the poison centers that more commonly recommended ipecac compared with those centers that did not. The authors concluded that although their data cannot exclude a benefit of ipecac in a very limited set of poisonings, any benefit remains to be proven.

There are a number of drawbacks to using ipecac. Adverse effects include lethargy, diarrhea, and persistent vomiting. Persistent vomiting can be especially troublesome because it may reduce the efficacy of other orally administered treatments for poisoning, such as activated charcoal, N-acetylcysteine, or agents used for whole-bowel irrigation. Second, ipecac is sometimes given, either without medical advice or based on inappropriate medical advice, when it is not needed (i.e., in the case of ingestion of a nontoxic agent) or when it is contraindicated. Examples of contraindications to ipecac include the following:

- Lack of or suppressed gag reflex
- Lethargy
- Seizures
- Following the ingestion of caustic agents, corrosive agents, ammonia, or bleach
- Chronic misuse: May lead to cardiomyopathy

Gastric lavage may occasionally be indicated for ingestion of noncaustic poisons that are not absorbed by activated charcoal, but only if less than 1 hour has elapsed since ingestion. Gastric lavage should not be attempted if the airway is not adequately protected.

Whole-bowel irrigation using a nonabsorbable osmotic agent such as a macrogol has also been used, particularly for substances that pass beyond the stomach before being absorbed (e.g., iron preparations or enteric-coated or modified-release formulations), but its role is not established.

Antidotes

Toxic Agent	Generic Name for Antidote	Brand Name for Antidote	Dose	Contraindications	Primary Side Effects	Key Monitoring	Med Pearl	Top 200
Mechanism of action — pure opioid antagonist that competes and displaces narcotics at opioid receptor sites								
Opioids	Naloxone	Narcan	Intravenous (IV), intramuscular (IM), subcutaneous (SC) 0.4 mg q2–3 min as needed; repeat dose q20–60 min	Hypersensitivity	• Tachycardia • Ventricular arrhythmia • Anxiety • Diaphoresis • Agitation	• Respiratory rate • HR • BP	• Adverse affects can occur secondarily to reversal (withdrawal) • IV route is preferred due to quick effect	No
Mechanism of action — acts as a competitive antagonist at opioid receptor sites								
Opioids	Nalmefene	Revex	IV: 0.25 mcg/kg followed by 0.25 mcg/kg at 2–5 minute intervals	Hypersensitivity	• Nausea • Tachycardia • Vomiting • Agitation	• Respiratory rate • Sedation • BP	6-Methylene analog of naltrexone	No
Mechanism of action — acts as a competitive antagonist at opioid receptor sites								
Opioids	Naltrexone	• Revia • Vivitrol	50 mg daily with 100 mg on Saturdays or 150 mg q3 days	• Acute opioid withdrawal • Failure to pass naloxone challenge • Positive urine drug screen for opioids	• Syncope • Headache • Arthralgia • Nausea • Vomiting	• Opioid withdrawal • Liver function test (LFT)	• Do not give until patient is opioid-free for 7–10 days • Alcohol and opioid dependence • Highest affinity for mu receptors	No
Mechanism of action — competitively inhibits the activity at the benzodiazepine recognition site on the GABA/benzo complex								
Benzodiazepines	Flumazenil	Romazicon	IV: 0.2 mg over 30 sec; repeat until conscious	Patients showing signs of serious cyclic antidepressant overdosage	• Palpitations • Hot flashes • Blurred vision • Vomiting • Ataxia • Agitation • Dizziness	• Benzo reversal may result in seizures in some patients • Return of residual effects of benzodiazepines	• If patient has not responded 5 min after receiving a cumulative dose of 5 mg, the sedation is likely not due to benzodiazepines • Reversal may affect nonbenzodiazepines (zaleplon, zolpidem)	No

Antidotes (cont'd)

Toxic Agent	Generic Name for Antidote	Brand Name for Antidote	Dose	Contraindications	Primary Side Effects	Key Monitoring	Med Pearl	Top 200
Mechanism of action – competitively inhibits alcohol dehydrogenase, an enzyme that catalyzes the metabolism of ethanol, methanol, and ethylene glycol								
• Methanol • Ethylene glycol	Fomepizole	Antizol	IV: loading dose 15 mg/kg, followed by 10 mg/kg q12 hrs × 4 doses	Hypersensitivity	• Headache • Nausea • Metallic taste • Drowsiness • Dizziness	• Fomepizole plasma levels should be monitored • Urinary ethylene glycol or methanol levels • Renal function		No
Mechanism of action – inhibits destruction of acetylcholine by acetylcholinesterase which prolongs effects of acetylcholine (anticholinergic drug overdose)								
Anticholinergic drugs	Physostigmine	Eserine	IV, IM, SC: 0.5–2 mg to start; repeat q10–30 min until response	• GI or genitourinary (GU) obstruction • Asthma, gangrene, severe cardiovascular disease	• Palpitation • Bradycardia • Restlessness • Seizure	• Heart rate • Respiratory rate		No
Mechanism of action – antigen-binding fragments (Fab) are specific for the treatment of digitalis intoxication								
Digoxin	Digoxin Immune Fab	DigiFab	40 mg will bind to 0.5 mg of digoxin or digitoxin	Hypersensitivity to sheep products	• Exacerbation of heart failure • Rapid ventricular response • Hypokalemia	• Serum potassium levels • BP • ECG	Digoxin levels will greatly increase with digoxin Fab use and are not an accurate determination of body stores	No
Mechanism of action – supplies a free thiol group which binds to and inactivates acrolein, the urotoxic metabolite of ifosfamide and cyclophosphamide								
• Cyclophosphamide • Ifosfamide	Mesna	Mesnex	IV: 60–80% of ifosfamide dose given TID to QID	Thiol compounds	• Platelet-count decrease • Dizziness • Anorexia • Headache	Urinalysis	Orphan drug; used for the prevention of hemorrhagic cystitis induced by ifosfamide	No

Antidotes *(cont'd)*

Toxic Agent	Generic Name for Antidote	Brand Name for Antidote	Dose	Contraindications	Primary Side Effects	Key Monitoring	Med Pearl	Top 200
Mechanism of action – cardioprotective by converting intracellularly to a ring-opened chelating agent that interferes with iron-mediated oxygen free radical generation								
Doxorubicin	Dexrazoxane	Zinecard	IV: 10:1 ratio of dexrazoxane: doxorubicin	Hypersensitivity	• Most adverse affects thought to be attributed to chemotherapy • Phlebitis	• Adds to myelosuppressive effects • LFTs		No
Mechanism of action – free thiol metabolite is available to bind to and detoxify reactive metabolites of cisplatin								
Cisplatin	Amifostine	Ethyol	IV	Hypersensitivity to amifostine or aminothiol	• Hypotension • N/V	• BP should be monitored every 5 min during the infusion • Serum calcium levels	Antiemetic medication is recommend prior to and in conjunction with amifostine	No
Mechanism of action – combines with strongly acidic heparin to form a stable complex (salt) neutralizing the anticoagulant activity of both drugs								
Heparin	Protamine	Protamine	• 1 mg of protamine nebulizes approx 100 units of heparin • Max: 50 mg	Hypersensitivity	• Hypotension • Flushing • Dyspnea	• Activated partial thromboplastin time (aPTT) • BP		No
Mechanism of action – promotes liver synthesis of clotting factors (II, VII, IX, X) which counteracts the mechanism of warfarin								
Warfarin	Vitamin K (phytonadione)	Mephyton	• Depends on international normalized ratio (INR) and bleeding risk factors; i.e., INR >10: hold warfarin and give 2.5–5 mg vitamin K, expect INR to be reduced within 24–48 hrs		• Cyanosis • Dizziness	• Prothrombin time (PT) • INR	• IM route should be avoided due to hematoma formation • SC is the preferred parenteral route	No

Antidotes *(cont'd)*

Toxic Agent	Generic Name for Antidote	Brand Name for Antidote	Dose	Contraindications	Primary Side Effects	Key Monitoring	Med Pearl	Top 200
Mechanism of action – reduced form of folic acid: supplies the necessary cofactor blocked by methotrexate								
Methotrexate	Leucovorin	Leucovorin	15 mg q6 hrs until levels normalize	• Pernicious anemia • B12-deficient megaloblastic anemias	• Rash • Anaphylactoid reactions • Thrombocytosis	Plasma methotrexate concentration	• Continue leucovorin until plasma methotrexate level <0.05 mmol/L • Decreased efficacy of cotrimoxazole against *Pneumocystis jiroveci* pneumonitis	No
Mechanism of action – absorbs toxic substances or irritants, thus inhibiting GI absorption								
Activated charcoal	Activated charcoal	Actidose	25–100 g/dose	• Unprotected airway • Non-intact GI tract • GI perforation • Intestinal obstruction	• Hypernatremia • Hypokalemia	• Constipation • Diarrhea	Sorbitol accelerates bowel evacuation	No
Mechanism of action – bind toxic agents in the biliary: forms a nonabsorbable complex with bile acids in the intestine; inhibits enterohepatic reuptake								
Leflunomide	Cholestyramine resin	• Questran • Questran Light	4 g–24 g/day administered up to 6 × day	• Complete biliary obstruction • Bowel obstruction	• Constipation • Nausea • Stomach pain • Gallstones • Bloating	Serum levels of poison	Arava (leflunomide) 8 g cholestyramine TID for 1–3 days; plasma level should reach <0.02 mg/L	No
Mechanism of action – exact mechanism of acetaminophen toxicity is unknown								
Acetaminophen	Acetylcysteine	• Acetadote • Mucomyst	140 mg/kg followed by 17 doses of 70 mg/kg q4 hrs	Hypersensitivity	• Drowsiness • Chills • Fever	• Aspartate aminotransferase (AST), alanine aminotransferase (ALT) • Bilirubin • PT • Serum creatinine	• Therapy should continue until acetaminophen levels are undetectable and there is no evidence of hepatotoxicity • Activated charcoal • 5–10 g:g acetaminophen	No

Antidotes (cont'd)

Toxic Agent	Generic Name for Antidote	Brand Name for Antidote	Dose	Contraindications	Primary Side Effects	Key Monitoring	Med Pearl	Top 200
Mechanism of action — blocks the action of acetylcholine at parasympathetic sites in the smooth muscle, secretary glands, and the central nervous system (CNS)								
Cholinergics	Atropine	AtroPen	• IM: 2 mg; may repeat with 2 additional doses q10 min • IV, IM: Dose for children is 0.02–1 mg/kg 5–10 min until effects are observed	No absolute contraindications in life-threatening poisoning	• Anaphylaxis • Nausea • Vomiting • Fatigue • Insomnia • Weakness • Cardiovascular changes	• Electrocardiogram (ECG) • Respiratory status • Metabolic panels • HR • BP	Dose until symptoms subside	No
Mechanism of action — stimulates adrenergic receptors resulting in relaxation of smooth muscle of the bronchial tree, cardiac stimulation and dilation of skeletal muscle vasculature								
Hypersensitivity reactions	Epinephrine	• Adrenalin • EpiPen • Twinject	0.2–0.5 mg IM or SC every 5–15 min until improvement	No absolute CI in life-threatening situation	• Angina • Anxiety • Flushing • Dyspnea	• Pulmonary function • HR • BP	IM administration in the anterolateral aspect of the middle third of the thigh is preferred	No
Mechanism of action — stimulates adenylate cyclase to produce increased cyclic AMP, which promotes hepatic glycogenolysis and gluconeogenesis								
Hypoglycemia	Glucagon	GlucaGen	IV, IM, or SC 1 mg, may repeat in 20 min as needed	• Hypersensitivity • Insulinoma • Pheochromocytoma	• Hypotension • Nausea	• BP • Blood glucose • ECG • HR	IV dextrose should be given as soon as available	No

Storage and Administration Pearls

- Protamine: Refrigerate, stable for 2 weeks at room temperature.
- Fomepizole: If solution becomes solid in the vial, warm carefully by running warm water over the vial.
- Naltrexone: Should be stored in the refrigerator. May be kept at room temperature for <7 days prior to use.
- Digoxin immune Fab: Should be refrigerated.
- Activated charcoal: Absorbs gas from air; store in closed container.

Patient Education Pearls

- Patient should stay calm and call the poison control center.
- If patient currently has ipecac in their home, it is better to dispose of it, according to the research.
- Most drugs do not have antidotes, so it is important to take medication as prescribed.

Learning Points

- It is important to memorize the phone number for the poison control center. The number should also be pasted on every telephone in your pharmacy.
- Storing ipecac in the home in case of acute poisoning is no longer recommended because of limited data suggesting any benefit. It is better to call the poison control center or 911 for advice.
- Few poisons have specific antidotes or methods of elimination; therefore, the mainstay of treatment for patients with suspected acute poisoning is supportive and symptomatic therapy.
- Flumazenil is the antidote for benzodiazepines.
- Do not confuse Fomepizole and flumazenil. At first glance they may seem similar, but they have completely different uses.
- Protamine is the antidote for heparin, and vitamin K is the antidote for warfarin. Protamine and vitamin K are not interchangeable and have different mechanisms of action. These two antidotes are used for both inpatient and outpatient treatment.

PRACTICE QUESTIONS

1. Which drug is used to decrease toxicities associated with cisplatin?

    (A) Amifostine
    (B) Physostigmine
    (C) Nalmefene
    (D) Fomepizole
    (E) Leucovorin

2. How many doses of activated charcoal are typically effective?

    (A) 1
    (B) 2
    (C) 3
    (D) 4
    (E) 5

3. Which of the following agents could correct an INR of 11.4?

    (A) Protamine
    (B) Vitamin K
    (C) Atropine
    (D) Glucagon

4. Atropine is used to treat which of the following?

    (A) Opioid toxicity
    (B) Hemorrhagic cystitis
    (C) Hypoglycemia
    (D) Cholinergic toxicity

5. Before starting naltrexone, which of the following should the patient achieve?

    (A) Normalization of blood pressure
    (B) Resolution of bradycardia
    (C) Negative urine drug screen
    (D) Normalization of platelet count

ANSWERS

1. **A**

Amifostine is used to prevent cisplatin toxicities associated with renal toxicity. Physostigmine (B) is used primarily to reverse toxic CNS effects caused by anticholinergic drugs. Nalmefene (C) is used as a partial reversal of opioid drug effects. Fomepizole (D) is used for methanol and ethylene glycol poisoning, and leucovorin (E) is used as an antidote for folic acid antagonist.

2. **A**

Activated charcoal typically requires only a single dose to be effective, particularly if it is given within 1 hour of toxin ingestion.

3. **B**

An elevated INR is a result of an overdosage of warfarin. Vitamin K is the reversal agent and is recommend for use in patients with an INR > 10 or significant bleeding. Protamine (A) can be used to reverse heparin; atropine (C) is used to reverse cholinergic toxicity; and glucagon (D) treats hypoglycemia.

4. **D**

Atropine is used to treat cholinergic toxicity. Nalaxone is used to treat opioid overdoses or respiratory depression associated with opioids (A). Hemorrhagic cystitis (B) secondary to ifosfamide is treated with mesna, and glucagon can be used to treat hypoglycemia (C).

5. **C**

Before starting naltrexone, a patient should be in an opioid-free state. Naltrexone is used to maintain an opioid free-state for patients and should not be used if they have not been opioid-free for 7–10 days.

Reproductive Health and Urologic Disorders

16

This chapter covers the following topics:

- **Pregnancy/lactation**
- **Contraception**
- **Hormone replacement therapy**
- **Erectile dysfunction**
- **Benign prostatic hyperplasia**
- **Urinary incontinence**

 Suggested Study Time: **60 minutes**

PREGNANCY AND LACTATION

Preconception Care

Adequate folic acid (400–800 mcg daily) is important for women to consume at least 1 month prior to pregnancy to aid in prevention of neural tube defects. Prenatal vitamins available for purchase over-the-counter (OTC) typically provide 600–800 mcg per serving, and prescription products typically provide 800 mcg (or more) per serving.

Patients on chronic medications who are planning to become pregnant should be educated about the potential for medication teratogenicity and encouraged to discuss the benefits and risks of treatment with their primary and specialty care providers.

Principles of Drug Use during Pregnancy and Lactation

Although it is ideal for patients to avoid pharmacologic agents during pregnancy, pharmacotherapy is often necessary. Reasons for taking pharmacologic agents during pregnancy include acute illness and chronic illnesses such as diabetes mellitus, hypertension, epilepsy, asthma, depression, anxiety, and bipolar disorder, among others.

Physiologic changes during pregnancy affect the actions and pharmacokinetics of many pharmacologic agents:

- Gastric motility decreases due to increasing progesterone levels.
- Increased plasma volume leads to increased volume of distribution for some drugs, increased cardiac output (CO), renal blood flow, and glomerular filtration rate (GFR), thereby increasing the renal excretion of many drugs.
- Decreased albumin levels can increase availability of highly albumin-bound drugs.
- Altered liver function can interfere with hepatic metabolism.

Cross-Placental Transfer

One consideration when deciding whether to prescribe a medication to a pregnant patient is the likelihood of that medication crossing the placenta; this helps determine the relative benefit:risk ratio of that medication during pregnancy. Crossing the placenta indicates exposure to the fetus and increased risk. Characteristics of pharmacologic agents that are more likely to cross the placenta include:

- Small size: Water-soluble agents with lower molecular mass (<500 Da) more readily cross the placenta, middle range (501–1000 Da) cross more slowly, and larger (>1,000 Da) will not cross.
- Fat solubility: Agents with greater lipophilicity are more likely to cross the placenta.
- Un-ionized.
- Minimal protein-binding: Lower protein binding translates to higher percentage of unbound/free drug available to cross the placenta.

Pregnancy Categories

The Food and Drug Administration pregnancy categories were developed to help clinicians quickly determine drug toxicity risk by assigning letters to medications based upon the available evidence (or lack of evidence) regarding risk of use during pregnancy.

- Category A: Adequate, well-controlled studies have failed to demonstrate a risk to the fetus in the first trimester of pregnancy, and there is no evidence of risk in later trimesters.

- Category B: Animal reproduction studies have failed to demonstrate a risk to the fetus, and there are as of yet no adequate, well-controlled studies in pregnant women.

- Category C: Animal reproduction studies have shown an adverse effect on the fetus and there are no adequate and well-controlled studies in humans, but potential benefits may warrant use of the drug in pregnant women despite potential risks.

- Category D: There is positive evidence of human fetal risk based on adverse reaction data from investigational or marketing experience or studies in humans, but potential benefits may warrant use of the drug in pregnant women despite potential risks.

- Category X: Studies in animals or humans have demonstrated fetal abnormalities and/or there is positive evidence of human fetal risk based on adverse reaction data from investigational or marketing experience, and the risks involved in use of the drug in pregnant women clearly outweigh potential benefits.

Properties of pharmacologic agents most likely to be excreted in breast milk include high degree of lipophilicity, basic, and water soluble with low molecular mass (<100 Da).

Sample Known Teratogens (Commonly Used)

General Class	Drug(s)	Effects
Alcohol	Dose-dependent/cumulative	Fetal alcohol syndrome, abnormal central nervous system (CNS) functioning
Antibiotics	Tetracyclines	Malformations of the teeth and bone
Anticoagulants	Warfarin	CNS and skeletal malformations, hemorrhage
Anticonvulsants	Valproate, carbamazepine	Neural tube defects
	Phenytoin	CNS malformations
Antihypertensives	ACE inhibitors, ARBs	Renal defects, restrict normal growth patterns
Antineoplastic	Any, thalidomide	Multiple, congenital malformations
Antiretrovirals	Efavirenz	Neural tube defects
Nonsteroidal anti-inflammatory medications (NSAIDs)	Ibuprofen, naproxen, ketoprofen, etc.	Premature closure of the ductus arteriosus
Prostaglandin	Misoprostol	CNS and limb malformations
Psychiatric medications	Lithium	Congenital cardiovascular defects
Retinoids	Isotretinoin	Multiple, congenital malformations

CONTRACEPTION

Definition

Contraception refers to the prevention of pregnancy and is accomplished pharmacologically through two general mechanisms: (*1*) inhibition of contact between sperm and egg, and (*2*) prevention of implantation of the fertilized egg in the endometrium. Available products most commonly contain estrogen, progestin, or both. The estrogen component suppresses follicle-stimulating hormone (FSH) and prevents the development of a viable follicle. The progestin component contributes to the production of thick cervical mucus and the involution of the endometrium, and blocks ovulation.

Therapy Selection

Available Prescription Therapies

- Combination estrogen and progestin
  - Monophasic
  - Multiphasic
- Progestin only
- Implantable
- Emergency contraception
  - Start within 72 hours of unprotected intercourse
  - Approved over-the-counter (OTC) if patient is >18 years of age
  - Plan B
    - » 2 tablets 0.75 mg levonorgestrel (taken q12 h × 2 doses)
  - Plan B One Step
    - » 1 tablet by mouth, levonorgestrel 1.5 mg
  - Ella (Rx only)
    - » Ulipristal acetate 30 mg by mouth within 120 hours of unprotected intercourse

Advantages and Disadvantages of Contraception

Product type	Advantages	Disadvantages
Combination products	Long history of superior efficacy; multiple formulations allow opportunity to try multiple-dose combination of estrogen/progestin components in different dosage forms (transdermal patch, oral, multiphasic, continuous); decreased length of menses; decreased incidence of cramping; decreased risk of ectopic pregnancy	Drug interactions present; need for backup contraception with missed pills
Progestin only	Can be used in safely patients that are breastfeeding, are >35 years of age, and/or have systemic lupus erythematosus or intolerable estrogen-related side effects	Slightly less effective; requires even stricter compliance than combinations; higher incidence of breakthrough bleeding; need for backup contraception with missed pills
Implantable	Longer-term efficacy	Not readily reversible; requires insertion at medical office

Adverse Effects Associated with Hormonal Imbalance

Estrogen Excess	Estrogen Deficiency	Progestin Excess	Progestin Deficiency
• Breast tenderness • Cyclic weight gain • Edema • Bloating • Hypertension • Melasma • Migraine • Nausea	• Vasomotor symptoms (hot flushes) • Spotting • Breakthrough bleeding (early) • Decreased libido • Dyspareunia	• Decreased libido • Depression • Fatigue • Weight gain • Acne • Hypomenorrhea • Vaginal candidiasis	• Heavy menstruation • Weight loss • Delayed menses • Spotting • Breakthrough bleeding (late)

Pharmacologic Contraceptives

Hormonal Contraceptives

Oral contraceptives

Monophasic/High-dose estrogen

Generic	Brand	Dose & Max	Contra-indications	Primary Side Effects	Key Monitoring Parameters	Pertinent Drug Interactions	Med Pearls	Top 200
Ethinyl estradiol/ norgestrel	• Ovral • Ogestrel	50 mcg E. estradiol/0.5 mg norgestrel	• Pregnancy • Breast cancer • History of deep vein thrombosis (DVT) or pulmonary embolism (PE) • Lactation (<6 wks postpartum) • Smoker >35 years of age	• Breast tenderness • Increased breast size • Nausea • Edema • Bloating • Cyclic weight gain • Headaches during active pills • Thrombophlebitis (rare) *Estrogen-excess side effects most common*	• Presence of adverse effects • Pregnancy	• Effect of oral contraceptive pill (OCP): • Antibiotics (ampicillin, sulfonamides, tetracycline) • Anticonvulsants (phenytoin, topiramate, barbiturates) • Protease inhibitors • Rifampin Need backup method of contraception during use and for at least 1 wk after; for chronic therapy with above medications use another form of contraception	Take 1 tablet daily at the same time of day for 21 days, followed by 7 days of inactive placebo pills	Yes
• Ethinyl estradiol/ • Ethynodiol diacetate	• Demulen 1/50 • Zovia 1/50	50 mcg E. estradiol/1 mg E. diacetate						No
Mestranol/ norethindrone	• Ortho-Novum 1/50 • Necon 1/50 • Norinyl 1/50	50 mcg mestranol/ 1 mg norethindrone						Yes

Pharmacologic Contraceptives *(cont'd)*

Generic	Brand	Dose & Max	Contra-indications	Primary Side Effects	Key Monitoring Parameters	Pertinent Drug Interactions	Med Pearls	Top 200
Monophasic/Low-dose estrogen								
Ethinyl estradiol and levonorgestrel	• Alesse • Aviane • Lessina • Levlite • Lutera • Sronyx	20 mcg E. estradiol, 0.1 mg levonorgestrel	• Pregnancy • Breast cancer • History of DVT or PE • Lactation (<6 wks postpartum) • Smoker >35 years of age	• Nausea • Vomiting • Breakthrough bleeding • Spotting • Melasma • Headache		Effect of OCP: • Antibiotics (ampicillin, sulfonamides, tetracycline) • Anticonvulsants (phenytoin, topiramate, barbiturates) • Protease inhibitors • Rifampin Need backup method of contraception during use and for at least 1 wk after; for chronic therapy with above medications use another form of contraception		No
	• Levlen • Levora • Nordette • Portia • Seasonale • Lo Ovral • Quasense • Jolessa	30 mcg E. estradiol, 0.15 mg levonorgestrel		• Weight change • Edema • Venous thromboembolism • Side effects associated with hormonal imbalance (see Table 2) • Presence of adverse effects			Seasonale is taken continuously for 84 days with 7 placebo pills; menses only q3 mo	No
Ethinyl estradiol and drospirenone	• Yasmin • Yaz • Beyaz (has added folate) • Safyral (has added folate) • Syeda • Gianvi • Loryna • Ocella • Vestura • Zarah	20–30 mcg E. estradiol, 3 mg drospirenone		• Potassium with drospirenone	Serum potassium		• Decreased duration of menses • Drospirenone is a structural analog to spironolactone	Yes
Ethinyl estradiol and norgestrel	• Cryselle • Low-Ogestrel	30 mcg E. estradiol, 0.3 mg norgestrel						Yes

Pharmacologic Contraceptives *(cont'd)*

Generic	Brand	Dose & Max	Contra-indications	Primary Side Effects	Key Monitoring Parameters	Pertinent Drug Interactions	Med Pearls	Top 200
Ethinyl estradiol and norethindrone acetate	• Loestrin 21 1/20 • Loestrin Fe 1/20 • Microgestin Fe 1/20 • Lo Loestrin Fe	10–20 mcg E. estradiol, 1 mg n. acetate						Yes
Ethinyl estradiol and norethindrone	• Ovcon 35 • Balziva • Femcon Fe	35 mcg E. estradiol, 0.4 mg norethindrone						Yes
	• Brevicon • Modicon • Neocon 0.5/35 • Nortrel 0.5/35	35 mcg E. estradiol, 0.5 mg norethindrone						Yes
	• Necon 1/35 • Norinyl 1/35 • Nortrel 1/35 • Ortho-Novum 1/35	35 mcg E. estradiol, 1 mg norethindrone						Yes
Ethinyl estradiol and desogestrel	• Kariva • Azorette • Mircette	10–20 mcg E. estradiol, 0.15 mg desogestrel						No
	• Emoquette • Apri • Desogen • Reclipsen	30 mcg E. estradiol, 0.15 mg desogestrel						No
Ethinyl estradiol and levonorgestrel	Seasonique Lo Seasonique	10–20 mcg E. estradiol, 0.15 mg levonorgestrel 10–20 mcg E. estradiol, 0.1 mg levonorgestrel						No
Ethinyl estradiol and norgestimate	• Ortho cyclen • Sprintec • MonoNessa • Previfem	35 mcg E. estradiol, 0.25 mg norgestimate						Yes

Pharmacologic Contraceptives *(cont'd)*

Generic	Brand	Dose & Max	Contra-indications	Primary Side Effects	Key Monitoring Parameters	Pertinent Drug Interactions	Med Pearls	Top 200
Biphasic								
Ethinyl estradiol and norethindrone	• Ortho-Novum 10/11 • Necon 10/11	35 mcg E. estradiol, 0.5–1 mg norethindrone	• Pregnancy • Breast cancer • History of DVT or PE • Lactation (<6 wks postpartum) • Smoker >35 years of age	• Nausea • Vomiting • Breakthrough bleeding • Spotting • Melasma • Headache • Weight change • Edema • Venous thromboembolism • Side effects associated with hormonal imbalance (see Table 2)	• Presence of adverse effects • Pregnancy	Effect of OCP: • Antibiotics (ampicillin, sulfonamides, tetracycline) • Anticonvulsants (phenytoin, topiramate, barbiturates) • Protease inhibitors • Rifampin Need backup method of contraception during use and for at least 1 wk after; for chronic therapy with above medications use another form of contraception	• Created to decrease overall hormone exposure • High incidence of breakthrough bleeding	Yes
Triphasic								
Ethinyl estradiol and norethindrone	• Tri-Norinyl • Necon 7/7/7 • Ortho-Novum 7/7/7 • Estrostep 21 • Estrostep Fe	35 mcg E. estradiol, 0.5–1 mg norethindrone	• Pregnancy • Breast cancer • History of DVT or PE • Lactation (<6 wks postpartum) • Smoker >35 years of age	• Nausea • Vomiting • Breakthrough bleeding • Spotting • Melasma • Headache • Weight change • Edema • Venous thrombo-embolism • Side effects associated with hormonal imbalance (see Table 2)	• Presence of adverse effects • Pregnancy	Effect of OCP (same as above)	• Many triphasics approved for treatment of acne as well • More difficult to deal with missed pills • Decreases overall hormone exposure	Yes
Ethinyl estradiol and desogestrel	Cyclessa	25 mcg E. estradiol, 0.1–0.15 mg desogestrel						No
Ethinyl estradiol and norgestimate	• Trinessa • Ortho-TriCyclen	35 mcg E. estradiol, 0.18–0.25 mg norgestimate						Yes
	• Orth-TriCyclen Lo	25 mcg E. estradiol, 0.18–25 mg norgestimate						
Ethinyl estradiol and levonorgestrel	• Enpresse • Tri-Levlen • Triphasil • Trivora	30–40 mcg E. estradiol, 0.075–0.125 mg levonorgestrel						No

Pharmacologic Contraceptives *(cont'd)*

Generic	Brand	Dose & Max	Contra-indications	Primary Side Effects	Key Monitoring Parameters	Pertinent Drug Interactions	Med Pearls	Top 200
Four-phasic								
Estradiol valerate and dienogest	Natazia	• Days 1–2: 3 mg estradiol valerate • Days 3–7: 2 mg estradiol valerate + 2 mg dienogest • Days 8–24: 2 mg estradiol valerate + 3 mg dienogest • Days 25–26: 1 mg estradiol valerate • Days 27–28: inactive	• Pregnancy • Lactation • Breast cancer • History of DVT or PE • Hepatic disease • Abnormal uterine bleeding • Vascular disease • Hypercoagulopathy			Effect of OCP: • Antibiotics (ampicillin, sulfonamides, tetracycline) • Anticonvulsants (phenytoin, topiramate, barbiturates) • Protease inhibitors • Rifampin Need backup method of contraception during use and for at least 1 wk after. For chronic therapy with above medications use another form of contraception.	• Only 4-phasic option available • Demonstrated increased efficacy for heavy menstrual bleeding	No
Transdermal								
Ethinyl estradiol and norelgestromin	Xulane	35 mcg E. estradiol and 0.15 mg norelgestromin	• Pregnancy • Breast cancer • History of DVT or PE • Lactation (<6 wks postpartum) • Smoker >35 years of age	• Nausea • Vomiting • Breakthrough bleeding • Spotting • Melasma • Headache • Weight change • Edema • Venous thrombo-embolism • Side effects associated with hormonal imbalance (see Table 2)	• Presence of adverse effects • Pregnancy	Same as OCP	• Safe with usual activities • Do not apply lotion to site of application • Improved compliance over oral • Apply weekly for 3 wks • Avoid if >90 kg	No

Pharmacologic Contraceptives *(cont'd)*

Generic	Brand	Dose & Max	Contra-indications	Primary Side Effects	Key Monitoring Parameters	Pertinent Drug Interactions	Med Pearls	Top 200
Other								
Ethinyl estradiol and etonogestrel	NuvaRing	• 0.015 mg E. estradiol and 0.12 mg etonogestrel released daily • Inserted by patient intravaginally q4 wks (active for 3 wks)	Negative pregnancy test needed for initiation	Same as OCP (systemic absorption occurs)	Same as OCP (systemic absorption occurs)	Same as OCP (systemic absorption occurs)	• May be removed before intercourse • Not to be used >4 mos after dispensed	Yes
Progestin-only contraceptives								
Oral								
Norethindrone	• Ortho Micronor • Errin • Jolivette • Nor-QD • Nora-BE • Camila	0.35 mg daily	Negative pregnancy test prior to initiation	• Libido depression • Fatigue • Weight gain • Acne • Hypomenorrhea	Presence of side effects	None	Can be used in breastfeeding women, those >35 who smoke, and those at risk of coronary heart disease (CHD)	No
Norgestrel	Ovrette	0.075 mg daily						No
Parenteral								
Medroxy-progesterone	• Depo-Provera • Depo-Subq Provera 104	150 mg/mL intramuscular (IM) q12 wks; or 104 mg SC q12 wks	• Must have negative pregnancy test to start therapy or to continue therapy if >14 wks since last injection • Breast cancer • Liver disease	• Weight gain • Decreased bone mineral density • Acne • Delayed return of fertility after discontinuation	Bone mineral density	None	• Supplement calcium and vitamin D due to potential bone loss • Do not use for >2 years unless unable to use other forms of contraception	Yes

Pharmacologic Contraceptives *(cont'd)*

Generic	Brand	Dose & Max	Contra-indications	Primary Side Effects	Key Monitoring Parameters	Pertinent Drug Interactions	Med Pearls	Top 200
Implantable/intrauterine								
Levonorgestrel	Mirena	• 20 mcg released daily • Intrauterine	• History or high risk of pelvic inflammatory disease (PID) or ectopic pregnancy	• Spotting • Breakthrough bleeding • Amenorrhea	• Presence of side effects • Pregnancy	None	Remains in place for up to 5 years	Yes
Levonorgestrel	Skyla	• 6 mcg released daily • Intrauterine	• Breast cancer • Abnormal uterine bleeding • High risk for sexually transmitted infections (STIs) (multiple sexual partners) • Uterine or cervical cancer	• Mastalgia • Headache • Abdominal pain • PID			Remains for 3 years	No
Etonogestrel	• Implanon • Nexplanon	• 68 mg subdermal implant in upper arm • Replace q3–5 yrs	History or high risk of pelvic inflammatory disease or ectopic pregnancy	• Amenorrhea • Infrequent menses • Weight gain			Not studied in women >130% ideal body weight	No
Nonhormonal								
Copper–T380	ParaGard	Intrauterine placement for up to 10 yrs	History or high risk of PID or ectopic pregnancy	• Heavy bleeding • Cramping	None	None	Can remain in place for up to 8–10 yrs with efficacy	No

Storage and Administration Pearls

- Store at controlled room temperature 20–25°C (68–77°F) in a dry area, protected from direct light.
- After use, discard NuvaRing away from children or pets.
- Store NuvaRing in refrigerator prior to use.

Patient Education Pearls

- Hormonal contraceptives do not prevent the transmission of STIs.
- Efficacy is high with strict adherence to therapy schedule.
- Establish a regular time to take OCP, preferably as a part of daily routine, such as brushing teeth.
- Plan a backup contraceptive method.
- Smoking with OCP poses significant risks and should be avoided.
- Contact physician immediately if any of the following occur:
  - Abdominal pain
  - Chest pain (severe), shortness of breath
  - Headache (severe), dizziness, weakness, or numbness
  - Eye problems (vision loss or blurring), speech problems
  - Severe leg pain (calf or thigh)
- Specific instructions for missed doses:

Doses Missed	Instructions for Patient
1	Take missed dose immediately and next dose at regular time
2 (during first 2 wks)	Take two doses daily for the next 2 days, then resume taking; use backup method for 7 days
2 (during third wk)	Sunday start: Take one dose daily until Sunday, dispose of current pack, then begin next pack without placebo pills. Backup method required for 7 days. Other: Dispose of current pack and begin new pack. Backup method required for 7 days.
3 or more	

HORMONE REPLACEMENT THERAPY

Definitions

- Menopause is the cessation of menses after the loss of ovarian follicular activity.
- Perimenopause refers to the period of time immediately prior to menopause and the 1 year following menopause onset.

Diagnosis

Diagnosis is made when amenorrhea occurs for a minimum of 12 consecutive months.

Signs and Symptoms

Symptoms are related primarily to lack of estrogen and include vaginal dryness, vaginal atrophy, hot flushes, and night sweats. Other potential symptoms include arthralgia, depression, migraine, mood swings, myalgia, and insomnia.

Guidelines

Estrogen and progestogen use in peri- and postmenopausal women: March 2007 position statement of the North American Menopause Society. *Menopause* 2007;14(2):168–82. www.guideline.gov/summary/summary.aspx?doc_id=10712&nbr=005575&string= hormone+AND+replacement.

Guideline Summary

- All women should undergo careful evaluation prior to initiation of hormone replacement therapy (HRT), including comprehensive history and physical, mammography, and, potentially, bone densitometry.
- The primary indication for HRT is vasomotor symptoms of hot flushes and night sweats.
- Local vaginal therapy is recommended when vaginal symptoms are the only complaint.
- Prevention of osteoporosis with HRT should be considered only for women with a very strong risk of osteoporosis and in whom other available therapies are not options.
- In women who are receiving HRT and who have an intact uterus, progestin is indicated as a means of reducing the risk of endometrial hyperplasia and cancer that exists with unopposed estrogen use in these patients.
- Due to an unclear evidence-based benefit:risk ratio, HRT is not recommended for use for any of the following indications: Cardiovascular disease, stroke prevention, hyperlipidemia, or dementia prevention.
- The Women's Health Initiative (WHI) indicated increased risks of venous thromboembolism, stroke, coronary disease, and breast cancer in women who receive HRT for an extended period of time.
- The current recommendation is to use HRT at the lowest effective dose for the shortest possible duration.
- Nonhormonal options are available for the treatment of vasomotor symptoms in patients with contraindications to hormone therapy or preference to avoid hormone therapy. Evidence-based options include venlafaxine, paroxetine, fluoxetine, and gabapentin. (These agents are detailed in drug tables in the neurological and psychiatric disorders chapters.) Brisdelle is a low-dose paroxetine product that is FDA approved solely for the treatment of vasomotor symptoms related to menopause.

Hormone Replacement Therapy

Generic	Brand	Dose & Max mg (frequency)	Contraindications	Primary Side Effects	Key Monitoring Parameters	Med Pearls	Top 200
Oral preparations							
Estrogens							
Conjugated equine estrogens	Premarin	0.3–2.5 mg daily	• Abnormal bleeding • Breast cancer • History of DVT or PE • Pregnancy	• Nausea • Fluid retention • Bloating • Headaches	Presence of side effects (especially vaginal bleeding or symptoms of VTE, stroke, or MI)	• Most studied • No generic equivalent • Should not be abruptly discontinued; taper	Yes
Synthetic conjugated estrogen	• Cenestin • Enjuva	0.3–1.25 mg daily	• Estrogen-dependent tumor • Cardiovascular accident (CVA) or myocardial infarction (MI) in past year • Thromboembolic disease	• Mood changes • Breast tenderness		• Long half-life • Most potent hepatic effects	No
Micronized estradiol	• Estradiol • Estrace • Gynodiol	0.5–2 mg daily		• Increased risk of venous thromboembolism (VTE), stroke, MI, breast cancer		• Should not be abruptly discontinued; taper	No
Estrone sulfate	• Estropipate • Ortho-Est • Ogen	0.625–6 mg daily					No
Esterified estrogens	Menest	0.3–2.5 mg daily				Should not be abruptly discontinued; taper	No
Progestins							
Medroxyprogesterone	Provera	2–10 mg daily		• Decreased libido • Cramping • Mood changes • Bloating • Nausea • Depression • Headache	Presence of adverse effects		Yes
Micronized progestin	Prometrium	100–200 mg daily				Primary use in patients with adverse effects associated with synthetic estrogens	No
Selective estrogen receptor modulator/Estrogen agonist–antagonist							
Ospemifene	Osphena	60 mg daily	Same as estrogens	Vasomotor symptoms		Drug interactions with azoles, rifampin	No

Hormone Replacement Therapy *(cont'd)*

Generic	Brand	Dose & Max mg (frequency)	Contraindications	Primary Side Effects	Key Monitoring Parameters	Med Pearls	Top 200
Combination oral preparations							
Conjugated equine estrogens and medroxyprogesterone	Prempro	0.3–0.625 mg estrogen/1.5–2.5 mg progestin	• Abnormal bleeding • Breast cancer • History of DVT or PE • Pregnancy • Estrogen-dependent tumor • CVA or MI in past year • Thromboembolic disease	• Nausea • Fluid retention • Bloating • Headaches • Mood changes • Breast tenderness • Increased risk of VTE • Stroke • MI • Breast cancer	Presence of side effects (especially vaginal bleeding or symptoms of VTE, stroke, or MI)		Yes
Conjugated equine estrogens and medroxyprogesterone	Premphase	0.625 mg/0 mg × 14 days then 0.625/5 mg × 14 days					No
Estradiol and drospirenone	Angelique	1/0.5 mg					No
Ethinyl estradiol and norethindrone acetate	FemHRT	2.5–5 mcg estrogen/0.5–1.0 mg progestin					No
Estradiol and norethindrone acetate	Activella	0.5–1.0 mcg estrogen/0.1–0.5 mg progestin					No
Estradiol and norgestimate	Prefest	1 mg/0 × 15 days then 1/0.09 mg × 15 days					No
Transdermal and topical preparations							
17β Estradiol transdermal	• Estraderm • Vivelle • Climara • Alora • Esclim	• 25–50 mcg/24 hours • Applied 1–2 × wk	• Abnormal bleeding • Breast cancer • History of DVT or PE • Pregnancy • Estrogen-dependent tumor • CVA or MI in past year • Thromboembolic disease	• Skin irritation • Nausea • Fluid retention • Bloating • Headaches • Mood changes • Breast tenderness • Increased risk of VTE • Stroke • MI • Breast cancer	Presence of side effects (especially vaginal bleeding or symptoms of VTE, stroke, or MI)	• Limited hepatic effects • Useful in patients with GI disturbances • Adverse effects less common in general	Yes
17β Reservoir	Estraderm	0.025–0.1 mg (2 ×/wk)					No
17β Gel	• Estrogel (q day) • Elestrin (q day) • Divigel (q day)	0.2–1 mg daily					No
17β Topical emulsion	Estrasorb (2 pkt q day)	0.05 mg daily					No
17β Transdermal spray	Evamist (initial: 1 spray q day, may increase to 2–3 sprays/day)	0.021 mg/spray					No

Hormone Replacement Therapy *(cont'd)*

Generic	Brand	Dose & Max mg (frequency)	Contraindications	Primary Side Effects	Key Monitoring Parameters	Med Pearls	Top 200
Vaginal preparations							
Conjugated estrogen cream	Premarin	1.25 mg applied vaginally from 1–2 × wkly to daily	• Abnormal bleeding • Breast cancer • History of DVT or PE • Pregnancy • Estrogen-dependent tumor • CVA or MI in past year • Thromboembolic disease	Systemic side effects possible but rare	• Presence of adverse effects • Efficacy	• Used in cases of vaginal symptoms only • Effective for stress incontinence	No
Estrone cream	Neo-estrone cream	1 mg/g					No
Estradiol ring	Estring	7.5 mcg/d × 90 days				Long-term use associated with endometrial hyperplasia	No
	Femring	5 mcg/d × 90 days					No
17β Cream	Estrace cream	2–4 g/d × 2–4 wk, 1 g/d × 1–3 wk				• Used in cases of vaginal symptoms only • Effective for stress incontinence	No
Estradiol tablet	Vagifem	2 × 25 mcg/wk					No

Drug Interactions

	Interacting Drug(s)	Result
Estrogen	CYP450 3A4 inducers: barbiturates, carbamazepine, rifampin, St. John's wort	↓ Effect of estrogen
	Hydantoins, thyroid hormone, anticoagulants (oral)	↓ Effect of interacting drug
	CYP450 3A4 inhibitors: azole antifungals, macrolide antibiotics, ritonavir, grapefruit juice, atorvastatin	↑ Effect of estrogen
	Corticosteroids, tricyclic antidepressants (potential increased toxicity)	↑ Effect of interacting drug
Progestin	Aminoglutethimide, rifampin	↓ Effect of progestin

Storage and Administration Pearls

- Store at controlled room temperature in a dry location.
- Dispose of patches in a safe place inaccessible to children or pets.

Patient Education Pearls

- Potential risks of HRT should be discussed thoroughly with every patient.
- Adverse effects may be decreased if a low dose is used for a short period of time.
- Contact physician promptly for any of the following: Abnormal vaginal bleeding, abdominal pain or tenderness, speech or visual disturbance, breast lumps, numbness in extremities, severe headache, vomiting, sharp pain in leg or chest, shortness of breath.

ERECTILE DYSFUNCTION

Definition

Erectile dysfunction (ED) is often referred to as impotence and is defined as the inability to achieve a penile erection suitable for sexual intercourse.

Diagnosis

Diagnostic workup of ED includes an assessment of the severity of the dysfunction, a complete history and physical, a review of medications, a physical examination, and selected laboratory tests (serum glucose, lipid profile, thyroid). Each component of the evaluation is used to rule out potential reversible causes of the ED.

Signs and Symptoms

The inability to achieve or maintain an adequate erection is the hallmark symptom; however, symptoms such as depression and anxiety are also commonly associated with ED.

Guidelines

Erectile Dysfunction Guideline Update Panel. The management of erectile dysfunction: an update. Linthicum, MD: American Urologic Association Education and Research, Inc.; 2006 May. www.guideline.gov/summary/summary.aspx?doc_id=10018&nbr=0053 32&string=erectile+AND+dysfunction.

Guidelines Summary

- Initial treatment for most patients will consist of therapy with a phosphodiesterase-5 (PDE5) inhibitor because these agents are known to be efficacious and are minimally invasive.
- PDE5 inhibitors are contraindicated in patients who are currently taking organic nitrates, due to a risk of significant, dangerous hypotension when these agents are used concomitantly.
- If a patient does not respond to therapy with a PDE5 inhibitor, alternate therapy options should be considered, including a different PDE5 inhibitor, alprostadil intraurethral suppositories, intracavernous injection, vacuum constriction devices, and penile prostheses.
- Lifestyle modification and treatment of underlying cause/secondary cause should also be encouraged (hypertension, diabetes, hyperlipidemia).

Drugs for Erectile Dysfunction

Mechanism of action – PDE5 inhibitors: enhance the activity of nitric oxide by inhibiting an enzyme (PDE5) responsible for its degradation; enhanced nitric oxide allows relaxed smooth muscles and increased vasodilation and blood flow to the penis following stimulation

Generic	Brand	Dose & Max	Contra-indications	Primary Side Effects	Key Monitoring Parameters	Pertinent Drug Interactions	Med Pearls	Top 200
Oral								
Sildenafil	Viagra	25–100 mg as needed (PRN) 0.5–4 hrs prior to sexual activity (max = 1 dose daily)	• Use with nitrates (continuous or intermittent) • Hypersensitivity • Nitric oxide donors	• Hypotension • Headache • Flushing • Dyspepsia • Priapism (not common) • Vision changes	• Efficacy • Presence of adverse effects • BP	***Nitrates—Combination results in potentially fatal hypotension. Avoid concomitant use within at least 24 hours; 48 hours with tadalafil.*** • Alpha-blockers: Potential significant reduction in BP; avoid combination or use lowest dose of each agent used with close monitoring • PDE5 inhibitors are metabolized by CYP450 3A4; therefore, inhibitors and inducers of this enzyme will affect PDE5 inhibitor levels accordingly	• Erection occurs only after physical and psychological stimulation	Yes
Tadalafil	Cialis	2.5–20 mg PRN prior to sexual activity; or 2.5–5 mg PO 1 × daily						Yes
Vardenafil	Levitra Staxyn (orally disintegrating tablet)	2.5–20 mg PRN ~1 hr prior to sexual activity						No
Avanafil	Stendra	50–100 mg daily; 0.5 hr prior to sexual activity						No
Topical								
Testosterone transdermal patch	• Testoderm • Testoderm-TTS • Androderm	2.5–6 mg patch applied daily	• Hypersensitivity • Carcinoma of the breast or prostate	• Elevated liver enzymes • Hyperlipidemia • Depression • Aggression	• Periodic liver function • Prostate-specific antigen (PSA) • Lipid panels	Increases the effects of anticoagulants and cyclosporine	• Only useful in ED due to hypogonadism • C–III	No
Testosterone gel	AndroGel 1%	AndroGel 1%: 50–100 mg daily; AndroGel 1.62%: 40.5–81 mg daily 5–10 g daily (morning) applied to shoulders, upper arm, or abdomen						Yes
Testosterone buccal	Striant	30 mg BID					Apply to gum, above incisor	No

Drugs for Erectile Dysfunction *(cont'd)*

Generic	Brand	Dose & Max	Contra-indications	Primary Side Effects	Key Monitoring Parameters	Pertinent Drug Interactions	Med Pearls	Top 200
Intramuscular								
Testosterone	• Depo-testosterone (cypionate) • Delatestryl (enanthate)	200–400 mg q2–4 wks	• Hypersensitivity • Carcinoma of the breast or prostate	• Elevated liver enzymes • Hyperlipidemia • Depression • Aggression	• Periodic LFT • PSA • Lipid panels	Increases the effects of anticoagulants and cyclosporine	Only useful in ED due to hypogonadism	No
Intraurethral								
Alprostadil	Muse	125–1,000 mcg pellets 5–10 min before intercourse	• Hypersensitivity • Urethral stricture • Chronic urethritis	• Urethral pain • Burning • Priapism • Hypotension	• Presence of adverse effects • Efficacy • BP periodically	None	Duration of effect is 30–60 min	No
Intracavernosal								
Alprostadil	• Caverject • Edex	1–40 mcg 5–20 min before intercourse injected intracavernosal	• Hypersensitivity • Sickle-cell trait • Multiple myeloma • Leukemia	• Pain at injection site • Erythema • Priapism • Hypotension	• Presence of adverse effects • Efficacy • BP periodically	None	Self-injection training should be done in physician's office	No

Storage and Administration Pearls

- Sildenafil should be taken at least 30 minutes prior to sexual activity and can be taken, at earliest, 4 hours prior.

- Vardenafil should be taken approximately 1 hour prior to anticipated activity.

- Tadalafil can either be taken prior to activity or as a scheduled daily dose.

- Alprostadil intraurethral: Store unopened foil pouches in a refrigerator at 2–8°C (36–46°F). Do not expose alprostadil urethral suppository to temperatures above 30°C (86°F). Alprostadil urethral suppository may be kept at room temperature (below 30°C [86°F]) for up to 14 days prior to use.

- Alprostadil intracavernosal: Prepare the solution immediately before use. Do not administer unless solution is clear. Do not add any drugs or other solutions to this solution. Discard any unused solution remaining in the cartridge.

Patient Education Pearls

- Testoderm TTS is applied to the arm, back, abdomen, or thigh.

- Testosterone gel is applied to shoulders, arms, or abdomen.

- Males using testosterone products should not allow direct contact between the testosterone product and a pregnant female, as teratogenic effects are possible.

BENIGN PROSTATIC HYPERPLASIA

Definition

Benign prostatic hyperplasia (BPH) is an enlargement of the prostate gland due to the proliferation of smooth muscle and epithelial cells. BPH often leads to lower urinary tract symptoms (LUTS) due to direct bladder outlet obstruction and increased smooth muscle tone/resistance from within the enlarged gland.

Diagnosis

Diagnosis of BPH primarily is made based upon symptoms. The American Urological Association Symptom Index (AUA-SI) and other similar symptom scores are used to determine the degree of impact the LUTS are having on an individual patient's quality of life and to guide therapy decisions.

Questions included in the AUA-SI include quantification of how frequently specific symptoms have occurred over the preceding month. Responses of higher frequency are assigned a higher point value. The overall score on the AUA-SI is a validated measure used to determine symptom severity and initiate patient-specific dialog regarding benefits and risks of treatment. In general, pharmacological therapy is considered for patients with moderate–severe symptoms (AUA-SI scores of >8).

Signs and Symptoms

Symptoms include LUTS such as urinary urgency, leaking, dribbling, hesitancy, frequency (especially nocturia), straining/weak stream, and incomplete bladder emptying.

Signs may include an enlarged prostate identified during a digital rectal exam (DRE) or an elevated prostate-specific antigen (PSA) in the serum.

Guidelines

American Urological Association Guideline: Management of Benign Prostatic Hyperplasia (BPH). Revised, 2010. http://www.auanet.org/education/guidelines/benign-prostatic-hyperplasia.cfm

Guidelines Summary

- Watchful waiting (no pharmacologic therapy) is appropriate for patients with mild symptoms (AUA-SI scores of <8).
- In general, pharmacologic therapy is considered for patients with moderate–severe symptoms (AUA-SI scores of ≥8).
- Alpha-antagonists are the treatment of choice for patients with LUTS and are used as monotherapy or in combination with 5-alpha reductase inhibitors or anticholinergics.
  - Nonselective agents such as terazosin and doxazosin are equally effective as the alpha 1A selective agents tamsulosin, alfuzosin, and silodosin.
  - Nonselective agents require slow dose titration and lower blood pressure; therefore, these agents should be used with caution in patients at risk of hypotension.
  - First-dose syncope and dizziness are common side effects, especially with nonselective agents. Dosing at bedtime can minimize this side effect, but patients should be educated to stand up slowly to avoid falls.
  - Intraoperative floppy iris syndrome (IFIS) is a potential side effect that can significantly complicate cataract surgery. Patients with planned cataract surgery should not initiate new alpha antagonist therapy until cataract surgery is complete.
- 5-alpha reductase inhibitors are appropriate as monotherapy or combination therapy with alpha antagonists in patients with enlarged prostate glands.
  - Although earlier guidelines suggested use in prostate glands >50 mL (50 g), newer studies have demonstrated benefits in patients with prostate glands >30 mL (30 g).
- Anticholinergic agents such as tolterodine may be considered in patient with LUTS (primarily irritative) and without an elevated postvoid residual (<250 mL). Please see the drug tables in the Urinary Incontinence section for specifics related to anticholinergic medications.

Phosphodiesterase-5 (PDE-5) inhibitors are now clinically indicated for daily use for the treatment of LUTS/BPH (tadalafil FDA approved) but are generally reserved for patients who have not responded to more conventional therapies. Because PDE-5 inhibitors exhibit a significant drug interaction with nonselective alpha antagonists, special care should be taken to monitor for and avoid this combination.

Drugs for BPH

Alpha antagonists (nonselective)

Generic	Brand	Dose & Max	Contra-indications	Primary Side Effects	Key Monitoring Parameters	Pertinent Drug Interactions	Med Pearls	Top 200
Doxazosin	Cardura	1–8 mg PO daily at bed time (HS)	Hypersensitivity	• Hypotension • Orthostasis • Syncope • Dizziness	• Blood pressure (BP) • Presence of orthostasis	• Phosphodiesterase inhibitors: combination may result in dangerous hypotension • Additive BP lowering with other antihypertensives	Dosed at HS to prevent dizziness/falls during the day	Yes
Terazosin	Hytrin	1–10 mg PO daily (HS)			• Efficacy		Not used often due to need for multiple daily dosing	Yes

Selective alpha 1A antagonists

Generic	Brand	Dose & Max	Contra-indications	Primary Side Effects	Key Monitoring Parameters	Pertinent Drug Interactions	Med Pearls	Top 200
Tamsulosin	Flomax	0.4–0.8 mg 1 × daily	Hypersensitivity	Headache, dizziness, orthostasis	• Presence of side effects • Efficacy • Periodic BP	Cimetidine increases tamsulosin levels	Expensive relative to nonselective agents	Yes
Alfuzosin	Uroxatral	10 mg PO daily	• Hypersensitivity • Moderate to severe hepatic disease	• Dizziness • Fatigue • Headache • Potential for hypotension (rare)	• Presence of side effects • Efficacy • Periodic BP	Levels with CYP3A4 inhibitors: ketoconazole, itraconazole, and ritonavir	• Hepatically eliminated • Tablets are extended-release; do not crush or chew	No
Silodosin	Rapaflo	4–8 mg PO daily	• Severe renal impairment (CrCl < 30 mL/min) • Severe hepatic impairment (Child-Pugh ≥10) • Concomitant administration with CYP3A4 inhibitors	• Postural hypotension • Retrograde ejaculation • Dizziness • Diarrhea • Headache	• Response to treatment • BP	• CYP3A4 inhibitors (ketoconazole, itraconazole, clarithromycin, ritonavir) increase plasma silodosin levels • Concomitant use with PDE5 inhibitors can cause significant hypotension	• Renal dose adjustment required • Inform ophthalmologist prior to eye surgery due to risk of intraoperative floppy iris syndrome	No

5α reductase inhibitors

Generic	Brand	Dose & Max	Contra-indications	Primary Side Effects	Key Monitoring Parameters	Pertinent Drug Interactions	Med Pearls	Top 200
Finasteride	Proscar	5 mg PO daily	• Female sex • Hypersensitivity	• Decreased libido • Erectile dysfunction • Gynecomastia	• Obtain PSA prior to therapy initiation • Agents can decrease PSA, thereby decreasing utility to detect cancer	None	• Should not be handled by pregnant women—teratogenic potential	Yes
Dutasteride	Avodart	0.5 mg PO daily	• Female sex • Hypersensitivity			• Metabolized by CYP450 3A4 • Unknown but suspected interactions with potent inhibitors and inducers	• Onset of effect can be up to 6 mos	Yes

Storage and Administration Pearls

- Alpha-blockers should be taken at bedtime to avoid side effects of syncope and ortho-stasis while awake.
- Nonselective alpha-antagonists should be taken at bedtime.
- Tamsulosin and silodosin should be taken with food.
- Alfuzosin cannot be crushed, chewed, or broken in half; tablets must be swallowed whole.

Patient Education Pearls

- Patients taking nonselective alpha-antagonists should be educated to take dose at bedtime and to rise slowly when waking to use toilet at night. Dizziness may occur and may require some time before patient feels steady on his or her feet. This side effect likely will be most pronounced immediately following dose changes and should subside over time.
- If receiving an alpha-blocker, rise slowly from seated position to avoid potential dizziness associated with the medication.
- If receiving an alpha reductase inhibitor, know that reaching full benefit of this medication may take up to 6 months. An adequate trial should be allowed.
- For alpha-antagonists, patients should be advised to tell their doctor about any planned cataract surgery.
- 5-alpha reductase inhibitors will take some time to demonstrate efficacy (up to several months).
- Women who may be pregnant or are of childbearing age should not handle 5-alpha reductase tablets. These medications can cause birth defects. The semen of men taking 5-alpha reductase inhibitors also may be harmful to women who are or could become pregnant.

URINARY INCONTINENCE

Definitions

This is a condition associated with the involuntary loss of urine. There are multiple subtypes of urinary incontinence differentiated by etiology. The major classifications are: (1) urethral underactivity (stress incontinence), (2) bladder overactivity (urge incontinence), and (3) urethral overactivity/bladder underactivity (overflow incontinence).

Diagnosis

Diagnosis is based primarily on patient complaints and a thorough history and physical.

Signs and Symptoms

Symptoms of stress incontinence include the loss of small amounts of urine during activities such as sneezing, coughing, laughing, or running. Symptoms of urge incontinence include urinary urgency and frequency that may be associated with the loss of large or small amounts of urine. Overflow incontinence is associated with the loss of a large amount of urine which may be accompanied by symptoms of frequency, nocturia, hesitancy, or weak urinary stream.

Guidelines

Because a nationally recognized guideline for the treatment of urinary incontinence does not currently exist, the following represents general recommendations for treatment of the various subtypes based on multiple primary and tertiary resources.

Summary of Treatment Recommendations

- General
  - Nonpharmacological therapy is important as either monotherapy or an adjunct to pharmacotherapy. Options such as Kegel exercises and scheduled voiding are common.
- Stress incontinence
  - Options for treatment include topical estrogen, alpha agonists, and tricyclic antidepressants. Alpha agonists carry the risk of elevating blood pressure and heart rate, and will be used only with caution in patients with pre-existing hypertension or heart conditions.
- Urge incontinence
  - Options for the treatment of urge incontinence include anticholinergic medications and imipramine.
- Overflow incontinence
  - Treatment options are varied based upon the determined etiology. Since many cases of overflow incontinence are secondary to benign prostatic hyperplasia (BPH), see BPH section for recommendations.

Drugs for Urinary Incontinence

Generic	Brand	Dose & Max	Contra-indications	Primary Side Effects	Key Monitoring Parameters	Pertinent Drug Interactions	Med Pearls	Top 200
Topical vaginal estrogen preparations: used in the treatment of stress incontinence (first-line) and urge incontinence (third-line); see HRT drug chart above for more detailed information								
Tricyclic antidepressants: imipramine and desipramine are the most commonly used in incontinence; used primarily in urge incontinence and stress incontinence; see drug charts in psychiatric disorders chapter for detailed information								
Anticholinergic/antimuscarinic agents								
Oxybutynin • Syrup	Ditropan	2.5–5 mg PO TID–QID	• Urinary retention • Gastric retention • Narrow-angle glaucoma	• Dry mouth • Dry eyes • Constipation • Urinary retention • Somnolence • Blurred vision • Increased intra-ocular pressure	Presence of adverse effects	Additive effects with other anticholinergic medications	Side effects less common with extended-release version and transdermal	Yes
• Extended-release	Ditropan XL	5–30 mg PO daily						
• Transdermal	Oxytrol	3.9 mg/day apply 2x/wk						
• Topical gel	Gelnique 3%	Apply 3 pumps (84 mg) once daily						
	Gelnique 10%	Apply contents of 1 sachet (100 mg /g) once daily						
Tolterodine Extended-release	Detrol	1–2 mg PO BID					Side effects less common with extended-release	Yes
	Detrol LA	2–4 mg PO 1×/day						
Darifenacin	Enablex	7.5–15 mg PO daily				• CYP450 3A4 inhibitors increase levels • Additive effects with other anticholinergic medications	Do not exceed 7.5 mg daily in combo with enzyme inhibitors	Yes
Solifenacin	Vesicare	5–10 mg PO daily						Yes
Fesoterodine	Toviaz	4–8 mg once daily				• CYP3A4 inhibitors increase levels • Doses above 4 mg not recommended concomitantly	• Dose adjusted for CrCl < 30 mL/min • Max dose of 4 mg daily with CYP3A4 inhibitors	Yes
Trospium	• Sanctura	20 mg BID	CrCl<30 mL/min					Yes
	• Sanctura XR	60 mg daily						

Drugs for Urinary Incontinence *(cont'd)*

Mechanism of action – beta-3 adrenergic receptor antagonist

Generic	Brand	Dose & Max	Contra-indications	Primary Side Effects	Key Monitoring Parameters	Pertinent Drug Interactions	Med Pearls	Top 200
Mirabegron	Myrbetriq	25–50 mg PO once daily	• Severe, uncontrolled hypertension (>180/110 mmHg) • Pregnancy	• Hypertension • Tachycardia • Headache • Urinary tract infections • Dizziness • Constipation • Xerostomia	• Blood pressure at baseline and periodically • Presence of adverse effects • Efficacy	• CYP2D6 substrate • Increases serum concentration of digoxin, thioridazine, pimozide, flecainide, propafenone, aripiprazole, and desipramine • Decreases serum concentration of tamoxifen and therapeutic effects of tramadol and metoprolol • Enhanced anticholinergic side effects with anticholinergic agents	• Newer agent with fewer anticholinergic side effects • Hypertension may limit use • Very expensive	No

Alpha agonists

Generic	Brand	Dose & Max	Contra-indications	Primary Side Effects	Key Monitoring Parameters	Pertinent Drug Interactions	Med Pearls	Top 200
Pseudoephedrine	Sudafed, many	30–60 mg PO q4–6 hours PRN (max = 240 mg/24 hrs)	• MAOI therapy • Hypersensitivity • Uncontrolled HTN	• Increased blood pressure • Increased HR	• Blood pressure and heart rate periodically • Blood sugar if diabetic	MAO inhibitors	• Increases blood pressure and heart rate • Use with caution in HTN or pre-existing cardiac conditions	No
Phenylephrine	Many	10–20 mg q4 hrs PRN		• Increased blood sugar • Irritability • Insomnia				No

Storage and Administration Pearls

- Store all medications at room temperature and out of the reach of children.

Patient Education Pearls

- Anticholinergic medications may make patient drowsy and experience dry mouth, dry eyes, blurred vision, or constipation.

PRACTICE QUESTIONS

1. Which of the following is most accurate regarding the coadministration of sildenafil and nitroglycerin?

   (A) There is no drug interaction between the two medications.

   (B) There is a minor drug interaction between the two medications. The patient should be counseled to monitor for signs and symptoms of the interaction.

   (C) There is a major drug interaction between these two agents, but they can be safely coadministered as long as doses are separated by at least 1 hour.

   (D) There is a major drug interaction between sildenafil and some forms of nitroglycerin. The specific formulation of nitroglycerin should be determined before the medications are taken.

   (E) There is a major, potentially life-threatening drug interaction between the two agents. Coadministration should be strictly avoided.

2. In which of the following clinical scenarios would hormone replacement therapy be contraindicated?

   (A) Breast cancer

   (B) Obesity

   (C) Stage III chronic kidney disease

   (D) Diabetes mellitus

   (E) History of hysterectomy

3. Which of the following is the correct trade name for tadalafil?

   (A) Viagra

   (B) Levitra

   (C) Cialis

   (D) Caverject

   (E) Proscar

4. Which of the following describes drugs most likely to cross the placenta?

   (A) High molecular mass (1,500 Da)

   (B) Highly protein bound

   (C) Highly lipophilic

   (D) Highly ionized

5. A 74-year-old man with benign prostatic hyperplasia (BPH) has taken terazosin for 6 months with some symptom improvement. He still complains of urinary urgency. His prostate size is 20 g and postvoid residual volume is 50 mL. Which medication is most appropriate in combination with his current treatment to address his symptoms?

    (A) Tolterodine
    (B) Dutasteride
    (C) Sildenafil
    (D) Saw palmetto

6. A 32-year-old woman with hypertension, headaches, and seasonal allergies expresses a desire to become pregnant. She is currently taking nifedipine 60 mg PO daily, lisinopril 10 mg daily, acetaminophen 500 mg 1–2 PRN Q 4–6 hours, and loratadine 10 mg daily. Which of the patient's medications is a known teratogen and should be discontinued prior to conception?

    (A) Nifedipine
    (B) Lisinopril
    (C) Acetaminophen
    (D) Loratadine

7. "Animal reproduction studies have failed to demonstrate a risk to the fetus, and there are as of yet no adequate, well-controlled studies in pregnant women." This statement describes which FDA pregnancy category?

    (A) Category A
    (B) Category B
    (C) Category C
    (D) Category D

8. A 24-year-old woman on a monophasic oral contraceptive informs you that she missed the last 2 doses of her contraceptive tablets in the first 2 weeks of the pack. In addition to using a back-up form of contraception for at least the next 7 days, which of the following is the most appropriate set of instructions to provide?

    (A) Take 1 extra dose today, the next dose at the regularly scheduled time, and resume 1 tablet daily.
    (B) Take 2 doses daily for next 2 days, then resume 1 tablet daily.
    (C) Take 1 tablet daily until Sunday, start a new pack without taking placebo pills.
    (D) Dispose of the current pack, wait until Sunday and restart a new pack on that day.

9. Which of the following contraceptives could be used safely in a 26-year-old woman who is 12 weeks postpartum and breastfeeding her baby?

   (A) Ortho Micronor
   (B) NuvaRing
   (C) Ovcon 35
   (D) Loestrin Fe

10. A 67-year-old man with BPH has an AUA-SI score of 10, prostate size of 15 g, and postvoid residual of 100 mL. He has a medical history of hypertension and cataracts and is scheduled to have cataract surgery in 2 weeks. Which of the following is the best recommendation?

   (A) Watchful waiting for 6 months
   (B) Initiate alfuzosin today
   (C) Initiate alfuzosin in 1 month
   (D) Initiate dutasteride today

ANSWERS

1. **E**

There is a major, life-threatening drug interaction between these two medications. When coadministered, the two agents can result in a life-threatening drop in blood pressure. All forms of nitroglycerin carry this risk, and coadministration should be avoided for *at least* 24 hours.

2. **A**

Hormone replacement therapy is contraindicated in patients with breast cancer due to the potential to exacerbate tumor growth. Obesity, kidney disease, and diabetes are not contraindications to hormone replacement therapy. Patients with a history of hysterectomy may take unopposed estrogen but do not need progestin.

3. **C**

Cialis is the trade name for tadalafil. Viagra is the trade name for sildenafil, Levitra is the trade name for vardenafil, Caverject is the trade name for alprostadil, and Proscar is the trade name for finasteride.

4. **C**

Greater fat solubility increases the likelihood that a drug will cross the placenta. Small molecular mass (<500 Da) agents are more likely to cross the placenta, as are drugs with lower degree of protein binding and drugs that are un-ionized.

5. **A**

Therapy with an anticholinergic drug such as tolterodine can be used in combination with alpha-blockers to treat symptoms of urinary urgency if the postvoid residual volume is below 250 mL. Dutasteride (B) is beneficial in combination with alpha-blockers in men with elevated prostate size (30–60 g or greater) and this patient's size is 20 g. Sildenafil (C) is appropriate for erectile dysfunction; however, phosphodiesterase inhibitors are reserved for patients that have not responded to conventional therapies, and tadalafil is the only currently FDA approved agent for LUTS associated with BPH. Saw palmetto (D) has limited evidence of benefit and would not be the best recommendation in this case.

6. **B**

ACE inhibitors such as lisinopril are pregnancy category D and are known to cause renal defects and restrict fetal growth patterns. Nifedipine (A) is classified as category C by the FDA but is endorsed and recommended by the ACOG guidelines as a potential first-line antihypertensive during pregnancy. Acetaminophen (C) and loratadine (B) have not demonstrated teratogenicity and are thought to be safe for use during pregnancy.

7. **B**

Category A: Adequate, well-controlled studies have failed to demonstrate a risk to the fetus in the first trimester of pregnancy (and there is no evidence of risk in later trimesters). Category B: Animal reproduction studies have failed to demonstrate a risk to the fetus and there are as of yet no adequate, well-controlled studies in pregnant women. Category C: Animal reproduction studies have shown an adverse effect on the fetus and there are no adequate and well-controlled studies in humans, but potential benefits may warrant use of the drug in pregnant women despite potential risks. Category D: There is positive evidence of human fetal risk based on adverse reaction data from investigational or marketing experience or studies in humans, but potential benefits may warrant use of the drug in pregnant women despite potential risks.

8. **B**

Taking 2 doses daily for the next 2 days, then resuming 1 tablet daily is appropriate. An extra dose today, then resuming 1 tablet daily (A) would be correct if the patient had missed only 1 dose but it will not provide enough contraceptive medication if she missed 2 doses. Starting a new pack on Sunday (C and D) would be appropriate if the patient had missed 3 or more doses or if she had missed 2 or more doses in the third week of the pack.

9. **A**

Progestin-only contraceptives such as Ortho Micronor are safe options during breastfeeding. NuvaRing (B), Ovcon 35 (C), and LoestrinFe (D) are all estrogen-containing contraceptives and cannot be used during breastfeeding.

10. **B**

The patient's AUA-SI score (≥8) warrants pharmacological treatment, thus watchful waiting (A) is incorrect. Alpha antagonists including alfuzosin (C) would be the appropriate first-line therapy; however, it should not be started until after the patient's cataract surgery. Alfuzosin has the potential to cause intraoperative floppy iris syndrome (IFIS) in patients undergoing cataract surgery. And 5 alpha reductase inhibitors such as dutasteride (D) are reserved for patients with prostate glands >30mL (30g); this patient's prostate size is 15g.

Solid Organ Transplant/ Immunosuppression

17

This chapter covers the following procedure:

- **Solid organ transplantation**

 Suggested Study Time: 30 minutes

SOLID ORGAN TRANSPLANTATION/IMMUNOSUPPRESSION

Definitions

Solid organ transplantation is a common treatment strategy for patients with organ failure. Immunosuppressive therapy is needed to prevent organ rejection and maintain graft function. Organs commonly transplanted include liver, kidney, heart, pancreas, and lung. Most commonly, transplants occur between individuals of the same species who are not genetically identical. These types of grafts are considered allograft transplants.

At the time of transplant, induction immunosuppression is needed to prevent acute graft rejection. *Hyperacute graft rejection* occurs within minutes to hours after the graft has been revascularized. *Acute graft rejection* usually occurs within the first 6 months after the transplant, but it may occur anytime post-transplant. Maintenance immunosuppression is then initiated and maintained for the life of the graft to reduce the risk of *chronic organ rejection*, which can occur months to years after transplant or acute rejection episodes. Chronic graft rejection may occur due to chronic inflammation or fibrotic vascular changes, which diminish the blood supply; over time, ischemia can lead to graft loss.

Induction therapy is used during the initial period post-transplant, when higher levels of overall immunosuppression are required to prevent acute graft rejection. Induction therapy requires selecting different combinations of therapies or using higher dosages of medications. Agents selected may include antibody therapies, intravenous (IV) corticosteroids, and other drugs. Maintenance therapy is used for the lifetime of the graft to reduce the risk of both acute and chronic organ rejection. Combinations of agents are selected and titrated to balance efficacy and toxicity.

Patients taking immunosuppressive therapies must be monitored for risk of infection, especially those who are taking multiple immunosuppressants, because overall immunosuppression is generally increased with the use of multiple immunosuppressive therapies. This encompasses any drug with immunosuppressive properties, including immunosuppressants used for oncologic or rheumatologic conditions.

Diagnosis

Diagnosis of acute organ rejection is dependent upon the specific organ that was transplanted. For acute renal allograft rejection, evidence of histologic changes, donor-specific antibodies, and antibody infiltration of endothelium are needed for diagnosis. Acute hepatic allograft rejection is diagnosed based on elevation of liver function tests and histologic changes.

Signs and Symptoms

Fever, malaise, and pain are nonspecific symptoms that may be seen with organ rejection. Hepatomegaly, abdominal pain, or jaundice may be present for hepatic rejection. Renal allograft rejection may present with rising serum creatinine levels, oliguria, graft pain, and hypertension.

Guidelines

There are no guidelines for immunosuppressive therapy. Regimens vary based on the organ, the patient population, and the transplant center.

Immunosuppressives

Generic	Brand	Dose & Max mg (frequency)	Contraindications	Primary Side Effects	Key Monitoring Parameters	Pertinent Drug Interactions	Med Pearls	Top 200
Mechanism of action — limits activity and volume of lymphatic system								
Prednisone		1–60 mg/day	• Hypersensitivity • Live vaccines • Systemic fungal infections	• Risk of infection • Hyperglycemia • Osteoporosis • Increased appetite • Irritability • Insomnia • Weight gain • Peptic ulcer disease • Hypertension	• S/S of graft rejection • S/S of infection • Glucose • BP • Electrolytes • Bone mass density • Intraocular pressure	• Live vaccines • CYP3A4 inducers and inhibitors • Other immunosuppressants	• Take with food • Taper if discontinuing high doses that have been used for long periods	Yes
Mechanism of action — inhibit inosine monophosphate dehydrogenase which blocks purine synthesis and lymphocyte function								
Mycophenolate mofetil	CellCept	PO and IV: 1–1.5 g BID	Hypersensitivity	• Diarrhea • Leukopenia • Anemia • Pain • Elevated LFTs • Increased SCr • Hypertension • Hypotension • Edema • Chest pain • Tachycardia • Headache • Insomnia • Rash • Increased risk of infection	• CBC • LFTs • SCr • S/S of graft rejection	• Live vaccines • Bile acid sequestrants • Cholestyramin • Other immunosuppressants	Take on an empty stomach	No
Mycophenolic acid	Myfortic	720 mg PO BID						No

Immunosuppressives *(cont'd)*

Generic	Brand	Dose & Max mg (frequency)	Contraindications	Primary Side Effects	Key Monitoring Parameters	Pertinent Drug Interactions	Med Pearls	Top 200
Mechanism of action – inhibit calcineurin (CNI) which inhibits the activation of T-cells and down regulation of interleukins and tumor necrosis factor-alpha								
Cyclosporine	• Neoral • Gengraf • SandIMMUNE	• PO: 7–10 mg/kg/day in 2 divided doses • IV: 3–7.5 mg/kg/day	Hypersensitivity	• Hypertension • Edema • Hypertrichosis • Hirsutism • Increased risk of infection • Tremor • Renal dysfunction • Dyslipidemia • Gingival hyperplasia	• Trough concentrations • BP • Renal function • Lipids • Electrolytes • S/S of infection	• Live vaccines • CYP 3A4 substrates • Inhibitors • Inducers • ACEI • Potassium sparing diuretics • Other immunosuppressants		No
Tacrolimus	• Prograf • Astagraf XL • Hecoria	• PO: 0.075–0.15 mg/kg/day in 2 divided doses • IV: 0.01–0.05 mg/kg/day continuous infusion	Hypersensitivity	• Hypertension • Edema • Chest pain • Headache • Insomnia • Pain • Fatigue • Diabetes mellitus • Dyslipidemia • Diarrhea • Abdominal pain • Renal dysfunction • Hepatic dysfunction • Increased risk of infection	• Renal function • Hepatic function • Electrolytes • Glucose • BP • Whole blood trough concentrations • S/S of graft rejection • S/S of infection	• Live vaccines • CYP 3A4 substrates • Inducers • Inhibitors • Potassium sparing diuretics • Other immunosuppressants	Must be consistent with taking medication with or without food	Yes

Immunosuppressives *(cont'd)*

Mechanism of action – inhibits mammalian target of rapamycin which inhibits the transduction of the signal generated by IL-2 binding to the IL-2 receptor which affects cell growth

Generic	Brand	Dose & Max mg (frequency)	Contraindications	Primary Side Effects	Key Monitoring Parameters	Pertinent Drug Interactions	Med Pearls	Top 200
Sirolimus	Rapamune	PO: 2–40 mg daily	Hypersensitivity	• Hypertension • Edema • Headache • Pain • Insomnia • Dyslipidemia • Constipation • Anemia • Renal dysfunction • Increased risk of infection	• LFTs • CBC • Lipids • BP • SCr • Serum drug concentrations • S/S of graft rejection • S/S of infection	• CYP3A4 inducers • P-gp inducers • Other immunosuppressants	Increased risk of nephrotoxicity if given in combination with CNIs	No
Everolimus	• Afinitor • Afinito • Disperz • Zortress	PO: 0.75–1 mg PO BID	Hypersensitivity	• Hypertension • Edema • Chest pain • Headache • Insomnia • Pain • Fatigue • Diabetes mellitus • Dyslipidemia • Diarrhea • Abdominal pain • Renal dysfunction • Hepatic dysfunction • Increased risk of infection • Impaired wound healing	• Renal function • Hepatic function • Electrolytes • Glucose • BP • Whole blood trough concentrations • S/S of graft rejection • S/S of infection	• Live vaccines • CYP 3A4 substrates • Inducers • Inhibitors • Grapefruit juice • Other immunosuppressants		No

Immunosuppressives *(cont'd)*

Generic	Brand	Dose & Max mg (frequency)	Contraindications	Primary Side Effects	Key Monitoring Parameters	Pertinent Drug Interactions	Med Pearls	Top 200
Antithymocyte globulin	Thymoglobulin (rabbit)	IV: 1.5 mg/kg/day for 7–14 days	• Hypersensitivity to antithymocyte globulin or rabbit proteins • Infection	• Chills • Fever • Headache • Malaise • Pain • Hypertension • Leukopenia • Thrombocytopenia • Dyspnea	• Lymphocytes • CBC with differential • Platelets • Vital signs • Signs and symptoms of graft rejection • Signs and symptoms of infection	• Live vaccines • Other immunosuppressants		No

Mechanism of action – selective T-cell costimulation inhibitor by binding to CD80 and CD86 receptors on antigen presenting cells

Generic	Brand	Dose & Max mg (frequency)	Contraindications	Primary Side Effects	Key Monitoring Parameters	Pertinent Drug Interactions	Med Pearls	Top 200
Belatacept	Nulojix	• 5–10 mg/kg dose • Rounded to the nearest 12.5 mg dosing increment	• Hypersensitivity • Seronegative or unknown Epstein-Barr virus status	• Risk of infection • Anemia • Leukopenia • Diarrhea • Constipation • Hypo- or hyperkalemia • Peripheral edema • Hypertension • Hypotension • Risk of post-transplant lymphoproliferative disorder (PTLD)	• S/S of graft rejection • S/S of infection or malignancy • Epstein-Barr virus status prior to therapy • Cognitive or neurological symptoms	• Live vaccines • Other immunosuppressants		No

Storage and Administration Pearls

- Refrigerate antithymocyte globulin powder (rabbit); do not freeze
- Stable for 24 hours if reconstituted at room temperature

Patient Education Pearls

- Avoid live vaccines in immunocompromised patients.
- Assess for signs of infection in immunocompromised patients.

Learning Points

Induction immunosuppression is administered at the time of transplant to prevent acute graft rejection.

- Maintenance immunosuppression is administered for the life of the graft to prevent chronic graft rejection.
- Immunosuppression increases the risk of infection in transplanted patients.
- Immunosuppressants may be administered as monotherapy or in conjunction with other immunosuppressants for solid-organ transplantation.
- Immunosuppression is increased with multiple immunosuppressive therapies, so pharmacists need to be aware of the risks to patients taking multiple immunosuppressants, even those for nontransplant indications.

PRACTICE QUESTIONS

1. Which of the following is an adverse effect associated with prednisone?

    (A) Hypoglycemia
    (B) Osteoporosis
    (C) Renal dysfunction
    (D) Thyroid dysfunction
    (E) Toxic epidermal necrolysis

2. Which of the following inhibits mammalian target of rapamycin?

    (A) Belatacept
    (B) Cyclosporine
    (C) Everolimus
    (D) Mycophenolate
    (E) Tacrolimus

3. Which of the following should be monitored for tacrolimus?

    (A) Blood glucose
    (B) Blood pressure
    (C) Drug levels
    (D) Hepatic function
    (E) All of the above

4. Which of the following should not be administered with cyclosporine?

    (A) Adacel
    (B) Engerix
    (C) Fluzone
    (D) Pneumovax
    (E) Zostavax

5. Which of the following must have Epstein-Barr serology tested before use?

    (A) CellCept
    (B) Nulojix
    (C) Prograf
    (D) SandIMMUNE
    (E) Thymoglobulin

ANSWERS

1. **B**

Long-term treatment with prednisone can result in osteoporosis, which necessitates screening of bone mineral density in those who chronically take prednisone. Prednisone causes hyperglycemia, so hypoglycemia (A) is incorrect. Prednisone is not associated with renal dysfunction (C), thyroid dysfunction (D), or toxic epidermal necrolysis (E).

2. **C**

Everolimus is an mTOR (mammalian target of rapamycin) inhibitor. Belatacept (A) is a selective T-cell costimulation inhibitor, and mycophenolate (D) inhibits inosine monophosphate dehydrogenase. Cyclosporine (B) and tacrolimus (E) are both calcineurin inhibitors.

3. **E**

Monitoring for tacrolimus includes blood glucose (A), blood pressure (B), trough concentrations (C), and hepatic function (D), as well as electrolytes, renal function, signs and symptoms of graft rejection, and signs and symptoms of infection.

4. **E**

Zostavax is a live attenuated vaccine that should not be used in patients taking immunosuppressive therapy due to the risk of disease occurrence caused by the vaccine. Adacel (Tdap) (A), Engerix (HepB) (B), Fluzone (influenza) (C), and Pneumovax (pneumococcal) (D) are inactivated vaccines and can be used in immunosuppressed patients.

5. **B**

Nulojix (belatacept) necessitates the patient to have virology test for the Epstein-Barr virus as patients without immunity (EBV seronegative) have an increased risk of posttransplant lymphoproliferative disorder.

Preventive Medicine 18

This chapter covers the following preventive health care measures:

- **Immunizations**
- **Weight loss**

 Suggested Study Time: **45 minutes**

IMMUNIZATIONS

Definitions

Vaccines provide immunization against multiple infectious diseases by stimulating an immune response and subsequent immunologic memory. Vaccines induce active immunity because they are composed of antigens that simulate exposure to an infectious disease caused by a virus or bacteria. Once the body identifies the foreign substance, the immune system creates antibodies to eliminate the pathogen.

Vaccines are categorized as live or inactivated. Live vaccines are made up of attenuated viruses or bacteria. Live vaccine pathogens have the ability to replicate in the body, but because they are weakened, they do not cause clinically significant disease. Immuno-compromised patients cannot safely receive live vaccines due to the potential for disease occurrence caused by the vaccine; immunocompromised patients include those with malignant neoplasms of the lymphatic system or bone marrow, patients with HIV or AIDS, and anyone receiving immunosuppression medications. Live vaccine can be given simultaneously or must be separated by at least 4 weeks to allow the body's immune response to adequately respond to the vaccine.

Inactivated vaccines are composed of inactivated or dead viruses or bacteria. There is no risk of contracting the disease from inactivated vaccines, but multiple doses may be needed to create or sustain immunity. Inactivated vaccine may be categorized as polysaccharides, polysaccharide conjugates, or toxoids. Polysaccharide vaccinations are not effective in those less than age 2 years due to the lack of memory B cell activity. There is also no additional immune response upon repeated vaccination for polysaccharide vaccines. Polysaccharide conjugated vaccines are polysaccharides linked to specific proteins which induces a better immune response in those less than 2 years of age. Toxoid vaccines are produced by the inactivation of a biological toxin.

Immunizations

Vaccine	Brand Name	Route	Contraindication	Adverse Effects	Target Population	Medication Pearls
Live vaccines						
Herpes zoster (shingles)	Zostavax	SC	• History of anaphylaxis to gelatin or neomycin • Immunosuppression or immunodeficiency	• Injection site reactions • Headache • Flu-like symptoms • Fever	Patients ≥60 years of age	Stored frozen
Live attenuated influenza	FluMist Quadrivalent	Intranasal	• Anaphylaxis to previous influenza vaccination • Hypersensitivity to egg protein • Children 2–17 years of age taking aspirin	• Runny nose • Nasal congestion • Fever • Sore throat • Headache • Decreased appetite • Weakness	All patients 2–49 years of age yearly	
Measles, mumps, rubella (MMR)	M-M-R II	SC	• Hypersensitivity to any vaccine component • Febrile illness • Immunosuppression or immunodeficiency • Pregnancy	• Injection site infections • Arthralgia • Myalgia • Rash	Children >12 months	
Rotavirus	• Rotarix • RotaTeq	Oral	• Hypersensitivity • History of intussusception • Severe combined immunodeficiency disease	• Fever • Diarrhea • Vomiting • Otitis media • Nasopharyngitis	• Infants and children 6–24 weeks (Rotarix) • Infants and children 2–32 weeks (RotaTeq)	
Varicella (chickenpox)	Varivax	SC	• Allergic reaction to vaccine, gelatin, or neomycin • Immunodeficiency or immunosuppression	• Injection site reaction • Rash • Fever • Malaise • Arthralgia	Children ≥12 months of age	

Immunizations *(cont'd)*

Vaccine	Brand Name	Route	Contraindication	Adverse Effects	Target Population	Medication Pearls
Inactivated vaccines						
Influenza	• Fluzone • Fluzone High-Dose • Fluarix • Fluarix Quadrivalent • FluLaval • FluLaval Quadrivalent • Fluvirin	IM or intradermal (Fluzone intradermal)	• Allergy to previous influenza vaccination • Allergy to eggs (except for Flucelvax)	• Fever • Malaise • Myalgia • Injection site reaction	All patients ≥6 months of age	Yearly vaccination to account for antigenic drifts and decreasing antibody levels over time
Diphtheria, tetanus, acelluar pertussis	• Daptacel • Infanrix (DTaP) • Adacel • Boostrix (Tdap) • Decavac (Td)		DTaP: serious allergic reaction to vaccine or encephalopathy within 7 days of previous vaccination	• Tetanus and diphtheria • Injection site reactions • Arthus reactions • Acellular pertussis: redness and swelling, fever	• DTaP: children 6 week–6 years of age • Tdap: single dose once >7 years of age or in third trimester of each pregnancy • Td: 1 dose every 10 years >11 years of age	Tdap is needed only once per lifetime, unless in each pregnancy
Human papillomavirus (HPV)	• Cervarix (HPV2) • Gardasil (HPV4)	IM	• Hypersensitivity • Allergy to yeast (Gardasil)	• Injection site reactions • Headache • Fever • Fatigue • Myalgia	• Females 9–26 years of age	If vaccinating males, HPV4 may be used
Streptococcus pneumoniae	• Pneumovax 23 (PPSV23) • Prevnar 13 (PCV13)	• IM: (PPSV23, PCV13) • SC: (PPSV23)	• Severe allergic reaction • Hypersensitivity	• Injection site reactions • Fever • Myalgia	• PCV13: children 2–59 months of age • PPSV23: patients >65 years of age, cigarette smokers, nursing home residents	• PPSV23 not indicated for children <2 years of age • Second dose of PPSV23 recommended for patients >65 years of age with previous dose given >5 years

Immunizations *(cont'd)*

Vaccine	Brand Name	Route	Contraindication	Adverse Effects	Target Population	Medication Pearls
Meningococcal	• Menomune (MPSV4) • Menveo (MCV4) • Menactra (MCV4)	• Menactra, Menveo: IM • Menomune: SC	• Hypersensitivity • Hypersensitivity to diphtheria toxoid (MCV4)	• Injection site reactions • Headache • Fever • Malaise	• MCV4: Adolescents 11–12 years of age with a booster dose after 5 years, can be used through age 55 • MPSV4: unvaccinated adults >56 years of age	MPSV4 should not be used in children <2 years of age
Hepatitis A	• Havrix • VAQTA	IM	• Hypersensitivity • Allergic reaction to vaccine or neomycin	• Injection site reactions • Fever	• Children 12–23 months of age • International travel other than Canada, Europe, Japan, New Zealand, or Australia • Men who have sex with men • Laboratory workers • Patients with chronic liver disease or clotting disorders	
Hepatitis B	• Engerix-B, Recombivax HB	IM	• Hypersensitivity • Allergy to previous hepatitis B vaccination	• Injection site reactions • Headache • Fatigue • Fever	• Infants at birth • Health care workers • International travel • Patients with multiple sexual partners • Diabetes mellitus • HIV • Liver disease • Renal disease	
Haemophilus influenza type B	• ActHIB • Hiberix • PedvaxHIB	IM	Hypersensitivity	Injection site reactions	All infants	Hiberix is used only as booster
Polio	IPOL	• IM • SC	Hypersensitivity	Injection site reactions	All infants >2 months of age	

Storage and Administration Pearls

- Tetanus, diphtheria, and acellular pertussis: Refrigerate, do not freeze; do not administer subcutaneously (SC)
- All influenza vaccinations: Refrigerate, do not freeze
- Varicella and herpes zoster: Must be kept frozen; unreconstituted powder must be used within 72 hours if refrigerated; reconstituted vaccine should be administered within 30 minutes or discarded
- HPV: Refrigerate, do not freeze; shake vial before administration
- MMR: May refrigerate or freeze vaccine; do not freeze diluent; vaccination should occur within 8 hours of reconstitution or be discarded
- PCV13 and PPSV23: Refrigerate, do not freeze
- Meningococcal: Refrigerate
- Hepatitis A and hepatitis B: Refrigerate, do not freeze; shake vaccination before administration
- Haemophilus influenza type B: Refrigerate, do not freeze; shake vaccination before administration
- Rotavirus: Refrigerate
- Polio: Refrigerate, do not freeze; shake vaccination before administration

WEIGHT LOSS

Definitions

Obesity is a chronic problem that increasing numbers of people are battling. Weight loss occurs with a net reduction in total caloric intake and may be accomplished with reduced calorie consumption or increased expenditure of energy.

To classify obesity, body mass index (BMI) is calculated as follows:

$$BMI = weight\ (kg)/[height\ (m)]^2$$

A BMI of <18.5 is considered underweight, and BMI of 18.5–24.9 is considered normal. People are considered overweight with a BMI of 25–29.9 and obese with BMI is >30. Obesity is furthered classified as stage I (BMI of 30–34.9), stage II (BMI of 35–39.9), and stage III (BMI ≥40).

Medications may be used to aid weight loss in conjunction with dietary and physical activity modifications. Weight must be monitored to ensure weight loss is occurring, or medication therapy should be modified or discontinued.

Guidelines

Jensen MD, Ryan DH, Donato KA, et al. Guidelines (2013) for managing overweight and obesity in adults. Obesity 2014;22(S2):S1–S410.

Guidelines Summary

Health care providers should evaluate a patient's BMI at each visit and create an individualized treatment plan. Weight loss plans need to include moderate caloric reduction, increased physical activity, and behavioral strategies that patients can use to sustain weight loss.

Drugs for Weight Loss

Generic	Brand	Dose	Contraindications	Primary Side Effects	Key Monitoring	Pertinent Drug Interactions	Med Pearls	Top 200
Mechanism of action – inhibits gastric and pancreatic lipase to inhibit dietary fat								
Orlistat	• Xenical • Alli (OTC)	• Xenical 120 mg TID with each meal • Alli 60 mg TID with each meal	• Hypersensitivity • Malabsorption • Pregnancy • Cholestasis	• Headache • Oily discharge/spotting • Fecal urgency • Back pain • Flatulence	• Weight • BMI • Glucose • Thyroid function	• Warfarin • Anticonvulsants • Cyclosporine • Vitamins A, D, E, K	Available OTC	No
Mechanism of action – stimulates hypothalamus to release NE (phentermine); suppresses appetite and increases satiety through inhibition of neuronal sodium channels and increased GABA activity (topiramate)								
Phentermine with topiramate	Qsymia	3.75 mg/23 mg–15/92 mg once daily	• Hypersensitivity to phentermine or sympathomimetics • Pregnancy • Hyperthyroidism • Glaucoma • MAOI use within 14 days	• Headache • Insomnia • Xerostomia • Constipation • Paresthesia • Pasopharyngitis	• Weight • HR • Serum bicarbonate • BP • SCr • Mood	• MAOIs • Orphenadrine • Amphetamines • carbonic anhydrase inhibitors		No
Mechanism of action – stimulates hypothalamus to release NE								
Phentermine	• Adipex-P • Suprenza	15–37.5 mg daily in 1–2 divided doses	• Hypersensitivity to phentermine or sympathomimetics • History of CVD • Pregnancy • Breast feeding • Hyperthyroidism • Glaucoma • MAOI use within 14 days • History of drug abuse	• Hypertension • Palpitation • Primary pulmonary hypertension • Euphoria • Dizziness • Insomnia • Psychosis • Constipation • Xerostomia • Tremor	• Weight • BP	• MAOIs • Carbonic anhydrase inhibitors • Linezolid • TCAs		Yes

Drugs for Weight Loss *(cont'd)*

Mechanism of action – activates 5HT2c receptors which stimulate POMC neurons that stimulate alpha-melanocortin-4 receptors which lead to increased satiety and decreased appetite

Generic	Brand	Dose	Contraindications	Primary Side Effects	Key Monitoring	Pertinent Drug Interactions	Med Pearls	Top 200
Lorcaserin	Belviq	10 mg BID	Pregnancy	• Headache • Hypoglycemia • Back pain • Upper respiratory tract infection	• Weight • CBC • Blood glucose • Prolactin levels • Mood • S/S of valvular heart disease	• Thioridazine • Antipsychotics • Ergot derivatives • Bupropion • Metoprolol • Tamoxifen • Serotonin modulators		No

Learning Points

- Live vaccines may be administered on the same day or must be separated by at least 4 weeks.
- Live vaccines should not be given to those with immunodeficiency or those who are receiving immunosuppression therapy.
- Caloric reduction and increased physical activity are mainstays for weight loss.
- Medications may be used to aid weight loss but should be used in conjunction with caloric reduction and increased physical activity.

PRACTICE QUESTIONS

1. Which of the following is indicated to prevent HPV infections?

   (A) Gardasil
   (B) Menomune
   (C) Prevnar 13
   (D) Rotarix
   (E) Zostavax

2. Which of the following is contraindicated in a patient taking tacrolimus?

   (A) Hepatitis B vaccine
   (B) Pneumococcal vaccine
   (C) Tdap vaccine
   (D) Varicella vaccine
   (E) All of the above

3. Which of the following should be monitored in a patient taking Qsymia?

   I. Weight
   II. Blood pressure
   III. Sedation

   (A) I only
   (B) III only
   (C) I and II only
   (D) II and III only
   (E) I, II, and III

ANSWERS

1. **A**

Gardasil is the vaccine that targets human papillomavirus types 6, 11, 16, and 18. Meno-mune (B) is the brand name of meningococcal vaccine. Prevnar (C) is the polysaccharide conjugate vaccine that targets pneumococcal disease. Rotarix (D) is the brand name for the rotavirus vaccine, and Zostavax (E) is the brand name for the herpes zoster vaccine.

2. **D**

Live vaccines are contraindicated in a patient receiving immunosuppressive therapies. Varicella is a live, attenuated vaccine that, if given to an immunocompromised patient, may cause infection with chickenpox. Vaccines against hepatitis B (A), pneumococcal (B), and Tdap (C) infection are all inactivated vaccines.

3. **C**

Qsymia is a combination of phentermine and topiramate. Due to the sympathomimi-etic activity of phentermine, blood pressure (II) should be monitored. Weight (I) is also monitored to ensure the effectiveness of the drug. Qysmia is associated with insomnia, so sedation (III) is generally not seen.

Clinical Lab Tests

19

This chapter covers clinical lab tests for the following:

- **Electrolytes and minerals**
- **Renal**
- **Hepatic**
- **Endocrine**
- **Cardiology**
- **Hematology**
- **Therapeutic drug levels**

 Suggested Study Time: **15 minutes**

Clinical lab tests are very important to pharmacists because they are commonly used to measure the safety and efficacy of medications. It is imperative that a pharmacist have a working knowledge of the most commonly used clinical lab tests in order to be able to recommend testing when necessary, and to interpret the results obtained. Education of the patient regarding clinical lab tests may also be a role of the pharmacist in some instances.

ELECTROLYTES AND MINERALS

Among the most common laboratory tests, electrolyte concentrations are used to detect and assess many medical conditions and are measured most commonly as part of a basic metabolic panel, or chem 7.

Substance	Normal Reference Range	Most Common Uses/Comments
Sodium	136–145 mEq/L	• May detect hypo- or hypernatremia • Used to monitor serum osmolality to determine total body water balance
Potassium	3.5–5.0 mEq/L	• May detect hypo- or hyperkalemia • Used primarily to monitor safety of medications and renal function
Chloride	96–106 mEq/L	• May detect hypo- or hyperchloremia • Used in evaluation of acid-based balance and to monitor for safety of medications
Magnesium	1.5–2.2 mEq/L	• May detect hypo- or hypermagnesemia
Calcium	8.5–10.8 mg/dL	• May detect hypo- or hypercalcemia • Used to monitor renal osteodystrophy • Requires correction with serum albumin <4 g/dL
Phosphate	2.6–4.5 mg/dL	• May detect hypo- or hyperphosphatemia • Monitored along with calcium for renal osteodystrophy

RENAL

The kidneys are the body's major filter of toxins. Thus, the renal system plays a large role in the maintenance of physiological homeostasis. The kidneys also serve the role of producing and activating substances that have an impact on red blood cell production, blood pressure regulation, and mineral metabolism.

The following represent the most commonly used lab assays for evaluation of renal function. Urinary sodium, potassium, and chloride as well as hematologic assays and electrolytes may also be used in the assessment.

Substance	Normal Reference Range	Comments
Serum creatinine (SCr)	0.7–1.4 mg/dL	• Excretion of creatinine closely estimates the glomerular filtration rate (GFR) • Elevated serum creatinine is indicative of decreased GFR • Serum creatinine is used in the Cockroft-Gault equation to calculate CrCl • May be inaccurate in the very elderly due to decreased muscle mass
Creatinine clearance (CrCl)	90–140 mL/min	• Estimate of GFR • Can be measured over 24 hours or calculated using serum creatinine and ideal body weight
Blood urea nitrogen (BUN)	8–20 mg/dL	• Used along with other labs to monitor hydration, renal function, protein tolerance, catabolism • Most commonly used in BUN:SCr ratio to determine hydration status and renal function
BUN:SCr	1:1–20:1	• >20:1 indicates dehydration in most patients
Urine microalbumin	<30 mg:g creatinine	• Microscopic protein that escapes into the urine when significant glomerular injury is present • Most commonly used to identify nephropathy in patients with diabetes

HEPATIC

The functions of the liver are numerous and varied. Some of the primary functions include the synthesis of bilirubin, coagulation factors, and albumin; amino acid and carbohydrate metabolism; and cholesterol synthesis. Along with these activities, the liver is also the primary site of metabolism for the majority of drugs and hormones. Hepatic assays are important in assessing the overall liver function and also in monitoring the safety of many medications.

The following represent the most commonly used lab assays for the assessment of hepatic function. Viral antigens and antibodies are not reviewed in this chapter.

Substance	Normal Reference Range	Comments
Albumin	3.5–5 g/dL	• Reflects liver's synthetic ability, nutritional status, and hydration; if low, should be factored into serum drug concentrations of highly protein bound drugs such as phenytoin
Total protein	5.5–8.3 g/dL	• Represents estimated sum of albumin and globulin measurements
Prothrombin time (PT)	10–13 seconds	• Represents the time needed for a series of events in coagulation cascade to occur • Helps to determine synthetic ability of liver; if elevated, indicates potential decreased production of clotting factors
Alkaline phosphatase (ALP)	Varies with assay used	• Used to detect hepatocellular injury but is not specific, so should be combined with other tests
Aspartate aminotransferase (AST)	8–42 IU/L	• Aminotransferases are the most frequently used assays in monitoring hepatic disease and are sensitive indicators of hepatic injury • Elevations indicate injury • Used often to monitor potential hepatic damage of medications
Alanine aminotransferase (ALT)	3–30 IU/L	
Total bilirubin	0.3–1 mg/dL	• Elevations may indicate hepatocellular injury, but test is not sensitive
Ammonia	30–70 mcg/dL	• Elevations indicate an inability of the liver to remove ammonia from the blood • Used to identify hepatic encephalopathy
Amylase	44–128 IU/L	• Most commonly used to diagnose acute pancreatitis
Lipase	<1.5 U/mL	• Most commonly used in the late diagnosis of acute pancreatitis (3–4 days postonset)

ENDOCRINE

Disorders of the endocrine system most commonly result from the deficiency or excess of a hormone. These hormones act as regulators within the body by stimulating or inhibiting biological responses. The most common endocrine disorder is diabetes mellitus (DM), which is discussed in detail in a previous chapter. Thyroid disorders are also common.

The assays listed below represent the most commonly used measurements to monitor diabetes and thyroid disorders, and the medications used to treat these disease states.

Substance	Normal Reference Range	Comments
Fasting plasma glucose (FPG)	70–100 mg/dL	• Most commonly used assay for diagnosis of DM; must be repeated on another day to confirm diagnosis • Patients may also self-monitor this value • Used for disease-state monitoring and adjustment of medication
2-Hour postprandial glucose	100–140 mg/dL	• May be measured as part of an oral glucose tolerance test (OGTT) or by the patient at home • Used for disease-state monitoring and adjustment of medication
A1c	4–6%	• Represents blood sugar over an approximate 90-day time frame • Most common lab test to monitor glycemic control in DM • May be inaccurate in cases of severe anemia • Not used in diagnosis of DM • Although 4–6% is normal range, <6.5–7% is the goal for a patient with DM • A1c correlation to plasma glucose: | A1c%	Mean Plasma Glucose (mg/dL)
---	---
6	126
7	154
8	183
9	212
10	240
11	269
12	298	
Free thyroxine (T4)	0.8–1.5 ng/dL	• Measures unbound T4 and is the most accurate representation of thyroid activity
Thyroid-stimulating hormone (TSH)	0.25–6.7 mcU/mL	• Low levels indicate hyperthyroid state; high levels indicate hypothyroid state • Used to monitor thyroid supplementation and need for dose adjustments

CARDIOLOGY

Laboratory tests are used both to detect and to monitor cardiac disorders. Because cardiovascular disease is the leading cause of death, it is imperative that pharmacists have a working knowledge of the markers used to evaluate these conditions.

The following measurements represent the most commonly used lab assays to detect acute cardiac conditions and to monitor chronic cardiac risk.

Substance	Normal Reference Range	Comments
Total cholesterol	<200 mg/dL	• Does not require that the patient fast but is most commonly measured as part of a complete fasting lipid panel • Not as useful as LDL and HDL in determining cardiovascular risk
Low-density lipoproteins (LDL)	Patient dependent-goals <160 mg/dL	• Highly atherogenic, known as "bad" cholesterol, used as the primary marker of cardiovascular risk • Higher values correlate with higher risk • Most often calculated rather than measured: LDL = Total cholesterol − HDL − Trigs/5 • Calculation inaccurate if triglycerides >400 mg/dL
High-density lipoproteins (HDL)	>40 mg/dL	• Antiatherogenic lipoprotein known as "good" cholesterol • Higher values associated with decreased cardiovascular risk
Triglycerides (Trigs)	<150 mg/dL	• High levels associated with cardiovascular risk • Very high levels associated with increased risk of pancreatitis
Troponin I	<1.5 ng/mL	• Elevated levels used to diagnose acute myocardial infarction (MI) • Elevation seen within 3–12 hrs and remain elevated for 5–10 days (I) or 5–14 days (T)
Troponin T	<0.1 ng/mL	
Creatine kinase–MB (CK–MB)	<12 IU/L	• Used to diagnose acute MI • Specific for cardiac tissue • Rises 3–12 hrs after onset and stays elevated for 2–3 days
B-type natriuretic peptide (BNP)	<100 pg/mL	• Secreted in response to cardiac stretching • Used to monitor heart failure
C-reactive protein (CRP)	≤1 mg/L	• Plasma protein synthesized by the liver • Biomarker of inflammation and cardiovascular risk
International normalized ratio (INR)	1.0	• Measure of coagulability • Goal is patient-dependent

HEMATOLOGY

The complete blood count (CBC) is among the most commonly ordered lab tests. The indices described below make up the CBC and are used to detect and monitor anemias and other hematologic disorders.

Indices	Normal Reference Range	Comments
Red blood cells (RBCs)	Males: 4.5–5.9 x 10^{12} cells/L Females: 4.1–5.1 x 10^{12} cells/L	• May be elevated in smokers
Hemoglobin (Hgb)	Males: 14–17.5 g/dL Females: 12.6–15.3 g/dL	• Indicates oxygen-carrying capacity of blood
Hematocrit (HCT)	Males: 42–50% Females: 36–45%	• Percentage of blood made up by erythrocytes; approximately 3 times Hgb
Mean cell volume (MCV)	80–96 fL/cell	• Hematocrit/RBC • Decreased in iron deficiency • Increased in vitamin B12 and folate deficiency
Mean cell hemoglobin concentration (MCHC)	33.4–35.5 g/dL	• Hgb/HCT • Decreased in iron deficiency
Reticulocyte count	0.5–2.5% of RBCs	• Reticulocytes are immature erythrocytes • Increased in blood loss (acute) • Decreased in iron deficiency and B12 and folate deficiency
RBC distribution width (RDW)	11.5–14.5%	• Variation in RBCs • Increased in iron deficiency
White blood cells (WBCs)	4.4–11 cells/mcL	• Made up of granulocytes and lymphocytes • Elevated in infection
Platelet count	150,000–450,000/mcL	• Important measure of coagulation

THERAPEUTIC DRUG LEVELS

Medications with narrow therapeutic indices and those with established therapeutic and/or toxic serum concentrations often require therapeutic drug monitoring. In general, serum concentrations are best obtained once the medication has reached steady state (in most cases a minimum of 5 elimination half-lives), just prior to an administered dose unless otherwise specified.

Drug	Therapeutic Concentration
Aminoglycosides: gentamicin, tobramycin	4–10 mcg/mL (peak) – efficacy, depending on the infection <0.5–2 mcg/mL (trough) – safety, for serious infections <1 mcg/mL (trough) – safety, for hospital-acquired pneumonia
Aminoglycosides: amikacin	25–40 mcg/mL (peak) – efficacy, for life-threatening infections 20–25 mcg/mL (peak) – efficacy, for serious infections 15–20 mcg/mL (peak) – efficacy, for urinary tract infections <8 mcg/mL (trough) – safety (the American Thoracic Society [ATS] recommends trough levels of <4–5 mcg/mL for patients with hospital-acquired pneumonia)
Vancomycin	20–40 mcg/mL (peak) – safety 5–10 mcg/mL (trough) – efficacy
Digoxin	0.5–1.5 ng/mL (inotropic effects) 0.8–2.0 ng/mL (chronotropic effects) >2 ng/mL (toxic)
Lidocaine	1.5–5 mcg/mL
Phenytoin	10–20 mcg/mL Must be corrected for hypoalbuminemia (Corrected phenytoin concentration = measured total concentration/[0.2*albumin] + 0.1)
Carbamazepine	4–12 mcg/mL
Valproic acid	50–100 mcg/mL
Phenobarbital	20–40 mcg/mL
Primidone	5–12 mcg/mL
Ethosuximide	40–100 mcg/mL
Cyclosporine	150–400 ng/mL
Lithium	0.6–1.5 mEq/L
Theophylline	10–20 mcg/mL

PRACTICE QUESTIONS

1. Which of the following lab tests is NOT used to monitor hepatic function?

    (A) Total protein
    (B) Ammonia
    (C) Prothrombin time
    (D) Alkaline phosphatase
    (E) Microalbumin

2. Which of the following is used to estimate glomerular filtration rate?

    (A) Ammonia
    (B) Blood urea nitrogen (BUN)
    (C) Serum creatinine
    (D) Urine microalbumin

3. Which enzyme is elevated within 3–12 hours of an acute myocardial infarction and remains elevated for up to 14 days?

    (A) Erythrocyte sedimentation rate (ESR)
    (B) Troponin I
    (C) Troponin T
    (D) Creatine kinase-MB (CKMB)

4. A peak vancomycin level is drawn. What is the best evaluation of the results?

    (A) 30 mcg/mL: Medication dose is safe.
    (B) 50 mcg/mL: Medication dose is safe.
    (C) 10 mcg/mL: Medication dose is effective.
    (D) 30 mcg/mL: Medication dose is effective.

5. A 60-year-old man (6'2", 220 lbs) with diabetes and history of venous thromboembolism (VTE) complains of redness and swelling in his left lower extremity. His current medications include warfarin 5 mg daily and metformin 1,000 mg BID. Lab results include serum creatinine 1.2 mg/dL, K 4.5, INR 2.5, WBC 15 cells/mcL, AST 18 IU/L, and ALT 20 IU/L. Based on the lab information available, what is the most likely cause of the patient's complaint?

    (A) VTE
    (B) Infection
    (C) Renal impairment
    (D) Liver impairment

ANSWERS

1. **E**

There are many tests used for the assessment of hepatic function. Total protein (A) represents the estimated sum of albumin and globulin that are produced by the liver. Ammonia (B) is removed from the blood by the liver, and elevations indicate the liver is not able to remove it. The prothrombin time (C) helps determine the liver's ability to make clotting factors under normal circumstances (without anticoagulant therapy). Alkaline phosphatase (D) is used to detect hepatocellular injury and is often combined with AST/ALT. Microalbumin (E) is actually a test of the kidneys and is elevated when glomerular injury is present. Therefore, (E) is correct.

2. **C**

The creatinine clearance is a close estimate to the glomerular filtration rate and is calculated using patient-specific factors including serum creatinine. Ammonia (A) is useful in evaluating liver function but not renal function. BUN (B) and urine microalbumin (D) are used for evaluating renal function but not, specifically, in estimating glomerular filtration rate.

3. **C**

Troponin T is elevated within 3–12 hours of an acute myocardial infarction (MI) and remains elevated for up to 14 days. ESR (A) is a marker of inflammation, but it is not specific to MI and does not rise rapidly in response to myocardial damage. While both Troponin I (B) and CKMB (D) increase within 3–12 hours of an acute MI, Troponin I remains elevated for a maximum of 10 days and CKMB for a maximum of 3 days, not 14 days.

4. **A**

It is appropriate to draw a peak level when assessing vancomycin safety. The safe therapeutic concentration range is 20–40 mcg/mL. Peak level of 50 mcg/mL (B) would be an unsafely high therapeutic concentration, while 10 mcg/mL (C) would be a low peak level and 30 mcg/mL (D) a normal peak level. None of the answer choices would be valuable for assessing efficacy of the medication, because peak levels are not used to assess efficacy. Troughs are used for that purpose. The reference range for troughs is 5–10 mcg/mL.

5. **B**

Elevated WBCs are indicative of infection. Although the patient has a history of venous thromboembolism (A), his INR is within the therapeutic/goal range for a patient with a history of VTE, making that less likely as the cause of his left lower extremity's redness and swelling. Etiology of renal impairment (C) is unlikely because the patient's calculated creatinine clearance is within normal range, and etiology of liver impairment (D) is unlikely because available liver enzymes (AST and ALT) are within the normal reference range.

Over-the-Counter Medications

20

This chapter covers the following drug classes:

- **Top 10 herbals and supplements**
- **Decongestants**
- **Antihistamines and proton pump inhibitors**
- **Cough suppressants**
- **Antidiarrheals**
- **Constipation medications**
- **Athlete's foot medications**

The text also provides an overview of basic treatment for common ailments treatable by pharmacists. This chapter also makes recommendations as to when self-treatment is not appropriate.

 Suggested Study Time: **75 minutes**

TOP 10 HERBALS AND SUPPLEMENTS

Definitions

Assessing herbals and supplements is important for medication therapy management. Data suggest that 1 in every 5 adults in the United States reports having used a natural product at least once in the previous 12 months.

The Dietary Supplement Health and Education Act of 1994 categorizes herbals, vitamins, protein bars, and shakes as dietary supplements. As a result, manufacturers are not required to demonstrate safety, purity, or efficacy of supplements. Labeling must include the FDA statement: "This statement has not been evaluated by the Food and

Drug Administration. This product is not intended to diagnose, treat, cure, or prevent any disease." Manufacturers cannot make specific claims on labels. The use of phrases such as "helps boost, support, enhance" are acceptable, though they essentially mislead the public and generate the need for healthcare assistance. It is important that you recommend only products that have undergone a standardization assurance.

Common Usage

- Saw palmetto
  - Used in men to improve symptoms of benign prostatic hyperplasia (BPH)
  - Meta-analysis data does not support clinical use
- Glucosamine and chondroitin
  - Used widely for treating osteoarthritis and joint structure support
  - Glucosamine: A precursor molecule important for maintaining elasticity, strength, and resiliency of the cartilage in articular (movable) joints
  - Chondroitin: A substance that promotes flexibility of cartilage
- Fish oils or omega-3 fatty acids
  - Used primarily for hypertriglyceridemia
  - Contain eicosapentaenoic acid (EPA) and docosahexaenoic acid (DHA), and are believed to be efficient in many people
- St. John's wort
  - Used for mild to moderate depression
  - Used in Europe for centuries for mild to moderate depression and its efficacy is comparable with tricyclic antidepressants; one study suggests it is no more effective than a placebo or sertraline in moderate to severe depression; it should not be used with other selective serotonin reuptake inhibitors (SSRIs).
- CoEnzyme Q10
  - Used for cardiovascular diseases, including angina, heart failure, and hypertension, and may help with myalgias due to statin therapy
- Melatonin
  - Used for insomnia, particularly when adjusting to shift-work cycles or jet lag
  - Naturally secreted from the pineal gland and appears to be the sleep-regulating hormone of the body; adults experience about a 37% decline in daily melatonin output between 20 and 70 years of age
- Echinacea
  - Used as an immune stimulant
  - Has been studied extensively in the area of flu and cold prevention/treatment

- Black cohosh
  - Used for women's health problems, especially postmenopausal symptom relief and painful menses
  - Should be avoided in pregnancy and lactation
- Ginger
  - Used primarily for motion sickness, dyspepsia, and nausea
  - Lacks sedative affects of other antinausea treatments
  - Has been studied in pregnant women at less than 17 weeks' gestation
- Ginkgo biloba
  - Used for vascular dementia, Alzheimer's, and ischemic stroke
  - The ginkgolides are potent platelet-activating factor (PAF) antagonists
- Ginseng
  - Used to treat diabetes mellitus
  - Thought to also help with decreasing mental and physical stress

Over-the-Counter Medications

Generic	Brand	Dose & Max mg (frequency)	Contra-indications	Primary Side Effects	Key Monitoring Parameters	Pertinent Drug Interactions	Med Pearls
Mechanism of action – inhibits production of dihydrotestosterone (DHT), inhibits receptor binding, and accelerates the metabolism of DHT							
Serenoa repens	Saw palmetto	Prostate: 160 mg BID	• Pregnancy or lactation • Age <12 years	Transient nausea, vomiting, and gastrointestinal (GI) distress	Improvements in BPH symptoms	• Oral contraception • Estrogens • Finasteride and dutasteride • Warfarin	• Data from meta-analysis does not support use
Mechanism of action – glucosamine is an amino-sugar that is naturally produced and is a key substrate in the synthesis of macromolecules for connective tissues; chondroitin absorbs water, adding to cartilage thickness, and is found in natural physiologic connective tissue; inhibits synovial enzymes that may contribute to cartilage destruction							
Glucosamine/ chondroitin	Osteo Bi-Flex	• Gluc: 500 mg TID • Chon: 400 mg TID	• Gluc: allergy to shellfish • Chon: Hx of bleeding	• GI discomfort • Increased glucose • Increased bleeding time	• Arthritis pain • Glucose • Aspirin • Warfarin	Gluc: insulin and oral diabetes medications	Chon: discontinue 14 days before dental procedure
Mechanism of action – inhibition of diacylglycerol transferase, reduction in hepatic synthesis of triglycerides							
Omega-3 fatty acids	Fish Oils	Triglycerides 500–3,000 mg/day	• Active bleeding • Hx of anticoagulants	• GI upset • Loose stools • Nausea • Decrease glucose • Lower BP	• Hypoglycemia • BP	• Warfarin • Aspirin • Antiplatelet agents	Mainly for treatment of triglycerides
Mechanism of action – increases concentrations of serotonin in the central nervous system (CNS) and may have some monamine oxidase (MAO) inhibition affects							
Hypericum perforatum	St. John's wort	300 mg TID	• Pregnancy • Severe depression • MAOI contraindications	N/V	• Depression symptoms • International normalized ratio (INR) if on warfarin	• CYP450 3A4 inducer • Cyclosporine, azoles, statins • Digoxin, lithium, serotonin modulators, oral contraceptives	Min of 4–6 wks of therapy is recommended before results seen
Mechanism of action – involved in adenosine triphosphate (ATP) generation and serves as a lipid-soluble antioxidant providing protection against free-radical damage within the mitochondria							
Ubiquinone	CoEnzyme Q10	20–300 mg/day	• Concurrent use with doxorubicin	• Abdominal discomfort • Headache • N/V	Bleeding time	Warfarin	

Over-the-Counter Medications *(cont'd)*

Generic	Brand	Dose & Max mg (frequency)	Contra-indications	Primary Side Effects	Key Monitoring Parameters	Pertinent Drug Interactions	Med Pearls
Mechanism of action—supplements the naturally deficient concentrations of melatonin							
N-acetyl-5-methoxy-tryptamine	Melatonin	1–5 mg at bedtime	Autoimmune disease	Morning sedation or drowsiness	INR with warfarin use	• CYP450 1A2 inhibitor • Theophylline • Caffeine • Clozapine 2C9 • Warfarin	Drugs that deplete vitamin B6 may inhibit the ability of the body to synthesize melatonin
Mechanism of action – may stimulate white blood cell function, including cell-mediated immunity							
Echinacea purpurea/angustifolia/pallida	Echinacea	50–1,000 mg TID on day 1, then 250 mg QID	• Use for more than 10 days in acute infections • Immunosuppressed patients • Pregnancy		• Electrolytes • Improvements in symptoms	• CYP450 3A4 inhibitor • Cyclosporine • Tacrolimus, sirolimus • Methotrexate • Corticosteroids	Prophylaxis therapy should be 3 wks on, 1 wk off
Mechanism of action – contains phytoestrogens, which mimic estrogen							
Cimicifuga racemosa	Black cohosh	20–40 mg BID	• Hx of estrogen-dependent tumors • Endometrial cancer • Pregnancy • Aspirin sensitivity	• N/V • Hypotension • Headaches • Hepatotoxicity	• BP • Serum hormones at baseline and 6 mos	• Oral contraceptives • Hormone replacement therapy (HRT) • Nonsteroidal anti-inflammatory drugs (NSAIDs) • Anticoagulants	
Mechanism of action – has local affects at the GI tract and in the CNS							
Zingiber officinale	Ginger	250 mg TID with food	Active bleeding	Very few side effects	Increased bleeding time	• Warfarin • Aspirin • NSAIDs	

Over-the-Counter Medications *(cont'd)*

Generic	Brand	Dose & Max mg (frequency)	Contra-indications	Primary Side Effects	Key Monitoring Parameters	Pertinent Drug Interactions	Med Pearls
Mechanism of action – the flavonoid component of gingko protects neurons and retinal tissue from oxidative stress and injury							
Ginkgo biloba	Ginkgo biloba	120–240 mg/day divided into 2–3 doses	• Pregnancy • Bleeding disorders • Seizures • 2 weeks prior to surgery	• GI effects • Headache • Dizziness • Skin reactions • Bleeding	• INR • Blood glucose	• Anticoagulants • Trazodone • NSAIDs • Anticonvulsants	
Mechanism of action – thought to reduce postprandial glucose levels and stimulate the release of insulin							
Panax quinquefolius	Ginseng	• Usual: 100–400 mg/day • Diabetics: up to 3 g/day, 2 hours before a meal	• Pregnancy • Patients taking warfarin	• Insomnia • Headache • Anorexia • CNS stimulation	• BP • Menstrual cycles	• Glucose-lowering drugs • Phenelzine • Anticoagulants • Antiplatelets • MAOIs	• Duration should be limited to 3 months • Can interfere with blood glucose lab tests

DECONGESTANTS

Definitions

Vasoconstrictive agents serve multiple roles in patient care including hemorrhoids, hypotension, ocular procedures and redness, and nasal congestion. Decongestants are the mainstay of therapy for colds and play an important role with allergic rhinitis. Nasal congestion can be treated with topical or oral adrenergic-agonist decongestants. Available agents include alpha- and beta-adrenergic agonists (pseudoephedrine), alpha1-adrenergic agonists (phenylephrine and naphazoline), and alpha-adrenergic agonists (oxymetazoline). This agonist effect causes vasoconstriction, which reduces the vascular blood supply to the sinuses, relieving intranasal pressure and reducing mucosal edema and mucus production. Decongestants are indicated for temporary relief of nasal congestion and cough associated with postnasal drip. They are no longer approved for sinusitis. Most recently, the FDA does not recommend over-the-counter (OTC) medications for children under the age of 2 years and includes decongestants because of the increased risk of death.

Signs and Symptoms

- Sinusitis
  - Tenderness over the sinuses; facial pain aggravated by postural changes; fever >101.5°F; tooth pain; halitosis; upper respiratory tract symptoms for >7 days with poor response to decongestants
- Common cold
  - Sore throat; nasal congestion; rhinorrhea; sneezing; common, low-grade fever; chills; headache; malaise; myalgia; cough
- Postnasal drip
  - Continued mucus accumulation in the back of the nose and throat leading to or giving the sensation of mucus dripping downward from the back of the nose

Guidelines

American Pharmaceutical Association. *Handbook of Nonprescription Drugs: An Interactive Approach to Self-Care*, 17th ed., 2011.

Adverse Effects

Appropriate FDA-approved doses should be used at all times since overdoses can cause excessive central nervous system stimulation and paradoxical depression. It is important to recognize any drug interactions that can occur with certain medications. The use of decongestants is contraindicated in patients taking MAO inhibitors. The main adverse effects of oral decongestants are cardiovascular stimulation and central nervous system stimulation.

Guidelines Summary

- A pharmacist may appropriately recommend a decongestant once the patient is excluded from the following:
  - Fever >101.5°F
  - Chest pain
  - Shortness of breath
  - Hypertension, arrhythmias, insomnia, and anxiety
  - Worsening of symptoms or development of additional symptoms during self-treatment
  - Concurrent underlying chronic cardiopulmonary disease
  - AIDS or chronic immunosuppressant therapy
  - Frail patients of advanced age
  - Children less than 2 years of age
  - Current medications such as MAOIs
- Topical decongestants should not be recommended for longer than 3 days due to the risk of rhinitis medicamentosa, a condition of rebound nasal congestion brought on by overuse of intranasal vasoconstrictive medications.

Decongestants

Oral decongestants

Mechanism of action – alpha-adrenergic stimulator with weak beta-adrenergic activity

Generic	Brand	Dose & Max mg (frequency)	Contra-indications	Primary Side Effects	Key Monitoring Parameters	Pertinent Drug Interactions	Med Pearls
Phenylephrine	• Neo-synephrine • Numerous others	• Topical: 1–2 sprays q4 hrs • Oral: 10–20 mg q4 hrs	• Uncontrolled hypertension • Ventricular tachycardia • Narrow-angle glaucoma • MAOI therapy within 14 days	• Restlessness • Hypertension • Tremor • Tachycardia • Insomnia	• BP • Pulse • Anxiety • Response to therapy	• MAOIs • Tricyclic antidepressants (TCAs) and methyldopa may enhance vasopressor effect	Avoid using with, or within 14 days of, MAOI therapy
Pseudoephedrine	• Sudafed • Numerous others	Oral: 240 mg/24 hrs					

Topical decongestants

Generic	Brand	Dose & Max mg (frequency)	Contra-indications	Primary Side Effects	Key Monitoring Parameters	Pertinent Drug Interactions	Med Pearls
Oxymetazoline	• Afrin • Numerous others	• Intranasal: 2–3 sprays BID • Ophthalmic: 1–2 drops q6 hrs	• Hypersensitivity • Narrow-angle glaucoma	• Hypertension • Palpitation • Stinging	• Rebound congestion • BP	MAOIs	Not recommended for longer than 3 days
Naphazoline	Naphcon	• Nasal: 1–2 drops q6 hrs • Ophthalmic: 1–2 drops q6 hrs				• MAOIs • TCAs and methyldopa may enhance vasopressor effect	

ANTIHISTAMINES AND PROTON PUMP INHIBITORS

Definitions

Antihistamines can be used for multiple roles in patient care, including contact dermatitis, allergic rhinitis, common colds, insomnia, heartburn, and nausea and vomiting.

Stimulation of histamine-1 receptors produces sneezing, pruritus, and mucus production. Histamine-2 receptors result in stomach acid production.

Antihistamines against H_1 receptors are classified as either sedating (first-generation, nonselective) or nonsedating (second-generation, peripherally selective). Second-generation antihistamines are nonsedating because they do not cross the blood-brain barrier. These agents are commonly used to treat allergic rhinitis and common cold symptoms. H_2 receptor antagonists (H2RAs) are used to decrease gastric acid secretion by inhibiting histamine production of parietal cells. These agents are used to treat heartburn. Another class of drugs used to treat heartburn is proton pump inhibitors (PPIs). PPIs have more potent and prolonged effects than H2RAs, and therefore are indicated in more frequent, severe heartburn. They work by inhibiting H/K/ATPase, or the proton pump, which irreversibly blocks gastric acid secretion.

Signs and Symptoms

- Contact dermatitis: Papules, vesicles, erythema, crusting, and oozing
- Allergic rhinitis: Nasal stuffiness, rhinorrhea usually clear, pruritus of nose, sneezing, watering eyes, nasal drainage
- Common colds: Nasal stuffiness, sneezing, scratchy throat, cough, hoarseness, headache, fever
- Insomnia: Difficulty initiating sleep at usual time and/or wakefulness during usual sleep cycle, daytime tiredness
- Heartburn: Stomach and chest pain, choking with swallowing, relief with solids or liquids

Guidelines

American Pharmaceutical Association. *Handbook of Nonprescription Drugs: An Interactive Approach to Self-Care*, 17th edition, 2011.

Guidelines Summary

- Contact dermatitis
  - Identify the cause: chemical, acids, solvent, fragrances, metals, poison ivy, etc.
  - Clean the area with mild soap and water.

- Refer patient to physician if the rash causes edema or invades the eyelids, external genitalia, anus, or massive areas of the body.
- Treatment includes topical treatment with hydrocortisone, bicarbonate pastes, and antihistamines.
■ Allergic rhinitis and common cold
  - Once the patient is excluded from the following, treatment recommendations can occur:
    » Symptoms of otitis media or sinusitis
    » Symptoms of lower respiratory tract infection
    » History of nonallergic rhinitis
■ Insomnia
  - Transient or short-term insomnia but no underlying problems are okay to self-treat.
  - Discuss good sleep hygiene practices—no caffeine after 5 P.M., no exercise in the evening.
  - If diphenhydramine is recommended, it should be taken at bedtime only as needed.
  - Patients who complain of continuing insomnia after 14 days of treatment should be referred to a physician.
■ Heartburn
  - Patient must be assessed for the following issues prior to self-treatment:
    » Frequent heartburn for more than 3 months
    » Heartburn while taking histamine-2 receptor agonist (H2RA) or proton pump inhibitor (PPI) or after initiating either one for 2 weeks
    » Nocturnal heartburn
    » Difficulty swallowing solid foods
    » Vomiting up blood or black material; or black, tarry stools
    » Chronic hoarseness, wheezing, coughing, choking
    » Unexplained weight loss
    » Pregnancy and nursing mothers
  - If the patient is a candidate, any of the following treatments are available—including antacids, which provide rapid relief versus the oral tablets, which have a slower onset of action.

Antihistamines

First-generation histamine H₁ antagonist

Mechanism of action – competes with histamine for H_1 receptor sites on effector cells in the GI tract, blood vessels, and respiratory tract

Generic	Brand	Dose & Max mg (frequency)	Contra-indications	Primary Side Effects	Key Monitoring Parameters	Pertinent Drug Interactions	Med Pearls
Clemastine	Tavist	• 1.34 mg TID (max = 8.04 mg/day)	• Narrow-angle glaucoma • Hypersensitivity	• Sedation • Anticholinergic effects • Dry mouth • Constipation • Blurred vision • Urinary retention	Mental alertness	Anticholinergic agents	Paradoxic reactions may be seen
Chlorpheniramine	Chlor-Trimeton	• 4 mg q4–6 hrs (max = 24 mg/day)					
Brompheniramine	• Dimetapp • Numerous others	1–2 tabs admin BID	• Hypersensitivity • MAOI within 14 days • Narrow-angle glaucoma • Breastfeeding • Peptic ulcer disease				
Diphenhydramine	• Benadryl • Sominex • ZzzQuil	• Allergic: 25–50 mg q6–8 hrs (max = 400 mg/day) • Insomnia: 50 mg at bedtime as needed	• Acute asthma • Hypersensitivity			• Acetylcholinesterase inhibitors • 2D6 substrates codeine, tramadol • Anticholinergic agents	
Doxylamine	Unisom	50 mg at bedtime as needed	Hypersensitivity				

Antihistamines (cont'd)

Second-generation histamine H$_1$ antagonist

Mechanism of action – long-acting tricyclic antihistamine with selectivity at H$_1$-receptor antagonistic properties; less blood-brain barrier penetration

Generic	Brand	Dose & Max mg (frequency)	Contra-indications	Primary Side Effects	Key Monitoring Parameters	Pertinent Drug Interactions	Med Pearls
Loratadine	Claritin	10 mg/day	Hypersensitivity	• Some sedation • Headache • Dizziness	• Relief of symptoms • Some sedation • Anticholinergic effects	Increased toxicity with CNS depressants and anticholinergics	Available in combination with pseudoephedrine
Cetirizine	Zyrtec	5–10 mg/day					
Azelastine	Astapro	Nasal spray: 1–2 sprays per nostril 2 × daily	Hypersensitivity	• Bitter taste • Nasal burning	Relief of symptoms		Prime before initial use or after 3 days of storage
Fexofenadine	Allegra	60 mg BID or 180 mg once daily	Hypersensitivity	• Headache • Fatigue	Relief of symptoms	Anticholinergic agents	Avoid taking with fruit juices

Antihistamines *(cont'd)*

Histamine H₂ antagonist

Mechanism of action — competitive inhibition of histamine at H_2 receptors of the gastric parietal cells, resulting in reduced gastric acid secretion

Generic	Brand	Dose & Max mg (frequency)	Contra-indications	Primary Side Effects	Key Monitoring Parameters	Pertinent Drug Interactions	Med Pearls
Cimetidine	Tagamet	400 mg/day (OTC)	Hypersensitivity	• Gynecomastia • Increased liver function tests (LFTs) • Stevens-Johnson syndrome	• LFTs • Serum creatine (SCr) • Complete blood count (CBC) • GI bleeding	• CYP450 inhibitor • 2D6, 1A2, 2C19 • ↓ absorption of acid dependent drugs	• Shorter half-life • Renal adjustment required
Ranitidine	Zantac-OTC	Tabs: 75 mg or 150 mg BID		• Arrhythmias • Dizziness • Leukopenia • Aplastic anemia	• Bone density • Relief of symptoms	↓ absorption of acid-dependent drugs	Renal adjustment required
Famotidine	• Pepcid AC • Pepcid Complete	OTC: 10–20 mg BID		• Headache • Dizziness		↓ absorption of acid-dependent drugs	• Renal adjustment required • Pepcid Complete contains calcium carbonate, magnesium
Nizatidine	Axid AR	75 mg BID		Thrombocytopenia		• CYP450 • Inhibits 3A4	Renal adjustment required

Mechanism of action – PPI; suppresses gastric basal and stimulated acid secretion by inhibiting the parietal cell H+/K ATP pump

Generic	Brand	Dose & Max mg (frequency)	Contra-indications	Primary Side Effects	Key Monitoring Parameters	Pertinent Drug Interactions	Med Pearls
Omeprazole	Prilosec OTC	20 mg/day	Hypersensitivity	• Increased LFTs • Headache • D/N	• Bone density • Relief of symptoms	• CYP450 • Inhibits: 1A2, 2C9, 2C19, 2D6, 3A4 • Induces: 1A2 • ↓ absorption of acid-dependent drugs	Treatment up to 14 days
Lansoprazole	Prevacid	15 mg/day		• Abdominal pain • Headache • Increased LFTS	• CBC • Liver function • Renal function • Bone density	• CYPC19 • Indinavir • Iron salts • Azoles • ↓ absorption of acid-dependent drugs	Treatment up to 14 days
Omeprazole and sodium bicarbonate	Zegerid	20 mg & 1,100 mg		Same as omeprazole	Relief of symptoms	• Omeprazole: same as above • Sodium bicarbonate: delavirine and nelfinavir • ↓ absorption of acid-dependent drugs	Sodium bicarbonate 1,100 mg = 300 mg = 13 mEq per capsule

COUGH SUPPRESSANTS

Definitions

A cough is caused by irritants or stimuli stimulating receptors located throughout the respiratory tract. The larynx is more sensitive than the trachea and bronchi. When activated, the receptors send signals through the brain-stem reflex pathway, the voluntary cerebral cortex pathway, or both. The signals eventually end up in the "cough center" of the medulla oblongata. The overall objective is to expel the irritant or stimuli.

Diagnosis

- A cough can be classified in the following ways:
  - Acute: duration less than 3 weeks
    - » Most commonly caused by a virus
  - Subacute: duration greater than 3 to 8 weeks
    - » Caused by infection, bacterial sinusitis, asthma
  - Chronic – duration longer than 8 weeks
    - » Smoking, post nasal drip, asthma, and gastroesophageal reflux disease (GERD)
- Angiotensin-converting enzymes (ACE) cause a dry cough in 20% or more of treated patients.
- Systemic and ophthalmic B-adrenergic blockers may cause cough in chronic obstructive pulmonary disease (COPD) patients.

Signs and Symptoms

- Productive
  - A wet or "chesty" cough, which expels secretions from the lower respiratory tract
  - Secretions may be clear, purulent, discolored, or malodorous
- Nonproductive
  - A dry or "hacking" cough that serves no useful physiologic purpose
  - Nonproductive coughs are caused by viral respiratory tract infections, atypical bacteria, GERD, cardiac disease, and some medications.

Guidelines

American Pharmaceutical Association. *Handbook of Nonprescription Drugs: An Interactive Approach to Self-Care*, 17th ed., 2011.

Guidelines Summary

- The primary goal of treating a cough is to reduce the number and severity of cough episodes.
- Codeine and dextromethorphan are the drugs of choice for nonproductive cough.
- Diphenhydramine is a better choice for coughs associated with allergies but is highly sedating.
  - Consider loratadine and/or cetirizine, as there is less sedation.
- Guaifenesin is marketed only as an expectorant and should not be used to treat effectively productive coughs.
- Patients should be excluded from self-treatment if they have any of the following:

Cough with thick yellow sputum or green phlegm	Fever >101.5°F	Unintended weight loss
Drenching nighttime sweats	Hemoptysis	History of asthma, COPD, CHF
Foreign-object aspiration	Cough greater than 7 days	Cough worsens during self-treatment

Cough Suppressants

Generic	Brand	Dose & Max mg (frequency)	Contra-indications	Primary Side Effects	Key Monitoring Parameters	Pertinent Drug Interactions	Med Pearls
Mechanism of action – serves as antitussive agent by depressing the medullary cough center							
Dextromethorphan	• Robitussin • Delsym • Several others	• Cough: 10–20 mg q4 hrs or 30 mg q6–8 hrs • ER: 60 mg BID (max = 120 mg/day)	Do not use within 2 wks of an MAOI	• Confusion • Irritability	Relief of symptoms	MAOIs	• Withdrawn from OTC market for children under age 2 • Chemically related to morphine; lacks narcotic properties except in overdose
Mechanism of action – expectorant; irritates the gastric mucosa and stimulates respiratory tract secretions, thereby increasing fluid volumes and decreasing mucous viscosity							
Guaifenesin	• Mucinex • Several other combination products	• IR: 200–400 mg q4 hrs • ER: 600–1,200 mg BID (max = 2.4 g/day)	Hypersensitivity	• Dizziness • Drowsiness • Kidney stone formation	Relief of symptoms	None	More effective with water intake
Mechanism of action – causes cough suppression by direct central action in the medulla; produces CNS depression							
Codeine phosphate		10–20 mg q4–6 hrs (max = 120 mg/day)	• Pregnancy • Hypersensitivity • Acute asthma	• N/V • Constipation • Sedation	• LFTs • CNS depression • Relief of symptoms	• CYP450 • 2D6 inhibitor • Alcohol	10% of a codeine dose is demethylated in the liver to form morphine

ANTIDIARRHEALS

Definitions

Diarrhea is defined as an abnormal increase in stool frequency or liquidity. Each individual has a different frequency, which is affected by many variables. The typical range of stool frequency can be three times per day to once every 2 days. More than three bowel movements per day is considered to be abnormal.

Diagnosis

- Diarrhea is defined and characterized by more than three bowel movements in 1 day.
- Diarrhea may be acute, persistent, or chronic in nature.
- Acute diarrhea is defined as an episode of less than 14 days' duration.
- Persistent diarrhea is diarrhea of 14-day to 4-week duration.
- Chronic diarrhea lasts more than 4 weeks.

Signs and Symptoms

- Abdominal pain, cramping, and frequency are signs.
- Stool is approximately 75% water and 25% solid material.
- Stool contains unabsorbed food residue and minerals, bacteria, desquamated epithelial cells.

Guidelines

American Pharmaceutical Association. *Handbook of Nonprescription Drugs: An Interactive Approach to Self-Care*, 17th edition, 2011.

Guidelines Summary

- Acute diarrhea can be managed with fluids, electrolyte replacement, dietary interventions, and nonprescription drug treatment.
- Persistent and chronic diarrhea requires medical care, and patients are not candidates for self-treatment if this is present.
- Patients should be excluded from self-treatment if any of the following apply:
  - <6 months of age
  - Severe dehydration
  - >6 months of age with persistent high fevers greater than 102.2°F
  - Blood, mucus, or pus in the stool
  - Protracted vomiting, severe abdominal pain
  - Pregnancy
  - Chronic or persistent diarrhea

Antidiarrheals

Generic	Brand	Dose & Max mg (frequency)	Contra-indications	Primary Side Effects	Key Monitoring Parameters	Pertinent Drug Interactions	Med Pearls
Mechanism of action – decreases pain through inhibition of central cyclooxygenase, which in turn inhibits prostaglandin synthesis							
Loperamide	Imodium	Initial: 4 mg, followed by 2 mg after each loose stool, up to 16 mg/day	• Abdominal pain without diarrhea • Children <2 yrs • Primary tx for acute dysentery, acute ulcerative colitis, and other colitis	• Constipation • Abdominal cramping • Abdominal distention	• CNS depression • Urinary retention • Paralytic ileus • Monitor for dehydration	• CYP450 • 2B6 substrate • May decrease levels of saquinavir	Toxicity can be treated with 100 g activated charcoal through nasogastric tube, and Naloxone
Mechanism of action – inhibits both antisecretory and antimicrobial and antiviral action; provides some anti-inflammatory action							
Bismuth	• Kaopectate • Pepto-Bismol	524 mg q30 min to 1 hr PRN; up to 8 doses/24 hrs	• Influenza or chickenpox due to risk of Reye's syndrome • Hx of GI bleed • Pregnancy: third trimester • Hypersensitivity to salicylates	• Discoloration of tongue and feces (grayish) • Impaction of feces • Hearing loss • Tinnitus		May decrease level and/or effects of tetracycline derivatives	
Mechanism of action – helps re-establish normal intestinal flora; suppresses the growth of potentially pathogenic microorganisms by producing lactic acid, which favors the establishment of an aciduric flora							
Lactobacillus	• Culturelle • Lactinex	• Culturelle: 1 caplet daily or BID • Lactinex: 4 tabs 3–4× daily	Hypersensitivity	Flatulence	Improvement	None	Lactinex must be stored in refrigerator
Lactase enzyme	• Lactaid • Lactrase	1–2 capsules taken with milk or meal	None	No common side effects reported at this time	Improving diarrheal symptoms	No known drug interactions	• Used in the treatment of lactose intolerance • Prevents osmotic diarrhea

CONSTIPATION MEDICATIONS

Definitions

Constipation is a symptom-based disorder that is described as a decrease in the frequency of fecal elimination characterized by the passage of hard, dry stools. The Rome III Criteria requires a patient to have experienced at least two of the following symptoms over the past three months: (1) fewer than three bowel movements per week; (2) straining; (3) lumpy/hard stools; (4) the sensation of an obstruction; (5) sensation of incomplete defecation; or (6) manual maneuvering required to defecate. Its occurrence increases as the patient ages in both men and women. However, it tends to be more commonly reported in women. Over half of the elderly population is affected by constipation. It is also a main complaint during pregnancy and after childbirth.

Constipation can be caused by various medical conditions, psychological and physiological conditions (menopause, dehydration), and lifestyle characteristics. There are several medications that can induce constipation, including: analgesics, antacids, anticholinergics, antidepressants, antidiarrheals, benzodiazepines, calcium channel blockers, iron supplements, monoamine oxidase inhibitors, opiates, parkinsonism agents, and sucralfate.

Diagnosis

- There are three clinical subgroups of constipation:
  - Normal transit constipation
    - » Most common form—59%
  - Slow transit constipation
    - » Accounts for 13%—delayed colonic transit
  - Pelvic floor dysfunction
  - Combination syndrome
- Less frequency of stooling than the "normal" 3–5 times/week
- Harder stool than "normal"
- Smaller stools than "normal"
- Colonoscopy if age >50, alarm signs, or additional symptoms present

Signs and Symptoms

- Lack of passing a bowel movement
- Very hard stools, lumpy stools
- Need for performing manual maneuvers to pass stools
- Anorexia, dull headache, low back pain, abdominal distention

Guidelines

American Gastroenterological Association Medical Position Statement: Guidelines on Constipation. *Gastroenterology* 2000;119:1761–78.

American Pharmaceutical Association. *Handbook of Nonprescription Drugs: An Interactive Approach to Self-Care*, 17th ed., 2011.

Cassagnol M, Saad M, Ahmed E, and Ezzo D. Review of Current Chronic Constipation Guidelines. *US Pharm* 2010;35(12):74–85.

Guidelines Summary

- Educate patient about high fiber and increased hydration in diet.
- Lifestyle modifications:
  - Encourage patients to avoid postponing defecation.
  - Monitor bowel habits with a daily diary.
  - Encourage patients to maintain moderate exercise.
- Patients should be excluded from self-treatment if they have any of the following:
  - Marked abdominal pain or significant distention or cramping
  - Marked or unexplained flatulence
  - Fever
  - Nausea and/or vomiting
  - Paraplegia or quadriplegia
  - Daily laxative use
  - Unexplained changes in bowel habits and/or weight loss
  - Bowel symptoms that persist for 2 weeks
  - History of irritable bowel disease
- Pharmacology begins with bulk-forming agents, proceeds to osmotic laxatives.
- If these options are not helpful, stimulant laxatives should be considered.
- Enemas, suppositories, and lubricants are also available as options.

Drugs for Constipation

Generic	Brand	Dose & Max mg (frequency)	Contraindications	Primary Side Effects	Key Monitoring Parameters	Pertinent Drug Interactions	Med Pearls	Top 200
Mechanism of action – bulk-forming by absorbing water in the intestine to form a viscous liquid that promotes peristalsis								
Psyllium	• Metamucil • Konsyl	1 tbsp TID 2–6 caps TID 1–2 wafers TID	• Fecal impaction • GI obstruction	• Abdominal cramps • Diarrhea	• Improvement • Diarrhea	• Warfarin • Digitalis • Diuretics	• Affects absorption of other meds • Take with full glass of water	No
Calcium polycarbophil	FiberCon	2–4 tabs daily						No
Methylcellulose	Citrucel	1–2 caps 6 ×/day 1 scoop TID						No
Mechanism of action – osmotic agent that causes water retention in the stool								
Polyethylene glycol 3350	MiraLax	17 g in 8 oz of water daily	• GI obstruction • Hypersensitivity	• Abdominal cramps • Diarrhea • Bloating	• Improvement • Diarrhea	None	Can reconstitute with 8 oz of water, juice, cola, or tea	No
Mechanism of action – stimulates peristalsis by directly irritating the smooth muscle of the intestine								
Senna	Senokot	2 tabs daily to 4 tab BID	• Fecal impaction • GI obstruction	• Abdominal cramps • Diarrhea • Bloating	• Improvement • Diarrhea	None		No
Bisacodyl	Dulcolax	5–15 mg daily				Milk and antacids may decrease the effect of bisacodyl		No
Mechanism of action – reduces surface tension of the oil-water interface of the stool, resulting in enhanced incorporation of water and fat and allowing for stool softening								
Docusate sodium	Colace	100 mg BID	• Concomitant with mineral	• Intestinal obstruction	• Improvement • Diarrhea	None	Take with full glass of water	No
Docusate calcium	Surlak	240 mg daily	• Fecal impaction • GI obstruction	• Diarrhea • Cramping				No
Mechanism of action – promotes bowel evacuation by causing osmotic retention of fluid which distends the colon with increased peristaltic activity								
Magnesium hydroxide	Phillips Milk of Magnesia	1–2 tbsp daily or BID	Hypersensitivity	Diarrhea	• Improvement • Diarrhea		Caution with impaired renal function	No
Mechanism of action – eases passage of stool by decreasing water absorption and lubricating the intestines								
Mineral oil	Fleet oil	1–2 tbsp at bedtime	• Colostomy • Ileostomy • Appendicitis • Ulcerative colitis	• Abdominal cramps • Diarrhea • Bloating	• Improvement • Diarrhea	May impair absorption of fat-soluble vitamins (A, D, K, E)	Aspiration is possible, especially in elderly population	No

ATHLETE'S FOOT MEDICATIONS

Definitions

Athlete's foot is a fungal infection called tinea pedis. The infection can range from mild itching to a severe inflammatory process characterized by fissuring, crusting, and discoloration of skin.

There are four types of tinea pedis.

- Chronic, intertriginous type
  - Most common form
  - Usually found in the lateral toe webs; however, infection is possible of spreading to the sole or instep of the foot
- Chronic, papulosquamous type
  - Found on both feet
  - Characterized by mild inflammation and diffuse, moccasin-like scaling
- Vesicular type
  - Occurs most often in the summertime
  - Characterized by small vesicles or vesicopustules near the instep and on the mid-anterior plantar surface
- Acute, ulcerative type
  - Caused from an overgrowth of gram-negative bacteria

Diagnosis

- Typically found in the lateral toe webs
- Can then spread to the sole or instep of the foot

Signs and Symptoms

- Fissuring and scaling
- Maceration in the interdigital spaces
- Malodor
- Stinging and burning sensation

Guidelines

American Pharmaceutical Association. *Handbook of Nonprescription Drugs: An Interactive Approach to Self-Care,* 17th edition, 2011.

Guidelines Summary

- Patients should be excluded from self-treatment if they have any of the following:
  - Causative factor unclear
  - Nails or scalp involved
  - Face, mucous membranes, or genitalia involved
  - Signs and symptoms of possible secondary bacterial infection
  - Excessive and continuous exudation, fever, malaise
- Apply a thin layer of medication to affected area for 2 weeks, even after the signs and symptoms disappear.

Athlete's Foot Medications

Generic	Brand	Dose & Max mg (frequency)	Contraindications	Primary Side Effects	Key Monitoring Parameters	Pertinent Drug Interactions	Med Pearls
Mechanism of action — squalene epoxidase inhibitor results in deficiency of ergosterol within the fungal cell							
Butenafine	• Lotrimin Ultra • Mentax	Apply daily	Hypersensitivity	• Burning • Contact dermatitis	Clinical signs of improvement	Minimal systemic absorption	• E. floccosum • T. mentagrophytes • T. rubrum
Terbinafine	Lamisil	Apply daily		• Erythema • Irritation • Stinging			
Mechanism of action — binds to phospholipids in the fungal cell membrane, altering cell wall permeability and resulting in loss of intracellular elements							
Clotrimazole	Lotrimin AF 1%	Cream; apply BID	Hypersensitivity	• Burning • Contact dermatitis	Clinical signs of improvement	Minimal systemic absorption	• E. floccosum • T. mentagrophytes • T. rubrum • Candida albicans
Miconazole	Micatin	Apply BID × 4 wks		• Erythema • Itching			
Mechanism of action — distorts the hyphae and stunts mycelial growth in susceptible fungi							
Tolnaftate	Tinactin	Spray: BID	Hypersensitivity	• Burning • Contact dermatitis • Erythema • Itching	Clinical signs of improvement	Minimal systemic absorption	• E. floccosum • T. mentagrophytes • T. rubrum
Mechanism of action — inhibits conversion of yeast to the hyphal form (active form) and interferes with fatty-acid biosynthesis							
Undecylenic acid	Fungi-Nail	Apply BID × 4 wks	None	High alcohol concentrations may cause burning	Clinical signs of improvement	Minimal systemic absorption	• Fungistatic against C. albicans, Tricophyton spp, and E. inguinale • Contains 5% undecylenic acid and 20% zinc undecylenate

Learning Points

- The Dietary Supplement Health and Education Act of 1994 categorizes herbals, vitamins, protein bars, and shakes as dietary supplements. As a result, manufacturers are not required to demonstrate safety, purity, or efficacy of supplements.

- Decongestants are the mainstay of therapy for colds and play an important role with allergic rhinitis.

- ACE inhibitors cause a dry cough in 20% or more of treated patients.

- Having more than three bowel movements per day is considered to be abnormal.

- Constipation can be caused by medications (anticholinergics, analgesics, benzos, sucralfate, calcium channel blockers, and more), menopause, dehydration, psychologic condition, depression, and more.

- When treating athlete's foot, a 2-week treatment period is typically required.

PRACTICE QUESTIONS

1. Which of the following conditions might St. John's wort be used to treat?

    (A) BPH
    (B) Depression
    (C) Diabetes
    (D) Hypertriglyceridemia
    (E) Lactose intolerance

2. Which of the following should be used for only 3 days to treat nasal congestion?

    (A) Diphenhydramine
    (B) Doxylamine
    (C) Loratadine
    (D) Naphazoline
    (E) Phenylephrine

3. Which of the following is considered a second-generation or less sedating antihistamine?

    (A) Brompheniramine
    (B) Chlorpheniramine
    (C) Doxylamine
    (D) Fexofenadine
    (E) Pseudoephedrine

4. Which condition can terbinafine be used to treat?

    (A) Athlete's foot
    (B) Constipation
    (C) Diarrhea
    (D) Lactose intolerance
    (E) Seasonal allergies

5. Which of the following is a stool softener that can be used to treat constipation?

    (A) Colace
    (B) Fibercon
    (C) Metamucil
    (D) Miralax
    (E) Sennakot

ANSWERS

1. **B**

St. John's wort is used to treat depression, as it increases the level of serotonin in the CNS. BPH (A) may be treated with saw palmetto, although meta-analysis data has not shown it to be useful. Diabetes (C) may be managed with the herbal supplement ginseng. Hypertriglyceridemia (D) may be treated with omega-3 fatty acids, and lactose intolerance (E) is treated with Lactaid.

2. **D**

Nasal decongestants—oxymetazoline and naphazoline—should be used for only 3 days to prevent rebound nasal congestion. Diphenhydramine (A), doxylamine (B), and loratadine (C) are oral antihistamines that can be used for more than 3 days and treat postnasal drip or allergic reactions. Phenylephrine (E) is an oral decongestant that can be used for more than 3 days.

3. **D**

Fexofenadine is a second-generation antihistamine and is less sedation that other first-generation antihistamines, including brompheniramine (A) and chlorpheniramine (B). Doxylamine (C) is a first-generation antihistamine used for the treatment of insomnia. Pseudoephedrine (E) is an oral decongestant.

4. **A**

Terbinafine is a topical antifungal used to treat athlete's foot. It should be applied to the affected area daily for at least 2 weeks, even after the condition appears to have cleared.

5. **A**

Colace is a stool softener and is used to prevent and treat constipation. Fibercon (B) and Metamucil (C) are bulk-forming laxatives that should be taken with a full glass of water. Miralax (D) is an osmotic laxative, and Sennakot (E) is a stimulant laxative.

Part Three

Pharmaceutical Sciences, Mathematics, and Biostatistics

Pharmaceutics

21

This chapter covers the following:

- Physical pharmacy
- Pharmaceutical dosage forms

 Suggested Study Time: **1.5 hours**

Pharmaceutics encompasses a number of disciplines, including dosage form design, biopharmaceutics, and pharmacokinetics. This chapter focuses on dosage form design (drug dosage forms, and the physical and chemical properties that allow these products to be manufactured).

A key concept to keep in mind is that patients don't simply take drugs, they take dosage forms: The active ingredient is not the only substance involved.

PHYSICAL PHARMACY

Physical pharmacy is a branch of pharmaceutics that deals principally with the physical and chemical properties of drugs. It is a highly mathematical subject, but the Board exam is not concerned with these aspects except as they relate to chemical kinetics. As you study, focus mainly on how specific properties of drugs make particular types of formulations more or less suitable. A simple example would be antibiotic suspensions that arrive at the pharmacy in dry powder form. The reason for this is that many antibiotics are chemically unstable in liquid formulations; if the water is added only at the time of dispensing, the drug will remain effective long enough for the patient to finish the bottle. If the product were manufactured as a liquid, the drug would be degraded by the time the bottle was processed, shipped, and stored in the pharmacy prior to dispensing.

Preformulation

Preformulation is an important stage of drug development where the pharmaceutical company characterizes the physicochemical properties of the drug. Preformulation allows the company to make the best decisions about how to formulate the drug into a usable dosage form.

Solubility and Lipophilicity

Every drug must be solubilized before it can be absorbed by the body. A drug must possess at least some aqueous solubility in order to be effective; poorly soluble compounds show incomplete and unpredictable absorption. However, at least some lipophilicity must also be present, as drugs must be able to pass through biological membranes in order to reach their sites of action. Salts or esters of drugs may be formed to increase or decrease the solubility, depending on the characteristics needed in a particular case. For example, the benzathine salt of penicillin G has a very low solubility, which causes the drug to dissolve slowly after injection, which prolongs the duration of action.

Dissolution rate is improved by decreasing particle size, which increases the surface area of the drug that comes into contact with the body fluids. A more in-depth treatment of factors that influence dissolution rate and absorption is contained in the biopharmaceutics chapter.

Ionization Behavior

Ionization behavior is one of the most important factors in drug development. It applies only if a drug is administered as a salt and therefore carries a positive or negative charge in solution. That is, when such a drug goes into solution, a fraction of the molecules dissociate into ions (i.e., charged compounds). The proportion of ionized to un-ionized drug is very important because the two behave very differently in the body:

- Ionized drug: More soluble, but cannot cross body membranes
- Un-ionized drug: Less soluble, but can cross body membranes

Salts are often preferred over the weak acid or base because they dissolve more quickly, are more stable on storage, and are easier to crystallize and handle during processing. Different salt forms may have very different properties, and pharmaceutical companies may intentionally modify drugs into more useful salts for a given purpose. Calcium salts, for example, show wide variation in absorption and possible efficacy.

Remember: Until the drug is absorbed across the body membranes it cannot get to the site of action, but it needs to go into solution before that can happen. The equilibrium between the more soluble ionized form and the more absorbable un-ionized form of the drug is crucial.

Henderson-Hasselbalch equation (below) can be used to calculate exact ratios of ionized to un-ionized drug, but the following table will give you a rough estimate of the ionization behavior of weak acids and bases when comparing pH of absorption site to the pKa. In most cases, you will be able to obtain a sufficiently accurate answer by using the table instead of the actual equation, saving valuable exam time.

$$pH = pK_a + \log\frac{[Salt]}{[Acid]} \text{ or } pH = pK_a + \log\frac{[ionized]}{[un\text{-}ionized]} \text{ if the drug is an acid}$$

$$pH = pK_a + \log\frac{[Base]}{[Salt]} \text{ or } pH = pK_a + \log\frac{[un\text{-}ionized]}{[ionized]} \text{ if the drug is a base}$$

Acid or base form is the un-ionized form and salt form is the ionized form of the corresponding acid or base. Accordingly, ionized and un-ionized can be substituted in the above equations in order to calculate the amount of ionization or un-ionization at a particular pH value. To identify which equation to use, you must first know if the drug in question is an acid or a base.

Ionization Behavior of Weak Acids and Bases

	Acidic Drug	Basic Drug
pH > pKa	More ionized	More un-ionized
pH = pKa	Equal	Equal
pH < pKa	More un-ionized	More ionized
Note that for pH more than 2 units away from pKa, expect almost complete ionization/un-ionization.		

It is impossible to tell if a drug is an acid or a base by looking only at the pKa. Some acids have higher pKa (phenytoin = 8.3) than do some bases (morphine = 8.0). You can tell if a drug is an acid or base, however, by what type of salt is used in its formulation. Weak acids form sodium, calcium, potassium, or other cationic salts; weak bases form hydrochloride or other anionic salts.

For example, warfarin is formulated as the sodium salt. Therefore, the drug warfarin is an acid. The positively charged sodium ion is used to displace the proton (i.e., hydronium ion or positively charged hydrogen) from the proton-donating acid in its formulation. In solution, warfarin disassociates from sodium into a negatively charged molecule (i.e., ionized form). If the solution is acidic (e.g., gastric fluid), a proton is likely to be donated back to the negatively charged warfarin to produce the uncharged drug (un-ionized form). Of course, this is a dynamic state in which the drug is going back and forth between the ionized and un-ionized form based on the pH of the environment. Determining this ratio provides information about the drug's solubility and its ability to cross biological membranes in any given environment. This is the power of the Henderson-Hasselbalch equation and of the table presented.

Stability

Physical, chemical, and microbiological stability are all very important in preformulation studies. While physical instability does not generally result in decreased drug concentration, it can lead to problems with dose uniformity and pharmaceutical elegance (eg., the mottled appearance that can develop in tablets over time, or the formation of a nonsuspendable sediment in a liquid dosage form). Polymorphism and anhydrous-to-hydrate conversions can be considered types of physical instability and are discussed in greater detail in the following section.

Chemical instability does result in loss of drug or excipient molecules. This can lead to either undertreatment, when a patient does not receive the full dose intended, or toxicity from toxic degradation products. In some cases, chemical instability can lead to microbiological instability if a preservative degrades and can no longer protect the formulation from bacterial or fungal overgrowth. The main types of degradation that occur in drug products are:

- Hydrolysis: Occurs in presence of water; typically no change in formulation appearance
- Oxidation: Occurs in presence of atmospheric oxygen; often results in insoluble precipitates or colored compounds
- Photochemical decomposition: Occurs on exposure to light; often results in colored compounds

Temperature, humidity, and light often hasten the degradation process, and drug companies use this fact to perform accelerated stability testing and to assign product expiration dates. Finished products must retain 90% of the labeled dose during their shelf life. Studies are performed at extreme storage conditions, and mathematical equations are used to extrapolate the degradation rate constants at normal conditions of storange. A good estimate, however, is that every 10°C rise in temperature doubles the rate constant.

Most drugs degrade by either zero- or first-order kinetics (see "Rate and Half-Life Equations" table, below). Drugs following zero-order degradation have a constant degradation rate that is independent of the drug concentration. First-order degradation, however, is concentration-dependent—the amount of drug degrading per unit of time is not constant. Suspensions degrade by pseudo–zero order kinetics, because only the drug molecules that are actually in solution are available for degradation. The concentration of drug in solution is in equilibrium with that in suspension, and the concentration of drug in solution is maintained at a constant level; suspended particles go into solution to replace the degraded drug. This continues as long as some solid is still present.

Rate and Half-Life Equations

Order	Rate Equation		Half-Life Equation
Zero	$C = C_0 - K_0 t$		$t_{1/2} = 0.5 \dfrac{C_0}{K_0}$
First	$\log C = \log C_0 - \dfrac{K_0 t}{2.303}$	$C = C_0 e^{-Kt}$	$t_{1/2} = \dfrac{\ln 2}{K_1} = \dfrac{0.693}{K_1}$

Where C is equal to concentration, C_0 is the initial concentration, K_0 is the zero-order degradation constant, t is time, $t_{1/2}$ is half-life, and K_1 is the first-order degradation constant.

With equations it is possible to calculate the concentration (or amount) of drug at any given time if its degradation rate constant is known. It is not, however, useful to memorize the first-order equation for the NAPLEX exam because the calculator provided does not include the exponential function on. Therefore, the only way to calculate the concentration (or amount) of drug at any given time is to estimate the amount by understanding what the degradation constants represent.

The first thing to do is identify if the question is related to a zero-order or first-order process. If a graphical representation is presented for any problem, a zero-order process will be linear with a constant degradation over time. Therefore, the units for zero-order degradation constants are in terms of amount per unit time (e.g., mg/hr). First-order degradation will be a nonlinear decline that is asymptomatic to the x-axis on a graph similar to a drug concentration-time curve seen in pharmacokinetics. The units of the first-order degradation constant are in terms of time^{-1} (e.g., yr^{-1}).

After identifying the process (zero or first order) of degradation, the second step is to estimate how much drug is remaining (or degraded) over some amount of time. This is simple for zero-order processes because a constant amount is being lost over time. For example, if the starting amount of drug is 1,000 mg and 10 mg per year is degraded (i.e., $K_0 = 10$ mg/yr), after 10 years it will have lost 100 mg of drug and have 900 mg remaining. Many zero-order degradation problems can rationalized without memorizing the equations in the table.

The estimation of amount of drug remaining following first-order degradation is not as straightforward and requires an in-depth understanding of the first-order degradation constant. The degradation constant is in terms of time^{-1}, as mentioned. This represents a percentage of drug lost per unit of time that is being presented. For example, a K_1 of 0.2 yr^{-1} indicates that 20% of the drug is lost every year. Thus, if the starting amount of drug is 1,000 mg of drug, 20% will be lost of that in the first year, or 200 mg, leaving 800 mg. The key in these estimations is to remember that in year 2, the starting amount is 800 mg because 200 mg was lost in year 1. To calculate the amount of drug lost after 2 years, subtract 20% of 800 mg (i.e., 160 mg) from 800 mg. Therefore, the amount of drug remaining after 2 years will be 800 mg minus 160 mg, for a total of 640 mg. This process must be repeated for year 3 and so on.

Solid-State Properties

Because most drugs are given as solid-dosage forms, many properties specific to the solid state are important in pharmacy.

Crystallization

Solids are present in crystalline or amorphous forms, or as a combination of the two. Crystalline forms show fixed geometric patterns, whereas the atoms in amorphous solids are randomly placed (as they would be in a liquid). The most important things to remember about crystalline versus amorphous solids for the purposes of this test are as follows:

- Crystalline solids have definite melting points, whereas amorphous solids melt over a range of temperature.
- Amorphous solids are more soluble than the corresponding crystalline forms.
- Solids tend to revert to the more stable crystalline form on storage.

Solvates are crystalline structures that contain trapped solvent; when the solvent is water, they are called hydrates. Typically, hydrates are less soluble than their anhydrous counterparts, whereas solvates are more soluble.

Polymorphism

Polymorphs are one of several crystalline structures that have the same chemical formula but show different physical properties. The properties they exhibit can vary substantially, however, and this leads to pharmaceutical companies patenting different polymorphic forms based on variations in solubility, bioavailability, solid-state stability, or processing behavior (such as improved powder flow or tablet compaction).

Metastable polymorphs will revert to the most stable form over time; in some instances, however, the metastable form might have more favorable properties than the stable form (e.g., better solubility). In those cases, even though it is not the most stable form, it may be the best one to market, provided the stability is at least acceptable.

The classic example of excipient polymorphism is cocoa butter, which is often used in suppository and troche formulations. Cocoa butter exists in four polymorphs, but only the β form is stable. When cocoa butter is heated above 34°C, some of the β form converts to unstable polymorphs. The unstable polymorphs are liquid at room temperature. The cocoa butter is never able to remain solid outside the refrigerator. This explains why chocolate or cocoa butter that has been overheated does not fully solidify when cooled.

Another pharmacy-related example of polymorphism is ritonavir (Norvir), a protease inhibitor used to treat HIV. Initially, it was thought to exist in only one polymorphic form, with relatively poor aqueous solubility. It was marketed in a soft gelatin capsule, which contained an ethanol/water cosolvent system. After drug approval, several batches failed quality control tests. It was discovered that a second polymorphic form with even lower solubility had formed, causing the drug to precipitate out of the cosolvent system. The product had to be reformulated to include Cremophor (polyethoxylated castor oil) as a solubilizing agent.

Rheology

Rheology is the science of flow properties, especially important when discussing liquid and semisolid dosage forms. During manufacturing, rheology is an important concept when mixing and packaging materials. Once the products reach the consumer, the rheology governs the removal of the product from its container, whether by pouring, extruding from a tube, or passing through a syringe needle.

Viscosity and fluidity are two common terms associated with rheology. Viscosity refers to the resistance offered when part of the liquid flows past another part; fluidity is essentially the opposite. Viscous liquids are thick and slow-moving; fluid liquids are thin and flow more readily.

Rheological behavior is divided into two main types: Newtonian flow and non-Newtonian flow. Newtonian materials do not change viscosity with changes in stirring speed; they do, however, become less viscous when heated. True solutions and pure liquid compounds such as water and oil are examples of Newtonian materials. Non-Newtonian materials do change viscosity when stirring speed changes. Three types of non-Newtonian behavior exist: Dilatant, plastic, and pseudoplastic. Dilatant materials become more viscous when stirred more rapidly, which can cause manufacturing equipment to malfunction. Plastic and pseudoplastic materials become more fluid when stirred. Plastic flow is best illustrated by a nonpharmacy example: Tomato catsup. It doesn't pour until shaken enough for contacts between adjacent particles to be broken but then acts much like a Newtonian material. Concentrated suspensions show similar behavior. Pseudoplastic flow differs in that flow can start immediately on stirring or shaking; the harder the bottle is shaken, the more fluid the material becomes. Polymer solutions often exhibit pseudoplastic flow.

Thixotropic products are a special case and are actually the ideal situation for pharmaceutical suspensions. They are viscous at rest but become fluid when shaken. Because of this, the suspension settles only slowly, but the liquid pours easily when shaken. After shaking stops, thixotropic products gradually become viscous again. Both plastic and pseudoplastic materials can show thixotropic behavior.

Testing

Numerous quality assurance tests exist for dosage forms, though only four will be discussed here. The four tests used for tablets and sometimes capsules are as follows: friability, hardness, disintegration, and dissolution testing.

Friability and hardness testing evaluate the ability of tablets to withstand manufacturing, packaging, and shipping. Hardness testing measures the force required to cause a tablet to break, and friability testing measures what percentage weight of a tablet is lost after it is tumbled for a specified amount of time in a friabilator. Tablets that are too soft or fragile will suffer too much damage during manufacturing and shipping to be useful, even if they have excellent dissolution and absorption behavior.

Disintegration testing is performed by placing tablets into mesh-bottomed cylinders that are immersed in a solution and agitated at a specified rate. The tablets are considered to have disintegrated when the particles are small enough to fall through the mesh screen. It is not a good measure of in vivo behavior, but is a frequently used quality-control measure for tablets.

A better measure of in vivo behavior is dissolution testing. Here, the tablets or capsules are immersed in appropriate dissolution liquids (typically, simulated gastric fluid) and samples are taken at specific time points to determine how much of the drug has gone into solution. While this test is still not a true predictor of in vivo behavior—because it does not demonstrate absorption—it is an improvement over disintegration testing, as the drug must go into solution with body fluids before being absorbed.

PHARMACEUTICAL DOSAGE FORMS

What things need to be considered when a drug company designs a dosage form for a particular drug? Some of the primary considerations are:

- Nature of the illness
- Manner in which the illness is treated
- Age of the patient
- Condition of the patient
- Stability of the drug

Suppose a patient suffers from motion sickness and is getting ready to go on a cruise. Would a tablet be the best dosage form in which their antinausea medication should be formulated? Probably not, as there is a risk that they could vomit and lose the medication before it had a chance to be absorbed by the body. For this reason, scopolamine is formulated into transdermal patches for motion sickness.

Some drugs can be used to treat different conditions based on their formulation and route of administration. An example is the antifungal product terbinafine (Lamisil). It is given as cream for surface conditions such as athlete's foot, and as tablets for more deep-seated fungal infections of the toenails and fingernails.

Age of the patient plays a large role in development of dosage forms. Young children and the elderly are much more likely than adults and teenagers are to have difficulty swallowing. Therefore, most medications for small children are marketed as easy-to-swallow dosage forms such as liquids and chewable or rapid-dissolve tablets. Other groups of patients may also lack the ability and willingness to swallow. Patients with psychiatric conditions will often refuse to swallow medication, and rapid-dissolve formulations or injections may be required to ensure that they receive treatment. Severely debilitated or comatose patients cannot swallow and may receive medicine through nasogastric tubes or by injection.

Oral Delivery: Solids

Solid dosage forms are the most commonly prescribed—over 80% of dosage forms are tablets or capsules. These products are convenient for the patient and are the preferred route for giving nonemergency medications. Some benefits of solid dosage forms are that they are already divided into accurate doses and are easy to handle. Taste is generally less of an issue than with liquid dosage forms and can be masked by coating the product, as long as the dosage is not designed to be chewed or dissolved in the mouth.

Solid products, however, are not perfect. If a very rapid response is needed, traditional tablets and capsules are not the best option because they take time to dissolve and become absorbed by the body. If formulated improperly, the absorption of the active ingredient(s) may be irregular or incomplete.

Traditional Release

The simplest type of solid dosage form is the powder. Powders taken orally have a few advantages: They are absorbed more rapidly than tablets and capsules because they do not have to undergo a disintegration step, they are easier to swallow than large tablets and capsules, and they are more chemically stable than liquids. It is easier to give large doses of drug in a powder than in a tablet. One gram of drug plus excipients is much easier to stir into water and swallow than it would be if formulated into a tablet.

One of the main drawbacks of powder as a dosage form is that it is very difficult to mask the taste or smell of unpleasant drugs when they are given in powder form. They are also highly inconvenient to handle and, if provided in bulk containers (such as Metamucil), may be subject to dose inaccuracy. Therefore, potent drugs should not be given as powders. If a drug is hygroscopic, it also should not be formulated into a powder dosage form as it will pick up too much moisture from the air. Finally, contrary to expectations, powders can be more expensive to produce than other solid dosage forms; there is a fairly substantial risk of explosion when working with large quantities of powder, and special handling equipment may be necessary to offset this risk.

Granules have many of the same advantages and disadvantages as powders. The primary difference between these two dosage forms is that granules are prepared agglomerations of smaller particles. They behave as single particles but are irregularly shaped and have a larger particle size than the associated powders. Granules therefore flow better than the powders and are more easily wetted by fluids, whether in manufacturing, in administration of the drug, or in the body. A simple example of the differences in properties of granulated versus powdered solids is sugar. Granulated (common table) sugar flows much more readily and dissolves easily in coffee or other liquids. Powdered sugar tends to clump, not flow freely, and dissolve slowly.

Granules are used more as a component of tablets and capsules than they are as dosage forms in their own right. They can be made by wet or dry methods. Wet granulation involves forming a dough of powder and liquid, pressing that dough through a mesh screen to form appropriately sized particles, and drying. In dry granulation, dry powders are compacted together, without the presence of liquid, into ribbons or oversized tablets that are then ground to size.

Capsules are a much more frequently dispensed type of solid dosage form and contain drug and excipients enclosed inside a gelatin, starch, or cellulose shell. They, like tablets, have many advantages over powders and granules. Since capsules are essentially unit-of-use products, they have excellent dose accuracy and the ability to mask the taste and smell of unpleasant drugs. They are also easy to administer, as the active ingredient does not need to be measured out. It is also easy to formulate products with multiple active ingredients. One advantage that capsules have over tablets is that they can be extemporaneously prepared in the pharmacy in instances where the prescriber requests a nonstandard dose of drug.

Capsules do have some disadvantages. They are permeable to moisture and may not be a suitable dosage form for moisture-sensitive drugs. They are also not suitable for water- or alcohol-based preparations, as those bases would dissolve the capsule shell. Some liquids, however, can be dispensed in capsules. Oil or nonaqueous water-miscible liquids such as polyethylene glycol (PEG) 400 can be used to dissolve or suspend drugs and vitamins that are then placed into soft gelatin capsules. Finally, gelatin may be inappropriate for certain patient populations who wish to avoid animal (particularly pork-based) products. In those cases, vegetarian capsule shells made of starch or cellulose may be substituted. Many dietary supplements and herbal products are manufactured in such capsules for this reason.

Tablets are the most frequently prescribed dosage form and are preferred for many reasons. In addition to the advantages they share with capsules, they are easy to make in a variety of shapes and colors, aiding in product identification. They are also inexpensive and quick to produce, especially when compared to most other dosage forms.

In order to make a drug into a tablet, however, the drug needs to be compressible. In other words, when force is placed on the powders in tableting equipment, they must be able to stick together sufficiently to make a durable tablet. Not all powders possess this property. If only small amounts of noncompressible active ingredient are needed, a compressible diluent can be used. Failing that, some materials can be granulated to improve compressibility. This does not work in all cases; if the material remains non-compressible, it may be best to formulate the product as a capsule instead of a tablet.

Types of Immediate-Release Tablets

Type of Tablet	Key Features	Example
Compressed	All ingredients contained in a single layer; designed to be swallowed whole; may or may not be coated	Various
Multi-compressed	Contain separate layers of drug, for various reasons (incompatibility of drugs, immediate- plus extended-release in the same tablet, etc.)	Mucinex (guaifenesin)
Chewable	Disintegrate rapidly when chewed; usually mannitol-based (pleasant mouth feel, sweet taste)	Children's vitamins Dilantin Infatabs (phenytoin)
Buccal	Dissolved in cheek cavity; may be designed to erode slowly or quickly	Fentora (fentanyl)
Sublingual	Dissolve under the tongue; erode quickly and are absorbed rapidly	Nitroglycerin tablets
Effervescent	Contain drug that dissolves rapidly after adding to water; results in carbonated liquid that masks taste	Alka Seltzer

Many immediate-release tablets are coated. This process can help mask unpleasant tastes and odors, as well as improve the appearance of the tablet, protect the drug from the atmosphere, and allow it to be swallowed more easily. The two types of coating used for immediate-release products are sugar and film coatings. Sugar coating produces a very attractive tablet that is typically much larger than the uncoated product, due to the several layers of sugar, color, flavor, and waterproofing shellac added. The process is very time-consuming, and batch variations are common in the coated tablets. The coatings are applied manually in coating pans, not mechanically, by highly skilled personnel. Film coatings are much thinner, and leave a coat of opaque, colored polymer on the surface of the tablet. Although they are customarily machine-applied, requiring less skill in application, many coating defects are possible:

- Picking and peeling: Film fragments flake from the tablet surface
- Orange-peel effect: Coating leaves rough surface on the tablet
- Mottling: Coating has uneven color distribution
- Bridging: Score lines or logos present on tablet are filled in by coating
- Erosion: Coating solution is in contact with tablet for too long and disfigures the core

Extended Release

Extended-release oral products maintain more constant blood levels of the drug than do immediate-release products. Because of this, patients can take the drugs less often (once or twice a day instead of up to four times), which improves adherence. Adverse effects are usually fewer and less severe, as the concentration of the drug in the blood does not vary as widely from peak and trough as much as with immediate-release products. There is a risk of dose-dumping, however, especially if the patient chews the medicine instead of swallowing it whole.

Drugs that are best suited for extended release are usually given in fairly small doses, as the practical limit for the amount of drug to be contained in an individual tablet or capsule is 500 mg. The drug should also not have either a particularly fast or slow rate of absorption: Drugs that absorb too quickly require too large a dose, and drugs that absorb slowly are inherently long-acting and an extended-release formulation is not needed. Because of the risk of dose-dumping, the drug should have a good margin of safety and be uniformly absorbed from the GI tract. Different methods of achieving extended release are given in the following table.

Types of Extended-Release Tablets and Coatings

Type of Tablet	Key Features	Example
Enteric coat	Coating remains intact until drug reaches small intestine; can protect drug from stomach acid and enzymes, or stomach from irritating drugs	Enteric-coated aspirin
Diffusion-controlled reservoir system	Beads or pellets are coated with polymer that releases drug at varying speeds; may involve several release rates	Theo-Dur (theophylline)
Diffusion-controlled matrix system	Drug is mixed into an inert plastic matrix; drug dissolves and leaves matrix	
Wax	Remains intact in GI tract and is eliminated in feces; inform patient that this is normal	Desoxyn Gradumet (methamphetamine)

Type of Tablet	Key Features	Example
Hydrophilic	Water causes matrix to swell; drug diffuses through gel layer, and may also be released as matrix erodes	Slo-Niacin (niacin)
Dissolution-controlled system	Rate of release affected by dissolution and tablet or bead erosion (some hydrophilic matrices fall into this category as well as diffusion-controlled)	Cardizem CD (diltiazem)
Ion-exchange resin	pH conditions of GI tract cause drug to be released from resin	Ionamin (phentermine resin)
Osmotically controlled system	Tablet pulls water into system, then releases drug at controlled rate by osmotic pressure; tablet shell eliminated in feces	Glucotrol XL (glipizide)
Complex formation	Drug is combined with other agents, forming a slowly soluble chemical complex	Rynatan allergy products

Rapid Release

Rapid-release products are becoming more important, particularly in the over-the-counter (OTC) industry. Because they can be taken without water, they are convenient for the patient, and they have a rapid onset of action. Some of the products are very soft, however, and they may require expensive protective packaging.

Types of Rapid-Release Solid Dosage Forms

Type of Product	Key Features	Example
Tablets	Product can contain large doses of drug	Claritin RediTabs
Strips	Dissolves before sick children can spit it out; cannot put large doses of drug into product	Triaminic Thin Strips
Lollipops	Absorbed through buccal mucosa	Fentanyl Actiq

Oral Delivery: Liquids

Oral liquid dosage forms have the same advantages as other oral products, with the additional advantage of being easy to swallow for small children and others who cannot easily swallow solid dosage forms. Several disadvantages exist as well. Liquids are less portable and convenient than solids. Incorrect doses are much more likely, as patients or caregivers could measure using an inappropriate measuring device (i.e., not all spoons are standard size), and product may be spilled before being consumed. Also, taste can be a large issue, as more of the drug will reach a patient's taste buds than with the same drug in a tablet or capsule.

Solvents

Water is the most common solvent for pharmaceutical products; purified water prepared by distillation, reverse osmosis, or ion-exchange treatment is acceptable for oral use. Other commonly used solvents include ethyl alcohol, glycerin, sorbitol, propylene glycol, and some edible oils. Typically, solvents other than water are included to improve solubility and, in some cases, add sweetness to the final product (glycerin, sorbitol, and propylene glycol). Only small amounts of sorbitol and glycerin should be present in a given dose of liquid, as they may act as osmotic laxatives in higher quantities.

Types of Liquids

Single-phase liquid dosage forms are all variants of the solution. One or more soluble substances are dissolved in one or more solvents, including water. Therefore, the drug(s) must be water-soluble and stable in aqueous solution. The presence of other excipients in varying amounts results in the following designations:

Types of Single-Phase Liquid Dosage Forms

Type of Product	Key Features	Examples
Syrups	• Contain sugar or sugar substitutes • Little or no alcohol • Thickeners improve mouth feel and physically conceal the drug from taste buds • Taste pleasant; often used with children	• Various cough/cold preparations
Elixirs	• By definition alcoholic, but some nonalcoholic commercial products are mislabeled as elixirs • Slightly sweet; artificial sweetener usually used since sucrose is not very soluble in alcohol • Less viscous than syrups	• Diphenhydramine • Phenobarbital • Digoxin
Tinctures	• 15–80% alcohol • Usually consist of drug extracted from plant material • Unpleasant taste; not commonly used today	• Laudanum (opium tincture; 1,000 mg morphine/100 mL) • Paregoric (camphorated opium tincture; 40 mg morphine/100 mL)
Spirits	• Alcoholic solutions of aromatic or volatile substances • High concentration of alcohol • Active ingredient may precipitate out when added to aqueous preparations	• Flavoring agents
Aromatic waters	• Aqueous solutions of volatile oils • Very dilute	• Flavoring and perfuming agents
Fluid extracts	• Similar to, but more potent than, tinctures • Used as drug source, not as dosage form	

Multiphase liquids are more complicated than single-phase liquids. They still possess most of the advantages and disadvantages of other liquid dosage forms but have the additional disadvantage of being nonhomogenous. Because of this, suspensions and emulsions should always have "Shake Well" labels attached.

Suspensions are multiphase products that contain finely divided solid particles distributed through the liquid phase. They can be used on the skin, used in the ear or eye, or given by intramuscular (IM) or subcutaneous (SC) injection, but are most commonly given by mouth. Some advantages exist over single-phase liquids: Drugs that have an unpleasant flavor are preferred as suspensions, since the drug does not interact with the taste buds as much when it is not dissolved. Also, drugs that have poor stability in water do not degrade as readily in suspension as they do in solution.

The primary concern with making suspensions is to have a particle size that is small enough to remain suspended in the dispersion medium of choice while not being so small that the particles start to attract each other and form clumps that will not resuspend. This can be achieved by two techniques, used separately or in combination: Use of structured vehicles and controlled flocculation.

- Structured vehicles: Increase viscosity and slow the sedimentation of suspended particles. Natural and synthetic polymer solutions are often used (cellulose gels, acacia, bentonite).
- Controlled flocculation: Add materials that promote loose aggregation of suspended particles, but that keep their surfaces apart, by charge or interaction of polymer chains. Settle, but loosely, and resuspend easily.

Emulsions are dispersions that consist of nonmiscible liquids. The dispersed phase is also called the internal phase, and the dispersion medium is called the external phase. These products are very thermodynamically unstable and require an emulsifying agent to keep them combined properly. A good nonpharmacy example is mayonnaise. Lemon juice or vinegar serves as the external phase, and the lecithin from the egg yolk emulsifies the product so that the oil that is added does not separate out.

Only oil-in-water (O/W) emulsions are used for oral dosage forms, as water needs to be in the external phase to be palatable to the patient; otherwise, all the patient would taste would be the oil in the outer portion of the product. Topical products can be either O/W or W/O. When prepared in the pharmacy, emulsions are made by rapid stirring in a mortar and pestle, shaking in a bottle (though only with reasonably thin oils), or using a hand blender, or by heating the phases separately and then mixing them. Three types of emulsifiers are used, depending on the product being made:

- Surfactants: Contain hydrophilic and hydrophobic portions, which remain at the interface of the oil and water phases to stabilize the product. Often used in combination.

- Hydrophilic colloids: Water-soluble polymers that form a film around oil droplets in O/W emulsions. Tend to increase viscosity of the product.
- Finely divided solids: Form a film of particles around the droplets of the dispersed phase, but allow interaction with the dispersion medium as well.

The exact quantity of surfactant needed can be determined by the hydrophilic-lipophilic balance (HLB) system. The HLB is a measure of the degree to which a given surfactant is hydrophilic or lipophilic. This number runs anywhere from 0 to 20. A value less than 10 indicates that the given surfactant is lipid soluble, and a value greater than 10 indicates that the given surfactant is water soluble. Surfactants and the ingredients to be emulsified have been assigned experimentally determined HLB numbers, and the exact amount of emulsifier needed can be determined algebraically if a formula has not already been determined.

Topical Delivery

Topical products are used for three primary reasons: To protect injured areas of the skin from the environment, to hydrate the skin, and to apply medication to the skin for local effect. In some cases, drug may reach the blood supply and be systemically absorbed; this is not desired with topical delivery. Systemic absorption of a drug applied to the skin is known as transdermal drug delivery and is discussed later in this chapter.

Powders and liquids are used as topical delivery systems, though not as frequently as semisolid preparations. Of the types of liquids mentioned in the oral delivery section, solutions, suspensions, and emulsions may all be used topically. Two external-use–only liquid products are:

- Liniments: Alcoholic solutions used to irritate the skin and relieve more deep-seated pain or discomfort (Heet, Absorbine Jr), or oleaginous emulsions used as emollients or protective agents. Liniments are applied by rubbing and are not suitable for application to bruised or broken skin.
- Collodions: Contain pyroxylin in an alcohol/ether base that evaporates, leaving an occlusive film on the skin; used to hold edges of incised wounds together.

Ointment Bases

Five types of ointment bases exist:

- Hydrocarbon/oleaginous: Greasy, petroleum-based products used for emollient effect (Vaseline, petrolatum)
- Anhydrous absorption: Greasy products that form W/O emulsions when aqueous solutions are added; can be used to incorporate solutions into an otherwise lipophilic base (hydrophilic petrolatum, anhydrous lanolin)

- W/O emulsion: Similar to anhydrous absorption bases, but already contain some water (hydrous lanolin, cold cream)
- O/W emulsion (water-removable): Creamy emulsions that are easily washed from the skin; may be diluted with water to form lotions (hydrophilic ointment, Lubriderm)
- Water-soluble: Greaseless, water-washable bases containing no oleaginous compounds; cannot add large amounts of water or will soften too much (polyethylene glycol ointment)

Particular bases are chosen on the basis of the desired rate of drug release, stability of the drug in the base, the need for an occlusive barrier, and ability to wash the ointment easily from the skin. When preparing ointments in a pharmacy, if a levigating agent is needed, it should be compatible with the type of ointment base used. For instance, mineral oil will mix well with any ointment base containing hydrocarbons (all except water-soluble bases). Water-miscible liquids such as glycerin and PEG will be more appropriate when using bases that contain water, such as water-soluble or emulsion bases. If solutions need to be incorporated into an ointment base, acceptable options are anhydrous absorption base or either type of emulsion base.

Other topical product definitions are:

- **Creams:** Terminology often used to describe emulsion bases; soft, cosmetically acceptable topical products
- **Pastes:** Very thick semisolids containing at least 20% solids by weight
- **Gels:** Jelly-like dispersions that are water-soluble, water-washable, and greaseless

Rectal, Vaginal, and Urethral Delivery

Rectal, vaginal, and urethral dosage forms such as suppositories and enemas are less frequently prescribed than many other types of dosage form, but they do have an important place in certain types of therapy. They can be useful for local therapy in rectal or vaginal conditions, or when protecting susceptible drugs from GI tract degradation or first-pass metabolism.

Rectal conditions amenable to local therapy with suppositories, enemas, or other rectally administered dosage forms include hemorrhoids, rectal itching, ulcerative colitis, and constipation.

Rectal suppositories can also be used to administer drug for systemic absorption. Usually, this is done when the patient cannot or will not take medication by mouth. Infants, small children, and severely debilitated patients cannot easily swallow. Patients with severe nausea (as a symptom of a condition such as gastroenteritis or migraine, or as a side effect of chemotherapy or anesthesia) cannot hold down oral antiemetics long enough for the medication to take effect; several medications (chlorpromazine, prochlorperazine, and trimethobenzamide) are given rectally to avoid this problem.

Vaginal dosing, including suppositories, creams, and other dosage forms, is usually used for local effect, either for treatment of local infections (clindamycin and -azole antifungals) or for contraception (nonoxynol-9). Hormone replacement may also be administered via vaginal cream or suppository, and will have local effects on the vaginal mucosa. Systemic absorption may be seen with higher estrogen doses.

Urethral suppositories are seldom seen. Alprostadil was approved in 1997 for use in impotence (as Muse urethral suppository) but is not commonly used now that oral medications are available and more readily acceptable to patients.

The most common bases used in suppositories are fatty bases similar to cocoa butter that melt at body temperature, and water-soluble bases such as polyethylene glycol and glycerinated gelatin bases that dissolve slowly in body fluids. Fatty bases are more soothing but do not mix well with body fluids and have a tendency to leak from body orifices. For this reason, they are not suitable for vaginal or urethral delivery. Water-soluble bases can be irritating to the mucosa because they take up water from the area. They are frequently used for vaginal or urethral delivery, but seldom for rectal. Different bases release drugs differently based on the water/oil partition coefficient of the base and of the drug. Lipophilic drugs are released slowly from oleaginous bases but more quickly from water-soluble bases. Hydrophilic drugs, on the other hand, are released extremely quickly from fatty bases but more slowly from water-soluble bases.

Pulmonary Delivery

The lung is an increasingly popular delivery site and is no longer reserved only for pulmonary conditions. The lungs possess a large surface area for drug absorption and a good blood supply that bypasses first-pass metabolism. Even though the first inhaled insulin (Exubera) was a market failure, it proved that large-molecule drugs could be delivered effectively via the lung for systemic use. Continued improvement in delivery devices should cause the field of pulmonary delivery to grow rapidly.

Metered-Dose Inhalers

Metered-dose inhalers (MDIs) are primarily used to deliver medications for the treatment of asthma and chronic obstructive pulmonary disease (COPD): Bronchodilators, steroids, and mast cell stabilizers. While MDIs are portable and able to deliver precise quantities of potent drugs, many patients have difficulty using them properly. MDIs have undergone rapid changes in the last few years, due in part to federal legislation restricting the use of chlorofluorocarbon (CFC) propellants due to their link to ozone depletion. Beginning in 2009, medical device exemptions will no longer be allowed for these propellants, so companies have redesigned their products as either hydrofluoro-alkane (HFA) propellant devices or dry-powder inhalers. Significant engineering challenges were involved in converting products to use these new delivery devices.

Dry-Powder Inhalers

Dry-powder inhalers (DPIs) avoid some of the difficulties with MDIs: They are generally easier for patients to use correctly, since the device can be primed before use and the patient does not have to coordinate breath with the device actuation. Ease of use, however, depends significantly on the particular type of device. One study indicated that 92% of patients learned to use the Diskus device correctly, whereas only 74% were able to learn proper use of the Turbohaler.

The Diskus device is a classic example of the discrete-dose style of DPI. Individual doses are contained in foil packets, protecting them from humidity and allowing for dose consistency if the device is dropped. Some discrete-dose devices are single-dose units, and the drug is added when the device is ready to be actuated (Rotahaler, Aerosilizer, Handihaler); this is often a necessity if a drug is heat-sensitive and must be kept refrigerated until use, such as Spiriva (tiotropium bromide). The Twisthaler, on the other hand, is an example of a reservoir device. All of the doses are contained in a central compartment; and if the device is dropped or exposed to humidity, all doses are affected. Of currently marketed products, only the Twisthaler and Flexhaler are reservoir devices.

Nebulizers

Nebulizers allow the drug to be delivered directly to the lung in high concentration and without the use of propellant. They are particularly useful for uncoordinated or unabled patients, including those who are intubated. Two types exist: Jet and ultrasonic. Jet nebulizers can be used with either solutions or suspensions, and operate by the Bernoulli principle: Compressed air from the machine flows at high speed over the medicated liquid, atomizing it and carrying it to the patient. Ultrasonic nebulizers can only be used with solutions. Ultrasonic nebulizers use the vibrations of high-frequency sound waves to move liquid from the machine through the face mask. Vibrations are timed to coincide with inhalation, so less medication is lost than with the jet nebulizers.

Nasal Delivery

Nasal delivery shares many of the advantages of pulmonary delivery: Drugs that are inactivated by the GI tract or that undergo first-pass metabolism are protected, and large-molecule drugs can be absorbed across the nasal mucosa. The nose has a dense vasculature, which aids in absorption. Viscosity enhancers and mucoadhesives are often included in the formulations to increase residence time, as nasal drainage can be a problem. In addition to the many drugs available via nasal delivery (e.g., oxytocin, desmopressin, calcitonin, and butorphanol tartrate), the route shows promise for vaccine delivery, with FluMist being the first approved example.

The most commonly used nasal products are saline solutions for dry nasal mucosa, nasal decongestants, and intranasal steroids. Nasal decongestants are adrenergic agents that constrict the nasal vasculature, shrinking the nasal mucosa and making breathing easier. Overuse can lead to a phenomenon called rhinitis medicamentosa (rebound congestion), so patients should be cautioned to use the products only as directed and for no longer than 3 to 5 days. Intranasal steroids are commonly prescribed for allergic rhinitis; they may be administered in pump spray containers or as metered-dose aerosols.

Parenteral Delivery

Injectable products have many advantages over other dosage forms but also have more potential complications. No drug is lost to first-pass metabolism or acid- or enzyme-mediated degradation in the GI tract, which makes injection a particularly useful route for protein drug delivery. The rate of delivery can be accurately controlled; and drug, nutrients, and fluids can be given when other routes cannot be used. However, injectable drugs must be prepared and administered by highly trained personnel and cannot be retrieved once given. Additionally, the products must be sterile, free from undesired particulate matter, and pyrogen-free.

Sterilization Methods Used in Industry

Method	How Does It Work?	Advantages	Disadvantages	Products Sterilized by This Method
Steam sterilization	Heat coagulates and kills microorganisms	• Method of choice when applicable • Lower heat than dry heat sterilization	• Cannot use with heat- or moisture-sensitive drugs • Autoclave can have cools spots	• Aqueous solutions in closed containers • Surgical instruments • Glassware
Dry heat sterilization	Heat coagulates and kills microorganisms	• Useful for moisture-sensitive material	• Cannot use with heat-sensitive drugs • Autoclave can have cool spots	• Glassware • Surgical equipment • Oleaginous materials • Powders • Moisture-sensitive material
Filtration	Bacteria and particulate matter are physically removed by membrane filters	• Inexpensive	• Technique failure • Membrane defects • Drug can absorb to membrane	• Small volumes of thin liquid • Heat-sensitive liquid formulations

Method	How Does It Work?	Advantages	Disadvantages	Products Sterilized by This Method
Ionizing radiation	Gamma radiation mutates and kills bacteria		• Expensive setup	• Sterilizing plastic medical devices
Gas sterilization	Ethylene and propylene oxide gases alkylate microbial protein	• Good for heat- and moisture-sensitive materials	• Possibility of toxic residue • Explosion hazard • Expensive setup • Cannot penetrate glass to sterilize material in sealed containers	• Heat-sensitive material • Moisture-sensitive material • Medical and surgical equipment wrapped in plastic

Multiple-dose injectable products must contain a preservative in order to ensure that the product remains sterile after the initial use. Large-volume, single-use products, however, cannot contain preservative, as the amount required to reach an effective concentration would lead to preservative-related toxicity. In addition to sterilization and preservation intended to decrease the likelihood of microbial growth in the product, steps must be taken to ensure that pyrogens (lipopolysaccharides from gram-negative bacterial cell walls that cause high fever, hypertension, and chills) are not present.

The main routes of injectable delivery are intravenous (IV), subcutaneous (SC), and intramuscular (IM). Intravenous products must be solutions or O/W emulsions (e.g., Intralipid, a component of total parenteral nutrition), as particulate matter could lead to phlebitis and other complications. SC and IM injections may be solutions or emulsions; however, they may also be suspensions, which exhibit slower absorption since the drug must go into solution in the tissue before being absorbed into the bloodstream. In some injectable suspensions, such as the contraceptive Depo-Provera (medroxyprogesterone acetate), release of medication can continue for several months, improving patient convenience. Some products are given by other injectable routes: Allergy tuberculosis testing is handled by intradermal injection; hydrocortisone is frequently injected directly into the joint (intra-articular) in arthritic patients; anesthesia is often injected into the epidural space (around the nerve roots of the spine); and anesthetics, some drugs used to treat meningitis, and some chemotherapy agents are injected into the intrathecal (subarachnoid) space (into the cerebrospinal fluid) to bypass the blood-brain barrier.

Ocular and Otic Delivery

Drug delivery to the eye is complicated by two factors: Drug loss due to blinking and lacrimal drainage, and poor drug penetration through the corneal membrane. Polymers are typically used as viscosity enhancers to prolong the retention time and reduce lacrimal drainage; some polymers, such as hyaluronic acid, have mild adhesive properties that prolong the retention time even further. Drop size reduction can also serve to improve ocular availability; only about 10 mcL of fluid remains in the conjunctival cul-de-sac after blinking, so dose volumes larger than this lead to waste.

Drug penetration into the eye can be improved by creating a prodrug that is more lipophilic than the original compound. It is then converted to the active substance by enzymes in the body.

Most ocular products are solutions, but suspensions, ointments, and gels may also be used. These dosage forms prolong drug contact with the eye and may be preferable in some situations. Drug contact may also be prolonged by the use of an ophthalmic insert (Pilocarpine Ocusert system); these small inserts are placed in the cul-de-sac of the eye and release the drug over a 7-day period, improving patient adherence with glaucoma therapy.

Ocular products must be sterile when dispensed, and all multidose products must contain preservative. This helps prevent serious ocular infections, which can lead to corneal ulcers and blindness.

Otic products are generally solutions or suspensions, which frequently contain glycerin or propylene glycol to increase the viscosity and maximize contact between the product and the ear canal. The hygroscopic nature of these solvents also helps them draw moisture out of the tissues, which can reduce inflammation and decrease the amount of moisture available for any microorganisms to grow. Most otic products fall into one of the following categories:

- Anti-infective and anti-inflammatory products: May contain analgesics and local anesthetics to reduce pain associated with otitis externa or otitis media
- Ear-wax removal agents: Contain surfactants (which emulsify ear wax) or peroxides (which release oxygen and disrupt the integrity of the ear wax), allowing easy removal

Transdermal Delivery

Transdermal delivery differs from topical delivery in that the drug is intended for systemic use. The drug molecules must therefore be small enough to penetrate the stratum corneum and reach the general circulation. Some transdermal ointments (nitroglycerin ointment) exist, but most products are available as transdermal delivery systems (patches).

Patches

Transdermal patches attach to the skin with adhesive and contain the drug either in a polymer matrix or in a drug reservoir covered by a rate-controlling membrane. An excess amount of drug is typically present to ensure that a concentration gradient exists, causing the drug to exit the patch and enter the skin passively. Patches provide more uniform blood levels than conventional release products and can improve patient compliance since, depending on the drug, they can be worn for 1 to 7 days. GI absorption problems and first-pass metabolism also are avoided. A wide range of drugs are now available in patches, including nitroglycerin, nicotine, and hormones (for birth control or hormone replacement therapy).

Ultrasound

Drug can be transported across skin by mixing it with a coupling agent and using ultrasonic energy to disrupt the stratum corneum and increase penetrability. This method of delivery is not common, but high-dose hydrocortisone can be delivered in this fashion.

Iontophoresis

This method of transdermal delivery is not widely used but is gaining popularity. It involves delivery of charged compounds across the skin by applying an electrical current. Since the skin is disrupted, larger molecules may pass than is possible with transdermal patches. Local anesthesia (Numby Stuff) and fentanyl (IONSYS) are available in small iontophoretic patches, and the method is being investigated to deliver protein drugs.

Learning Points

- A drug cannot work until it is absorbed. It cannot be absorbed until it is dissolved.
- Ionized, hydrophilic drugs dissolve more readily; un-ionized, lipophilic drugs are absorbed more easily.
- Focus on why a particular dosage form might work better for a particular condition or with a particular drug.
- Consider nonoral routes for drugs that undergo extensive first-pass metabolism.
- At this time, protein drugs can be given only by injectable or pulmonary routes. There is future potential with nasal delivery.

PRACTICE QUESTIONS

1. Which of the following dosage forms must be sterile?

    (A) Ophthalmic suspension
    (B) Oral suspension
    (C) Topical suspension
    (D) Suspension for rectal administration
    (E) Otic suspension

2. A 15-year old patient with ADHD who had been stable on a dose of 10 mg BID of Focalin is transitioning to Focalin XR 20 mg QD. After 2 weeks, he returns to the doctor complaining of distractedness during school and a jittery feeling in the morning an hour or two after taking his medication. When asked how he is taking his medication, he states that due to difficulty swallowing he has been opening the capsules of Focalin XR and mixing them with chunky applesauce, which he chews before swallowing. How do you explain the patient's current symptoms?

    (A) The new dose of Focalin XR is too high and should be reduced.
    (B) The patient is experiencing dose-dumping because he is opening the capsules.
    (C) The patient is experiencing dose-dumping because he is chewing the capsule contents with the applesauce.
    (D) The severity of the patient's ADHD has increased and he is suffering from a new-onset anxiety disorder.
    (E) The patient is experiencing dose-dumping because the capsule contents are interacting with the applesauce.

3. What environmental advantage do HFA inhalers have over CFC inhalers?

    (A) They contain less packaging.
    (B) They are less likely to lead to ozone depletion.
    (C) They do not contain mercury.
    (D) They are a pump spray instead of an aerosol spray.
    (E) They do not use petroleum-based mineral oil as an emulsifier.

4. An insulin injection decomposes at a rate of 0.15 yr^{-1}. How many units of an initial 100-unit solution remain after 3 years?

    (A) 70 units
    (B) 67 units
    (C) 65 units
    (D) 63 units
    (E) 61 units

5. Using the graph below, indicate which of the following statements is true.

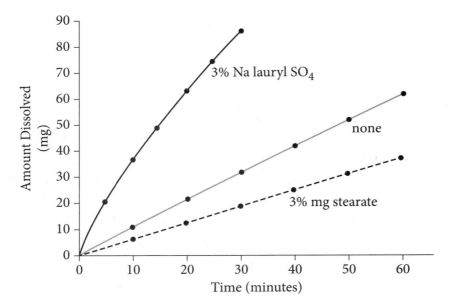

Figure 1. Effect of lubricant on dissolution rate of salicylic acid contained in the compressed tablets.

(A) Sodium lauryl sulfate appears to decrease the rate of dissolution.

(B) At 10 minutes, approximately 10 mg of salicylic acid have dissolved when formulated with sodium lauryl sulfate.

(C) The rate of dissolution of tablets containing magnesium stearate is greater than the control.

(D) The dissolution rate for tablets with sodium lauryl sulfate follows zero-order kinetics.

(E) None of the above statements is true.

6. What approximate percentage of phenytoin sodium (pK_a = 8.3) is un-ionized at a physiological pH of 7.3?

(A) 99%

(B) 90%

(C) 45%

(D) 10%

(E) 1%

ANSWERS

1. **A**

All ophthalmic dosage forms must be sterile, and either packaged in single-dose containers or formulated to contain a preservative. Sterility is not required for any of the other routes, as the drug is being applied either to an epithelial surface (topical, otic) or to the GI mucosa (oral, rectal). These surfaces are not sterile in their natural state, and dosage forms applied to them need not be sterile.

2. **C**

Focalin XR derives its extended-release properties from a coating on the beads contained within the capsule. It is therefore appropriate to open the capsule and consume the contents with food or in liquid; applesauce is specifically mentioned in the manufacturer instructions as appropriate. However, crushing or chewing the beads destroys the coating, causing dose-dumping. The patient's jitteriness in the morning and inattention later in the day are symptomatic of too high a dose being absorbed in the morning, and too little medication remaining in his system later in the day.

3. **B**

HFA inhalers were designed to replace CFC inhalers, which are being phased out due to the Montreal Protocol and the effect of CFCs on ozone depletion. HFA inhalers are similar in size to CFC inhalers. Neither type of product contains the other excipients mentioned in the question.

4. **E**

The first step toward answering this problem is to determine if this is a zero-order or first-order degradation process. The units of the degradation rate constant are in time^{-1}, which indicates a nonlinear process and, therefore, a first-order degradation. The rate constant is given as 0.15 yr^{-1}, indicating that 15% of the insulin injection is lost every year. In year 1, 15% of the initial 100 units are lost, leaving 85 units. In year 2, 15% of the remaining 85 units are lost; that is, 12.75 units (85×0.15) are lost, and $85 - 12.75 = 72.25$ units remain after year 2. In year 3, 15% of the 72.25 units are lost, or 10.84 units (72.25×0.15), and $72.25 - 10.84 = 61.41$ units remain after year 3. This result is rounded to the answer 61 units.

5. D

The rate of dissolution follows zero-order kinetics. This can be observed on the graph because there is a linear relationship between the amount dissolved (y-axis) and time (x-axis). Because this graph is on a linear scale (i.e., it is NOT a log or natural log scale) and the relationship is linear, it is a zero-order process. Choice (A) is incorrect because the rate of dissolution (or any rate) is directly related to the slope of a line. A steeper slope indicates a faster rate. Because sodium lauryl sulfate had a steeper slope than control, it indicates that those tablets dissolved faster. The same concept applies to choice (C), which is incorrect. Choice (B) is also incorrect: Drawing a straight line up from 10 minutes on the x-axis to the line indicating sodium lauryl sulfate demonstrates that approximately 40 mg of the salicylic acid has dissolved, not 10 mg.

6. B

The first step to answer this question is to determine if phenytoin is an acidic or basic drug. Phenytoin is formulated with sodium; this indicates that phenytoin is a weak acid. The sodium ion replaces a proton on the phenytoin molecule in its salt formulation and disassociates in solution. Once phenytoin is identified as an acid, it is clear that the following equation applies:

$$pH = pK_a + \log\frac{[Salt]}{[Acid]}$$

The salt in the numerator is the ionized form of the drug; the denominator indicates the drug itself, which is un-ionized. The next step is to fill in the pH and pKA given in the equation and change the ratio to be ionized over un-ionized as follows:

$$7.3 = 8.3 + \log\frac{ionized}{un\text{-}ionized}$$

To solve this equation, first, move all numeric values to one side of the equation:

$$-1 = \log\frac{ionized}{un\text{-}ionized}$$

Second, get rid of the log function by taking each side of the equation to the power of 10:

$$10^{-1} = 10\log\frac{ionized}{un\text{-}ionized}$$

The 10 to a log power on the right side of the equation cancels out, and converting from scientific notation gives the following:

$$0.1 = \frac{ionized}{un\text{-}ionized}$$

Note that this is a good time to review general principles of using logarithmic functions and scientific notation. These functions will not be available on the NAPLEX calculator; understanding the simple principles is needed to calculate these problems.

Any number on either side of an equation can be divided by 1 without altering the math, thus the 0.1 on the left side of the equation can be divided by 1 to give ratios on both side of the equation:

$$\frac{0.1}{1} = \frac{ionized}{un\text{-}ionized}$$

This equation can be read need to add the 0.1 to the 1 (total drug parts = 1.1). This shows that 0.1 of a total of 1.1 is ionized and 1 of 1.1 is un-ionized. The question asks for the percentage un-ionized, so divide 1 by 1.1. The result is a value of 90.9%, which is approximately 90%.

Biopharmaceutics

22

This chapter covers the following:

- **Drug liberation and absorption**
- **Drug distribution**
- **Drug metabolism**
- **Drug excretion**

 Suggested Study Time: **2–3 hours**

Biopharmaceutics deal with the relationship between the physicochemical properties of a drug; the dosage form in which the drug is available; and its route of administration, with the rate and extent of its absorption and elimination from the body. It is the science that links together traditional pharmaceutics (physical pharmacy and dosage form design) with pharmacokinetics. The acronym LADME (liberation, absorption, distribution, metabolism, and excretion) is often used to describe the main processes addressed by biopharmaceutics.

DRUG LIBERATION AND ABSORPTION

A key concept to remember is that drugs are administered as dosage forms, not individual chemicals. Once taken, they must first be liberated from the dosage form in question and absorbed into the bloodstream before they become available in the systemic circulation. The exception is intravenously administered drugs, as they are delivered directly into the systemic circulation.

Liberation from a dosage form can be as simple as powder from a capsule being released from the capsule shell after ingestion, or as complicated as the slow release of drug from a tablet or transdermal patch matrix. Oral compressed tablets are the most commonly dispensed dosage form; in this case, liberation of the drug requires disintegration of the tablet into smaller drug particles that then undergo dissolution.

If a drug is not already in solution within the dosage form (as in an oral syrup or elixir), it must first undergo dissolution. Undissolved drug particles cannot cross biological membranes and are therefore trapped at their location of administration. For oral dosage forms, this means the gastrointestinal (GI) tract; any drug that is not absorbed is lost in the feces. In the case of an eyedrop given in suspension form, the drug particles remain on the corneal surface until the drug either dissolves and passes through the corneal membrane or is lost via lacrimal drainage. Similarly, topical products remain on the skin surface, and intramuscular and subcutaneous injections remain in the tissues until the drug is dissolved in the body fluids.

The rate and extent to which the drug contained in the dosage forms described above is absorbed into the systemic circulation is the **bioavailability**. This property plays a very important role in the biopharmaceutics and pharmacokinetics of drugs. The liberation and dissolution of a drug can be affected by processing factors and excipients, which can in turn affect bioavailability. Other factors affecting bioavailability are addressed later in this chapter.

One physicochemical property that can affect bioavailability is particle size. Decreasing the particle size of a drug formulation increases the surface area, which leads to more rapid dissolution. This is an important factor for drugs with low water solubility; finely milling or micronizing drugs such as griseofulvin and nitrofurantoin can dramatically improve their oral bioavailability.

Many excipients can affect product bioavailability. Some examples are listed in the table below.

Excipients That Affect Product Bioavailability

Excipient Category	Examples	Effect on Drug Particles	Effect on Bioavailability
Disintegrants	Starch, microcrystalline cellulose	Breaks tablet into smaller particles, increases dissolution	Possible increase
Surfactants	Tweens, Spans	Low concentration: Decrease surface tension and increase dissolution rate	Possible increase
		High concentration: Form micelles with drug inside, decrease dissolution	Possible decrease
Lubricants	Magnesium stearate	Has tendency to waterproof particles in large concentration, making them less soluble	Possible decrease

Drug Transport Across Membranes

There are several ways for drugs to cross body membranes that you should be aware of: Passive diffusion, carrier-mediated transport, endocytosis, and drug efflux. In passive diffusion, the drug crosses cell membranes based on a concentration gradient, moving from regions of higher concentration to areas of (relatively) lower concentration. For this mechanism to be practical, the drug must be small enough to be absorbed across cells and lipid-soluble enough to interact with the cell membranes. The rate of transport is described by Fick's first law of diffusion:

$$\frac{dC}{dt} = \frac{DA(C_s - C)}{h}$$

While it is unlikely that the exam will require you to perform calculations based on this equation, you should be familiar with the items that affect it: The concentration gradient ($C_S - C$), the thickness of the membrane being crossed (h), the surface area of the membrane (A), and the diffusion coefficient of the drug (D).

As would be expected, drugs diffuse more slowly through thicker membranes. Body locations with larger surface area tend to promote faster diffusion, as there is more available membrane through which the drug molecule can diffuse. The small intestine is thus a prime location for drug absorption, as the surface area is very large due to the presence of villi and microvilli.

Another key factor to remember is that the GI membranes are more permeable to the drug in the un-ionized form. It would therefore be expected that weakly acidic drugs would be better absorbed in the highly acidic environment of the stomach. In an acidic environment, a weakly acidic drug would be primarily in its un-ionized form. However, solubility of weakly acidic drugs increases as the drug moves from the stomach to the intestines. The reason that weakly acidic drugs are commonly better absorbed in a more basic environment such as the duodenum is not the pH of the environment. The aforementioned factors that affect drug absorption play a bigger role, such as a decreased membrane thickness and increased surface area of the small intestine. Furthermore, even though the un-ionized form of a drug is more permeable to cell membranes, the ionized form of the drug is more soluble. Therefore, basic drugs will be more soluble in the highly acidic environment of the stomach. Because of this, poorly soluble, weakly basic drugs may be poorly absorbed if taken with drugs that reduce gastric acid secretion. Ketoconazole and dipyridamole both exhibit reduced rate and extent of absorption when taken with H_2 blockers such as cimetidine or with proton pump inhibitors such as omeprazole. This phenomenon of solubility and permeability is governed by Henderson-Hasselbalch equation, as explained in the Ionization Behavior section of chapter 21.

Not all drugs are absorbed by passive diffusion; many undergo carrier-mediated transport processes. Active transport, which requires input of energy and occurs against a concentration gradient, is the most common type. Unlike passive diffusion, the process can be saturated or competitively inhibited by chemically similar substrates. Many drugs are transported via transport systems designed to move amino acids and vitamins across cell walls (see table on next page). Some drugs undergo simultaneous passive diffusion and active transport.

Active Transport Mechanisms for Drugs in the Body

Transporter	Drugs Transported
Peptide	• Penicillins • Cephalosporins • ACE inhibitors
Nucleoside	• Anticancer/antiviral nucleosides
Amino acid	• L-dopa • Methyldopa

Facilitated diffusion is another carrier-mediated transport process; it differs from active transport in that it occurs only from high to low concentrations. As with active transport, the transporter may bind to structurally similar inhibitors, which will decrease the transport rate of the drug. If the inhibitor is present in high concentration, the transporter may become saturated. Furosemide, morphine, and dopamine are examples of drugs that undergo facilitated diffusion.

Macromolecules are most likely to cross cell membranes by endocytosis, a process in which substances are transported across cell membranes by formation of vesicles. Most endocytosis is receptor-mediated; nonreceptor-mediated endocytosis is called either phagocytosis (engulfment of solid particles) or pinocytosis (engulfment of liquid), and is often seen in the GI tract and lungs. Protein and peptide drugs such as insulin, erythropoietin, and growth hormone are transported in this fashion. Polio and other oral vaccines are absorbed from the GI tract by phagocytosis, a specific type of endocytosis that is not receptor mediated.

The final method of drug transport with which you should be concerned is drug efflux. In this case, transporters pump drugs and other substances out of cells rather than into them. P-glycoprotein is the key efflux protein, and is linked to multidrug resistance in tumor cells. In this case, resistance occurs because the transporter pumps drug back out of the tumor site before it can accumulate to an effective concentration. P-glycoprotein is also expressed on the intraluminal surface of the gastrointestinal tract. In this location, it pumps substrates out of the plasma and back into the intestinal lumen, resulting in a reduced net absorption (and bioavailability) of some drugs. Digoxin, steroids, and immunosuppressive agents are just a few of the drugs that can be affected in this way. There is significant overlap between drugs that are inhibitors of the cytochrome P450 3A (CYP3A) isoenzyme and inhibitors of P-glycoprotein. Therefore, many drugs that are known inhibitors of the CYP3A can decrease the absorption and plasma concentrations of digoxin despite the fact that digoxin is not a CYP3A substrate. The amiodarone–digoxin interaction is a clinically relevant example of an interaction involving P-glycoprotein that results in decreased plasma digoxin concentrations.

Barriers to Drug Absorption

Several factors can affect drug absorption. The drug not only must dissolve initially but also should stay in solution during the absorption process. The pH of the GI tract varies significantly, and a drug that is in solution at the low pH of the stomach may be less soluble in the higher pH of the small intestine. Food intake can affect absorption and bioavailability in a variety of ways, including increasing the pH in the stomach, which can in turn affect the drug dissolution and absorption (increasing dissolution and absorption for weak acids, and decreasing both for weak bases). Chemical stability may be affected as well, which can in turn lower the amount of drug available for absorption.

Food-Related Absorption and Bioavailability Variations

Process	Explanation	Examples
Food-drug complexation	Can bind and make drug insoluble; prevent absorption	Tetracycline complexes with calcium and iron in food and supplements
Alteration of pH	Food acts as buffer in stomach; increases pH	• Increases dissolution (and subsequent absorption) of weak acids • Decreases dissolution of weak bases
Gastric emptying	Foods (especially fatty ones) and some drugs slow gastric emptying and delay drug onset	
Gastric acid secretions	• Pepsin may increase drug metabolism • Bile salts increase dissolution of poorly soluble drugs, but can form complexes with other drugs	Bile acid-drug complexes: Neomycin, kanamycin, nystatin
Competition for specialized absorption mechanisms	Competitive inhibition of drugs by nutrients with similar chemical structures	
Increased volume and viscosity of GI contents	Presence of food can lead to: • Slower drug dissolution • Slower diffusion of dissolved drug from GI tract	
Food-induced changes in first-pass metabolism	Increased bioavailability due to inhibited cytochrome P450 (primarily CYP3A)	Grapefruit juice ingestions lead to increased bioavailability of: • Cyclosporin • Saquinavir • Verapamil

Food-Related Absorption and Bioavailability Variations *(cont'd)*

Process	Explanation	Examples
Food-induced changes in blood flow	• Giving some drugs with food increases bioavailability due to increased blood flow to the GI tract and liver following a meal • A larger fraction of drug escapes first-pass metabolism because the enzyme system becomes overwhelmed	Drugs with metabolism sensitive to rate of presentation to liver: • Propranolol • Hydralazine

DRUG DISTRIBUTION

Once in the bloodstream, some drug may be bound to the plasma proteins while the remainder remains unbound. A key point to remember is that only drug that is unbound can pass out of the plasma to reach the site of action. The amount of drug that is bound to plasma protein is in dynamic equilibrium with the amount that is not.

Volume of Distribution

In the average 70-kg (~155-lb) patient, blood volume is approximately 5 L and total body water is about 40 L. After absorption, a drug will distribute into the body fluids; since the total amount of drug placed into the body is known and the concentration of drug in the plasma can be measured, the volume of fluid through which the drug seems to have distributed throughout the body can be determined. This volume is referred to as the *apparent* volume of distribution, because it is not a physical volume. Rather, it is a calculated number, dependent on physicochemical properties of the drug, which helps compare the behavior of different drugs. Thus, the apparent volume of distribution may be a much larger value than what is physiologically possible (i.e., $\geq 1,000$ L). This indicates that the drug either is primarily distributed into extravascular tissue or is highly protein bound. This phenomenon can be visualized by the following equation to determine a drug's apparent volume of distribution (V_d):

$$V_d = \frac{dose}{C_p}$$ when dose = IV bolus and C_p is unbound plasma drug concentration measured immediately after injection

Plasma Protein Binding

Most drugs exhibit protein binding, and this greatly affects their volume of distribution. Proteins are large molecules that cannot leave the capillaries; therefore, the drug-protein complex remains in the plasma. However, since the concentration of protein-bound drug is not usually measured, protein binding results in lower free plasma concentration of the drug, increasing the apparent volume of distribution. As protein binding is reversible, equilibrium exists between bound and free drug. As free drug distributes out of the bloodstream, bound drug is released from plasma proteins to maintain the equilibrium.

Although plasma proteins are relatively nonspecific in their binding behavior, the different proteins do tend to bind to different types of drug:

- Albumin: Weak acids
- α_1-acid glycoprotein: Weak bases
- Lipoproteins: Basic and neutral drugs
- Globulins: Steroids, vitamins, metal ions

Dosing a highly protein-bound drug based only on physiological volumes (plasma volume, interstitial volume, or total body water) may not produce a high enough concentration at the site of drug action to yield an adequate pharmacological response. Therefore, a higher dose may need to be given. The protein-drug complex can also act as a drug reservoir, prolonging action of the drug in the body. These factors must be considered when determining dose and dosing frequency. Certain disease states can alter the levels of plasma proteins significantly enough to require drug dose adjustments. Additionally, if a patient is receiving several drugs that all bind to the same plasma protein, one drug may displace another, leading to higher-than-expected drug concentrations and possible toxicity. This is most important in drugs that are more than 95% bound, particularly if they have a narrow therapeutic index. Warfarin (99% bound) is an excellent example of this. Even a minor displacement of protein-bound warfarin (e.g., 99% to 98% bound) would double the unbound and therefore the effective concentration of warfarin from 1% to 2%. However, there are few examples of clinically relevant drug interactions related to displacing plasma protein binding.

Some Disease States and Physiological Conditions That Affect Plasma Protein Concentration

Decrease plasma protein concentration	• Liver disease • Trauma (albumin) • Surgery (albumin) • Burns • Renal failure (albumin) • Hyperthyroidism • Age (neonate, geriatric) • Pregnancy
Increase plasma protein concentration	• Hypothyroidism • Schizophrenia • Rheumatoid arthritis • Renal failure (α_1-acid glycoprotein) • Trauma (α_1-acid glycoprotein) • Surgery (α_1-acid glycoprotein)

DRUG METABOLISM

Drugs are eliminated from the body by two processes: Metabolism and excretion. Metabolism, also referred to as biotransformation, leads to the chemical conversion of drug to active or inactive compounds called metabolites. These metabolites are generally more polar (and hence more water-soluble) than the parent drugs. This allows the metabolites to be more efficiently cleared in the urine. Not all drugs undergo metabolism.

Metabolism is most likely to occur in organs that contain high levels of enzymes. Many microsomal enzymes, including the cytochrome P450 (CYP450) mixed-function oxidases, are found in the liver, which is the primary site of biotransformation. Metabolizing enzymes are found in many other locations of the body, and significant biotransformation of some drugs can occur in the intestinal tract, kidney, and brain. Drugs administered via nasal, pulmonary, or dermal routes often also show significant biotransformation in the nasal tissue, lung, or skin.

One concern with oral delivery of certain drugs is presystemic, or first-pass, metabolism. Because the venous outflow of the GI tract travels directly to the liver via the portal vein, drugs administered via the GI tract are susceptible to hepatic metabolism before they reach the systemic circulation. Bioavailability is decreased, so the drug must be given either in a higher dose or by a delivery route that bypasses the GI tract. Nitroglycerin, for example, is almost completely degraded by first-pass metabolism and is therefore usually formulated as sublingual tablets or spray, or transdermal ointment or patches. Oral extended-release capsules are also available and are believed to work by saturating the hepatic enzymes responsible for metabolism and by producing metabolites that possess some activity.

Phase I Reactions

Metabolism is classified into Phase I and Phase II reactions. In many cases, a drug may undergo metabolism by competing pathways, leading to multiple metabolites. The metabolites may in turn undergo metabolism. Some of these metabolites may possess therapeutic activity. Some medications are deliberately administered as inactive prodrugs, and the therapeutic component results from the metabolism of the prodrug. Formulating a medication as a prodrug can improve its pharmaceutical, pharmacodynamic, or pharmacokinetic properties.

Phase I reactions are so named because they generally occur before Phase II reactions. However, in some instances, drugs are solely metabolized by Phase II reactions. They are nonsynthetic and introduce or expose a functional group. The primary types of Phase I reactions are oxidation, reduction, and hydrolysis. Oxidation is the most common type of metabolism, and many of these reactions are catalyzed by enzymes in the CYP superfamily.

Phase II Reactions

Phase II reactions are synthetic reactions. They are often called conjugation reactions, as a reactive group on the drug is attached to a polar molecule or group originating inside the body. This generally leads to a polar, water-soluble metabolite. While most drugs undergo Phase I metabolism prior to Phase II, this is not required provided the drug already possesses one or more reactive groups.

Examples of Phase II reactions are listed in the table on the next page, with glucuronidation being the most common example. Since these reactions involve enzymes, the reactions may be capacity limited. If the concentration of drug approaches or exceeds the metabolic capacity of the enzyme, nonlinear drug metabolism may be observed.

Two types of conjugation reactions (methylation and acetylation) lead to metabolites that are less polar, and therefore less soluble, than the original compound. Less soluble metabolites will have extended elimination half-lives. This can extend the duration of action in cases where an active metabolite is formed, such as *N*-acetylprocainamide. Toxicity may also occur from increased blood or tissue levels of toxic metabolites. For example, at high concentrations the acetylated metabolites of sulfonamides can precipitate in the kidney tubules and lead to kidney damage and crystalluria.

Phase II Reactions

Type of Phase II Reaction	Drugs Metabolized by This Route
Glucuronidation	• Chloramphenicol • Meprobamate • Morphine
Sulfation	• Acetaminophen • Estradiol • Methyldopa • Minoxidil
Amino acid conjugation	• Salicylic acid
Acetylation	• Isoniazid • Procainamide • Sulfonamides • Hydralazine
Methylation	• Catecholamines • Niacinamide • Thiouracil
Glutathione conjugation	• Chlorambucil

Factors Affecting Biotransformation

Several factors can affect metabolizing enzyme activity in the body. Disease state, age, gender, or chemical and nutritional exposure to a variety of substances can lead to enzyme inhibition or enzyme induction. Genetic variability also plays a role. Drug–drug interactions are a common result of the metabolic process, as most marketed drugs are metabolized by multiple pathways, and drugs that inhibit or induce enzyme activity can affect the metabolism of many other drugs.

Enzyme Inhibition

Enzyme inhibition describes the situation when an enzyme is prevented from binding with its substrate. The substrate is therefore unable to be properly metabolized, and plasma concentrations rise, possibly to toxic concentrations. In cases where a prodrug must be activated by metabolism, enzyme inhibition may limit, delay, or prevent drug activity. Enzyme inhibitors can act by competitive or noncompetitive means.

Drugs that are metabolized by the same metabolic pathways frequently act as competitive inhibitors to each other. Drug metabolites, herbal products, and foods can also act as enzyme inhibitors. Compounds containing imidazole, pyridine, or quinolone groups in particular are often found to be enzyme inhibitors. The table below contains an incomplete list of common enzyme inhibitors.

One of the most widely known drug–food interactions results from enzyme inhibition. Grapefruit juice is an inhibitor of CYP3A, the isozyme responsible for metabolism of a host of drugs, including macrolide antibiotics, benzodiazepines, calcium channel blockers, and HIV protease inhibitors. While a single portion is unlikely to lead to problems, patients receiving drugs metabolized by this isozyme should be cautioned to avoid grapefruit juice.

Drugs Involved in Inhibition of Metabolic Enzymes

CYP1A2	CYP2C9	CYP2C19	CYP2D6	CYP3A
fluvoxamine	fluconazole	cimetidine	bupropion	indinavir
ciprofloxacin	amiodarone	esomeprazole	fluoxetine	nelfinavir
		lansoprazole	paroxetine	ritonavir
		omeprazole	quinidine	clarithromycin
		pantoprazole	duloxetine	itraconazole
		fluoxetine	sertraline	ketoconazole
		fluvoxamine	terbinafine	nefazodone
		indomethacin	amiodarone	saquinavir
		isoniazid	cimetidine	telithromycin

CYP1A2	CYP2C9	CYP2C19	CYP2D6	CYP3A
		ketoconazole	chlorpromazine	erythromycin
		oxcarbazepine	clomipramine	fluconazole
		probenecid	doxepin	grapefruit juice
		topiramate	haloperidol	verapamil
		voriconazole	methadone	diltiazem
				cimetidine
				amiodarone

Enzyme Induction

Enzyme induction is essentially the opposite of enzyme inhibition. Enzyme inducers stimulate enzyme activity, which leads to decreased plasma concentrations of the enzyme's targets. In most cases, this means a decrease in both activity and adverse effects of the drug. If active or toxic metabolites are produced, however, drug activity and toxic effects may be increased. A number of commonly prescribed drugs induce metabolic enzymes, as do ethanol, tobacco, marijuana, and certain herbal products, most notably St. John's wort. This can lead to clinically significant drug interactions. For example, triazolam is extensively metabolized by CYP3A4. St. John's wort, rifampin, and several seizure medications (carbamazepine, phenytoin, and phenobarbital) induce this isozyme. Using any of these agents with triazolam or other drugs metabolized by 3A4 may lead to significantly reduced plasma concentrations and therapeutic effect. The table below lists some of the most common inducers of drug metabolism. Although there are exceptions, the inducers commonly affect all of the inducible CYP enzymes including CYP1A2, CYP2B6, CYP2C9, CYP2C19, and CYP3A.

Some drugs undergo a phenomenon called auto-induction, wherein they stimulate their own metabolism. Carbamazepine is a key example of a drug of this type. Due to auto-induction, long-term administration of carbamazepine can lead to decreased blood concentrations and therapeutic activity.

Drugs Involved in Induction of Metabolic Enzymes

Seizure medications	• Carbamazepine • Phenytoin • Phenobarbital • Secobarbital
Tuberculosis medications	• Rifampin • Isoniazid

Genetic Variability

Genetic polymorphisms lead to a number of metabolism-related issues. Extensive and poor metabolizers exist for particular drugs. Dosage adjustments must be made in order to avoid subtherapeutic consequences or toxic effects, depending on the population into which a patient falls.

CYP enzymes in particular are highly polymorphic. The following table lists select drugs metabolized by the most common CYP enzymes. CYP2D6 in particular can be problematic, as individuals can be classified as poor, intermediate, extensive, and ultra-rapid metabolizers. The percentage of poor metabolizers varies somewhat by ancestry, comprising approximately 5–10% of Caucasians, 4–6% of Blacks, and 1% of Asians. One of the drugs metabolized by CYP2D6 is codeine; in this case, poor metabolizers receive less benefit from the drug, as codeine must be metabolized into morphine to take effect. Pharmacists should be aware of this variability, since poor metabolizers may be falsely labeled as drug-seekers when in fact codeine is an ineffective analgesic for them. These patients should instead be placed on analgesics not activated by CYP2D6, such as morphine itself.

Common Drugs Metabolized by Pathway

CYP1A2	CYP2C9	CYP2C19	CYP2D6	CYP3A
caffeine	warfarin	omeprazole	codeine	clarithromycin
theophylline	phenytoin	esomeprazole	dextromethorphan	erythromycin
	glipizide	lansoprazole	hydrocodone	quinidine
	glyburide	pantoprazole	oxycodone	midazolam
		citalopram	fluoxetine	alprazolam
		voriconazole	haloperidol	diazepam
		clopidogrel	venlafaxine	cyclosporine
			paroxetine	tacrolimus
			duloxetine	cisapride
			risperidone	amlodipine
			propranolol	diltiazem
			metoprolol	nifedipine
			tamoxifen	verapamil
				atorvastatin
				lovastatin
				simvastatin
				estradiol
				carbamazepine

Glucose-6-phosphate dehydrogenase is an enzyme with over 300 reported polymorphic variants, leading to individuals possessing low, normal, or increased levels of the enzyme. As this enzyme protects red blood cells from oxidative stress, low levels combined with certain environmental or pharmacological stresses—such as eating fava beans or taking certain drugs—can lead to life-threatening hemolytic anemia. Prevalence of this deficiency is highest among those of African, Asian, and Mediterranean ancestry, with more severe variants occurring in Mediterranean populations. The high gene frequency in certain populations is believed to be related to its protective effect against malaria.

Substances to Be Avoided in Glucose-6-Phosphate Dehydrogenase Deficiency

- Oxidant drugs
    - Primaquine
    - Chloroquine
- Sulfonamides
- Quinolones
- Aspirin
- Probenecid
- Vitamin K
- Nitrofurantoin
- Fava beans
- Mothballs

Acetylation is another important instance of genetic variability in drug metabolism. Rapid-metabolizing and slow-metabolizing polymorphic variants of *N*-acetyl-transferase-2 can have therapeutic implications for several drugs, most notably the tuberculosis drug isoniazid. Slow acetylators do not metabolize the drug quickly, and must be given lower doses in order to prevent toxic effects. Rapid acetylators require substantially higher doses, and therapeutic failure rates are more common than with normal or slow acetylators.

DRUG EXCRETION

The other process by which the body eliminates substances is excretion. Unlike metabolism, excretion eliminates the substances without further chemical change. The kidney is the primary organ involved, and most substances are excreted in the urine. Polar, water-soluble drugs are usually excreted unchanged; lipophilic drugs are generally excreted as metabolites. There are three components to renal excretion:

1. Glomerular filtration:
    - Blood passes through the capillary network (glomerulus) inside Bowman's capsule.

- Fenestrated endothelium allows paracellular transport of most solutes (other than macromolecules) into Bowman's capsule.
- Filtrate (including drug) moves from Bowman's capsule into renal tubules.
- All nonprotein-bound, small-molecule drugs undergo glomerular filtration; the concentration of drug or metabolite in the filtrate will be equal to the concentration of unbound drug in the plasma.

2. Tubular reabsorption:
   - Many nutrients and ions are actively reabsorbed into the bloodstream.
   - Water is reabsorbed, and filtrate becomes more concentrated as it moves along the tubule.
   - No transporters exist for reabsorption of drug; passive diffusion process is dependent on filtrate pH. Acidic (citrus fruits, cranberry juice, aspirin) and basic (milk products, sodium bicarbonate) foods and drugs can alter urine pH enough to affect reabsorption.
     » In alkaline urine: Acidic drugs are ionized → less reabsorbed → more readily excreted
     » In acidic urine: Basic drugs are ionized → less reabsorbed → more readily excreted
     » Pentobarbital (weak acid) overdose: Treated by alkalinizing urine with sodium bicarbonate injection

3. Tubular secretion:
   - This occurs simultaneously with tubular reabsorption.
   - This removes certain substances from the blood and secretes them back into the filtrate.
   - This occurs against the concentration gradients and is an energy-requiring process that uses protein transporters.
   - Only ionized drugs are bound to and secreted by the transporter proteins; drugs that are highly ionized at pH 7.4 will be secreted to a greater extent.
   - Plasma protein binding has little effect on this process; transporters can strip drug off of protein.
     » Competitive process; can lead to drug interactions
       - Saturable process; at high dose, process plateaus → less drug excreted → higher plasma concentration than expected

The rate of renal excretion of drugs is the net result of the above processes. It depends on blood flow in addition to the physicochemical properties of the drugs in question. More rapid blood flow through the nephron generally leads to an increase in all three processes, with an overall higher drug excretion rate. Glomerular filtration rate (GFR) is normally about 120 mL/min, but may vary widely with the patient's age, body weight, and disease state. GFR for an individual is determined by calculating the clearance of creatinine, an endogenous substance that is not reabsorbed or secreted. This value gives an indication of kidney function.

Renal clearance is a measure of the efficiency of renal excretion in removing unchanged drug in the urine. It is an indirect measurement expressed by the following equation, where C_U and V_U are concentration of drug in the urine and volume of urine formation per unit time:

$$CL_r = \frac{excretion\ rate\ in\ urine}{plasma\ concentration} = \frac{C_U V_U}{C_p}$$

Nonrenal Excretion

Drugs may also be excreted by the liver into the bile; at this point, one of two things can happen:

- Biliary excretion: Bile (including drug) is emptied into the small intestine, where it is eventually excreted from the body in the feces.
- Enterohepatic recycling: The drug is partially reabsorbed from the intestines (based on pKa and partition coefficient) and re-enters the bloodstream. Drugs undergoing this process may show a secondary peak in plasma concentration; with multiple dosing regimens, the blood-concentration curve can be altered significantly.

Some drugs are excreted into other fluids, though this is usually not a significant route:

- Saliva: Swallowed, leading to salivary recycling; routine and noninvasive way of monitoring for concentrations of certain drugs
- Breast milk: Mostly occurs by passive diffusion (primarily of weak bases); can lead to drug transfer to breastfeeding infants
- Sweat: Small volume, so not a significant mode of drug excretion; could become a convenient method for detecting use of illegal or restricted drugs (cocaine, amphetamines, morphine, and ethanol)
- Expired air: Significant route of excretion for volatile drugs (anesthetics, ethanol); drug volatility is more important than polarity for this method of excretion

Learning Points

- The prime body location for drug absorption is the small intestine, due to the high surface area; the drug must be dissolved in order to be absorbed. Factors affecting dissolution in the small intestine (i.e., pH) may prevent this from being the prime absorption location for a particular drug.

- Only drugs that are unbound to plasma protein can pass from the plasma to reach the site of action.

- Enzyme inhibition can often lead to toxicity; enzyme induction can lead to inadequate blood concentrations of drug.

- Genetic variations in CYP metabolism lead to fast and slow metabolizers of a variety of drugs; dosage adjustments or alternate therapies must be made in some cases.

- Tubular reabsorption decreases drug and metabolite concentration in the urine, while tubular secretion increases the amount. Water-soluble, ionized drugs are more likely to be excreted.

PRACTICE QUESTIONS

1. A single IV dose of a drug is given and the AUC is calculated. After an adequate washout period, a single oral dose of the same drug is given. If the doses are the same size, which of the following results is possible?

   I. $AUC_{PO} = AUC_{IV}$
   II. $AUC_{PO} > AUC_{IV}$
   III. $AUC_{PO} < AUC_{IV}$

   (A) I only
   (B) II only
   (C) I and II
   (D) II and III
   (E) I, II, and III

2. The quality control test required for tablets, intended to reflect the release of the drug, is the

   (A) weight variation test.
   (B) content uniformity test.
   (C) dissolution test.
   (D) disintegration test.
   (E) friability test.

3. A 15-year-old patient taking Focalin XR for his ADHD is experiencing inattention later in the day. He admits that after having a cold 2 weeks ago, he started taking 2 g of vitamin C per day to "boost his immune system." What do you think is causing his symptoms?

   (A) He is experiencing vitamin C toxicity.
   (B) The vitamin C is acidifying his urine, causing decreased excretion of Focalin XR.
   (C) The vitamin C is acidifying his urine, causing increased excretion of Focalin XR.
   (D) The vitamin C is inducing CYP2D6, causing increased metabolism of Focalin XR.
   (E) The vitamin C is inhibiting CYP2D6, causing increased metabolism of Focalin XR.

4. Which of the following is the most likely clinical outcome in a CYP2D6 poor metabolizer being treated for pain?

   (A) Hallucinations associated with morphine
   (B) Failed pain management with codeine
   (C) Respiratory depression with hydrocodone
   (D) Failed pain management with hydromorphone
   (E) None of the above would be expected

5. In cases of overdose of the sodium salt of a chemotherapeutic drug, the rate of excretion of the drug may be increased by which of the following?

    (A) Intravenous administration of ammonium chloride
    (B) Intravenous administration of calcium chloride
    (C) Acidifying the urine
    (D) Intravenous administration of sodium bicarbonate
    (E) Intravenous administration of monosodium phosphate

6. Acidification of the urine in a patient taking aspirin can be expected to do which of the following?

    (A) Increase the rate of excretion of the drug
    (B) Increase the blood concentrations of the drug
    (C) Cause hydrolysis of the drug
    (D) Lower the blood concentration of the drug
    (E) Have no effect on the concentration of the drug

ANSWERS

1. E

Because the bioavailability of a drug administered intravenously is 1, by definition, the oral bioavailability of a dosage form containing the same drug may be as high as the IV bioavailability (assuming complete absorption and no first-pass metabolism). It will usually be lower than the IV dose. However, because bioavailability can never be greater than 1, the oral bioavailability may never exceed the IV bioavailability. The AUC_{PO} may, therefore, be less than or equal to the AUC_{IV}, but never greater.

2. C

The quality control test intended to reflect the absorption of the drug is the dissolution test. It is only an approximation; going into solution is the last step before absorption. Weight variation and content uniformity tests assess the distribution of the active ingredients across the tablets and ensure that each dose is approximately the same weight. The disintegration test evaluates how quickly or slowly a tablet disintegrates; disintegration is a necessary step prior to dissolution. The friability test determines how well tablets will hold up to handling.

3. C

Focalin (dexmethylphenidate) is a weakly basic drug primarily excreted via the renal route. Acidification of the urine will cause trapping of the ionized form of the drug in the urine, increasing urinary excretion. Although some quantity of Focalin is metabolized by CYP2D6, vitamin C does not induce this enzyme. Symptoms of vitamin C toxicity do not include inattention.

4. B

The parent drug codeine has minimal analgesic effectiveness. It primarily exerts it analgesic effect through activation to morphine by cytochrome P450 2D6 (CYP2D6). Therefore, a poor metabolizer of CYP2D6 would have negligible morphine concentrations and would likely lack a clinically effective analgesic effect from codeine.

5. D

Because the drug is formulated as a sodium salt, the drug must be a weak acid. The positive charge of the sodium ion replaces the hydronium ion of the acid through an ionic bond. Placing the drug in its ionized form to facilitate the excretion and limit reabsorption. To ionize a weak acid, the pH of the ultrafiltrate should be raised with a basic solution. Sodium bicarbonate is the only basic solution provided that can be used clinically and that raises the pH of the ultrafiltrate.

6. **B**

Aspirin is a weak acid. As the pH of the environment is lowered, weak acids will be primarily in the un-ionized form. Remember that acids are proton donors (i.e., hydronium ion donors). In an acidic environment, weak acids are surrounded by other proton donors; thus they are more likely to have the hydronium ion and be without charge. The uncharged drug molecule is more lipophilic and can cross biological membranes. Hence, in its un-ionized form, the drug will be without charge and can undergo passive reabsorption to increase blood concentrations.

Pharmacokinetics

23

This chapter covers the following:

- **Plasma drug concentration profiles**
- **Theoretical compartments**
- **Basic pharmacokinetic parameters**
- **Oral dosing**
- **Multiple drug dosing**
- **Multiple dosing factor and accumulation factor**
- **Nonlinear pharmacokinetics**

 Suggested Study Time: **2 hours**

Pharmacokinetics is the mathematical study of drug concentration in the body. It is dependent on the absorption, distribution, metabolism, and excretion (ADME) discussed in this book's biopharmaceutics chapter and is the quantitative description of what happens to the drug in the body. Clinical pharmacokinetics applies the concepts directly to individual patients, making individualized drug therapy and therapeutic drug monitoring possible.

Many equations are employed in pharmacokinetics. The more complicated of these equations are unlikely to be used in calculations on the NAPLEX due to time constraints, but you should be familiar with their concepts because they could form the basis for theoretical questions. Study for this section of the exam should focus primarily on being able to perform calculations related to the basic pharmacokinetic parameters discussed below and being able to properly interpret graphs of blood concentration data. Calculations involving drugs most likely to be monitored clinically (e.g., digoxin, phenytoin, and so on) are the most important to focus on.

PLASMA DRUG CONCENTRATION PROFILES

Plasma-drug-concentration-versus-time curve charts are used extensively in pharmacokinetics. A known dose of drug is given to a patient, and blood samples are taken at various time intervals following drug administration. The concentration of drug in plasma following IV and oral administration is measured and plotted in the following figure. The shape of the curve depends on the relative rates of absorption, distribution, and elimination of the drug.

Plasma-Level-versus-Time Curves for Intravenous and Oral Drug Administration

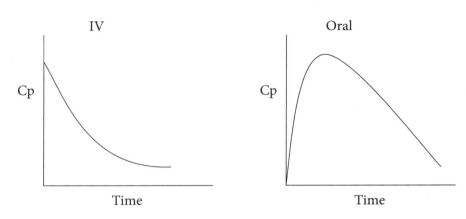

The preceding graphs represent drug plasma concentration versus time profiles following an IV bolus and oral administration of a mock drug. At time 0 (leftmost point on the X-axis) following IV administration, the drug will reach its maximum plasma concentration (*Cmax*). Therefore, the time to maximum plasma concentration (*Tpeak* or *Tmax*) is at time 0 following an IV bolus. The only route of administration that can be delineated from the concentration-time curve alone is an IV bolus due to the *Cmax* occurring at time 0.

The time 0 on the oral concentration-time profile does not display measurable plasma concentrations. This is true for any route of administration for which absorption into the systemic circulation is required (e.g., sublingual, inhalational, subcutaneous, and so on). Following the lag time for absorption, a rise in drug plasma concentration is seen until it reaches a plateau, which represents the *Cmax* on the oral curve. The time of this plateau (i.e., *Cmax*) is the *Tpeak*. At the Tpeak, there is a brief time period where this is no net change in drug plasma concentration. This represents the time when the rate of drug absorption is equal to that of elimination. Beyond the *Cmax*, elimination will be greater than absorption and is represented by a decline in the drug plasma concentration.

THEORETICAL COMPARTMENTS

From a pharmacokinetic perspective, the body is considered to consist of compartments, inside each of which the drug can be considered evenly distributed. These compartments are interconnected, and the drug moves between them at defined rates. Although compartments are completely theoretical (consisting of groups of tissues with similar blood flow and drug affinity, not actual body regions), they serve a useful purpose in simplifying calculations. Several models exist, but only two are likely to be considered on the NAPLEX:

- One-compartment model:
  - Body consists of one homogenous central compartment.
  - Drug distributes rapidly and uniformly to this compartment.
- Two-compartment model:
  - Central compartment is still present, and includes highly perfused organs (e.g., liver, kidneys).
  - There is a slow distribution of drug into a peripheral compartment that consists of poorly perfused tissue (e.g., muscles, connective tissue).

One-Compartment Model

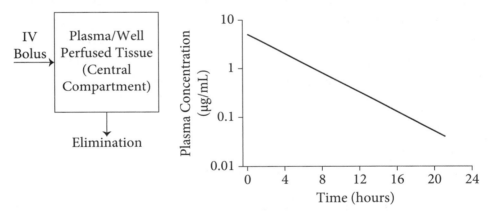

The basic structure of a one-compartment drug is displayed on the left, with a corresponding drug log concentration-time curve on the right. At time 0, the drug is administered into the central compartment. This can be observed on the concentration-time curve by the *Cmax* at time 0. The central compartment represents plasma and tissue that the drug rapidly distributes. The slope of the concentration time curve on a log or natural log scale is directly proportional to the first-order elimination rate constant and therefore the drug half-life. The elimination rate constant can be calculated by taking the difference of the natural log of two concentrations and dividing by the difference of the two corresponding times.

Two-Compartment Model

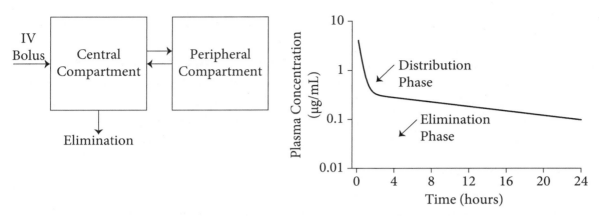

The general structure of a two-compartment model is displayed on the left of the figure above. The right side of the figure represents the log concentration-time profile following an IV bolus of a two-compartment drug. As displayed on the concentration-time curve, there are two distinct slopes labeled as the distribution phase and the elimination phase. The *Cmax* following an IV bolus in a two-compartment model is still at time 0. However, the slope of the line at time 0 is representative of both the elimination from the central compartment and slow distribution into peripheral tissue. This phase, commonly called the *distribution phase* of the drug, is not directly representative of elimination. Therefore, it is inappropriate to calculate an elimination rate constant or half-life while a drug is in the elimination phase. Once drug accumulates in the peripheral tissue to a point of equilibrium (i.e., drug diffuses from peripheral tissue back into the central compartment), the change in the concentration-time curve is solely due to the elimination of the drug. The half-life of the drug can be calculated only in this phase.

BASIC PHARMACOKINETIC PARAMETERS

Most calculations you are likely to see on the NAPLEX involve the parameters listed below.

Bioavailable Fraction

Bioavailable fraction (F) is the portion of dose administered that reaches the systemic circulation. For IV administration, $F = 1$. Drug given by any other route can have a bioavailable fraction ranging from 0 to 1; the bioavailable fraction will never be greater than 1. Two factors can decrease the bioavailable fraction of a drug:

- Incomplete absorption
- First-pass metabolism

The equation governing the bioavailable fraction is given below. *fa* represents the fraction of administered dose absorbed into the bloodstream, and *ffp* represents the fraction of absorbed drug escaping first-pass metabolism.

$$F = ffp \cdot fa$$

Hepatic Extraction Ratio

The hepatic extraction ratio (E) is the fraction of drug in the blood that is metabolized during each pass of blood through the liver.

$$(1 - E) = ffp$$

High-E drugs are extensively metabolized by the liver enzymes. Low-E drugs are metabolized by enzymes with relatively low affinity for the drug. Knowing a drug's E value is useful in predicting the effects of first-pass metabolism, disease states, and drug–drug interactions on the metabolism of the drug.

Plasma Concentrations

The plasma concentation of the drug (C) can be determined by a number of equations. The most basic version, for a drug following a one-compartment model, is given below in three formats.

$$C = C_0 e^{-kt}$$
$$\ln C = \ln C_0 - kt$$
$$\log C = \log C_0 - \frac{kt}{2.3}$$

When calculating plasma levels following an intravenous (IV) bolus dose, these are the equations you should use. The NAPLEX exam does not have an exponential or log function on the available calculator, so these equations likely have little use on the exam.

Elimination Rate Constant

The first-order elimination rate constant, k, represents the fraction of drug eliminated per unit time, and thus has units of reciprocal time (i.e., hr^{-1}). It can be obtained graphically (see figure below) or from the drug half-life:

$$k = \frac{\ln 2}{t_{1/2}} = \frac{0.693}{t_{1/2}}$$

Graphical Calculation of Elimination Rate Constant

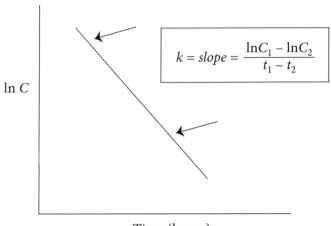

$$k = slope = \frac{\ln C_1 - \ln C_2}{t_1 - t_2}$$

ln C

Time (hours)

Half-Life

The elimination half-life of a drug is the time required for its serum concentration to decrease by half. It can be obtained mathematically or graphically:

$$t_{1/2} = \frac{\ln 2}{k} = \frac{0.693}{k}$$

Half-life can also be calculated from clearance and volume of distribution (see sections below). While these parameters do not influence or depend on one another, half-life depends on both of them:

$$t_{1/2} = 0.693 \cdot \left(\frac{Vd}{CL} \right)$$

Clearance

Clearance refers to the efficiency of the body in removing drug from the blood. The liver and kidney are the primary organs involved, and body clearance refers to the sum of the hepatic and renal clearances, plus any clearance from other organs, usually negligible:

$$CL = CL_h + CL_r$$

Some drugs are cleared primarily by one organ (propranolol has a hepatic clearance of 840 mL/min and a total clearance of only 848 mL/min), while others show more mixed clearance (procainamide has a hepatic clearance of 268 mL/min and a renal clearance of 303 mL/min). Knowledge of drug clearance can help determine when dosage adjustments are needed in patients with liver or kidney disease. Using the above examples, patients with kidney disease would need dose adjustments for procainamide but not for propranolol. Patients with liver disease would need dose adjustments for both drugs.

If clearance increases, the drug is more efficiently removed from the body and the drug half-life decreases.

Population clearance values are typically based on body weight; clearance corresponds to ideal body weight (IBW):

- Tall, lean individuals have larger eliminating organs à higher clearance than a shorter lean person.
- Adipose tissue does not affect the size of eliminating organs, thus actual body weight should not be used to determine clearance in obese patients (use IBW).

$$IBW\ (males) = 50kg + [2.3 \cdot (\#\ of\ inches\ of\ height > 60")]$$
$$IBW\ (females) = 45kg + [2.3 \cdot (\#\ of\ inches\ of\ height > 60")]$$

Volume of Distribution

Apparent volume of distribution (V_d) describes the volume of body fluids required to account for all drugs in the body. As mentioned in the biopharmaceutics chapter, it is not a real volume but a calculated number that helps to compare the behavior of different drugs. Several equations can be used to calculate V_d, depending on the information you have available:

$$V_d = \frac{dose}{C_{peak}} = \frac{F \cdot D_0}{AUC \cdot k} = \frac{CL \cdot t_{1/2}}{0.693}$$

Volume of distribution has the following effect on half-life:

- Small V_d:
  - Drug mostly located in blood
  - Liver and kidneys can only clear drug in blood
  - Fewer passes needed to rid body of drug
  - Shorter half-life
- Large V_d:
  - Drug is extensively distributed into extravascular tissues
  - More passes are required to clear drug from body
  - Longer half-life

Area under the Curve

Area under the curve (AUC) is a measure of the extent of drug exposure. It is defined as the area under the drug plasma level – time curve from $t = 0$ to infinity. It can be calculated by the trapezoidal rule (unlikely to appear on the NAPLEX, due to time constraints), or by the other listed equations, and has units of concentration/time. S is the salt factor for a given drug formulation and refers to the percentage of administered product that is the active moiety (the acid or base, not the salt). A commonly used example of a drug with a salt factor is aminophylline ($S = 0.8$), as compared to theophylline ($S = 1$).

Trapezoidal rule:

$$AUC = \frac{C_{n-1} + C_n}{2}(tn - t_{n-1})$$

Other equations:

$$AUC = \frac{F \cdot S \cdot D_0}{CL} = \frac{F \cdot D_0}{k \cdot V_D}$$

AUC is often directly proportional to dose, such that increasing the dose of a drug from 500 mg to 1,000 mg will lead to a two-fold increase in AUC. This is not always the case, however. If a pathway for drug elimination becomes saturated, as can happen with the enzyme-dependent metabolism of certain drugs (such as phenytoin and salicylates), increasing the dose can lead to a disproportionately large increase in AUC.

ORAL DOSING

Most immediate-release oral dosage forms follow a first-order absorption model, as do some nonoral dosage forms such as suppositories and intramuscular (IM) injections. When plotting log C versus time (see figure below), the following equation of the "y = mx + b" format applies:

$$\log C = \log \frac{F \cdot K_a \cdot D}{V_D(k_a - k)} = \frac{kt}{2.3}$$

First-Order Drug Plasma-Level-versus-Time Curve

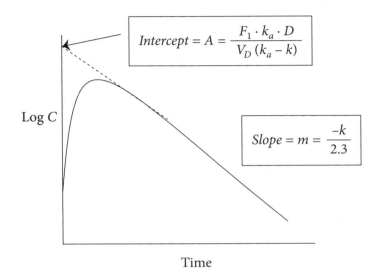

The above equation may also be expressed as:

$$C = \frac{F \cdot K_a \cdot D}{V_D(k_a - k)} = (e^{-kt} - e^{-k_a t}) \quad \text{or} \quad C = Ae^{-kt} - Be^{-k_a t}$$

The absorption rate constant, k_a, cannot be measured directly. It can be calculated by several methods, which are fairly lengthy mathematical processes and are unlikely to be tested on the NAPLEX. General questions about the methods could be asked, however.

- Method of residuals (feathering, peeling)
  - The difference between the extrapolated line in the above graph and the point directly below it on the absorption portion of the curve (the residual) is plotted versus time.
  - The slope of this line is equal to $-k_a / 2.3$.
- Wagner-Nelson method
  - Plots fraction of drug unabsorbed versus time
  - Can use blood level and/or urinary excretion data
- Loo-Riegelman method
  - Plots percent of drug unabsorbed versus time
  - Used for two-compartment model drugs
  - Must give drug intravenously and orally in order to obtain all necessary information

MULTIPLE DRUG DOSING

Most drugs are not given as single doses but are administered in multiple doses over prolonged periods of time. Since plasma concentrations must be maintained within certain levels in order to achieve maximum effectiveness and to limit toxicity (minimum effective concentration [MEC] and minimum toxic concentration [MTC]), drug accumulation must be considered. Knowing the basic pharmacokinetic parameters for a given drug (k, V_d, and/or CL), as well as the dose (D) and dosing interval (τ), it is possible to predict the plasma concentration at any time after beginning the dosage regimen.

The most common model used in calculating drug concentrations in the setting of multiple-dosage regimens is that of superposition. It assumes that early doses do not affect the pharmacokinetics of subsequent doses, and that the blood concentrations after subsequent doses will overlay the previous doses. In other words, the blood concentration after each dose can simply be added to the level remaining in the system from prior doses. First-order elimination kinetics are assumed.

If the same dose of drug is given at a fixed-dose frequency, eventually the plasma concentration curve reaches a plateau and a steady-state plasma concentration is reached (C_{SS}). At this point, the rate of the drug entering the body equals the rate of drug leaving the body. Blood concentrations are constant from interval to interval, provided the patient's pharmacokinetic parameters do not change and the dose and dosing interval stay the same. Ninety percent of the steady-state concentration is attained after three half-lives; after five half-lives, 97% is attained. These numbers are very important to remember as they will allow you to estimate some answers on the NAPLEX. Calculation of C_{SS} is discussed soon, but two other terms must be accounted for first.

MULTIPLE DOSING FACTOR AND ACCUMULATION FACTOR

The extent of accumulation can be predicted by using the multiple dosing factor (MDF), where N = the number of doses:

$$MDF = \frac{1 \cdot e^{-N \cdot k \cdot t}}{1 - e^{-k \cdot t}}$$

Single-dose equations can be converted to multiple-dose equations simply by multiplying each exponential term that contains time as a variable by the MDF.

At steady state, the MDF simplifies to the following accumulation factor (AF):

$$MDF = \frac{1}{1 - e^{-k \cdot t}}$$

As the equation for *AF* shows, two things affect how much drug accumulates between the first dose and a dose at steady state:

- Elimination constant or half-life
- Dosing interval

We cannot control the half-life; it is dependent on the drug in question. However, the dosing interval can be adjusted in order to increase or decrease the drug accumulation factor. A simple estimation of this can be described by:

- Dosing interval < drug half-life → C_{SS} will be much higher than the concentration after the first dose.
- Dosing interval = drug half-life → C_{SS} will be twice as high as the concentration after the first dose.
- Dosing interval > drug half-life → C_{SS} will be similar to the concentration after the first dose (because the drug is almost completely washing out before the next dose is given).

Peak-to-Trough Ratio

Multiple intermittent dosing results in peak and trough drug concentrations. As will be discussed, a dose and dosing interval (τ) are calculated to achieve a desired steady-state plasma concentration average ($C_{SS,avg}$). The $C_{SS,avg}$ represents the average concentration between the peak and trough. The peak (P) to trough (T) ratio can be useful in determining the fluctuation of drug concentrations for a given dose and dosing interval. This is calculated by the following equation:

$$P : T = e^{+k(t - T_{max})}$$

Shorter dosing intervals for a particular dose will lead to a decreased *P:T* ratio, meaning that less fluctuation in peak-to-trough is occurring.

The peak-to-trough ratio can be especially useful when predicting the effect of switching a patient from a regular to a sustained-release formulation. T_{max} represents time to peak concentration within the dosing interval; it is smaller for immediate-release formulations than for sustained-release, as the drug is liberated and absorbed more quickly, and so the peak concentration occurs sooner.

Loading Doses

Loading doses are often used to achieve target plasma drug concentrations as quickly as possible. These large initial doses (which may be given as either a single dose or divided doses over a specified period of time) are especially important in life-threatening conditions such as myocardial infarction, status asthmaticus, and status epilepticus. Loading doses should not be used when there is not an urgent need to achieve target blood concentrations immediately or the patient cannot be supervised for possible toxicity. Loading doses for narrow-therapeutic-index drugs should ideally occur within a clinical setting.

Loading doses that are given slowly can be calculated by the equation given below. If given rapidly (by bolus injection, for example), the volume of the central compartment (V_c) should be used instead of V_d. Lidocaine is an example of a drug that would require a fast loading dose, due to its use in the treatment of life-threatening arrhythmias.

$$F \cdot Loading\ dose = C_{ss(target)} \cdot V_d$$

Loading doses are commonly given by the IV route, so the F will be equal to 1 in these cases. If an oral loading dose is being administered, the bioavailability of the drug MUST be taken into consideration. The target concentration will be given along with the drug's V_d. Therefore, this is a simple and important equation to know for the NAPLEX exam.

If the patient already has drug in his or her system, this needs to be taken into consideration. Simply take the desired concentration ($C_{ss(target)}$) and subtract out the concentration already in the system. Just be sure the units are identical when performing this calculation.

When patients are within 20% of their IBW, total body weight (TBW) should be used when calculating loading dose. For obese patients, the decision to use IBW versus TBW depends on the drug and its ability to partition into adipose tissue.

- Drug fully partitions into fat: V_d will increase with weight gain; use TBW
  - Example: Lidocaine
- Drug does not partition into fat: V_d does not change with weight gain; use IBW
  - Example: Digoxin
- Drug that partially partitions into fat: an intermediate value should be used
  - Example: Theophylline

Constant IV Infusion

Constant-rate infusions do not generate fluctuations in plasma concentrations. Determining the rate for such infusions is relatively simple:

1. Determine the target steady-state plasma concentration.
2. Find the appropriate population CL.
3. Look up S (if drug is a salt).
4. Calculate infusion rate (R). (The infusion rate is in units amount per time [e.g., mg/min].)

$$R = \frac{CS \cdot CL}{S}$$

In most instances, S will be equal to 1 and can be ignored. Clearance adjustment factors may be available for some drugs. Some conditions that may have corresponding clearance adjustments include patient age, smoking status, and concurrent use of certain drugs. If available, these factors should be used in order to better predict blood concentrations in the individual patient.

If a drug is infused at a faster rate, a higher steady-state concentration will result. However, the time to steady-state is based on half-life and will remain the same. In order to achieve and maintain immediate steady-state concentrations:

- Give IV loading dose.
- Begin IV infusion.

Intermittent IV Infusion

Short IV infusions separated by the time required for drug elimination are often given to prevent high drug concentration and associated adverse effects. The drug may not reach steady-state in such cases.

$$C = \frac{R}{V_d \cdot k}(1 - e^{-kt})$$

The rate of infusion is equal to the dose/infusion period. After the infusion has stopped, drug concentration at a particular time can be determined by the following equation, given the concentration at the time the infusion was stopped.

$$C = C_{stop}(1 - e^{-kt})$$

These equations are not important to memorize for the NAPLEX exam because they contain an exponential function. However, the principles should be noted.

Intermittent Oral Dosing

Dose rate in intermittent oral dosing is calculated in a similar fashion to IV infusions. Remember to take F into account with oral dosing, however, since bioavailability may not be equal to IV products. The equation to calculate a dosing rate (dose divided by dosing interval, τ) for an intermittent infusion or oral dosing to a desired steady-state plasma concentration is displayed:

$$\frac{F \cdot Dose}{\tau} = C_{SS}, avg \cdot CL$$

where F is the bioavailability (equal to 1 for IV infusion), dose is the amount administered, τ is the dosing interval, Css, avg is the average steady-state plasma concentration, and CL is the clearance. This is an important equation that can be used to calculate maintenance dosing of drugs to desired steady-state concentrations.

NONLINEAR PHARMACOKINETICS

So far, this chapter has referred to general pharmacokinetic principles. These principles are applicable to most drugs without significant modification, and they result in linear mathematical models. Several assumptions are made when different or multiple doses are given:

- Drug clearance remains constant.
- Doubling the dose à doubled C and AUC.

These assumptions are not always accurate. With some drugs, giving a single low dose of the drug leads to the expected linear pharmacokinetics. However, when higher doses are given, or when the medication is taken chronically, the drug no longer fits the linear pharmacokinetic profile.

Pharmacokinetic Relationships: Linear versus Nonlinear

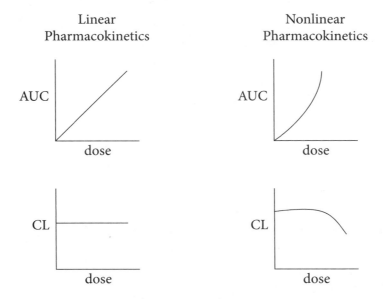

Nonlinear pharmacokinetics generally occur when one or more enzyme- or carrier-mediated systems are saturated. These systems are often referred to as capacity-limited.

- Active drug absorption: Absorption of riboflavin involves saturable gut wall transport
- Drug distribution: Saturable protein binding of salicylates
- Drug metabolism: Saturable metabolism of phenytoin
- Drug excretion: Active secretion of penicillin G

Most elimination processes can be saturated if enough drug is given. Certain drugs (phenytoin in particular) show nonlinear behavior even at normal drug doses.

For drugs exhibiting nonlinear behavior, dose increases lead to half-life increases, and AUC is not proportional to the amount of bioavailable drug. The behavior is described by the Michaelis-Menten equation:

$$\frac{dC}{dt} = \frac{V_{max} - C_{SS}}{K_M + C_{SS}}$$

V_{max} (the maximum elimination rate) and K_M (the Michaelis constant, equal to one-half the concentration at V_{max}) are dependent on both the drug and the enzyme system. Two general situations can apply:

- $C \gg K_m$; rate of change simplifies to V_{max}, a constant $\rightarrow$ zero-order kinetics
- $C \ll K_m$; rate of change is concentration dependent $\rightarrow$ first-order kinetics

In order to determine K_m and V_{max}, steady-state concentrations are measured as the result of two different doses given at different times. Recall that at steady-state, the rate of drug metabolism is assumed to be the same as the rate of drug input. In other words, the change in concentration over time is equal to the dosing rate (DR). As most non-linear calculations that you will encounter involve phenytoin, remember that the salt factor (S) for phenytoin sodium is 0.92, and the dose must be multiplied by this number when the salt form (capsules and injection) is used.

$$DR = \frac{V_{max} - C_{SS}}{K_M \cdot C_{SS}}$$

K_m may be obtained in two ways:

1. Graph the data and obtain K_m from the slope.
2. Solve simultaneous equations using two dosing rates and respective C_{SS} (algebraic determination; see below).

$$DR_1 = V_{max} - Km \cdot \frac{DR_1}{C_{ss1}}$$

$$-(DR_2 = V_{max} - Km \cdot \frac{DR_2}{C_{ss2}})$$

Subtracting the second equation from the first, V_{max} will drop out and the equation can be solved for K_m.

V_{max} may be obtained in two ways as well:

1. Graph the data, and determine the y-intercept from the graph.
2. Use the dosing rate, C_{ss}, and the newly calculated K_m to solve mathematically.

Graphical data, if available, is the faster way to obtain K_m and V_{max}.

Graphical Determination of K_m and V_{max}

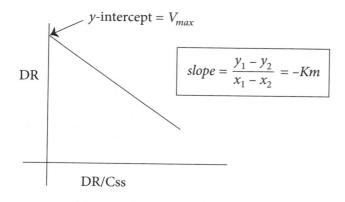

y-intercept $= V_{max}$

DR

$$slope = \frac{y_1 - y_2}{x_1 - x_2} = -Km$$

DR/Css

Learning Points

- Ninety percent of steady-state blood concentrations are achieved after three half-lives; 97% after five half-lives.

- Increasing the infusion rate will lead to higher steady-state concentrations, but the drug will not reach steady state more quickly.

- The main parameters you should be able to calculate are half-life, k, CL, V_d, plasma concentration (simple cases), and R.

- When calculating loading doses, the tendency of drug to partition into fat must be considered when determining whether to use TBW or IBW for obese patients (use TBW for drugs that partition heavily into fat).

- Increasing the dose for nonlinear drugs such as phenytoin increases the half-life and can increase AUC above what would be expected for drugs exhibiting linear behavior. Pharmacokinetic monitoring is especially important in such cases.

PRACTICE QUESTIONS

1. A patient is being started on IV digoxin. What plasma concentration of digoxin would you expect after a loading dose of 0.75 mg? Patient weight = 65 kg · V_d = 6 L/kg

   (A) 167 mcg/L
   (B) 2.6 mcg/L
   (C) 125 mcg/L
   (D) 1.95 mcg/L
   (E) 11.5 mcg/L

2. What is the half-life of procainamide in a patient whose total clearance is estimated to be 18 L/h and the volume of distribution is 140 L?

   (A) 10.8 hours
   (B) 7.4 hours
   (C) 5.4 hours
   (D) 4.6 hours
   (E) 2.7 hours

3. An investigational drug was intravenously injected into a patient, and serum samples were obtained at specific time intervals, displayed in the table below. What is the half-life of this drug?

Time Following IV Administration (min)	Serum Drug Concentrations (mg/dL)
10	8.6
20	7.5
30	6.5
60	4.2
80	3.2
100	2.4
120	1.8

   (A) 58 minutes
   (B) 48 minutes
   (C) 38 minutes
   (D) 28 minutes
   (E) 18 minutes

4. Which of the following statements is true regarding the administration of theophylline depicted in the following graph?

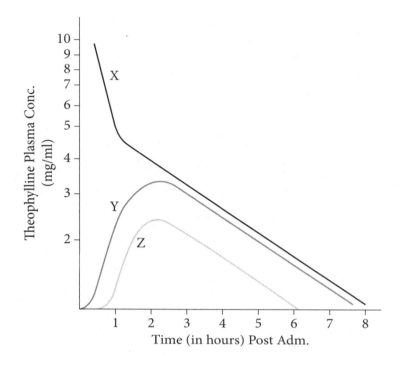

This graph illustrates the time course of the mean plasma theophylline (administered as the ethylenediamine salt) concentrations when 0.5 g is administered (X) intravenously, (Y) as a retention enema, and (Z) as an oral tablet.

(A) The elimination half-life of theophylline is 3.5 hours.
(B) Theophylline is eliminated from the body by zero-order kinetics.
(C) The bioavailability of theophylline is not affected the route of administration.
(D) The retention enema and oral tablet are bioequivalent to each other.
(E) None of the above statements is true.

5. A patient taking 40 mg of propranolol PO enters the hospital and is switched to propranolol IV. What would be an appropriate dose in milligrams, considering the drug undergoes approximately 90% first-pass effect?

(A) 4
(B) 20
(C) 40
(D) 80
(E) 120

6. The apparent V_d of gentamicin in a patient is 8 L. What dose of the antibiotic should be given to a patient with a current plasma concentration of 2 mg/L when a 6 mg/L concentration is desired?

(A) 48 mg
(B) 40 mg
(C) 32 mg
(D) 12 mg
(E) 6 mg

7. 250 mg of an antibiotic with a half-life of 9 hours is given every 6 hours to a patient with a clearance rate of 1.54 L/hr. What is the steady-state concentration of this drug assuming 80% is absorbed?

(A) 64.2 mg/L
(B) 51.3 mg/L
(C) 33.3 mg/L
(D) 21.6 mg/L
(E) 3.7 mg/L

ANSWERS

1. **D**

Use $C = \dfrac{dose}{V_d} = \dfrac{0.75\ mg}{\dfrac{6L}{kg} \cdot 65\ kg} = \dfrac{1{,}000\ mcg}{1\ mg} = \dfrac{1.95\ mcg}{L}$

2. **C**

$t\frac{1}{2} = 0.693 \cdot \dfrac{V_d}{CL}$

$t\frac{1}{2} = 0.693 \cdot \dfrac{140}{18} = 5.4\ \text{hours}$

3. **B**

The elimination rate constant can be directly calculate by first calculating the slope of the line on a natural log scale. The slope is equal to the negative value of the elimination rate constant. Theoretically any two time points and concentrations in the table can be used, but in practice it is important that you avoid choosing points in a distribution phase. It advisable to choose the later time points, as shown below.

$-k = slope = \dfrac{\ln C_1 - \ln C_2}{t_1 - t_2}$

$-k = slope = \dfrac{\ln 3.2 - \ln 1.8}{80 - 120}$

$k = 0.0144$

$t\frac{1}{2} = \dfrac{0.693}{k} \approx 48\ \text{minutes}$

This answer can also be estimated by simply looking at the time it takes for any given concentration to decrease by half. For example, it took 40 minutes (difference between 120 and 80) for the concentration to go from 3.2 to 1.8. This is just a little less than half, so you know that the half-life of the drug must be slightly >40 minutes. Indeed, the calculated half-life was 48 minutes. This is a good method to check your calculations.

4. **A**

The half-life can be estimated from any of the three administration routes because the elimination phases are parallel to each other and have similar slopes. This indicates that they have identical elimination rate constants and half-lives. The key is to find identify two concentrations (one that is half the value of the other) in the elimination phase of any of the routes. The half-life of theophylline can be estimated from the IV curve (*X* in the graph) because concentration 4 mg/mL and 2 mg/mL are in the elimination phase in the curve. To estimate the half-life, use a straight edge to extrapolate from 4 mg/mL on the y-axis to the IV curve (*X* on the graph) and then down from that point to the time (x-axis value) that theophylline was at 4 mg/mL. This time is approximately 2 hours following IV administration. Do the same extrapolation for the 2 mg/mL concentration. The time of the 2 mg/mL concentration is approximately 5.5 hours. Therefore, between 2 and 5.5 hours (or 3.5 hours) after IV administration, the concentration of theophylline decreased by half its value from 4 mg/mL to 2 mg/mL. Therefore, choice (A) is a true statement. Choice (B) is false because the elimination of theophylline is linear on the log-axis, indicating a first-order process. Choice (C) is false because the bioavailability is clearly altered by the route of administration. This can be seen by the vastly different AUCs given the same total dosages of each route. Choice (D) is false because the C_{max} and AUCs are different between the retention enema and the oral dose. These, along with T_{max}, must be similar to demonstrate bioequivalence.

5.   **A**

If 90% of the oral drug is lost to a first-pass effect, then the bioavailability (F) cannot be greater than 10%. Therefore, one would administer 10% of the oral dose by the IV route; 10% of 40 mg is 4 mg.

6.   **C**

$$F \cdot Loading\ dose = C_{SS\ (target)} \cdot V_d$$

In this case, an IV drug is being administered, so F is equal to 1. Additionally, there is drug onboard at 2 mg/L with a target of 6 mg/L. These concentrations can be subtracted from each other to get the concentration for the $C_{SS(target)}$ value.

6 mg/L (desired C_{SS}) – 2 mg/L (onboard C) = 4 mg/L

$$F \cdot Loading\ dose = 4 \cdot 8 = 32\ mg$$

7.   **D**

$$\frac{F \cdot Dose}{\tau} = C_{SS,avg} \cdot CL$$

$$\frac{0.8 \cdot 250\ mg}{6\ hours} = C_{SS,avg} \cdot 1.54\ L/hr$$

$$C_{SS,avg} = 21.6\ mg/L$$

Calculations

This chapter covers the following:

- **Problem-solving techniques**
- **Fundamentals of units and measurement**
- **Density, specific gravity, and specific volume**
- **Reducing and enlarging formulas**
- **Percentage, ratio strengths, and parts per million**
- **Dosage calculations**
- **Dilution, concentration, and alligation**
- **Electrolyte solutions**
- **Compounding calculations**

Suggested Study Time: **2 hours**

This section contains a quick review of the types of calculation questions likely to be covered on the NAPLEX. Practice is the key to this section. Keep in mind that you will be restricted to using a basic calculator (provided by testing centers).

If you would like additional review, older editions of pharmacy calculation text books will be helpful—the techniques involved have not changed. Two suggestions are *Pharmaceutical Calculations* by Ansel and Stoklosa, and *Pharmaceutical Calculations* by Zatz and Teixeira.

PROBLEM-SOLVING TECHNIQUES

Ratio-Proportion and Dimensional Analysis

There are two techniques that can be used to solve most pharmaceutical calculations: Ratio-proportion and dimensional analysis. Either of these techniques is acceptable, and you should use whichever one you find most comfortable.

Ratio-proportion is a one-step calculation technique that is probably the easiest to use for simple (one- or two-step) calculations. In this process, you set up a likeness between a fraction involving known quantities and one that includes your unknown, and solve the equation by cross-multiplying. An example is given below, illustrating how to convert 3 fluid ounces to milliliters:

$$\frac{30\ mL}{1\ fl\ oz} = \frac{x\ mL}{3\ fl\ oz}$$

$$(30\ mL)(3\ fl\ oz) = (x\ mL)(1\ fl\ oz)$$

$$\frac{(29.6\ mL)(3\ fl\ oz)}{(1\ fl\ oz)} = x\ mL$$

While ratio-proportion is often the most intuitive method, and is something with which you have been familiar since early grades of school, it has no inherent error-checking and it is not ideal for multistep calculations. When using ratio-proportion for multistep problems, you will have to write down intermediate steps; rounding intermediate answers reduces your accuracy, and writing them down takes time. Both of these can be problems when taking exams, so dimensional analysis might be preferred for these reasons.

To avoid rounding errors, keep as many decimal points as possible until the last step in the calculation. If the question is fill-in-the-blank style, it will instruct you how many decimals points to take the final answer. An advantage of the ratio-proportion method is that it is more logical than using a dimensional analysis, which is primarily set up based on units alone.

Dimensional analysis is a technique, often used in chemistry and other sciences, which allows you to set up long calculations in a single step. Using the short example given above, the problem would be solved:

$$3\ fl\ oz \bullet \frac{(30\ mL)}{(1\ fl\ oz)} = 90\ mL$$

As you can see, the fluid ounces cancel out and leave you with the correct units of milliliters. This serves as an internal error-check and is especially helpful in longer, more complex problems. Also, it saves you from having to write down intermediate steps, and helps prevent "kitchen-sink" syndrome (using every bit of information given, whether it will help solve the problem or not). Finally, it avoids the problem of rounding too early; you round once, when the problem is finished.

When you have completed a calculation, regardless of the method you choose, always ask yourself if the answer makes sense. You won't always be able to determine this, but in many cases you can tell if something has gone wrong in your calculation just by looking at the final answer. For example, it would be impractical to have an IV drip rate of 1,000 mL/min, or a dose rate of 52 tablets per day. If your answer doesn't make sense, check your calculation to find out where you went wrong.

Estimation

Estimation is not always appropriate; when working in pharmacy, you want the most accurate answer possible, especially when working with drugs with narrow therapeutic indices, or for dosing of infants and children. However, for exam purposes you will often be able to eliminate several, if not all, incorrect options by using estimates, particularly of some of the conversion factors listed in the upcoming section. This could allow you more time to focus on other portions of the exam. Use estimation with caution, however, especially if several foils are very similar to each other.

FUNDAMENTALS OF UNITS AND MEASUREMENT

The metric system is the standard system used for science worldwide. It is not, however, the only system used in pharmacy. The avoirdupois, or "common," system is the customary measure in the United States, and most patients will communicate with you in this system. Because of this, you will have to convert between systems of measurement. Unfortunately, cross-system conversions are inherently inexact. Convert from one system of measurement to another only once in a problem, not multiple times, and use the most direct conversion possible. Otherwise, the measurement error will be compounded.

A few key facts about systems of measurement are given below:

- Avoirdupois refers to solid measures only (pounds and ounces).
  - 1 pound = 16 ounces
- Common or household liquid measurements start with the teaspoon:
  - 3 teaspoons (tsp) = 1 tablespoon (T)
  - 2 T = 1 fluid ounce (fl oz) = 1/8 cup
  - 1 cup = 8 fl oz
  - 1 pint = 16 fl oz (or 2 cups)

- 1 quart = 32 fl oz (or 4 cups)
- 1 gallon = 128 fl oz (or 16 cups)

■ Apothecary measures, the measures pharmacists originally used (drams, grains, and scruples), are no longer used.

- Some medications (aspirin is one) were traditionally measured in grains, and you may still see strength listed this way; Roman numerals are used instead of Arabic (65 mg = 1 grain [gr]; a gr V aspirin tablet = 325 mg).

- The apothecary system adopted the common or household liquid measurements of pint, quart, and gallon.

- Note that the apothecary system has pounds and ounces. These are not the same size as avoirdupois pounds and ounces, and are seldom—if ever—used. The grain, however, is the same size in the avoirdupois and apothecary systems.

Some of the more common conversion factors are given below:

Avoirdupois System	Metric System
1 lb	454 g
2.2 lb	1 kg
1 oz	28.4 g (30 g is an acceptable estimate)
1 grain	64.8 mg (65 g is an acceptable estimate)

Apothecary System	Metric System
1 tsp	5 mL
1 T	15 mL
1 fl oz	29.6 mL (30 mL is an acceptable estimate)
1 cup	240 mL
1 pint	473 mL
1 quart	946 mL
1 gallon	3,785 mL

DENSITY, SPECIFIC GRAVITY, AND SPECIFIC VOLUME

Density describes the relationship between the mass of a substance and the volume it occupies. This is a helpful concept in pharmacy, as it allows you to convert between measures of mass and measures of volume. This is most useful with liquid ingredients used in compounded formulations. In compounded recipes, you may see liquid amounts expressed as either weight or volume and, depending on the recipe and the equipment you have available, it might be easier to measure in one form over the other. For instance, viscous liquids might be hard to get out of a graduated cylinder and, if you don't have a dosing syringe in which to measure the liquid, it might be better to weigh the product in a weigh boat.

Density should be treated like a conversion factor, since you are converting between mass and volume. The following example will illustrate:

450 mL of phenol weighs 482.56 g. What is its density? Express your answer in g/mL.

$$\frac{482.56\,g\,phenol}{450\,mL} = 1.07\,g/mL$$

Specific gravity (SG) is a related concept, one that many pharmacy students find confusing. SG is simply the density of a substance relative to a reference substance (usually water). It is a unitless number, because it is equal to density divided by density—the units cancel out. Since water has a density of 1 g/mL, the SG will be numerically identical to the density expressed in g/mL. However, the SG of a substance is the same regardless of what units it was calculated from, so it allows you to compare the relative masses of equal volumes of substances. Also, some sources will list SG instead of density, so you need to be familiar with it to understand these sources. An example is given below:

150 mL of formaldehyde weighs 121.82 g. What is its specific gravity?

$$\frac{\dfrac{121.82\,g\,formaldehyde}{150\,mL}}{\dfrac{1\,g\,water}{1\,mL}} = 0.81$$

Thus, formaldehyde has an SG of 0.81, which is the same as the density if presented in g/mL. It is recommended to convert SG problems into g and mL as a first step in the calculation.

REDUCING AND ENLARGING FORMULAS

Most compounding formulas are for stock quantities, and how much the formula makes is rarely the amount you are actually wishing to prepare. However, it is simple to reduce or enlarge the formula to make the amount you need, provided you keep the ingredients in the same proportion with one another. In many ways, this is similar to doubling a recipe when you are cooking for a crowd. Compounding recipes come in two formats:

1. The amount of product produced is specified (formula makes 1,000 mL, for instance).
2. The quantity of each ingredient is specified, either in measured units or in parts. You figure out how much product will be made.

Say you wish to make 50 capsules from the following recipe:

Rx   Ketoprofen 2.5 g

   Phenyltoloxamine citrate 6 g

   Caffeine 6 g

   Lactose 70.5 g

   M et div caps 200

First of all, how many doses is this recipe for? "M et div" means "mix and divide," so the recipe is for the entire amount of capsules (200), not for a single capsule. What do you do now? You can either reduce each ingredient by the same proportion (which is easy to figure out but involves lots of writing) or create a single conversion factor and apply it to each ingredient. Since you want 50 capsules and your recipes makes 200, your conversion factor would be 50 capsules/200 capsules = 0.25. Multiplying each ingredient by 0.25 yields:

2.5 g ketoprofen × 0.25	=	0.625 g
6 g phenyltoloxamine citrate × 0.25	=	1.5 g
6 g caffeine × 0.25	=	1.5 g
70.5 g lactose × 0.25	=	17.625 g

This method also works well if you do not have enough of a particular ingredient in stock. Say you have only 4 g of caffeine and want to use the above recipe, which calls for 6 g. You can reduce the recipe to fit the amount of your limiting ingredient. Simply multiply each ingredient by the conversion factor of 4 g/6 g = 0.667.

If you have a recipe that does not have a total amount calculated, you will need to add up the amounts represented by each ingredient to find your total. Remember that you must add like to like, using density if needed in order to make sure that all amounts are specified in the same units (usually either g or mL).

Finally, some recipes are given in parts rather than measurements. If total parts are given (total is listed on the recipe, or one or more ingredients is listed as "qs" or "ad"):

- Set total parts to the amount you want to make
- Solve for the value of one part
- Multiply the size of one part by the number of parts for each ingredient

If total parts are not given:

- Add the number of parts for each ingredient to obtain the total number of parts in the recipe
- Proceed as above

Try this example:

> Rx *Bacitracin*   *105 parts*
>   *Neomycin*   *35 parts*
>   *Polymyxin B*   *5 parts*
>   *Petrolatum*   *qs 10,000 parts*

Calculate the quantities of all ingredients to make 30 grams

In this case, 30 g/10,000 parts = 0.003

Multiplying this factor times the other ingredients gives:

> 105 parts bacitracin × 0.003 = 0.315 g = 315 mg
> 35 parts neomycin × 0.003   = 0.105 g = 105 mg
> 5 parts polymyxin B × 0.003 = 0.015 g = 15 mg

The petrolatum needed may be found by subtracting the masses of the other ingredients from the 30 total grams desired:

> 30 g total – 0.315 g bacitracin – 0.105 g neomycin – 0.015 g polymyxin B = 29.565 g petrolatum

PERCENTAGE, RATIO STRENGTHS, AND PARTS PER MILLION

Since drugs are administered as dosage forms that contain more than just the active ingredient, the amount of the active ingredient needs to be expressed. There are several ways to do this:

- Amount per individual dosage form (capsule, tablet, suppository)
- Concentration per dosing volume (oral liquids, certain topical products)
- Percent
- Ratio strength
- Parts per million or billion

Percent describes the number of parts of active relative to 100 parts of the total. In pharmacy, simply stating % is incomplete; you must attach the appropriate descriptor from the following list:

- % w/w: g of active per 100 g of product
- % w/v: g of active per 100 mL of product
- % v/v: mL of active per 100 mL of product

Examples:

(1) A 10% w/v = 10 g of drug in every 100 mL of the total

(2) A 10% w/w = 10 g of drug in every 100 g of the total

You may also see concentrations expressed in milligram percent. In this case, the amount in the numerator, usually assumed to be in grams, is expressed in milligrams instead: 0.001% w/w = 1 mg% w/w.

Ratio strength is another way of expressing concentration, in terms of parts of active related to any number of parts of the whole. Ratio strength is usually expressed in terms of 1 part of active relative to the total number of parts of the product, as opposed to percent, which is any number of parts of active relative to 100 parts of product. For example, 5% means 5 parts per 100, or 5:100, or 1:20. Ratio strength is used for low-concentration solutions, and triturations of high-potency powders (e.g., 1:75 trituration of estradiol).

Express 1 g of epinephrine in 1 L of solution as a percent strength and as a ratio strength.

First convert the units to g and mL:

$$1 \text{ L} = 1{,}000 \text{ mL}$$

To convert to **percentage strength**, set the denominator on the right side of the ratio-proportion equation to 100 and calculate for the numerator.

$$\frac{1\,g\ epinephrine}{1{,}000\ mL} = \frac{g\ active}{100\ mL\ product} = 0.1\%\ w/v$$

To convert to **ratio strength**, set the numerator on the right side of the ratio-proportion equation to 1 and calculate for the denominator.

$$\frac{1\,g\ epinephrine}{1{,}000\ mL} = \frac{1\ active}{X\ mL\ product} = 1:1{,}000\ w/v$$

Using another example:

How much sodium benzoate do you need to preserve 10 L of a solution at a concentration of 1:10,000?

$$\frac{1\,g\ sodium\ benzoate}{10{,}000\ mL} \times \frac{1{,}000\ mL}{1 L} \times 10\,L = 1\,g$$

Parts per million (ppm) is a special case of ratio strength. Instead of fixing the numerator as 1, in this case you fix the denominator constant as 1,000,000. Parts per billion (ppb) and trillion (ppt) are handled in the analogous fashion. These are used to express very small concentrations; for example, the EPA action level for lead in drinking water is 15 ppb (or 0.015 mg/L).

DOSAGE CALCULATIONS

Pharmacists frequently need to calculate the size of a dose or total amount of medication to dispense, even for noncompounded prescriptions. The following general equation applies:

Number of doses × size of dose = total amount

Example:

How many milliliters of a liquid medicine would provide a patient with 2 teaspoons three times a day for 7 days?

$$2\ tsp \times \frac{3\ doses}{day} \times 7\ days \times \frac{5\ mL}{tsp} = 210\ mL$$

DILUTION, CONCENTRATION, AND ALLIGATION

In some cases, you may receive a prescription in which you need to either dilute a product you have on hand or make a product more concentrated. These problems can generally be solved by:

1. Using the equation: (quantity) × (concentration) = (quantity) × (concentration)
2. Determining the quantity of active ingredient needed and then calculating the quantity of the available solution (usually a concentrated stock solution), which will provide the needed amount of active ingredient

When some ingredients are given as ratio strength, you can convert them to percentage strength before setting up the proportion. Whenever proportional parts enter the calculation, you should reduce them to their lowest terms before beginning (i.e., reduce 75 parts:25 parts to 3 parts:1 part). In both cases, this will simplify your calculations. Example:

If 250 mL of a 15% v/v solution of methyl salicylate in alcohol are diluted to 1,500 mL, what will be the percentage strength of this diluted solution?

250 mL × 15% = 1,500 mL × X%   X = 2.5% v/v

Stock Solutions

Stock solutions are strong solutions of known concentration that allow the pharmacist to conveniently prepare weaker solutions. They are generally prepared on a w/v basis and their concentration is expressed as a ratio strength. Example:

How many milliliters of a 1% stock solution of certified red dye should be used in preparing 2,000 mL of an antiseptic that is to contain 1:5,000 of the certified red dye as a coloring agent?

First, how many grams of red dye are needed in the 2,000 mL of antiseptic solution?

$$\frac{1\ g\ red\ dye}{5,000\ mL} = \frac{1\ g\ red\ dye}{2,000\ mL}$$

$x\ g\ red\ dye = 0.4\ g$

Next, how much of the 1% stock solution of red dye contains this amount of dye?

$$\frac{1\ g\ red\ dye}{100\ mL} = \frac{0.4\ g\ red\ dye}{x\ mL}$$

$x = 40\ mL$

Alligation

Alligation is a method of solving problems that involves mixing multiple products that have different percentage strengths. Two types of alligation exist: Alligation medial and alligation alternate.

Alligation Medial

This method allows the calculation of the weighted average percentage strength of a mixture of two or more substances of known quantity and strength. The technique is best shown via illustration:

What is the percentage strength (v/v) of alcohol in a mixture of 3,000 mL of 40% (v/v) alcohol, 1,000 mL of 60% (v/v) alcohol, and 1,000 mL of 70% (v/v) alcohol?

$$
\begin{aligned}
40 \times 3,000 &= 120,000 \\
60 \times 1,000 &= 60,000 \\
70 \times 1,000 &= 70,000 \\
\hline
\text{Totals: } 5,000 &= 250,000
\end{aligned}
$$

$250,000\ /\ 5,000 = 50\%$ (v/v)

Alligation Alternate

This method allows calculation of the number of parts of two or more components of a given strength when they are mixed to prepare a mixture of a desired strength. Cross-wise subtraction is used to determine the amounts needed of each component. This method can be used regardless of how concentration is expressed (mg/mL, ratio, parts, %). Example:

In what proportion should 20% benzocaine ointment be mixed with an ointment base to produce a 2.5% w/w benzocaine ointment?

Since there is no active drug in the ointment base, its strength can be expressed as 0%. To complete this problem, set up a table with the high concentration (i.e., 20%) in the upper left corner and the low concentration (i.e., 0%) in the lower left corner. The desired concentration (i.e., 2.5%) is placed in the center column between the low and high concentrations. Note that the desired concentration must always be a value between the high and low concentrations. Subtract crosswise to calculate the parts of the low and high concentration solutions to be mixed. Always subtract in a manner that will get you a positive value in the right column. In this example, 20% − 2.5% = 17.5 parts. Because this value is in the lower row of the table, it indicates that this is the parts of the low concentration to add to the mixture. In a similar fashion, 2.5 is the value of the parts for the high concentration. See the table below for the appropriate setup of this problem.

Strengths to Be Mixed	Desired	Difference in Strength Mixed (crosswise subtraction of absolute values)
20%		2.5 parts (2.5−0) of 20% ointment
	2.5%	
0%		17.5 parts (20 − 2.5) of ointment base

So 2.5 parts of the 20% w/w ointment should be added to 17.5 parts of the ointment base. Remember that the values are subtracted crosswise, but the identities of the substances are read across.

The standard alligation problem on the NAPLEX will provide you with not only the concentrations of both starting amounts and the desired concentration to be made, as described above, but also the total amount that is to be dispensed. Thus, the final step is to take the total amount to be dispensed and calculate the amounts of each ingredient based on the parts that were calculated above. For example, if 12 g were to be dispensed in the problem above, you would use the parts as shown below.

Parts of high concentration: 2.5 parts

Parts of low concentration: 17.5 parts

Total parts (i.e., high plus low concentration): 20 parts

To calculate the amount of the *high* concentration to be mixed:

$$\frac{2.5\ parts}{20\ parts} = \frac{x\ g}{12\ g}$$
$$x = 1.5\ g$$

To calculate the amount of the *low* concentration to be mixed:

$$\frac{17.5\ parts}{20\ parts} = \frac{x\ g}{12\ g}$$
$$x = 10.5\ g$$

Another method is to simply take the total amount to be dispensed (i.e., 12 g) and subtract out the amount of the high concentration to be mixed (i.e., 1.5 g), which was calculated in the first step. That is, 12 g − 1.5 g = 10.5 g, which is the amount of the low concentration to add. This is a good method for checking calculations, because there are two ways to calculate the last amount to be added.

Therefore, to get 12 g of a 2.5% w/w benzocaine ointment, mix 1.5 g of a 20% concentration with 10.5 g of the ointment base (0% concentration).

ELECTROLYTE SOLUTIONS

Electrolyte solutions are frequently prescribed for patients who have lost an essential ion through disease, as they play a critical role in maintaining normal body function. Sometimes the necessary amount of the appropriate salt will be stated on the prescription, but often the prescription will ask for a quantity of the needed ion in chemical units, and the pharmacist will need to calculate how much of the salt will contain the desired amount. Milliequivalents are the most common unit used.

Millimoles and Milliequivalents

A review of several chemistry concepts will be useful before beginning milliequivalent calculations.

- Moles (mol): Measurement of the amount of a substance; Avogadro's number of particles (6.023×10^{23})
- Atomic weight: Found on the periodic table; 1 mol of that atom weighs that many grams (also, 1 mmol of that atom weighs that many mg)
- Molecular weight (MW): The sum of all the atomic weights for all of the atoms in the molecule. 1 **mole** of the molecule will weigh the value of the molecular weight in **grams**. However, in electrolyte solutions and osmolarity calculations, it is necessary to convert to millimoles. This can be done easily by taking the amount of the substance in milligrams and dividing by the molecular weight to get the answer in millimoles. This can be visualized in the following important equations:

$$moles = \frac{Amount\ (grams)}{Molecular\ weight}$$

$$millimoles = \frac{Amount\ (milligrams)}{Molecular\ weight}$$

- Molar solution: The molarity of a solution is the moles of solute in every 1 L of solution. This is an important concept on the NAPLEX, as questions can ask for the answer in terms of molarity and, on the last step of the problem, calculate how many moles there are in 1 L for the solutes in the problem.

- Stock solutions often expressed this way
- 0.1 M = 0.1 mol of solute/1 L solution

What is the molar concentration of a 5% w/v $MgCl_2$ solution? MW $MgCl_2$ = 95.

The 5% concentration indicates that there are 5 g of $MgCl_2$ per every 100 mL. The question is asking for the molar concentration, so directly calculate the moles per every 100 mL solution by the following:

$$\frac{5 \text{ g } MgCl_2}{95} = 0.053 \text{ moles per } 100 \text{ mL}$$

It is recommended to indicate the volume of solution in each step of the problem, as indicated earlier. Because the answer needs to be in molar concentration, the moles per liter can be calculated as follows:

$$\frac{0.053 \text{ moles}}{100 \text{ mL}} = \frac{x \text{ moles}}{1,000 \text{ mL}} = 0.53 \text{ mol/L} = 0.53 \text{ M}$$

or using dimensional analysis:

$$\frac{1 \text{ mol } MgCl_2}{95 \text{ g } MgCl_2} \times \frac{5 \text{ g } MgCl_2}{100 \text{ mL}} \times \frac{1,000 \text{ mL}}{1 \text{ L}} = 0.53 \text{ mol/L} = 0.53 \text{ M}$$

What if you are interested in moles of atoms instead of moles of molecules? In this case, you need to look at the molecular formula. If there is more than one of an atom in a molecule (such as the chloride in the example above), you need to adjust your formula. In that example, you have 1 mol of $MgCl_2$, which contains 1 mol of Mg^{+2} and 2 mol of Cl^-. If you don't have a molecular formula, you can figure one out by balancing charges, provided you know the valencies of the ions involved. The table below displays the valence of the most common ions. This information will likely not be provided on the NAPLEX.

Valence	Ions
+1	Sodium, potassium, lithium
+2	Barium, calcium, magnesium, zinc
+3	Aluminum
+1 or +2	Copper
+2 or +3	Iron, manganese
−1	Acetate, chloride, bicarbonate
−2	Sulfate, carbonate
−1, −2, or −3	Phosphate, citrate

In the magnesium chloride example, Mg^{+2} is divalent; it takes two Cl^- to make as much negative charge as one Mg^{+2}. Therefore, the correct formula is $MgCl_2$, not MgCl. NaCl, however, is made up of two monovalent ions, so the charges are equal.

Electrolytes are commonly prescribed in terms of equivalents rather than mass. What does this mean? One mol of hydrogen has 1 mol of positive charge. One equivalent of an ion is the amount required to replace (in positively charged ions) or react with (in negatively charged ions) 1 mol of hydrogen. Monovalent ions (Cl^-, Na^+, K^+, NH_4^+, OH^-) therefore have 1 Eq/mol. Divalent ions like Ca^{+2} are 2 Eq/mol, as it takes 2 mol of hydrogen to replace the charge carried by 1 mol of calcium.

The concept of equivalents is important in pharmacy when dispensing electrolytes or small drug molecules as salts. For example, a prescription that is written for 40 mg of potassium chloride does not contain the same amount of elemental potassium as a prescription written for 40 mg potassium acetate. The reason is that the 40 mg in each prescription is the total weight of potassium and the salt form (i.e., chloride or acetate). Since acetate has a larger molecular weight than chloride, it contributes more to the 40 mg, and therefore, the patient will receive less potassium in this prescription compared with 40 mg of potassium chloride. This concept is also true for drugs for which the amount of drug dispensed is the weight of the drug itself and also the salt that is formulated. However, drugs are much larger molecules than electrolytes. Thus the percentage of salt is so small that switching salt formations of drugs has limited clinical applicability. The only clinical relevance would be for drugs with a narrow therapeutic index or a small molecular weight.

To overcome this problem for electrolytes, the prescriptions will be written in terms of milliequivalents (mEq). For example, a prescription that calls for 40 mEq of potassium chloride will contain the same amount of elemental potassium as a prescription that calls for 40 mEq of potassium acetate.

To calculate mEq, simply calculate the millimoles of the substance and multiply by the valence of either the positive or negative of the molecular formula. For example, if $MgCl_2$ is the compound of interest, you would multiply the millimoles by a factor of 2. The factor of 2 is due to the fact that Mg has 2 positive charges and Cl has a negative charge with two of them giving a total negative charge of 2. Remember that the charges of the positive side and the negative side must equal zero.

Use the following equation to calculate mEq:

$$milliequivalents\ (mEq) = \frac{Amount\ (milligrams)}{Molecular\ weight} \times valence$$

Example:

How much potassium citrate powder (MW = 324.41) would we weigh to compound 1 dose of the following prescription?

Rx   *Potassium citrate, 20 mEq, tid*

Recall that potassium has a valence of +1 and citrate has a –3, so the formula must have 3 potassium ions for every citrate or $K_3(C_6H_5O_7)$.

$$20\ mEq = \frac{x\ mg}{324.1} \times 3$$
$$x = 2,160\ mg$$

Therefore, 20 mEq of potassium citrate provides 20 mEq of potassium and 20 mEq of citrate. This means that a quantity of 2,160 mg of potassium citrate would provide 20 mEq of potassium and 20 mEq of citrate. The important thing to keep track of with this method is the amount and molecular weight being used. Since we used the molecular weight of potassium citrate (and not just potassium or citrate alone), the amount calculated in milligrams is the weight of both potassium and citrate together. One could calculate the actual amount of potassium in a dose by replacing the molecular weight of potassium citrate with the atomic weight of potassium (i.e., 39.1). NAPLEX questions may provide either the full molecular weight or an atomic weight of one of the components. Remember: Using an atomic weight of one of the components of the prescription means committing to use that atomic weight. However, the milliequivalents will be the same value for the total compound and each of the components.

Osmolarity and Isotonicity

Osmotic pressure is the pressure that exists across a semipermeable membrane due to the free movement of solvent but not solute. Because cell membranes are semipermeable, this concept is important in patients. When administering parenteral drugs, you must balance the osmolarity of your medication with the osmolarity of the body. If not, tissue damage, pain, and possibly death can result due to cells swelling or shrinking with the movement of solvent.

Solutions are considered isotonic when each one has the same osmotic pressure; in pharmacy and medicine, the reference solution is the plasma (280–300 mOsm/L). Hypertonic solutions have higher osmotic pressure than this; hypotonic solutions have lower osmotic pressure. Some other facts you should remember about osmotic pressure are:

- It is a colligative property, based on the number of particles in solution.
- It can be calculated directly, using dissociation constants.
  - NaCl dissociates into sodium and chloride 80% in aqueous solution.

- For every 100 particles, 80 will have dissociated (making 160 particles) and 20 will not → 180 particles (20 + 160).

$$\frac{180 \; particles \; after \; dissociation}{100 \; particles \; before \; dissociation} = 1.8 = i$$

- It can be calculated by its effect on other colligative properties, including freezing point, boiling point, and vapor pressure.

  - All colligative properties vary together.
  - A solution with the same freezing point as a reference solution will have the same osmolarity as that reference solution.

- To calculate the milliosmoles (mOsm) in a given solution, multiply the millimoles by the theoretical number of particles that the compound would dissociate into in solution. For example, to calculate the mOsm in an $MgCl_2$ solution, the millimoles would be multiplied by a factor of 3. Theoretically, $MgCl_2$ would dissociate into 1 magnesium and 2 chloride ions in solution. If the dissociation constant is provided in the problem, it would provide a more accurate calculation and should be used as displayed in the equation.

$$mOsm = \frac{Amount \; (mg)}{Molecular \; weight} \times \begin{array}{c} Theoretical \; number \; of \; particles \\ (or \; disassociation \; constant) \end{array}$$

- The NAPLEX may ask for answers to be written in terms of milliosmolarity. Remember: When the suffix "-arity" is at the end of a word in chemistry, it indicates the need to calculate an amount in 1 L of solution. In other words, to calculate milliosmolarity you need to calculate the amount of milliosmoles in the quantity of solution in the problem and convert to 1 L at the end.

Try this example:

A solute dissociates 50% in aqueous solution. Assuming each molecule of the solute dissociates into two parts, give the dissociation constant (i).

$$\frac{100 \; dissociated \; particles + 50 \; undissociated \; particles}{100 \; particles \; before \; dissociation} = 1.5 = (i)$$

You can use the ratio form of the dissociation constant as a conversion factor. If $i = 1.5$, 1 mol = 1.5 Osm, and 1 mmol = 1.5 mOsm.

Try another example: Calculate the osmolarity of NS in mOsm/L MW NS = 58.5 and $i = 1.8$.

NS = normal saline = 0.9% w/v NaCl in water

$$\frac{0.9 \; g}{100 \; mL} = \frac{x \; g}{1,000 \; mL}$$

$x = 9\,g$ or $9,000\;mg$ of NaCl per liter

$$x\;mOsm = \frac{9,000\;mg}{58.5} \times 1.8$$

$x = 276.9\;mOsm$ per liter

Because NS is nearly isotonic with plasma, it is useful for comparison. If we know that a product is isotonic to NS, it will be isotonic to body fluids as well. Sodium chloride equivalents are therefore useful, and are for expression of the amount of NaCl it would take to exert the tonic effect of a particular active ingredient. Some baseline assumptions are:

- The tonic effects of solutes are additive and independent.
- The total tonic effect in the solution is the sum of the effect of each solute.

The following steps can be followed when adjusting tonicity:

1. Determine how much NaCl it would take to exert the tonic effect already seen in the solution.
2. Calculate how much NaCl is required to make the solution isotonic if NaCl is the sole tonicity agent. Compare this to the amount already present (step 1). Proceed only if the total amount of NaCl equivalent already present is less than the amount needed (i.e., solution is currently hypotonic).
3. *Amount needed = Goal amount – Amount you already have*
   a. If adjusting tonicity with NaCl, use amount in step 3.
   b. If adjusting tonicity with another substance, figure out how much of your substance is needed to deliver the required tonic effect, using the E value (1 g of substance has the same tonic effect as E g of NaCl).

If one of your ingredients is already isotonic, you can disregard that volume as you calculate your values.

For example, how much boric acid (E = 0.52) should be added to make 15 mL of a 3% w/v pilocarpine HCl (E = 0.24) eye drop solution isotonic?

Following the steps given above:

1. $\dfrac{3\,g\;pilocarpine}{100\;mL} \times 15\;mL = 0.45\,g\;pilocarpine$

   $0.45\,g\;pilocarpine \times \dfrac{0.24\,g\;NaCl(eq)}{1\,g\;pilocarpine} = 0.108\,g\;NaCl(eq)$

2. $\dfrac{0.9\,g\;NaCl}{100\;mL} \times 15\;mL = 0.135\,g\;NaCl$

3. $0.135\,g - 0.108\,g = 0.027\,g\,NaCl$

$$0.027\,g\,NaCl \times \frac{1\,g\,boric\,acid}{0.52\,g\,NaCl(eq)} = 0.05192\,g = 0.052\,g\,boric\,acid$$

Another way to describe and calculate osmolarity and isotonicity is freezing-point depression. As mentioned above, this is a colligative property that varies along with other colligative properties of a solution. Some things to remember:

- Plasma freezes at –0.52°C.
- Solutions isotonic to plasma (such as NS) will also freeze at –0.52°C.
- Pure water freezes at 0°C. Therefore, an amount of solute that will make the solution isotonic depresses the freezing point by 0.52°C.

Given the following prescription, how much NaCl must be added to make the solution isotonic? The freezing point of a 1% w/v solution of procaine HCl is –0.122°C.

Rx	Procaine HCl	2% w/v
	NaCl	qs
	Sterile water	qs 30 mL

First, what would be the effect of a 2% w/v solution?

$$\frac{1.22°C}{1\%} \times 2\% = 0.244°C$$

The desired freezing point – The depression from the ingredients already in the formulation = The additional depression needed:

$$-0.52°C - (-0.244°C) = -0.276°C$$

So, the required concentration of sodium chloride is:

$$-0.276°C\,\frac{0.9\%\,NaCl}{-0.52°C} = 0.48\%\,NaCl \quad or$$

$$30\,mL\,\frac{0.48\,g\,NaCl}{100\,g\,NaCl} = 0.144\,g\,NaCl$$

COMPOUNDING CALCULATIONS

Use of Prefabricated Dosage Forms in Compounding

When compounding, the source of active ingredient will often be prefabricated dosage forms (tablets, capsules, ointments). When performing such calculations, it is important to remember that if your calculation determines that you need 1.3 tablets as your source drug, you must actually crush 2 tablets and then weigh out a proportional amount of the resultant powder. Remember, a tablet contains far more ingredients than just the drug, so take that into account in your calculations.

> Rx   Aspirin   300 mg
>   Lactose   qs
>
> M.ft. cap DTD #60

Using 325-mg aspirin tablets (weighing 430 mg each) as the source drug, how many tablets are needed to compound this prescription? How much of the crushed powder should be weighed out?

$$\frac{300\,mg\,ASA}{capsule} \times 60\,capsules \times \frac{tablet}{325\,mg\,ASA} = 55.38\,tablets \rightarrow 56\,tablets$$

$$55.38\,tablets \times 430\,mg\,total\,tablet\,weight = 23{,}813\,mg = 23.813\,g$$

Suppository Calculations

The density factor method is often used when preparing suppositories. The density factor expresses the relationship between the mass of an ingredient and the volume of suppository base it displaces. Therefore, a drug will have a different density factor in each suppository base.

$$density\,factor = \frac{weight\,of\,drug}{weight\,of\,base\,displaced}$$

If a pharmacist needs to prepare six 30-mg phenobarbital suppositories in cocoa butter, how many grams each of cocoa butter and phenobarbital should be weighed? Density factor of phenobarbital in cocoa butter is 1.2. Blank suppositories (base only) weigh 2 g.

If one suppository contains 30 mg drug (0.03 g), it will replace:

$$\frac{0.03\,g\,drug}{1.2\,g} = 0.025\,g\,cocoa\,butter$$

$2\,g - 0.025\,g = 1.975\,g\,cocoa\,butter\,/\,suppository \times 6\,suppositories =$
$11.85\,g\,cocoa\,butter$

$0.03\,g \times 6\,suppositories = 0.18\,g\,phenobarbital$

Reconstitution Calculations

Some medications, particularly antibiotics for oral suspension or parenteral use, come as powders for reconstitution. While the container or package will include instructions for reconstitution, including what and how much diluent to use, occasionally the prescriber will need to manipulate the final concentration of the drug. Some simple calculations can help you make these adjustments to provide a more dilute or concentrated product. First, a simple example:

Cefadroxil powder for oral suspension comes in a strength of 250 mg/5 mL. The reconstitution instructions are to add 70 mL of purified water to yield a final solution volume of 100 mL. How many grams of cefadroxil powder are in the bottle?

$$\frac{250\,mg\,cefadroxil}{5\,mL\,suspension} \times 100\,mL = 5{,}000\,mg = 5\,g$$

There are a few interesting things to pay attention to here. First, this is an easy example of a question that gives more information than you need to solve the problem (while the 70 mL is necessary for reconstitution, it is not needed to answer this particular question). Be sure to pay attention and use the correct numbers when extra information is given. Second, if you add only 70 mL of water, how do you get 100 mL of total suspension? The powder takes up space in the final product. This volume is called the powder volume: It is a calculated quantity, not corresponding to the physical volume. The powder volume may be greater than, equal to, or less than zero, depending on the drug and the way it was prepared.

When preparing a final concentration that is different from the package directions, you must first calculate the powder volume. The powder volume is equal to the difference between the diluent volume and the final solution volume. Take the following case:

Rx   Biaxin 100 mg/5 mL suspension
        Sig: 1 tsp PO q 12 hr × 10 days

Biaxin comes as a powder for reconstitution with instructions to prepare a final concentration of 125 mg/5 mL by adding 55 mL diluent to make a final volume of 100 mL. The amount of active ingredient in the bottle is 2,500 mg, and the powder volume = total volume – diluent, so 100 mL – 55 mL = 45 mL.

$$2{,}500\,mg\,Biaxin\,\frac{5\,mL}{100\,mg\,Biaxin} = 125\,mL\,total$$

$$125\,mL\,total - PV = 125\,mL - 45\,mL = 80\,mL$$

Adding 80 mL of diluent will produce 125 mL of solution with a concentration of 100 mg/5 mL.

Drip Rate Calculations

IV medications are regulated by one of the following methods:

- Drip chambers
  - Deliver drops of defined volume.
  - Flow is adjusted by the nurse to a set number of *whole* drops per minute.
  - Standard sets are 10 gtt/mL or 15 gtt/mL.
  - Pediatric and critical care drugs may use microdrop infusion sets: 60 gtt/mL.
- Infusion pumps
  - Deliver a rate of mL/hr.
  - Round to the nearest 0.1 mL.

17 mL of concentrated vancomycin solution is added to a 100-mL piggyback bag of NS. This solution is to be infused over 1 hour. What is the infusion rate?

$$\frac{17\,mL\,vancomycin + 100\,mL\,NS}{60\,min} = 117\,mL/60\,min = 117\,mL/hr$$

What is the infusion rate in drops/min if the drug is administered using an infusion set that delivers 10 gtt/mL?

$$\frac{117\,mL}{60\,min} \times \frac{10\,gtt}{mL} = 19.5\,gtt/min = 20\,gtt/min$$

Enteral Nutrition

Some or all of the patient's nutritional needs are provided by use of orally or enterally administered nutritional products, usually through feeding tubes. Enteral nutrition (EN) products are commercially available, and limited calculations are needed. If the patient can tolerate it, EN is usually recommended over parenteral nutrition (PN).

Parenteral Nutrition

Most of the calculations on the NAPLEX exam regarding nutrition will be related to the parenteral route. The cost of TPN therapy is usually 10 times more expensive than EN, with greater possibilities of metabolic and/or infectious complications. Common abbreviations follow:

- **TPN = total parenteral nutrition:** Provides fluid, macronutrients (i.e., dextrose, amino acids, and fatty acids), electrolytes, and micronutrients (i.e., vitamins and trace elements).

- **TNA = total nutrition admixture:** Contains all of the macro and micronutrients in a single bag. The terms TNA and TPN are often used synonymously in clinical practice, although there are technical differences.

Calculations Involving Calories

The usual term is Calorie (with a capital C), which is equal to 1 kilocalorie. Therefore, Calories and kilocalories are synonymous. However, many texts do not use a capital C when referring to Calories. Therefore, whenever Calorie is written (with or without the capital C), do not do any metric conversions.

To calculate the caloric requirements for a hospitalized patient, first calculate that patient's basal energy requirement. There are equations to calculate basal energy expenditure based on several patient demographics. The stressed adult in a hospital likely will require additional energy depending on several factors. The calculated basal energy expenditure is then multiplied by a stress factor (usually between 1 and 2) to obtain a total energy expenditure (TEE).

The normal adult requires 25–35 Cal/kg/day. Once the TEE is calculated, the Calories are provided to the patient through dextrose and fatty acids. Amino acids also provide Calories, but those Calories generally are used to meet to the TEE in a TPN. The Calories provided by a TPN can be estimated as follows:

Dextrose in the hydrated form (D_5W, $D_{70}W$, etc.)	3.4 Cal/g
Carbohydrates	4 Cal/g
Fats	9 Cal/g
Protein	4 Cal/g

Dextrose in water is the hydrated form and is used in TPN. Although dextrose is a carbohydrate, water molecules are attached to the dextrose to make it more soluble. The water molecules add weight without adding calories, and they dilute the Calorie per gram ratio from 4 to 3.4. Therefore, when calculating caloric content of a TPN, 3.4 Cal/g should be used for the dextrose content.

Dextrose cannot be used alone to meet TEE because there are essential fatty acids. To prevent essential fatty acid deficiency, particularly a deficiency of linoleic acid, which cannot be synthesized in the body, fats are incorporated into TPNs usually two to three times weekly.

Fats are provided through infusion of oil emulsions. Fatty oil emulsions are approximately isotonic, have a milky appearance, and can be infused into peripheral blood vessels. Every milliliter of 10% fat emulsion has 1.1 Calories, whereas every milliliter of 20% fat emulsion has 2 calories. The emulsions contain glycerol, which provides Calories in addition to the fats. Therefore, there is no easy way to calculate the caloric content of the emulsions and require the memorization of the caloric content per milliliter described.

Calculations Involving Amino Acids

The average adult requires approximately 1 g/kg/day of amino acids. Amino acids are included in TPN primarily to provide protein and nitrogen supplementation. Nitrogen is an important element in the diet that is a precursor to DNA synthesis and other important metabolic functions. On average, 16% of an amino acid solution is nitrogen content.

Try this example:

How many milliliters of an 8.5% amino acid solution are required to provide 20 g of nitrogen?

$$\frac{16 \ g \ nitrogen}{100 \ g \ amino \ acids} = \frac{20 \ g \ nitrogen}{x \ g \ amino \ acids}$$

$$x = 125 \ g \ amino \ acids$$

$$\frac{8.5 \ g \ amino \ acids}{100 \ mL} = \frac{125 \ g \ amino \ acids}{x \ mL}$$

$$x = 1{,}470 \ mL$$

Of importance is the Cal/g nitrogen ratio. The desired ratio is 125/1 up to 150/1. That is, a formula should provide at least 125 Calories for each gram of nitrogen being infused. This amount is needed to provide for normal energy expenditure and calories to aid in the anabolic conversion of nitrogen sources into lean body mass.

Calculations Involving Electrolytes and Micronutrients

There are not many sources of calculations regarding TPN on the NAPLEX outside of the macronutrients described above. Electrolyte calculations have been described in this chapter related to milliequivalents. For TPN, the most important concept regarding electrolytes is clinical considerations. This includes limiting potassium and sodium in patients with renal, hepatic, or cardiac dysfunction. Similarly, there are not calculations involving vitamins or trace elements as these are added to TPNs via commercially available products.

Compounding Considerations for TPNs

Both calcium and phosphate are essential components of TPN formulas. Sources of calcium include the chloride and gluconate salts. Phosphorous is supplied as combinations of mono- and disodium phosphates or mono- and dipotassium phosphates. The exact ratio depends on the pH of the solution.

Depending upon the relative concentrations of the soluble calcium salts and the phosphate salts, a chemical reaction may occur forming the very **insoluble dibasic calcium phosphate** ($CaPO_4$). This fine, white precipitate may form slowly and be difficult to visualize, especially if a milky fatty oil emulsion is also included in the TPN.

Methods for lessening the incompatibility problem:

1. Keep Ca and PO_4 concentrations below certain limits (solubility curves are available for various mixtures).
2. Agitate the mixture after each ingredient addition.
3. Add Na or K phosphates first and calcium salt last.
4. Add the Na or K phosphates to the amino acid solution, and the calcium salt to the dextrose solution; then, mix by shaking.
5. Use a 0.2 micron filter for nonfat emulsion formulas; a 1.2 micron filter is needed for fatty oil emulsions.

Learning Points

- Always perform a "sanity" check on your answer. Does it make practical sense? If not, recheck your numbers.
- Remember crucial conversion factors (or at least approximations of these): 1 fluid oz = 30 mL, 2.2 lb/kg (*not* the reverse; remember, your weight is always a smaller number when measured in kilograms; if you get an answer to the contrary, you flipped your conversion).
- Valence of a molecule is equal to the total number of negative charges *or* the total number of positive charges, not the two numbers added together.
- When using prefabricated dosage forms as a drug source, fractions of a dosage form must always be rounded up to the next nearest whole.
- Drops must be rounded to the nearest whole drop. You cannot measure partials.

PRACTICE QUESTIONS

1. How many milliliters of water should be mixed with 240 mL of syrup containing 85% w/v sucrose to make a syrup containing 60% w/v sucrose?

   (A) 80 mL
   (B) 100 mL
   (C) 160 mL
   (D) 240 mL
   (E) 340 mL

2. If 10 mL of a solution are to contain 3 mEq of sodium ion, how many 1-g sodium chloride (MW 58.5) tablets would be required to compound 250 mL of solution?

   (A) 2
   (B) 3
   (C) 4
   (D) 5
   (E) 6

3. You have been asked to prepare 500 mL of a benzalkonium chloride solution. The concentration of the solution you prepare must be such that if 20 mL of your solution are diluted to a liter, a 1:1,470 solution is formed. How many milliliters of a 17% benzalkonium chloride solution will you need to compound the solution?

   (A) 17 mL
   (B) 20 mL
   (C) 100 mL
   (D) 147 mL
   (E) 500 mL

4. A pharmacist has 75 grams of 3% w/w zinc oxide paste in stock, to which she adds 5 g of pure zinc oxide. What is the percent concentration of zinc oxide in the final product?

   (A) 2.4% w/w
   (B) 3% w/w
   (C) 7.25% w/w
   (D) 9.06% w/w
   (E) 9.67% w/w

5. How many milligrams of boric acid are needed to compound the following prescription? (The E values are as follows: zinc chloride 0.62, phenacaine HCl 0.17, and boric acid 0.52.)

Rx	Zinc chloride	0.2%
	Phenacaine HCl	1%
	Boric acid	qs
	Purified water qs	60 mL

(A) 92 mg
(B) 189 mg
(C) 339 mg
(D) 364 mg
(E) 698 mg

6. How many milligrams of sodium chloride are needed to compound the following prescription? (The E value of phenylephrine HCl is 0.32.)

Rx	Phenylephrine HCl	0.5%
	Sodium chloride	qs
	Purified water qs	30 mL

(A) 48 mg
(B) 86 mg
(C) 150 mg
(D) 222 mg
(E) 270 mg

7. How many mL of a 1% stock solution of epinephrine HCl are needed for the following prescription?

| Rx | Epinephrine HCl sol. 1:500 | 60 mL |

(A) 0.012 mL
(B) 0.12 mL
(C) 1.2 mL
(D) 12 mL
(E) 120 mL

8. Calculate the percentage (v/v) of witch hazel in the following prescription. Round to one decimal place.

Rx	Sulfur ppt	15 g
	Witch hazel	45 mL
	Alcohol	
	Calamine lotion qs	120 mL

   (A) 12.5%
   (B) 25%
   (C) 27.3%
   (D) 37.5%
   (E) 45%

9. A prescription calls for penicillin suspension to be administered: 1.5 teaspoonfuls PO TID for 12 days. How many mL of the suspension should be dispensed?

   (A) 23 mL
   (B) 54 mL
   (C) 90 mL
   (D) 270 mL
   (E) 810 mL

10. A 40-pound child is to receive Dilantin 2.5 mg/kg PO BID. How many mL of Dilantin suspension (125 mg/5 mL) should be dispensed for a 30-day supply?

   (A) 55 mL
   (B) 109 mL
   (C) 240 mL
   (D) 265 mL
   (E) 528 mL

11. A patient who weighs 167 pounds is receiving phenylephrine at a dose of 2 mcg/kg/min. How many mg of phenylephrine does the patient receive over 2 hours?

   (A) 0.30 mg
   (B) 9.1 mg
   (C) 18.2 mg
   (D) 40 mg
   (E) 5,060 mg

12. A formula for 2,000 levothyroxine tablets contains 274 mg of levothyroxine. How many mcg of levothyroxine are in each tablet?

    (A) 0.137 mcg
    (B) 1.37 mcg
    (C) 13.7 mcg
    (D) 137 mcg
    (E) 1,370 mcg

13. The formula for an analgesic ointment is 10 g menthol, 95 g benzocaine, 5 g camphor, 40 g mineral oil, and 850 g petrolatum. How many grams of benzocaine are needed to prepare 5 lbs. of this product?

    (A) 0.22 g
    (B) 215.7 g
    (C) 238.3 g
    (D) 253.7 g
    (E) 1,045 g

14. A solution of iodine in chloroform has a strength of 1.4% (w/v). How many mL of chloroform must be evaporated from the original 180 mL to adjust the iodine concentration to 2.4%?

    (A) 50 mL
    (B) 75 mL
    (C) 105 mL
    (D) 125 mL
    (E) 155 mL

15. How many grams of zinc oxide should be mixed with 8% zinc oxide ointment to make 250 g of a 12% zinc oxide ointment? Round your answer to one decimal place.

    (A) 10.9 g
    (B) 18.5 g
    (C) 37.9 g
    (D) 100 g
    (E) 239.1 g

16. A patient is to receive 2 mEq of sodium chloride per kilogram of body weight. If the patient weighs 186 lbs., how many milliliters of a 0.9% solution of sodium chloride (MW = 58.5) should be administered?

    (A) 11 mL
    (B) 321 mL
    (C) 550 mL
    (D) 1,099 mL
    (E) 5,320 mL

17. How many milliosmoles of calcium chloride (MW = 147) are represented in 200 mL of a 10% (w/v) calcium chloride solution?

    (A) 8.8 mOsm
    (B) 136 mOsm
    (C) 272 mOsm
    (D) 408 mOsm
    (E) 816 mOsm

18. If an ointment contains 60% (w/w) of polyethylene glycol 400 (specific gravity = 1.13), how many mL of polyethylene glycol are needed to prepare 1 kg of ointment?

    (A) 53 mL
    (B) 68 mL
    (C) 354 mL
    (D) 531 mL
    (E) 678 mL

19. How many mL of water should be added to 50 mL of zephiran chloride 1:750 solution to obtain a 1:10,000 strength solution?

    (A) 100 mL
    (B) 200 mL
    (C) 250 mL
    (D) 617 mL
    (E) 667 mL

20. You receive a prescription for fluticasone HFA 440 mcg BID with instructions to dispense a 90-day supply. Fluticasone HFA is available commercially as 220 mcg/metered dose with 120 doses per inhaler. How many inhalers should be dispensed for a 90-day supply?

    (A) 1 inhaler
    (B) 2 inhalers
    (C) 3 inhalers
    (D) 4 inhalers
    (E) 6 inhalers

21. You receive a prescription for insulin glargine 65 units once daily with instructions to dispense a 30-day supply. Insulin glargine is available commercially as 100 units/mL in 10-mL vials. How many vials should be dispensed for a 30-day supply?

    (A) 1 vial
    (B) 2 vials
    (C) 3 vials
    (D) 4 vials
    (E) 5 vials

22. You receive a prescription for oxycodone/acetaminophen 5/500 mg 1–2 tablets every 4–6 hours PRN pain. Based upon a maximum daily acetaminophen dose of 4 grams, how many tablets should be dispensed for a 30-day supply?

    (A) 60 tablets
    (B) 120 tablets
    (C) 240 tablets
    (D) 360 tablets
    (E) 480 tablets

23. An elixir contains 250 mg of active ingredient per 5 mL. You receive a prescription for 500 mg PO twice daily with instructions to dispense 120 mL of the elixir. How many days would the elixir last if taken as prescribed?

    (A) 4 days
    (B) 6 days
    (C) 8 days
    (D) 10 days
    (E) 12 days

24. A pediatric ferrous sulfate suspension contains 75 mg/1.5 mL (20% elemental). What dose (in mL) would provide the patient with 30 mg of elemental iron?

    (A) 0.3 mL
    (B) 0.6 mL
    (C) 1.5 mL
    (D) 3 mL
    (E) 6 mL

25. You are asked to compound a prescription for 120 mL of calamine lotion. The following formula is available.

Rx	Calamine	80 g
	Zinc oxide	80 g
	Glycerin	20 g
	Bentonite magma	250 mL
	Calcium hydroxide topical solution to make	1,000 mL

How many grams of calamine should be used to prepare the quantity specified?

(A) 0.96 g
(B) 8 g
(C) 9.6 g
(D) 80 g
(E) 96 g

26. You receive a prescription for 60 g of zinc oxide ointment. The following formula is available.

Rx	Zinc oxide	1 part
	Starch	1 part
	Petrolatum	2 parts

How many grams of zinc oxide should be used to prepare the quantity specified?

(A) 1 g
(B) 10 g
(C) 15 g
(D) 30 g
(E) 45 g

27. Approximately how many liters of a 0.9% aqueous solution can be made from 30 grams of sodium chloride?

(A) 1 L
(B) 2 L
(C) 3 L
(D) 4 L
(E) 5 L

28. You receive a prescription for 500 mL of a 0.5% w/v solution of drug A. You have on hand 10% w/v solution of drug A. What volume of your available solution should be diluted with water to make the 500 mL prescription?

   (A) 5 mL
   (B) 10 mL
   (C) 15 mL
   (D) 20 mL
   (E) 25 mL

29. A prescription is written for a total quantity of 100 mEq of NaCl. You have normal saline (0.9%) solution on hand. What volume should be dispensed? (MW NaCl = 58.5)

   (A) 58.5 mL
   (B) 65 mL
   (C) 527 mL
   (D) 585 mL
   (E) 650 mL

30. A medication order calls for 75 mL of a 0.8 mEq potassium/mL solution. How many grams of potassium chloride should be used to prepare the quantity specified? (MW KCl = 74.5)

   (A) 4.5 g
   (B) 7.5 g
   (C) 45 g
   (D) 75 g
   (E) 450 g

31. A medication order calls for 10 mL of a 1% tobramycin (E = 0.07) ophthalmic solution. You have on hand tobramycin 40 mg/mL solution. How much NaCl should be added to make the solution isotonic with tears?

   (A) 7 mg
   (B) 33 mg
   (C) 83 mg
   (D) 100 mg
   (E) 400 mg

32. You receive a prescription for amoxicillin 100 mg/5 mL. You have on hand amoxicillin 125 mg/5 mL powder for reconstitution. The label calls for the addition of 63 mL of water to make 80 mL of the 125 mg/5 mL suspension. What volume of water should be added to prepare the concentration specified?

    (A) 68 mL
    (B) 70 mL
    (C) 83 mL
    (D) 88 mL
    (E) 100 mL

33. What volume of a 10% w/v stock solution should be diluted with water to make 500 mL of a 0.25% w/v solution?

    (A) 12.5 mL
    (B) 25 mL
    (C) 50 mL
    (D) 125 mL
    (E) 200 mL

34. A prescription for lansoprazole suspension is written as follows.

Rx	Lansoprazole	3 mg/mL
	Sodium bicarbonate 8.4% ad	150 mL
	Sig. 5 mL BID	

    How many lansoprazole 30 mg capsules are needed to compound the prescription?

    (A) 10 capsules
    (B) 15 capsules
    (C) 30 capsules
    (D) 45 capsules
    (E) 60 capsules

35. What is the caloric requirement for a 52-year-old female patient with a calculated basal energy expenditure of 1,200 Calories and a stress factor of 1.5 due to a fever?

    (A) 1,200
    (B) 1,400
    (C) 1,600
    (D) 1,800
    (E) 2,000

36. The caloric requirement for a 62-year-old male patient is 1,950 Calories. If 250 mL of a 10% IV fat emulsion product were to be used daily, how many milliliters of $D_{70}W$ would need to be administered to meet his caloric requirements?

(A) 493 mL
(B) 704 mL
(C) 855 mL
(D) 1,220 mL
(E) 1,675 mL

ANSWERS

1. **B**

$$240\,mL \times \frac{85\,g\,sucrose}{100\,mL} = 204\,g\,sucrose$$

$$204\,g\,sucrose \times \frac{100\,mL}{60\,g\,sucrose} = 340\,mL\,total\,volume$$

$$340\,mL\,total\,volume - 240\,mL\,85\%\,w/v\,sucrose\,syrup = 100\,mL\,of\,water\,to\,add$$

2. **D**

$$250\,mL \times \frac{3\,mEq\,Na^+}{10\,mL} \times \frac{1\,mmol\,Na^+}{1\,mEq\,Na^+} \times \frac{1\,mmol\,NaCl}{1\,mmol\,Na^+} \times \frac{58.5\,mg\,NaCl}{1\,mmol\,NaCl} \times$$

$$\frac{1\,g}{1,000\,mg} \times \frac{1\,tablet}{1\,g} = 4.4\,tabs = 5\,tabs$$

If you are using a partial tablet, you must always round up. If you use 4.4 tablets, you will actually expend 5 tablets from inventory, use 4.4 for your product, and discard the remainder of the fifth tablet.

3. **C**

Final solution: 1 L of 1:1,470 BC $1,000\,mL \times \frac{1\,g\,BC}{1,470\,mL} = 0.68\,g\,BC$

This solution was produced by diluting 20 mL of the solution you made. Therefore, the solution you made has 0.68 g of BC in every 20 mL.

$$500\,mL \times \frac{0.68\,g\,BC}{20\,mL} = 17\,g\,of\,BC$$

You need 17 g of benzalkonium chloride. How many milliliters of a 17% w/v stock solution will be required to deliver 17 g?

$$17\,g \times \frac{100\,mL}{17\,g} = 100\,mL\,stock\,solution$$

4. **D**

$$75\,g\,ung \times \frac{3\,g\,ZnO}{100\,g\,ung} = 2.25\,g\,ZnO$$

$$\frac{(2.25+5)\,g\,ZnO}{(75+5)\,g\,ung} = \frac{7.25\,g\,ZnO}{80\,g\,ung} = \frac{9.0625\,g\,ZnO}{100\,g\,ung} = 9.0626\%\,w/w$$

5. **E**

Step 1: Determine the weight of all chemicals present in this prescription.

Zinc chloride: $\dfrac{0.2\ g}{100\ mL} = \dfrac{x}{60\ mL}$

$$x = 0.12\ g$$

Phenacaine: $\dfrac{1\ g}{100\ mL} = \dfrac{y}{60\ mL}$

$$y = 0.6\ g$$

Step 2: Multiply each weight by the listed E value of the chemical.

Zinc chloride: $0.12\ g \times 0.62 = 0.0744\ g$

Phenacaine: $0.6\ g \times 0.17 = 0.102\ g$

Step 3: Add the weights from Step 2. The sum is the amount of NaCl currently present in this prescription.

$$0.0744\ g + 0.102\ g = 0.1764\ g$$

Step 4: Determine the theoretical amount of NaCl that would be necessary to make this prescription isotonic if no other chemical were present.

$\dfrac{0.9\ g}{100\ mL} = \dfrac{p}{60\ mL}$

$$p = 0.54\ g$$

Step 5: Subtract the value in Step 3 from the value in Step 4 to determine the amount of NaCl that needs to be added to make this prescription isotonic.

$$0.54\ g - 0.1764\ g = 0.3636\ g$$

Step 6: Determine the amount of boric acid that would be used instead of NaCl to make this prescription isotonic.

$\dfrac{0.3636\ g\ NaCl}{q} = \dfrac{0.52\ g\ NaCl}{1\ g\ boric\ acid}$

$$q = 0.698\ g \times 1{,}000 = \mathbf{698\ mg}$$

6. **D**

Step 1: Determine the weight of all chemicals present in this prescription.

$$\text{Phenylephrine: } \frac{0.5\ g}{100\ mL} = \frac{x}{30\ mL}$$

$$x = 0.15\ g$$

Step 2: Multiply each weight by the listed E value of the chemical. The product is the amount of NaCl currently present in this prescription.

Phenylephrine: $0.15\ g \times 0.32 = 0.048\ g$

Step 3: Determine the theoretical amount of NaCl that would be necessary to make this prescription isotonic if no other chemical were present.

$$\frac{0.9\ g}{100\ mL} = \frac{y}{30\ mL}$$

$$y = 0.27\ g$$

Step 4: Subtract the value in Step 2 from the value in Step 3 to determine the amount of NaCl that needs to be added to make this prescription isotonic.

$$0.27\ g - 0.048\ g = 0.222\ g \times 1{,}000 = \textbf{222 mg}$$

7. **D**

The concentration of the epinephrine solution is presented as a ratio strength. A concentration of 1:500 translates into 1 g/500 mL. The first step in solving this problem is to determine the amount of epinephrine (in grams) that would be contained in 60 mL of the solution.

$$\frac{1\ g}{500\ mL} = \frac{x}{60\ mL}$$

$$x = 0.12\ g\ epinephrine$$

Next, set up a ratio-proportion to determine the volume of the 1% epinephrine stock solution needed to obtain the 0.12 grams of epinephrine.

1% stock solution:

$$\frac{1\ g}{100\ mL} = \frac{0.12\ g}{y}$$

$$y = \textbf{12 mL}$$

8. **D**

To determine the percentage of witch hazel, you must calculate the amount of witch hazel in 100 mL of the compound. According to the problem, there are 45 mL of witch hazel in 120 mL of calamine lotion in this prescription. To solve this problem, set up a ratio-proportion.

$$\frac{45\ mL}{120\ mL} = \frac{x}{100\ mL}$$

$$x = \textbf{37.5\%}$$

9. **D**

First, calculate the number of teaspoons to be administered on a daily basis.

$$1.5\ tsp/dose \times 3\ doses/day = 4.5\ tsp/day$$

Next, set up a ratio-proportion to determine the total volume (in mL) of penicillin suspension to be administered (assuming 1 teaspoon = 5 mL).

$$\frac{4.5\ tsp}{x} = \frac{1\ tsp}{5\ mL}$$

$$x = 22.5\ mL$$

Finally, multiply this daily volume by 12 days to determine the total volume of suspension (in mL) that should be dispensed.

$$22.5\ mL/day \times 12\ days = \textbf{270 mL}$$

10. **B**

Using dimensional analysis, multiply the weight-based dose by the weight of the child (being sure to convert the weight into kilograms), then by 2 (since the weight-based dose is being given twice daily), and then by 30 (to account for the 30-day supply). You can see below that all the units cancel out except for mg. The answer in this first step is the total number of milligrams of Dilantin that will be dispensed for this child for a 30-day supply.

$$\frac{2.5\ mg}{kg\ dose} \times 40\ lb \times \frac{1\ kg}{2.2\ lb} \times \frac{2\ doses}{day} \times 30\ days = 2{,}727.27\ mg$$

Next, using the concentration of Dilantin suspension of 125 mg/5 mL given in the problem, set up a ratio-proportion to determine the volume of this suspension to be dispensed that will contain 2,727.27 mg.

$$\frac{125\ mg}{5\ mL} = \frac{2{,}727.27\ mg}{x}$$

$$x = \textbf{109 mL}$$

11. **C**

Set up the problem using dimensional analysis: Multiply the weight-based dose by the weight of the patient, being sure to convert into kilograms; convert the units of time to hours; and convert the dose from micrograms to milligrams, since that is what the question is asking. You can see below that all the units cancel out except for mg.

$$\frac{2\ mcg}{kg/min} \times 167\ lb \times \frac{1\ kg}{2.2\ lb} \times \frac{60\ min}{1\ hr} \times 2\ hr \times \frac{1\ mg}{1{,}000\ mcg} = \textbf{18.2 mg}$$

12. **D**

Given that there are 274 mg of levothyroxine in 2,000 tablets, set up a ratio-proportion to determine how many milligrams are in 1 tablet. Then multiply this answer (in milligrams) by 1,000 to arrive at the answer in micrograms.

$$\frac{274\ mg}{2{,}000\ tablets} = \frac{x}{1\ tablet}$$

$$x = 0.137\ mg \times 1{,}000\ mcg/mg = \textbf{137 mcg}$$

13. **B**

The first step is to determine the total amount of the analgesic ointment that will be made given the formula provided.

$$10\ g + 95\ g + 5\ g + 40\ g + 850\ g = 1{,}000\ g\ ointment$$

Next, convert the total amount of ointment to be prepared, 5 pounds, into grams.

$$5\ lb \times \frac{454\ g}{1\ lb} = 2{,}270\ g$$

Finally, set up a ratio-proportion to determine how much benzocaine is needed to prepare 2,270 g of ointment, given that 95 g of benzocaine is used to prepare 1,000 g of the same ointment.

$$\frac{95\ g\ benzocaine}{1{,}000\ g\ ointment} = \frac{x}{2{,}270\ g\ ointment}$$

$$x = \textbf{215.7 g}$$

14. **B**

In this problem, the solution of iodine in chloroform is being concentrated (rather than diluted). The $Q_1C_1 = Q_2C_2$ method can be used to solve the problem. The volume that is solved for x is the amount of the 2.4% solution that would be made.

$$(1.4\%)\,(180\ mL) = (2.4\%)\,x$$

$$x = 105\ mL \text{ (this is the amount of 2.4\% solution)}$$

However, the question asks how much chloroform *must be evaporated from* the original 180 mL to adjust the iodine concentration to 2.4%. Therefore, this amount (105 mL) must be subtracted from the original amount (180 mL) to determine how much solution must be evaporated.

$$180\ mL - 105\ mL = \textbf{75 mL must be evaporated}$$

15. **A**

Alligation:

High Concentration [A]		Parts of High Concentration Ingredient [D]
	Desired Concentration [C]	
Low Concentration [B]		Parts of Low Concentration Ingredient [E]

Parts of high-concentration ingredient [D] = [C] – [B]

Parts of low-concentration ingredient [E] = [A] – [C]

Zinc Oxide Ointment:

Assume pure zinc oxide = 100%

100%		12 − 8 = 4 parts
	12%	
8%		100 − 12 = 88 parts Total = 92 parts

Quantity of 100% zinc oxide ointment needed:

$$\frac{4\ parts}{92\ parts} = \frac{x}{250\ g}$$

$$x = \textbf{10.9 g}$$

16. **D**

The first step is to multiply the weight-based dose by the weight of the patient using dimensional analysis, being sure to convert the weight into kilograms.

$$\frac{186\ lb}{} \times \frac{1\ kg}{2.2\ lb} \times \frac{2\ mEq}{kg} = 169.1\ mEq$$

At this point, the milliequivalent formula below can be used to determine the weight of sodium chloride (in mg) present in 169.1 mEq. Remember that the valence of sodium chloride (NaCl) is 1. The molecular weight of sodium chloride was given to you in the problem (58.5).

$$mEq = \frac{amount\ (mg)}{molecular\ weight} \times Valence$$

$$169.1 = \frac{x}{58.5} \times 1$$

$$x = 9{,}891.8\ mg\ /1{,}000 = 9.89\ g$$

Once the weight of sodium chloride is known, a ratio-proportion can be used to determine the volume of 0.9% sodium chloride solution to be administered. Remember that a 0.9% solution of sodium chloride contains 0.9 g of sodium chloride in 100 mL of solution.

Volume of 0.9% NaCl needed:

$$\frac{0.9\ g}{100\ mL} = \frac{9.89\ g}{x}$$

$$x = \mathbf{1{,}099\ mL}$$

17. **D**

The first step is to determine how much calcium chloride (in grams) is contained in 200 mL of a 10% (w/v) solution. Set up a ratio-proportion to solve this step.

$$\frac{10\ g}{100\ mL} = \frac{x}{200\ mL}$$

$$x = 20\ g\ CaCl_2$$

At this point, the milliosmole formula below can be used to determine how many milliosmoles are represented by 20 grams of calcium chloride. Remember that calcium chloride dissociates into 3 species. The molecular weight of calcium chloride was given to you in the problem (147).

$$mOsm = \frac{amount\ (mg)}{molecular\ weight} \times Theoretical\ number\ of\ particles$$
$$(or\ dissociation\ constant)$$

$$mOsm = \frac{20,000\ mg}{147} \times 3$$

$$mOsm = \textbf{408 mOsm}$$

18. **D**

The first step is to determine how much of the polyethylene glycol 400 would be needed to prepare 1 kg (or 1,000 g) of ointment, starting with a 60% (w/w) polyethylene glycol 400 ointment. A ratio-proportion can be set up to solve this problem.

$$\frac{60\ g}{100\ g} = \frac{x}{1,000\ g}$$

$$x = 600\ g\ of\ polyethylene\ glycol\ 400\ needed$$

Next, set up a ratio-proportion with this information to determine the volume of polyethylene glycol solution needed to prepare this compound. Remember that the specific gravity of a substance represents weight/volume in grams per milliliters.

Specific gravity (SG) = wt/vol

$$\frac{1.13\ g}{1\ mL} = \frac{600\ g}{y}$$

$$y = \textbf{531 mL}$$

19. **D**

This is a dilution problem that involves ratio strengths. The first step is to determine how much zephiran chloride (in grams) is contained in 50 mL of a 1:750 solution. This can be determined by setting up a ratio-proportion.

$$\frac{1\ g}{750\ mL} = \frac{x}{50\ mL}$$

$$x = 0.067\ g$$

Since the solution will be diluted to a 1:10,000 solution, the next step is to determine what volume of this solution would contain 0.067 g of zephiran chloride. Again, this can be determined by setting up a ratio-proportion.

$$\frac{1\ g}{10,000\ mL} = \frac{0.067\ g}{y}$$

$$y = 666.67\ mL$$

This dilution process involved going from 50 mL of a 1:750 solution to 666.67 mL of a 1:10,000 solution. However, 666.67 mL is not the final answer, as the question asked how many milliliters of water *should be added* to arrive at this amount. Thus, the final step of the problem is to subtract the initial volume from the total volume to arrive at the answer.

$$666.67\ mL - 50\ mL = 616.67\ mL = \textbf{617 mL of water needs to be added}$$

20. **C**

Solve this problem using dimensional analysis: Multiply the number of doses per day (2) by the strength of each prescribed dose (440 mcg); by the strength per metered dose (220 mcg/dose) and the number of doses per inhaler (120) to factor in the available dosage form; and by the number of days needed (90). Each fraction should be set up such that all the units cancel out except for inhalers.

$$2 \times \frac{440\ mcg}{1\ day} \times \frac{1\ dose}{220\ mcg} \times \frac{1\ inhaler}{120\ doses} \times 90\ days = \textbf{3 inhalers}$$

21. **B**

Solve this problem using dimensional analysis: Multiply the number of units the patient will need each day (65) by the number of units in each milliliter of insulin (100); by the number of milliliters per vial (10); and by the number of days needed (30). Each fraction should be set up such that all the units cancel out except for vials.

$$\frac{65\ units}{1\ day} \times \frac{1\ mL}{100\ units} \times \frac{1\ vial}{10\ mL} \times 30\ days = 1.95\ vials$$

Therefore, **2 vials** should be dispensed.

22. **C**

Solve this problem using dimensional analysis: Convert the maximum daily dose (4 g/day) to milligrams, and multiply by the strength of each tablet (500 mg) and the number of days needed (30). Each fraction should be set up such that all the units cancel out except for tablets.

$$\frac{4\ g}{1\ day} \times \frac{1,000\ mg}{1\ g} \times \frac{1\ tablet}{500\ mg}\ 30\ days = \textbf{240 tablets}$$

23. **B**

Solve this problem using dimensional analysis: Multiply the strength of the elixir (250 mg/5 mL) by the desired dose (500 mg); by the number of doses per day (2); and by the quantity dispensed (120 mL). Each fraction should be set up such that all units cancel out except for days.

$$\frac{250\ mg}{5\ mL} \times \frac{1\ dose}{500\ mg} \times \frac{1\ day}{2\ doses} \times 120\ mL = \textbf{6 days}$$

24. **D**

First, use dimensional analysis to determine the amount of elemental iron per milliliter. Multiply the strength of the available suspension (75 mg/1.5 mL) by the percent of elemental iron (20%).

$$\frac{75 \; mg \; ferrous \; sulfate}{1.5 \; mL \; suspension} \times \frac{20 \; mg \; elemental \; iron}{100 \; mg \; ferrous \; sulfate} = 10 \; mg \; elemental \; iron/mL$$

Then, set up a ratio-proportion to calculate the volume of the suspension needed to obtain the 30 mg of elemental iron, and cross-multiply to solve the problem.

$$\frac{10 \; mg \; elemental \; iron}{1 \; mL} = \frac{30 \; mg \; elemental \; iron}{x}$$

$$10x = 30 \; mL$$

$$x = 30 \, / \, 10 = \textbf{3 mL}$$

25. **C**

One approach to solving this problem is to identify the factor that represents the relationship between the desired quantity (120 mL) and the quantity specified in the compounding recipe (1,000 mL), then multiply by this factor to determine the appropriate amount of each ingredient. In this case, the relationship can be expressed by dividing 120 mL by 1,000 mL, yielding a factor of 0.12.

$$\frac{120 \; mL}{1,000 \; mL} = 0.12 \; (factor)$$

Next, multiply the relevant ingredient—in this case, 80 g of calamine—by this factor to calculate the appropriate amount.

$$80 \; g \; calamine \times 0.12 = \textbf{9.6 g}$$

26. **C**

First, determine the ratio of zinc oxide to the total recipe by finding the sum of the parts: 1 part + 1 part + 2 parts = 4 parts. So the ratio of parts zinc oxide to total parts is 1:4. Next, set up a ratio-proportion to calculate how much zinc oxide is contained in a total weight of 60 grams, and cross-multiply to solve.

$$\frac{1 \; part \; zinc \; oxide}{4 \; parts \; total} = \frac{x \; g \; zinc \; oxide}{60 \; g \; total}$$

$$4x = 60$$

$$x = 60 \, / \, 4 = \textbf{15 g}$$

27.   **C**

The first step in solving this problem is to set up a ratio-proportion representing the relationship between the desired %w/v (0.9%) and the available weight of the product (30 g).

$$\frac{0.9\ g}{100\ mL} = \frac{30\ g}{x}$$

$$0.9x = 3{,}000\ mL$$

$$x = 3{,}000\ /\ 0.9\ mL$$

$$x = 3{,}333\ mL$$

The problem asks for liters, so convert from milliliters to liters to solve the problem.

$$3{,}333\ mL \times \frac{1L}{1{,}000\ mL} = \textbf{3.33 L}$$

28.   **E**

The first step is to calculate how much of drug A (in grams) is contained in 500 mL of a 0.5% w/v solution. Solve this step using dimensional analysis.

$$\frac{0.5\ g\ drug\ A}{100\ mL} \times 500\ mL = 2.5\ g\ drug\ A$$

Next, set up a ratio-proportion to determine the volume of the available 10% w/v solution needed to obtain the desired weight of drug A (2.5 g), and cross-multiply to solve the problem.

$$\frac{10\ g}{100\ mL} = \frac{2.5\ g}{x\ mL} = \textbf{25 mL}$$

29.   **E**

Sodium and chloride are monovalent ions, so 1 mol = 1 equivalent. The first step in solving this problem is to determine the number of grams of NaCl per mEq. Because there is 1 mol per equivalent, this is a simple calculation: Divide the molecular weight (which is equal to the EqW) by 1,000 to determine g/mEq.

$$MW\ NaCl = 58.5$$

$$EqW = \frac{58.5\ g}{1}$$

$$1\ mEq = \frac{58.5}{1{,}000} = 0.0585\ g$$

Next, multiply the weight by the desired number of mEq (100) to determine the total weight needed.

$$100 \; mEq = 0.0585 \; g \times 100 = 5.85 \; g \; NaCl \; needed$$

Finally, set up a ratio-proportion indicating the relationship between the available concentration (0.9% for normal saline) and the desired weight of NaCl (5.85 g), and cross-multiply to solve the problem.

$$\frac{0.9 \; g}{100 \; mL} = \frac{5.85 \; g}{x}$$

$$0.9x = 585$$

$$x = 585 \; / \; 0.9 \; = \; \textbf{650 mL}$$

30. **A**

Because KCl is made up of monovalent ions, the molecular weight is equal to the EqW. Divide the number by 1,000 to determine the weight/mEq.

$$MW \; KCl = 74.5$$

$$EqW = \frac{74.5 \; g}{1}$$

$$1 \; mEq = \frac{74.5}{1{,}000} = 0.0745 \; g$$

From here, the problem can be solved using dimensional analysis: Multiply the desired concentration (0.8 mEq/mL) by the weight/mEq (74.5 g/mEq) and by the total quantity desired (75 mL). Each fraction should be set up such that units cancel out except for grams.

$$\frac{0.8 \; mEq}{1 \; mL} \times \frac{0.0745 \; g}{1 \; mEq} \times 75 \; mL = \textbf{4.5 g}$$

31. **C**

First, calculate the total amount of tobramycin in the desired product by multiplying the %w/v by the given volume.

$$1\% \; solution = \frac{1 \; g \; tobramycin}{100 \; mL} \times 10 \; mL = 0.1 \; g \; tobramycin$$

Then, multiply the weight of the active ingredient by the E value of the active ingredient (0.07) to determine the weight of NaCl required to exert the tonic effect represented in the solution.

$$0.1 \; g \; tobramycin \times \frac{0.07 \; g \; NaCl(eq)}{1 \; g \; tobramycin} = 0.007 \; g \; NaCl(eq)$$

Next, use the %w/v of normal saline (0.9%) to calculate the total amount of NaCl needed to make the solution isotonic if this were the sole tonicity agent.

$$\frac{0.9 \ g \ NaCl}{100 \ mL} \times 10 \ mL = 0.09 \ g \ NaCl$$

Finally, subtract the amount of NaCl already present in the tobramycin (0.007 g) from this total amount (0.09 g) to determine how much should be added.

$$0.09 \ g \ - \ 0.007 \ g \ = \ 0.083 \ g \ NaCl \times \frac{1,000 \ mg}{1 \ g} = \textbf{83 mg}$$

32.   **C**

First, set up a ratio-proportion to calculate the total weight of medication in the bottle.

$$\frac{125 \ mg}{5 \ mL} = \frac{x}{80 \ mL}$$

$$5 \ mL \times x \ mg = 125 \ mg \times 80 \ mL$$

$$x = 2,000 \ mg \ amoxicillin$$

Then, set up another ratio-proportion to determine the total volume needed to provide the desired concentration.

$$\frac{100 \ mg}{5 \ mL} = \frac{2,000 \ mg}{y}$$

$$100 \ mg \times y = 2,000 \ mg \times 5 \ mL$$

$$y = 100 \ mL$$

Next, calculate the volume of the dry powder to be used in this prescription by subtracting the amount of water added from the total end volume.

volume of dry powder = 80 mL − 63 mL = 17 mL

Finally, determine the amount of water to add for reconstitution by subtracting the volume of dry powder calculated in the previous step from the total volume needed.

100 mL − volume of dry powder (17 mL) = water to add = **83 mL**

33. **A**

This problem can be solved by setting up a simple ratio-proportion indicating the relationship between the available stock solution and the desired volume and concentration of the new solution.

$$(10\%) \times (x\ mL) = (0.25\%) \times (500\ mL)$$

$$10x = 125$$

$$x = 125\ /\ 10\ =\ \textbf{12.5 mL}$$

34. **B**

First, determine the total weight of drug needed by multiplying the concentration (3 mg/mL) by the given volume (150 mL).

$$\frac{3\ mg}{1\ mL} \times 150\ mL\ =\ 450\ mg\ lansoprazole\ needed$$

Next, divide the total weight needed by the available capsule strength (30 mg) to determine the number of capsules needed.

$$450\ mg\ /\ 30\ mg\ capsules = total\ number\ of\ capsules\ needed\ =\ \textbf{15 capsules}$$

35. **D**

The patient's total caloric requirement can be calculated by multiplying the patient's estimated basal energy expenditure by the stress factor. The patient has an estimated basal energy expenditure of 1,200 and a stress factor of 1.5.

$$1,200 \times 1.5 = \textbf{1,800 Calories}$$

36. **B**

The fatty acid emulsion and dextrose are used in the TPN to meet the patient's caloric requirement. To calculate the amount of dextrose that is needed to meet the caloric requirement, first calculate the calories obtained from the fatty acid emulsion. The fatty acid emulsion contains 1.1 Cal/mL.

Therefore,

$$\frac{1.1\ Calorie}{1\ mL} = \frac{x\ Calorie}{250\ mL}$$

$$x = 275\ Calories\ from\ the\ fatty\ acid\ emulsion$$

Next, calculate the calories needed from the dextrose solution by subtracting the fatty acid emulsion calories from the total caloric need. The number of calories required from dextrose would be:

$$1{,}950 - 275 = 1{,}675 \; Calories$$

Then, calculate the amount of dextrose needed to meet the requirements.

$$\frac{3.4 \; Calories}{1 \; g} = \frac{1{,}675 \; Calories}{x \; g}$$

$$x = 493 \; g \; of \; dextrose$$

Finally, convert the amount of dextrose into milliliters of solution.

$$\frac{70 \; g \; dextrose}{100 \; mL} = \frac{493 \; g}{x \; mL}$$

$$x = \textbf{704 mL of } \mathbf{D_{70}W}$$

Biostatistics

25

This chapter contains the following:

- **Descriptive statistics: Summarizing the data**
- **Statistical test selection**

Suggested Study Time: **60 minutes**

Statistics play an important role in the development and interpretation of clinical trials. Biostatistics is defined as the application of statistics to biological data. The NAPLEX exam tests fundamental statistical knowledge. Many times the questions are not math based problems but are conceptual in nature. This chapter covers the most important definitions in biostatistics and proper uses of the most common statistical tests.

Statistics can be broken into two fundamental parts: descriptive and inferential.

Descriptive statistics are used to organize, summarize, categorize, and display data. If an entire population were to be studied, one would need only to summarize the data. However, in almost all cases, an entire population cannot be studied, and inferential statistics is needed from a sample of the population. **Inferential statistics** is used make predictions (i.e., infer) about a large amount of information (population) based on a sample. Ultimately, inferential statistics is used in decision making in many fields, including regulatory drug approval and clinical drug usage.

DESCRIPTIVE STATISTICS: SUMMARIZING THE DATA

Central Tendency

A population or sample from that population can generate a lot of data that need to be simplified. One of the most basic forms of descriptive statistics is to take a large amount of information and simplify that into one or two values that can provide information regarding the tendency of the data. **Central tendency** is a general term used to describe the distribution of a set of values or measurements and the simplification to a single value near a point in the dataset that represents where the largest portion of data are located. The following are the most commonly used central tendency measures.

Median (*m*): The median is the value directly in the middle of the ranked values in a dataset; that is, 50% of all ranked values are smaller than the median and the other 50% of ranked values are larger. The median is **not** influenced by extreme values (outliers). The median is useful in situations in which there are unusually low or high values that would render the mean unrepresentative of the data.

Mean ($\overline{X}$ or μ): The mean is the average of all observations in a dataset. The mean is the most commonly used measure of central tendency because it has properties that make it useful for statistical analyses. It is influenced by extreme values (outliers) and is most useful when the data are symmetrically distributed without outliers (i.e., normal distribution).

Mode: The mode is the value with the greatest frequency of occurrence. It is not generally used because it is often not representative of the data, particularly when the dataset is small.

Variability

The central tendency (e.g., median, mean) does not provide any information about the variability in a given dataset. An additional measure that describes the variability in a dataset is, therefore, generally provided with a central tendency measure to better describe the dataset. The following are the most commonly used measures of variability.

Standard Deviation (SD or σ): The standard deviation is the most common measure of the variability around the mean. It is used with a mean because it is most informative when the dataset is normally distributed, as described below. *The mean and standard deviation are commonly used together as the most informative measures of central tendency and variability of a dataset, respectively.*

Standard Error of the Mean (SEM): The standard error of the mean is defined as the variability of the sample means. It is calculated as the SD divided by the square root of the sample size. This will always be smaller than the sample SD. It is sometimes reported in the scientific and medical literature and is an intermediary step in calculating confidence intervals.

Absolute Range: The absolute range is simply the difference between the largest and smallest observation in a dataset. A disadvantage is that the range is based solely on two observations and is likely not representative of the whole dataset. Absolute range is particularly susceptible to outliers.

Interquartile Range (IQR): Quartiles are calculated in a way similar to the median, which splits a dataset into two equally sized groups. Quartiles split the data into four approximately equal sized groups. The interquartile range is the range between the lower and upper quartiles. Like the median, the interquartile range is not influenced by unusually high or low values and is particularly useful when data are not symmetrically distributed.

The **interquartile range** is the difference between the upper and lower quartiles:

- The lower Quartile (Q_L or Q_1) is the 25th percentile; that is, 25% of the data are below the value of Q_1.
- The upper Quartile (Q_U or Q_3) is the 75th percentile; that is, 75% of the data are below the value of Q_3.

A dataset with a large number of outliers is best described by a median and IQR as opposed to a mean and SD. These datasets are often displayed graphically with box-plots. **Boxplots** are one-dimensional graphs that can be drawn from the range, IQR, and median, as displayed here.

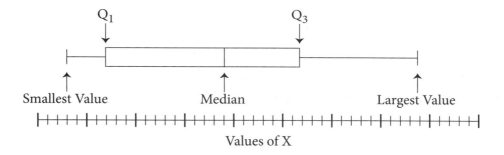

Distributions

Statistical test selection relies heavily on the distribution of data. These distributions can be summarized by a central tendency and variation around that center. The most important distribution is the normal or Gaussian curve. This "bell-shaped" curve is symmetric, with one side the mirror image of the other.

The distribution of any dataset can be assessed visually using a **histogram**, displayed below. The x-axis represents the actual values in the dataset which, for pharmacy, are usually measures made of patients enrolled in a clinical trial (e.g., systolic blood pressure, creatinine clearance, LDL concentrations, etc.). The y-axis represents the frequency of the value or the number of patients who had a value within a defined range. An example of a histogram is displayed here.

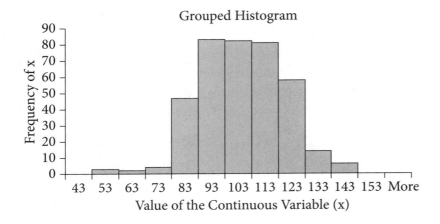

As the sample size (n) displayed in the histogram above approaches the population size (N), the lines on the graph become smooth and look more like the graph described below for normally distributed data:

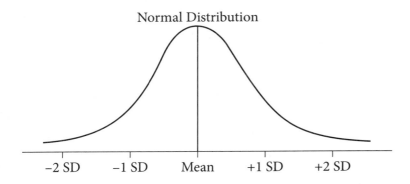

There are important attributes of the Normal Distribution shown above that can be useful in a number of problems on the NAPLEX. Importantly, the data is symmetric about the mean, as shown by the vertical line in the graph. This means that 50% of the values will be greater than the mean and 50% of the values will be less than the mean. Because this is the definition of a median, the mean and median are equal values in a normal distribution. The informative power of the normal distribution comes from the value of the standard deviation:

- The mean ± 1 SD contains 68% of the values in the dataset (or population)
- The mean ± 2 SD contains 95% of the values in the dataset (or population)
- The mean ± 3 SD contains 99.7% of the values in the dataset (or population)

The following graph displays two normal curves with the same means but different standard deviations:

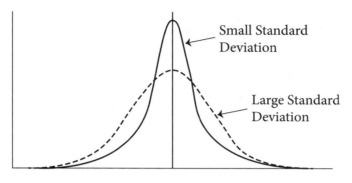

Small Standard Deviation

Large Standard Deviation

© Kaplan 2015.

Example:

Patients (N = 100) enrolled in a clinical trial have a mean ± SD creatinine clearance of 110 ± 20 mL/min. Approximately how many patients have creatinine clearance values between:

- 90 and 130 mL/min?

    Answer: The value of 90 mL/min is 1 SD away from the mean in the negative direction, and the value of 130 mL/min is 1 SD away from the mean in the positive direction. Approximately 68% of the values will be ± 1 SD away from the mean; therefore, 68% of the sample size of N = 100 gives an answer of 68 patients.

- 70 and 110 mL/min?

    Answer: The value of 70 mL/min is 2 SD away from the mean in the negative direction, and the value of 110 mL/min is the value of the mean. Approximately 95% of the values will be ± 2 SD away from the mean. Because the question is asking for only 2 SD in the negative direction and the normal distribution is symmetrical, it will be half the value of 95%. Half of 95% is 47.5%. Therefore, approximately 47.5% of the sample size of N = 100 patients will have values in this range. The answer would be approximately 48 patients have creatinine clearance values in this range.

Not all curves are normally distributed. Sometimes the curve is skewed either positively or negatively. A positive skew has the tail to the right with mean greater than the median. A negative skew has the tail to the left and the median greater than the mean.

For skewed distributions, the median is a better representation of central tendency than is the mean, and the IQR is a better measure of the variability than is the SD, as shown below:

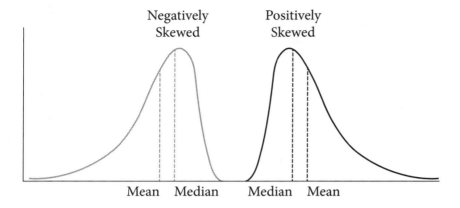

INFERENTIAL STATISTICS: SUMMARIZING THE DATA

The main goal of several studies in the pharmacy literature is to compare measurements from two groups of study patients: a group that receives a standard drug (e.g., control) and a group that receives an investigational drug. Even if both groups are administered placebo, it is highly unlikely that an identical mean and standard deviation of any value will be obtained for both groups. This is due to inherent variability in humans, among other sources, and is termed sampling error. The purpose of inferential statistics is to determine if the observed differences in the measures between the two groups of patients is due to chance (i.e., sampling error) or if one drug is really better than the other.

The following table summarizes important definitions regarding statistical inference.

General Statistical Definitions

Hypotheses	Hypothesis	Theoretical statement that the study is intended to test
	Null hypothesis	States that there is no difference between the study and control groups
	Alternative hypothesis	States that the null hypothesis is incorrect; there is a difference between the study and control groups
Variables	Independent variable	Known variable(s)
	Dependent variable	Variable with a value dependent upon the value of an independent variable
Error	Type I error	Rejecting a true null hypothesis: Finding a difference between the study and control groups that does not exist
	Type II error	Accepting a false null hypothesis: Failing to detect a difference between the study and control groups that does exist

Tests	Parametric	Requires prior knowledge of the nature of the data under examination; data must fall under a normal (Gaussian) distribution and be measured on an interval or a ratio scale
	Nonparametric	Does not require prior knowledge of the distribution of the observations; data need not follow a normal or Gaussian distribution
Miscellaneous definitions	Accuracy	Measure of how close a measured value is to the expected value
	Precision	Measure of how close a particular measured value is to the other values in a set of measurements; does not imply proximity between measured values and the expected value
	Sample	Data set taken under homogenous conditions; a subset of a population
	Population	Entire group from which a sample is taken
	Gaussian (or normal) distribution	A bell-shaped distribution Given a large enough sample size, the Central Limit Theorem states that the distribution of means will follow this type of distribution even if the population is not Gaussian. • 68% of values fall within $\pm$ 1 SD of the mean • 95% of values fall within $\pm$ 2 SD of the mean • 99.7% of values fall within $\pm$ 3 SD of the mean

Several additional statistical concepts are included below, in slightly greater detail. Many of these concepts apply regardless of the statistical test chosen.

Confidence Intervals

Statistical decisions are made based on sampling from a larger population. The true values for the population may be above or below the sample values. For example, the sample mean is unlikely to be the same value as the actual mean of the entire population. Therefore, confidence intervals are calculated from the sample to provide a range of values that is likely to contain the actual population value. The most common confidence interval used is the 95% confidence interval. This interval implies that you are 95% confident that the actual mean value of the population lies within this range of values. The 5% of uncertainty is the same concept as described with the p-value below. Therefore, 95% confidence intervals can be used to determine statistical significance with a Type I error rate of 5%, as demonstrated below.

Example:

The following graph displays the 95% confidence intervals for blood pressure measurements following the administration of three drugs. The closed circle represents the sample mean estimate in each group, and the error bars encompass the values of the 95% confidence interval. Which drugs are statistically different from each other?

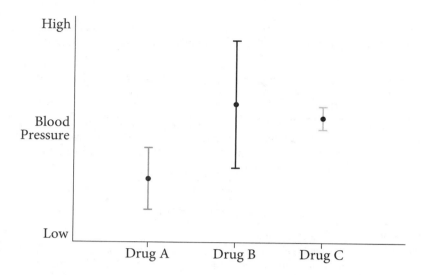

© Kaplan 2015.

Answer: When comparing two groups, any overlap of confidence intervals indicates that the groups would have a p-value > 0.05 and are not significantly different. Therefore, if the graph represents 95% confidence intervals and each drug is compared with the others, Drugs B and C are no different in their effects, and Drug B is no different from Drug A. Drug A lowers blood pressure to a greater statistically significant extent than Drug C. Of note, comparing these drugs individually to one another as in this example would increase the Type I error rate >5%, as will be discussed (see ANOVA).

Relative Risk and Odds Ratios

A relative risk (RR) is the ratio of the probability of an event occurring in a treatment (i.e., exposed) group to the probability of the event occurring in a control (i.e., nonexposed) group, as displayed in the equation below:

$$RR = \frac{p(exposure\ group)}{p(nonexposed\ group)}$$

Example:

In a local hospital over the last year, the frequency of patients with heart failure developing myopathy among those taking statins was 5 out of 100, and among patients not taking statins, it was 2 out of 100 patients. Calculate the relative risk.

Answer:

$$RR = \frac{5/100}{2/100} = 2.5$$

This implies that patients with heart failure who are taking statins were 2.5 times more likely to develop myopathy than patients who were not taking statins. Clearly, there are many variables in a study that could affect the relative risk beyond that of the statin use. Multivariate regression is commonly used in these types of analyses to account for variables beyond the exposure itself. Similar to the relative risk, an **odds ratio** is also a measure of association between an exposure and an outcome. An odds ratio will provide a similar estimate to that of a relative risk, but the calculation is not as intuitive. However, the odds ratio has a mathematical advantage and is commonly reported because it is used in logistic regression to account for study variables beyond the exposure.

It is important to be able to make statistical determinations when provided with confidence intervals for relative risks and odds ratios. Simply put, if the 95% confidence interval contains 1, there is no statistically significant effect of the treatment (i.e., exposure). This is demonstrated in the following table for three hypothetical measures:

Relative Risk or Odds Ratio	Confidence Interval	Interpretation
1.98	(1.45–2.53)	Statistically significant (increased risk)
1.25	(0.78–1.53)	No statistical difference (risk the same)
0.45	(0.22–0.68)	Statistically significant (decreased risk)

© Kaplan 2015.

Understanding Statistical Inference

The table at the beginning of this chapter introduced the definitions of hypothesis testing that are used after a research question has been identified. The null and alternative hypotheses are tested after the study has been conducted and the data have been collected. The process of running these statistical tests will not be covered on the NAPLEX. However, it is important to be able to interpret the results of the statistical tests. Interpreting statistics is quite simple because most statistical tests convert the output to a single p-value, which always has the same meaning. Therefore, to interpret the output of statistical tests, understanding the p-value is critical. Beyond the p-value, it is important to know what types of statistical error can be made and the power of a given test to determine significance. Finally, for the NAPLEX you will need to know the most commonly used statistical tests and their appropriate uses. All these important topics will be described in detail here.

p-Value and Statistical Significance

The p-value is the probability that the difference measured between your study group and the control group is the result of random chance rather than a true difference. The p-value is expressed as a value between 0 and 1; therefore, the higher the p-value, the more likely it is that a difference in sample means was due to chance and that a drug had no effect.

When the p-value is low (e.g., <5%), it indicates that it was unlikely that the difference was due to chance; therefore, the drug had a statistically significant effect.

The null hypothesis may be rejected if there is a sufficiently small probability that it is true. A significance level (or α) of 0.05 is most commonly chosen, although it should be chosen based on the relative consequences of making a Type I or Type II error in the particular study setting. When a 0.05 significance level is chosen, if $p \leq 0.05$, a statistically significant difference in treatment effect exists between the control and treatment groups. If $p > 0.05$, the results of the study are considered to be not statistically significant, meaning no difference exists between the treatment and control groups. Choosing a larger significance level, like $p = 0.1$, gives a higher probability of rejecting a true null hypothesis (Type I error, or false positive test).

Types of Statistical Error

As defined in the table at the beginning of this chapter, there are two types of error that can be made at the end of a statistical test. The significance level (i.e. alpha, α) is commonly set to 0.05. This means that there is a 5% chance that a **Type I error (α error)** will be made during hypothesis testing. A Type I error is the conclusion that there is a statistical difference when in reality there is not one. Of course, you cannot know from a given experiment if you made a Type I error or not. You can only know the rate at which they occur (i.e., 5%).

The other type of error is **Type II error (β error)**, which is the conclusion that there is not a difference between groups when, in reality, there is a difference. A Type II error can only be made when the p-value is > 0.05 and the conclusion is made that there is no statistical difference between groups. As in a Type I error, one cannot know from a single experiment if a Type II error has been made, but can only calculate the frequency of the error. The Type I error rate is set at 5%, but the Type II error rate varies depending on the variable being measured and the study itself (see "Power and Sample Size"). Type II error rates are commonly designed to be <10% or 20%. The factors that affect Type II error are the same that effect study power.

Power and Sample Size

The power of a study is the ability to detect a difference between study groups if one actually exists. Study power is indirectly related to the likelihood of making a Type II (β) error. Therefore, as study power increases, the likelihood of concluding that there is not a difference when one actually does exist decreases. Therefore, as power increases, Type II error rate decreases. The following factors affect the power of a study:

- **Sample size (*n*):** The closer the sample size is to the actual population size, the easier it is to detect a difference.

- **Difference between the actual population means:** It will be easier to detect a difference between drugs with large effects versus the control or comparator. For example, it is much easier to show that a β-blocker will lower blood pressure compared to a placebo than it would be compared to an ACE inhibitor.
- **Variability around the population means (and sample means):** The more variable effect there is, the harder it is to show a difference. For example, if a drug only works in a small percentage of the population, it will be difficult to show statistical significance in a sample from the entire population.
- **Significance Level, α:** The Type I error rate directly alters the Type II error rate. This is one reason why the significance level is traditionally set at 5%. If one wanted to decrease the Type I error rate and set it at 1%, it would increase the Type II error rate and, thereby, decrease the power of the study.

Of the factors just listed, the only way to decrease Type II error (increase power) without increasing Type I error is to increase the sample size. The researcher does not have control over the other factors (except the Type I error rate, which should not be changed). Therefore, increasing sample size increases one's power to detect a difference without altering the Type I error rate. Sample size calculations are commonly made before initiating a study. They are made by calculations including the four factors listed. The Type I error rate is set at 5%, and the Type II error rate is determined by the researcher, usually 10% or 20% (to give 90% to 80% power, respectively). The difference in the means is commonly chosen based on clinical significance. For example, if a 45% reduction in blood pressure is considered to be clinically significance, then it would be appropriate to base the sample size on a 45% different in the means. Finally, the variability is often estimated based on previous research with the same drug or animal studies if human studies have not been conducted.

At the conclusion of a study, if the p-value is > 0.05, the actual study power can be calculated. This is done by simply using the actual values of the factors listed about the study (e.g., the sample size, variability, and mean difference). Of course, it would only make sense to calculate the power of a study if the p-value was > 0.05. If the p-value is < 0.05, it is impossible to make a Type II error. Only a Type I error could have been made with a p-value < 0.05, and the power of the study would be irrelevant.

Correlation

Correlation measures the degree of a linear relationship between two variables. Correlation is often represented by the correlation coefficient (r), which can range in value from −1 to +1. A correlation coefficient of 0 indicates no linear relationship between variables. A coefficient of −1 reflects a perfect inverse relationship between variables, while a value of +1 reflects a perfect direct relationship.

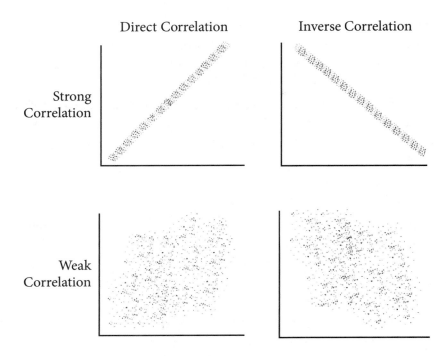

© Kaplan 2015.

A key point to remember is that an observed correlation between two variables does not imply that there is a causal link between the two variables. For example, warm weather causes an increase in both the crime rate and the incidence of sunburn. Crime rate and sunburn incidence will therefore be positively correlated; however, crime does not cause sunburn and sunburn does not cause crime.

Another important point to consider is that correlation coefficient assumes a normal distribution of measured values; if this assumption is incorrect, the coefficient is not relevant.

STATISTICAL TEST SELECTION

The first thing that must be done when determining what statistical test should be employed is to identify the dependent variable and the scale of measurement that will be used for this variable. The scale of measurement may be numeric, ordinal, or nominal.

Tests Appropriate for Numerical Scales of Measurement

Numeric scales (also called interval or ratio scales) of measurement are used when the measured values are numbers. Examples include height, weight, or blood pressure level. When the data follows a Gaussian distribution, parametric statistical tests should be used.

- Two independent groups: ***T-test***
- Two dependent groups: ***Paired t-test***

- Three or more independent groups: *ANOVA*
- Three or more dependent groups: *Repeated measures ANOVA*

T-test

The *t-test* is one of the most commonly used statistical tests. It compares means obtained from the numeric data of two groups that are independent of each other. This is commonly used in the pharmacy literature to compare the outcomes of numeric data (e.g., clinical measures, drug concentrations, etc.) in a sample of patients who received an experimental drug versus a different (i.e., independent) sample of patients who received a control drug.

Paired T-test

A paired *t*-test is used when the same sample is being used to compare the experimental and the control drug; that is, this test is appropriate when numeric data is being compared between two dependent groups. This is commonly referred to as a cross-over design and is the appropriate statistical test for numeric or interval data.

ANOVA

When a third group (or more) is added to a study design for comparison, it is not appropriate to perform multiple *t*-tests. For example, an experimental drug to lower blood pressure is being compared to a group of patients taking β-blockers and another group of patients taking angiotensin-converting enzyme (ACE)-inhibitors. In this study design, one cannot perform a *t*-test to compare the experimental drug to the β-blocker group and then perform another *t*-test to compare the ACE-inhibitor group. Each time a *t*-test is performed there is a 5% chance of a Type I error; making multiple comparisons increases this rate of Type I error greater than 5%. Therefore, if three or more groups are being compared, it is appropriate to use Analysis of Variance (ANOVA). An ANOVA will generate one p-value from the three groups. If the p value is < 0.05, it states that at least one drug was different than another at lowering blood pressure. Importantly, the Type I error rate is maintained at 5% for an ANOVA.

To determine which drug has a statistically significant effect, additional tests are needed. These statistical tests are referred to as *post-hoc tests*. The most commonly used post-hoc test is Tukey's test. The Bonferroni and Scheffe's tests are also post-hoc tests that can be used to determine which groups were statistically different if an overall p value from the ANOVA was less than 0.05. If a p-value is > 0.05 following an ANOVA, no further tests are needed.

Repeated Measures ANOVA

The repeated measures ANOVA is the equivalent of using a paired *t*-test instead of a *t*-test. It, therefore, can be used in crossover studies when there are three or more study periods following appropriate wash-out of the drug between each period. This test is referred to as *repeated measures* because it is commonly used when the same measures are being made in patients throughout a study. For example, in many statin clinical trials, the low density lipoprotein (LDL) lowering ability of the statins is not determined at only one point but at several points (e.g., 1, 3, 6, 12, 18, and 24 months). To determine if significant LDL lowering occurred in patients during these time intervals, a repeated measures ANOVA must be used. The Dunnett's test is the post-hoc test that should be used if an overall p-value < 0.05 is obtained.

When the data does not follow a Gaussian distribution, the same tests used for ordinal data should be employed.

Tests Appropriate for Ordinal Scales of Measurement

Ordinal scales of measurement are used when characteristics have an underlying order to their values but the numbers used are arbitrary (e.g., Likert scales). Various non-parametric tests (e.g., Mann-Whitney U and Wilcoxon Signed-Rank) are used for analyzing such data. Ordinal scales also are used for numeric data that is not distributed normally and that has a small sample size. The following are situations in which a nonparametric test should be considered:

- The outcome is ordinal and the sample is clearly not normal.
- There are values that are too high or too low to obtain accurate measures. It is impossible to analyze such data with a parametric test because the exact value is not determined.
- The sample size is small and the sample is not approximately normally distributed. Data transformation can be done by taking the logarithm of the values. This is common for biological data, which often has outliers in the positive direction (i.e., skewed to the right).

The following table lists parametric tests for normally distributed data and the corresponding nonparametric test for ordinal or non-normally distributed data.

Parametric Versus Nonparametric Statistics

Parametric Tests	Nonparametric Equivalent
T-test ⟶	Wilcoxon-Rank Sum (Mann Whitney U)
Paired t-test ⟶	Wilcoxon Sign Rank (Sign Test)
ANOVA ⟶	Kruskal-Wallis Test
Repeated measures ANOVA ⟶	Friedman Test

Note: The Wilcoxon-Rank Sum is the post hoc test for the Kruskal-Wallis Test

Tests Appropriate for Nominal Scales of Measurement

Nominal scales are used for characteristics that do not have numerical value (such as gender or race). The Chi-square test and its variants are used to test the null hypothesis that proportions are equal, or that factors or characteristics are not associated with each other.

Learning Points

- Smaller p-values associated with a statement reflect a greater likelihood that the statement accurately reflects a difference between groups. Larger p-values mean that the difference detected between groups is more likely to have been due to random chance.

- Power is the ability of a study to detect an actual effect. Power can be increased by increasing the number of patients enrolled in a study. Inadequate power may result in a study failing to detect a difference that actually exists between groups.

- The mean is the numerical average of the entire range of data; the mode is the central point in the data distribution. In a pure Gaussian distribution, the median will be equal or very close to the mode; large variance between median and mode may reflect non-Gaussian distribution or significant outlying data.

- ANOVA and t-tests are appropriate only for numeric data in a Gaussian distribution. Nonparametric tests are appropriate for numeric data in a non-Gaussian distribution, as well as for ordinal data. Chi-square tests should be used for nominal data.

PRACTICE QUESTIONS

1. The median value of a data set is the

    (A) mathematical average of all the values in the data set.
    (B) value equidistant from the extremes of a distribution.
    (C) average of the difference between each value in the set and the mean.
    (D) most commonly occurring value in the data set.
    (E) distance between the smallest and largest values in the data set.

Questions 2–3 refer to the following graph.

Total serum cholesterol concentrations were measured in 175 patients with coronary artery disease. The measured serum cholesterol concentrations are displayed in the grouped frequency distribution histogram using 10 equal intervals, shown below.

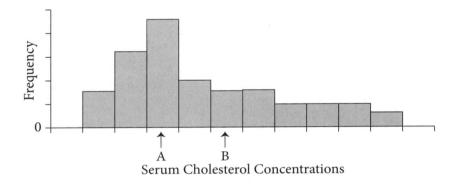

2. The class interval as indicated by "B" in the above histogram most likely contains which of the following measures for this dataset?

    (A) Median
    (B) Mean
    (C) Mode
    (D) Standard deviation
    (E) Range

3. Which of the following is the best description of the distribution of this sample dataset?

    (A) Normal
    (B) Positively skewed
    (C) Negatively skewed
    (D) Gaussian
    (E) None of the above

4. A study reports that the mean ± SD peak plasma concentration of a drug is 1.0 ± 0.1 mg/dL in a study consisting of 1,000 patients. Approximately how many patients had values >1.1 mg/dL?

   (A) 840
   (B) 680
   (C) 320
   (D) 160
   (E) 16

5. A clinical study was performed and serum glucose concentrations were measured in 14 diabetic patients following 1 week of an investigational treatment to directly compare it to the decrease following glipizide treatment in a crossover trial. Statistics were performed and a p-value of 0.45 was obtained. Which of the following is (are) the most likely form of statistical error that the researchers could have made?

   (A) Type I error
   (B) Type II error
   (C) Type I or Type II error
   (D) Neither Type I or II error could be made because the results were NOT significant
   (E) Neither Type I or II error could be made because the results were significant

6. In most clinical studies, the Type I error rate is set to 0.05 before the study is performed. This indicates that the research group has a 5.0% chance of making a Type I error. If a research group were to set α at 0.01, corresponding to a Type 1 error rate of only 1.0%, which of the following statements would be true?

   (A) A smaller sample size could be used.
   (B) The study power would increase.
   (C) There would be an increased α error rate.
   (D) There would be an increased β error rate.
   (E) None of the above statements are true.

Questions 7–8 refer to the following table.

A clinical study enrolled 70 patients who were randomized to receive either lisinopril or ramipril (n = 35 per drug). The table shows measures obtained at the end of the study period in patients who received lisinopril and ramipril.

After Drug Treatment (End of Study Period)	Lisinopril n = 35	Ramipril n = 35
Disease states	—	—
Diabetes alone	29%	20%
Atherosclerosis alone	23%	31%
Diabetes and atherosclerosis	43%	34%
Neither disease	5%	15%
Mean serum cholesterol concentrations (mg/dL)	118 ± 4.0	116 ± 4.0
Sex (% male)	62%	46%

Data are presented as percentage of mean ± SD.

7. Which of the following statistical tests would be most appropriate to use to compare the serum cholesterol concentrations in the ramipril versus the lisinopril group?

    (A) *T*-test
    (B) Paired *t*-test
    (C) Chi-square test
    (D) Wilcoxon sign rank test
    (E) ANOVA

8. Which of the following statistical tests would be most appropriate to use to compare the percentage of males in the ramipril versus the lisinopril group?

    (A) *T*-test
    (B) Paired *t*-test
    (C) Chi-square test
    (D) Wilcoxon sign rank test
    (E) ANOVA

ANSWERS

1. **B**

The median value is the value equidistant from the extremes of the data set. The mathematical average of the values in the data set (A) is the mean. The average of the difference between each value and the mean (C) is the standard deviation. The most commonly occurring value in the data set (D) is the mode. The distance between the smallest and largest values in the data set (E) is the range.

2. **B**

The mean is the most likely measure listed in the position marked by "B" on the graph. The mean is susceptible to outliers, and this dataset is skewed to the right, which means that there are outliers in the positive direction. The mean is pulled from the real central tendency of the data marked by "A" on the graph. The "A," most likely, is represented by the median, which is not susceptible to outliers and is the best measure of central tendency for skewed data.

3. **B**

The dataset is positively skewed because there are outliers on the graph in the positive direction. This pulls the mean to the right of the central tendency as described in the answer to question number 2.

4. **D**

1.1 mg/dL is 1 SD away from the mean, and the question is asking for values greater than that. With 68% of the dataset ± 1 SD away from the mean, the remaining 32% is outside of this range. Because normally distributed data is symmetrical, there is 16% of the dataset on the two sides that encompass data greater or less than 1 SD away from the mean. Thus, 16% of 1,000 patients equals 160, which is the answer.

5. **B**

The p-value is > 0.05; therefore, the authors would conclude that the differences observed between the investigational drug and glipizide are due to chance and that the investigational drug was not different than glipizide. Because the authors conclude that there is no difference, the only possible type of error is Type II (β) error. A Type II error is a conclusion that there is no difference when one actually exists. Given the small sample size of this study, the likelihood of a Type II error is likely very high. A Type I error cannot be made because there is no conclusion that a difference exists between the investigational drug and glipizide.

6. **D**

Setting the Type I (α) error rate to 0.01 instead of the traditional 0.05 would increase the Type II (β) error rate. The Type II error is inversely related to power; therefore, the study's power to detect a difference would be smaller. This would mean that a larger sample size would be needed to detect a difference if one actually exists.

7. **A**

The ramipril and lisinopril groups are independent of each other because this study is not a crossover design. Cholesterol concentrations are interval data, thus considered numeric; therefore, the most appropriate test for two independent groups with numeric data is a *t*-test. The sample size is >30, so the data does not have to be normally distributed. If the sample size were small and not normally distributed, the nonparametric Mann–Whitney U test should be used.

8. **C**

The sex of the patients is considered a nominal variable, which is often referred to as *categorical* because the patients can be placed into categories. Each patient is either a male or a female and cannot be classified as both. The fact that the percentages are provided instead of the actual number of males in each group does not change the fact that the data is categorical. The most appropriate statistical test for this type of categorical data is the chi-square test.

Part Four

Resources and Policy

Drug Information

26

This chapter provides an overview of common tertiary literature resources that can be used as drug information resources for pharmacists:

- **General drug information resources**
- **Pharmacotherapy resources**
- **Internal medicine resources**
- **Drug interaction resources**
- **Adverse drug reaction resources**
- **Pharmacology resources**
- **Compounding and pharmaceutics resources**
- **Drug identification resources**
- **Foreign drug information**
- **Pediatric drug information resources**
- **Pregnancy and lactation resources**
- **OTC drug resources**
- **Natural product resources**

 Suggested Study Time: **30 minutes**

GENERAL DRUG INFORMATION RESOURCES

American Hospital Formulary Service (AHFS) Drug Information (published by the American Society of Health-System Pharmacists [ASHP])

- Provides Food and Drug Administration (FDA)-approved and off-label uses
- Each monograph contains general drug information (e.g., pharmacology, pharmacokinetics, side effects, toxicology, drug interactions, dosing, administration, available preparations)

Drug Facts and Comparisons

- Provides information on:
  - Prescription/over-the-counter (OTC) drugs
  - Investigational/orphan drugs
- Each monograph contains general drug information
- Also provides helpful comparison tables

United States Pharmacopeia Drug Information (USP DI)

- Volume I: Drug Information for the Healthcare Professional
  - Provides general drug information
  - Various appendices (poison control centers, drug-induced side effects, selected therapeutic guidelines, drug identification color inserts)
- Volume II: Advice for the Patient: Drug Information in Lay Language
  - Provides supplemental information for patient counseling
- Volume III: Approved Drug Products and Legal Requirements
  - Provides information on therapeutic equivalence (contains FDA Orange Book), labeling/storage/packaging requirements, and pharmacy law

Physicians' Desk Reference (PDR)

- Contains FDA-approved package insert information
  - Does not provide unlabeled drug uses
- Also contains a colored insert (for drug identification) and manufacturer information

Drug Information Handbook (Lexi-Comp)

- Provides general drug information
- Contains useful charts, tables, and treatment algorithms
- Also available in specialty versions (pediatrics, geriatrics, psychiatric, oncology)

Red Book

- Provides the following information on prescription and OTC drugs:
  - Cost data (average wholesale price [AWP])
  - National Drug Code (NDC) numbers
  - Formulations available (dosage forms, sugar-free/alcohol-free preparations)
  - Drug identification (colored inserts)
  - Manufacturer

PHARMACOTHERAPY RESOURCES

Pharmacotherapy: A Pathophysiologic Approach (DiPiro)
- Provides the following information regarding various disease states: Pathophysiology, etiology, clinical presentation, diagnosis, treatment

Applied Therapeutics: The Clinical Use of Drugs (Koda-Kimble)
- Focuses on treatment of disease states
- Case-based format

INTERNAL MEDICINE RESOURCES

Harrison's Principles of Internal Medicine
- Focuses on pathophysiology, etiology, clinical presentation, and diagnosis
- Provides an overview of treatment; does not provide detailed information on drugs or dosing recommendations

Cecil Textbook of Medicine
- Not as comprehensive as Harrison's

Washington Manual of Medical Therapeutics
- Provides a general overview of disease states and treatment

Merck Manual of Diagnosis and Therapy
- Provides a quick summary of disease-state information (etiology, pathophysiology, clinical presentation, diagnosis, prognosis, treatment)

DRUG INTERACTION RESOURCES

Hansten and Horn's Drug Interaction Analysis and Management
- Provides the following information on drug interactions: Summary of interaction, proposed mechanism, significance, risk factors, treatment options

Drug Interaction Facts (published by Facts and Comparisons)
- Provides similar information as *Hansten and Horn's*

ADVERSE DRUG REACTION RESOURCES

Meyler's Side Effects of Drugs

- Provides critical review of literature regarding drugs' side effects: Effects on organ systems, interference with lab/diagnostic tests, withdrawal, and overdose
- Provides 2 indexes for ease of reference:
  - Drugs
  - Side effects

PARENTERAL DRUG COMPATIBILITY/STABILITY RESOURCES

Handbook on Injectable Drugs (published by ASHP)

- Previously known as Trissel's
- Provides information regarding compatibility/stability of parenteral drugs
- Also provides information on commercially available dosages, volumes, and sizes

King Guide to Parenteral Admixtures

- Provides similar information as *Handbook on Injectable Drugs*

PHARMACOLOGY RESOURCES

Goodman & Gilman's: The Pharmacological Basis of Therapeutics

- "Gold standard" pharmacology reference
- Provides very thorough discussion of the pharmacology of drugs; also provides information on the drugs' pharmacokinetics, pharmacodynamics, and toxicology

COMPOUNDING AND PHARMACEUTICS RESOURCES

Merck Index

- Different from the *Merck Manual*
- Provides chemical and pharmacologic information on drugs (e.g., chemical name, molecular formula, structure, molecular weight, solubility, drug class, toxicity, data, manufacturer)

Remington: The Science and Practice of Pharmacy

- Provides information on numerous issues concerning pharmacy practice (e.g., pharmaceutical calculations, chemistry, radioisotopes, compounding techniques/ ingredients)

DRUG IDENTIFICATION RESOURCES

American Drug Index

- Cross-referenced by brand, generic, and chemical names
- Also provides available dosage forms/strengths and manufacturer information

IDENTIDEX (available through MICROMEDEX)

- Identifies drug after entering in imprint on tablet/capsule

Other useful resources are the color inserts in the following guides:
- *USP DI Volume I*
- *PDR*
- *Red Book*

FOREIGN DRUG INFORMATION RESOURCES

Martindale: The Complete Drug Reference

- Provides information on drugs used throughout the world

Index Nominum: International Drug Directory

- Provides similar information as *Martindale*

PEDIATRIC DRUG INFORMATION RESOURCES

The Harriet Lane Handbook

- Pocket guide that provides brief overview (especially diagnosis and treatment) of common disease states in children

Pediatric Dosage Handbook (Lexi-Comp)

- Provides drug information specific to the pediatric population

General drug information resources (e.g., MICROMEDEX, AHFS) also provide general pediatric dosing information.

PREGNANCY AND LACTATION RESOURCES

Drugs in Pregnancy and Lactation (Briggs)

- "Gold standard"
- Focuses on safety of drugs in pregnancy and lactation

La Leche League (www.llli.org)

- Provides practitioners and patients with clinical and practical information on all aspects of breastfeeding

OTC DRUG RESOURCES

Handbook of Nonprescription Drugs: An Interactive Approach to Self-Care (published by the American Pharmacists Association)

- Provides etiology, pathophysiology, clinical presentation, and treatment of disease states that may be amenable to self-care
- Provides comprehensive information on OTC products (e.g., side effects, drug interactions, dosing, dosage forms, patient counseling)

PDR for Nonprescription Drugs

NATURAL PRODUCTS RESOURCES

Natural Standard

- "Gold standard"
- Comprehensive database

PDR for Herbal Medicines
Complete German Commission E Monographs
PDR for Nonprescription Drugs, Dietary Supplements, and Herbs

Comparison of Tertiary Drug Information Resources

Reference	Monograph: Basic Info	Approved Uses	Unapproved Uses	Drug Interactions	Language for Patients	Manufacturer Contact Information	Product ID	Cost	Dosage Form Availability	Pathophysiology	Disease State Management	Treatment of Drug Overdoses	Foreign Drug Identification	IV Drug Compatibility	Chemical Properties	Generic Availability	Compounding Information	Lactation Information	Mechanism of Action
American Hospital Formulary Service Drug Information (AHFS)	X	X	X	X					X			X			X	X		X	X
Physicians' Desk Reference (PDR)	X	X		X		X	X		X			X			X			X	X
Drug Information Handbook (Lexi-Comp)	X	X	X	X					X			X				X		X	X
Facts and Comparisons	X	X	X	X					X			X				X		X	X
Martindale: The Complete Drug Reference													X						
USP DI Drug Information for the Healthcare Provider (Vol I)	X	X	X	X			X		X			X						X	X
USP DI Advice for the Patient: Drug Information in Lay Language (Vol II)					X														
USP DI Approved Drug Products and Legal Requirements (Vol III)		X																	
Pharmacotherapy: A Pathophysiologic Approach (DiPiro's)										X	X	X							X
Remington: The Science and Practice of Pharmacy															X		X		
Handbook on Injectable Drugs (Trissel's)									X					X					
King Guide to Parenteral Admixtures														X					

Reference	Monograph: Basic Info	Approved Uses	Unapproved Uses	Drug Interactions	Language for Patients	Manufacturer Contact Information	Product ID	Cost	Dosage Form Availability	Pathophysiology	Disease State Management	Treatment of Drug Overdoses	Foreign Drug Identification	IV Drug Compatibility	Chemical Properties	Generic Availability	Compounding Information	Lactation Information	Mechanism of Action
Goodman and Gilman's: The Pharmacological Basis of Therapeutics																			X
Harrison's Principles of Internal Medicine										X	X	X							
Drug Interactions Analysis and Management (Hansten and Horn's)				X															
Drug Interaction Facts				X															
Harriet Lane Handbook	X	X		X							X							X	
Drugs in Pregnancy and Lactation (Briggs)																		X	
Red Book						X	X	X	X										

Learning Points

- Learn drug information resources by various categories. Once you know the kind of information that you need, you can select the most appropriate reference.
- Do not memorize the table above; it can be used to assess your general knowledge of tertiary literature sources.
- Remember the differences between primary, secondary, and tertiary literature:
  - Primary literature: Original journal articles (research reports, case reports, editorials); serves as information for development of secondary and tertiary literature resources
  - Secondary literature: Indexing and abstracting services (e.g., MEDLINE, IPA, EMBASE, Cochrane)
  - Tertiary literature: Textbooks and review articles; summarize and interpret primary literature

PRACTICE QUESTIONS

1. A physician calls to ask the pharmacist about the mechanism of action of a new drug that has been approved for hypercholesterolemia. Which of the following references is/are most appropriate for obtaining this information?

  I. AHFS Drug Information
  II. Facts and Comparisons
  III. USP DI Volume III

  (A) I only
  (B) III only
  (C) I and II only
  (D) II and III only
  (E) I, II, and III

2. A patient comes to your pharmacy and gives you a prescription for an ointment that needs to be compounded. Which of the following references would be most appropriate to obtain information regarding the preparation of this ointment?

  (A) *Martindale: The Complete Drug Reference*
  (B) *Pharmacotherapy: A Pathophysiologic Approach*
  (C) *Physicians' Desk Reference*
  (D) *Remington: The Science and Practice of Pharmacy*
  (E) *Harriet Lane Handbook*

ANSWERS

1. **C**

AHFS Drug Information (I) and Facts and Comparisons (II) both contain general drug information in monograph format, so choice (C) is correct. USP DI Volume III (III) contains information on approved drug products (generic availability) and legal requirements.

2. **D**

Remington would be the most appropriate reference to obtain information regarding compounding of an ointment, so choice (D) is correct. *Martindale* (A) provides information on foreign drugs. *Pharmacotherapy: A Pathophysiologic Approach* (B) is a general pharmacotherapy resource. *Physicians' Desk Reference* (C) is a general drug information resource. *Harriet Lane Handbook* (E) is a pediatric drug information resource.

Health Policy

27

This chapter covers the following areas of health policy:

- **HIPAA**
- **FDA regulatory process**
- **The Joint Commission accreditation process**
- **Medication therapy management**

 Suggested Study Time: **30 minutes**

HIPAA

The Health Insurance Portability and Accountability Act (HIPAA) of 1996 was established to guarantee patients access to health care after leaving a job and to regulate the electronic transmission of medical information. Given the risk of disclosure of patient health information, the HIPAA privacy rule provides regulations regarding how covered entities can use and exchange protected health information (PHI). Covered entities include health care plans, health care providers, and health care clearinghouses.

PHI consists of any type of identifiable health information that pertains to the following:

- Past, present, or future medical or mental health conditions
- Provision of health care
- Payment of health care services

The Office for Civil Rights (OCR) enforces the HIPAA privacy rule. The OCR is responsible for investigating any complaints, conducting compliance reviews of covered entities, and providing education about the regulations. Once a complaint is generated, the OCR gathers facts pertaining to the case to determine whether a violation occurred.

If the investigation determines that a violation has occurred, the OCR notifies the covered entity named in the complaint. If a compliance issue on the part of the covered entity is found to be valid, the OCR will work with the entity to resolve the complaint. If the covered entity does not fulfill its responsibility in rectifying the complaint, the OCR may impose civil monetary penalties, which are collected and deposited into the U.S. Treasury.

All pharmacies are considered a covered entities and must comply with HIPAA regulations. Regulations mandate covered entities to inform patients how their PHI may be used; this includes information about both treatment and payment of services. All pharmacies are also required to provide a paper notice to the public of measures taken to ensure patient privacy. The privacy notice must be:

- Available to everyone, regardless of whether they are patients of the pharmacy.
- Provided to the patient no later than the date of first service, including services conducted electronically. In the event of an emergency, the notice may be provided as soon as possible. Pharmacies can elect to send the notice to all patients at once or give it to each patient as he or she comes in for services.
- Available at the pharmacy for anyone who requests a copy.
- Displayed in a noticeable location in the store for patients to read.

FDA REGULATORY PROCESS

In the United States, the regulation and approval of new drugs is founded on the New Drug Application (NDA) process. Before any drug may be made commercially available, it is subject to the NDA process to ensure its safety and efficacy. The NDA is a standardized process that documents research from animal and human studies about each new drug.

When a new compound is in development, the sponsor's main goal is to determine whether the drug is safe for human use and whether it has pharmacologic activity for clinical use. Once the sponsor decides to test the compound in humans, the compound changes legal status and becomes a drug under the Federal Food, Drug, and Cosmetic Act, and the sponsor must file an Investigational New Drug (IND) application with the FDA.

The IND application contains the following information:

- Pharmacology and toxicology data from animal studies to demonstrate that the drug is safe to test in humans.
- Manufacturing information to ensure the stability, safety, and consistency of the drug throughout the manufacturing process.

- Clinical protocols and investigator information to detail trial design and safety precautions for study patients.

- Agreement to adhere to clinical protocols and IND regulations to ensure adherence to regulations.

There are three types of IND applications:

- An **investigator IND application** is submitted by the investigator who initiates and conducts the clinical trials and also oversees the administration and use of the investigational drug. An IND can be used to request approval of either an unapproved drug or a new indication for an existing drug.

- An **emergency-use IND** allows the FDA to authorize the use of an investigational drug for emergency use when time is too short to allow the full NDA process. It also permits individuals to use the drug who would not have been included in clinical trials because they do not meet the study criteria.

- A **treatment IND** is submitted to request authorization to distribute an investigational drug that has shown clinical promise for a serious condition while the remaining clinical trials and FDA review are conducted.

After gathering the data from the IND studies, the sponsoring entity can submit an NDA to the FDA for review. The FDA review evaluates the drug's safety and efficacy for the proposed indication in order to confirm that the benefits outweigh the risks of the medication. The FDA also reviews the medication labeling to ensure that it includes the proper information. Finally, the FDA reviews manufacturing protocols to confirm that adequate quality controls are in place for safe drug preparation.

Types of Clinical Trials

Four types of clinical trials are used in the IND and NDA application process:

- **Phase I** trials are the first studies of investigational new drugs in humans and are focused on drug safety. These trials generally are conducted in small numbers of healthy subjects to determine pharmacologic, pharmacokinetic, and adverse drug reaction information. Dose-ranging data also may be obtained during this phase.

- **Phase II** trials are controlled studies conducted in large numbers of patients to evaluate clinical efficacy. These trials often enroll hundreds of patients in order to test the effectiveness of the drug in patients with certain health conditions and support clinical indications.

- **Phase III** trials are controlled studies conducted in larger numbers of patients (potentially hundreds or thousands) to evaluate clinical efficacy that can be extrapolated to the general population. Information from Phase III trials contributes to drug labeling and provides guidance for use in clinical practice. The trials may compare the investigational drug to a placebo or to another standard of care.

- **Phase IV** trials are conducted after a drug has been approved for clinical use. These trials conduct post-marketing surveillance to collect information about the use of the medication in various populations and the prevalence of long-term use or rare side effects.

Orphan Drug Products

Orphan drug products are medications that aid in the diagnosis or treatment of rare diseases or conditions. The Office of Orphan Product Development promotes and provides incentives to encourage companies to develop new products for conditions that affect an extremely small number of people.

THE JOINT COMMISSION ACCREDITATION PROCESS

The Joint Commission is a private, nonprofit organization that sets the standards by which health care quality is measured. Accreditation by the Joint Commission means that health care facilities have demonstrated compliance with the standards of performance in meeting the needs of their patients. To maintain accreditation, health care facilities periodically undergo an extensive on-site review by a Joint Commission team of professionals. The review evaluates the facility's performance in all areas that affect patient care; accreditation is awarded based on how well the facility met the standards.

MEDICATION THERAPY MANAGEMENT

Medication therapy management (MTM) is a process in which a health care professional monitors a patient's medications in order to improve the patient's therapeutic outcomes. MTM provides patient-specific services that promote the best outcomes for each individual and reduce medication related problems. MTM can be conducted in any setting, either face-to-face manner or electronically. Services can be provided by a pharmacist or health care provider and are covered under Medicare Part D.

MTM services may include the following:

- Assessment of the patient's health status
- Comprehensive medication review to identify medication-related problems
- Creation of a medication treatment program, which may add new therapy or modify existing therapy

- Patient education and counseling resources to optimize therapeutic outcomes and patient adherence
- Medication monitoring for efficacy and safety parameters
- Documentation of services
- Coordination of services with other health care providers

Learning Points

- HIPAA was established to ensure patient privacy and regulate the electronic transmission of medical information.
- All pharmacies are considered covered entities and must comply with HIPAA regulations.
- To gain FDA approval of a drug, the sponsor must submit an NDA to the FDA for review.
- Information for an IND is collected from Phase I, II, and III trials.
- The Orphan Drug Act provides incentives for drug companies to create medications to treat rare diseases.
- MTM is the provision of patient-specific services to optimize pharmacotherapy outcomes.

PRACTICE QUESTIONS

1. An orphan drug product might apply to which of the following disease states?

   (A) Asthma
   (B) Diabetes mellitus
   (C) Gaucher's disease
   (D) Hypertriglyceridemia
   (E) Hypertension

2. Which of the following statements is true regarding protected health information (PHI)?

   (A) PHI applies only to current health conditions.
   (B) PHI excludes information about future treatment.
   (C) PHI excludes mental health diagnoses.
   (D) PHI includes de-identified information.
   (E) PHI includes the payment of health services.

3. Which of the following statements is true regarding MTM services?

   I. MTM services must be performed by pharmacists.
   II. MTM services focus on patient-specific outcomes.
   III. MTM services may include modification of medication therapy.

   (A) I only
   (B) III only
   (C) I and II only
   (D) II and III only
   (E) I, II, and III

4. Which of the following is included in an investigational new drug application?

   (A) Pharmacology data
   (B) Manufacturing information
   (C) Toxicology data
   (D) Clinical trial protocols
   (E) All of the above

5. The Joint Commission does which of the following?

   (A) Accredits health care facilities
   (B) Approves investigational new drugs
   (C) Ensures electronic patient privacy
   (D) Creates drug products for rare diseases
   (E) Provides payments to health care facilities

ANSWERS

1. **C**

Orphan drugs are those drugs that aid in the diagnosis or treatment of rare diseases. Gaucher's disease is a rare disease and would be eligible for the creation of a medication through the Orphan Drug Product Act. Disease states that affect millions of people, such as asthma (A), diabetes mellitus (B), hypertriglyceridemia (D), and hypertension (E), would not be granted orphan drug product status.

2. **E**

Protected health information (PHI) includes the payment of health services. PHI consists of any type of identifiable health information that pertains to a patient's past, present, and future medical or mental health conditions and treatments (A and B), and to both the provision and payment of health care services. Mental health diagnoses (C) are not excluded, and PHI does not apply to de-identified information (D).

3. **D**

MTM provides patient-specific services to improve pharmacotherapy outcomes (II). It may include a variety of services, such as assessment of patient health, comprehensive medication therapies, and optimization of pharmacotherapy regimens, which may include modification of drug therapy (III). Although MTM is often provided by pharmacists (I), it can be delivered by other health care professionals.

4. **E**

An Investigational New Drug (IND) application is submitted to provide information that the new drug may be used safely in humans. An IND contains preclinical pharmacology data (A) from animal and toxicology trials (C), manufacturing information (B) to ensure consistency and safety of the drug product, information about clinical trial protocols (D), and investigator information.

5. **A**

The Joint Commission accredits health care facilities, ensuring that they meet the standards of care to provide optimal patient care. Facilities undergo periodic visits to ensure standards are being consistently met.

Part Five

Full-Length Practice Test

Full-Length Practice Test

To mimic the realistic conditions of the NAPLEX, allow yourself a total of **4 hours and 15 minutes** to complete all 185 questions. Take a 10-minute break at the 2-hour time point.

While every test-taker is different, the average candidate takes 2.5 to 3 hours to complete the exam. There are no bonus points for finishing early.

The computer-adaptive format of the exam requires that you **answer all questions in the order in which they are presented**. You cannot skip a question or return to a previous question to review your answer. Again, to make this practice test as realistic as possible, **do not** return to the previous question to change your answer.

ANSWER GRID

1. Ⓐ Ⓑ Ⓒ Ⓓ Ⓔ
2. Ⓐ Ⓑ Ⓒ Ⓓ Ⓔ
3. Ⓐ Ⓑ Ⓒ Ⓓ Ⓔ
4. Ⓐ Ⓑ Ⓒ Ⓓ Ⓔ
5. Ⓐ Ⓑ Ⓒ Ⓓ Ⓔ
6. Ⓐ Ⓑ Ⓒ Ⓓ Ⓔ
7. Ⓐ Ⓑ Ⓒ Ⓓ Ⓔ
8. Ⓐ Ⓑ Ⓒ Ⓓ Ⓔ
9. Ⓐ Ⓑ Ⓒ Ⓓ Ⓔ
10. Ⓐ Ⓑ Ⓒ Ⓓ Ⓔ
11. Ⓐ Ⓑ Ⓒ Ⓓ Ⓔ
12. Ⓐ Ⓑ Ⓒ Ⓓ Ⓔ
13. Ⓐ Ⓑ Ⓒ Ⓓ Ⓔ
14. Ⓐ Ⓑ Ⓒ Ⓓ Ⓔ
15. Ⓐ Ⓑ Ⓒ Ⓓ Ⓔ
16. Ⓐ Ⓑ Ⓒ Ⓓ Ⓔ
17. Ⓐ Ⓑ Ⓒ Ⓓ Ⓔ
18. Ⓐ Ⓑ Ⓒ Ⓓ Ⓔ
19. Ⓐ Ⓑ Ⓒ Ⓓ Ⓔ
20. Ⓐ Ⓑ Ⓒ Ⓓ Ⓔ
21. Ⓐ Ⓑ Ⓒ Ⓓ Ⓔ
22. Ⓐ Ⓑ Ⓒ Ⓓ Ⓔ
23. Ⓐ Ⓑ Ⓒ Ⓓ Ⓔ
24. Ⓐ Ⓑ Ⓒ Ⓓ Ⓔ
25. Ⓐ Ⓑ Ⓒ Ⓓ Ⓔ
26. Ⓐ Ⓑ Ⓒ Ⓓ Ⓔ
27. Ⓐ Ⓑ Ⓒ Ⓓ Ⓔ
28. Ⓐ Ⓑ Ⓒ Ⓓ Ⓔ
29. Ⓐ Ⓑ Ⓒ Ⓓ Ⓔ
30. Ⓐ Ⓑ Ⓒ Ⓓ Ⓔ
31. Ⓐ Ⓑ Ⓒ Ⓓ Ⓔ
32. Ⓐ Ⓑ Ⓒ Ⓓ Ⓔ
33. Ⓐ Ⓑ Ⓒ Ⓓ Ⓔ
34. Ⓐ Ⓑ Ⓒ Ⓓ Ⓔ
35. Ⓐ Ⓑ Ⓒ Ⓓ Ⓔ
36. Ⓐ Ⓑ Ⓒ Ⓓ Ⓔ
37. Ⓐ Ⓑ Ⓒ Ⓓ Ⓔ
38. Ⓐ Ⓑ Ⓒ Ⓓ Ⓔ
39. Ⓐ Ⓑ Ⓒ Ⓓ Ⓔ
40. Ⓐ Ⓑ Ⓒ Ⓓ Ⓔ

41. Ⓐ Ⓑ Ⓒ Ⓓ Ⓔ
42. Ⓐ Ⓑ Ⓒ Ⓓ Ⓔ
43. Ⓐ Ⓑ Ⓒ Ⓓ Ⓔ
44. Ⓐ Ⓑ Ⓒ Ⓓ Ⓔ
45. Ⓐ Ⓑ Ⓒ Ⓓ Ⓔ
46. Ⓐ Ⓑ Ⓒ Ⓓ Ⓔ
47. Ⓐ Ⓑ Ⓒ Ⓓ Ⓔ
48. Ⓐ Ⓑ Ⓒ Ⓓ Ⓔ
49. Ⓐ Ⓑ Ⓒ Ⓓ Ⓔ
50. Ⓐ Ⓑ Ⓒ Ⓓ Ⓔ
51. Ⓐ Ⓑ Ⓒ Ⓓ Ⓔ
52. Ⓐ Ⓑ Ⓒ Ⓓ Ⓔ
53. Ⓐ Ⓑ Ⓒ Ⓓ Ⓔ
54. Ⓐ Ⓑ Ⓒ Ⓓ Ⓔ
55. Ⓐ Ⓑ Ⓒ Ⓓ Ⓔ
56. Ⓐ Ⓑ Ⓒ Ⓓ Ⓔ
57. Ⓐ Ⓑ Ⓒ Ⓓ Ⓔ
58. Ⓐ Ⓑ Ⓒ Ⓓ Ⓔ
59. Ⓐ Ⓑ Ⓒ Ⓓ Ⓔ
60. Ⓐ Ⓑ Ⓒ Ⓓ Ⓔ
61. Ⓐ Ⓑ Ⓒ Ⓓ Ⓔ
62. Ⓐ Ⓑ Ⓒ Ⓓ Ⓔ
63. Ⓐ Ⓑ Ⓒ Ⓓ Ⓔ
64. Ⓐ Ⓑ Ⓒ Ⓓ Ⓔ
65. Ⓐ Ⓑ Ⓒ Ⓓ Ⓔ
66. Ⓐ Ⓑ Ⓒ Ⓓ Ⓔ
67. Ⓐ Ⓑ Ⓒ Ⓓ Ⓔ
68. Ⓐ Ⓑ Ⓒ Ⓓ Ⓔ
69. Ⓐ Ⓑ Ⓒ Ⓓ Ⓔ
70. Ⓐ Ⓑ Ⓒ Ⓓ Ⓔ
71. Ⓐ Ⓑ Ⓒ Ⓓ Ⓔ
72. Ⓐ Ⓑ Ⓒ Ⓓ Ⓔ
73. Ⓐ Ⓑ Ⓒ Ⓓ Ⓔ
74. Ⓐ Ⓑ Ⓒ Ⓓ Ⓔ
75. Ⓐ Ⓑ Ⓒ Ⓓ Ⓔ
76. Ⓐ Ⓑ Ⓒ Ⓓ Ⓔ
77. Ⓐ Ⓑ Ⓒ Ⓓ Ⓔ
78. Ⓐ Ⓑ Ⓒ Ⓓ Ⓔ
79. Ⓐ Ⓑ Ⓒ Ⓓ Ⓔ
80. Ⓐ Ⓑ Ⓒ Ⓓ Ⓔ

81. Ⓐ Ⓑ Ⓒ Ⓓ Ⓔ
82. Ⓐ Ⓑ Ⓒ Ⓓ Ⓔ
83. Ⓐ Ⓑ Ⓒ Ⓓ Ⓔ
84. Ⓐ Ⓑ Ⓒ Ⓓ Ⓔ
85. Ⓐ Ⓑ Ⓒ Ⓓ Ⓔ
86. Ⓐ Ⓑ Ⓒ Ⓓ Ⓔ
87. Ⓐ Ⓑ Ⓒ Ⓓ Ⓔ
88. Ⓐ Ⓑ Ⓒ Ⓓ Ⓔ
89. Ⓐ Ⓑ Ⓒ Ⓓ Ⓔ
90. Ⓐ Ⓑ Ⓒ Ⓓ Ⓔ
91. Ⓐ Ⓑ Ⓒ Ⓓ Ⓔ
92. Ⓐ Ⓑ Ⓒ Ⓓ Ⓔ
93. Ⓐ Ⓑ Ⓒ Ⓓ Ⓔ
94. Ⓐ Ⓑ Ⓒ Ⓓ Ⓔ
95. Ⓐ Ⓑ Ⓒ Ⓓ Ⓔ
96. Ⓐ Ⓑ Ⓒ Ⓓ Ⓔ
97. Ⓐ Ⓑ Ⓒ Ⓓ Ⓔ
98. Ⓐ Ⓑ Ⓒ Ⓓ Ⓔ
99. Ⓐ Ⓑ Ⓒ Ⓓ Ⓔ
100. Ⓐ Ⓑ Ⓒ Ⓓ Ⓔ
101. Ⓐ Ⓑ Ⓒ Ⓓ Ⓔ
102. Ⓐ Ⓑ Ⓒ Ⓓ Ⓔ
103. Ⓐ Ⓑ Ⓒ Ⓓ Ⓔ
104. Ⓐ Ⓑ Ⓒ Ⓓ Ⓔ
105. Ⓐ Ⓑ Ⓒ Ⓓ Ⓔ
106. Ⓐ Ⓑ Ⓒ Ⓓ Ⓔ
107. Ⓐ Ⓑ Ⓒ Ⓓ Ⓔ
108. Ⓐ Ⓑ Ⓒ Ⓓ Ⓔ
109. Ⓐ Ⓑ Ⓒ Ⓓ Ⓔ
110. Ⓐ Ⓑ Ⓒ Ⓓ Ⓔ
111. Ⓐ Ⓑ Ⓒ Ⓓ Ⓔ
112. Ⓐ Ⓑ Ⓒ Ⓓ Ⓔ
113. Ⓐ Ⓑ Ⓒ Ⓓ Ⓔ
114. Ⓐ Ⓑ Ⓒ Ⓓ Ⓔ
115. Ⓐ Ⓑ Ⓒ Ⓓ Ⓔ
116. Ⓐ Ⓑ Ⓒ Ⓓ Ⓔ
117. Ⓐ Ⓑ Ⓒ Ⓓ Ⓔ
118. Ⓐ Ⓑ Ⓒ Ⓓ Ⓔ
119. Ⓐ Ⓑ Ⓒ Ⓓ Ⓔ
120. Ⓐ Ⓑ Ⓒ Ⓓ Ⓔ

ANSWER GRID

121. Ⓐ Ⓑ Ⓒ Ⓓ Ⓔ
122. Ⓐ Ⓑ Ⓒ Ⓓ Ⓔ
123. Ⓐ Ⓑ Ⓒ Ⓓ Ⓔ
124. Ⓐ Ⓑ Ⓒ Ⓓ Ⓔ
125. Ⓐ Ⓑ Ⓒ Ⓓ Ⓔ
126. Ⓐ Ⓑ Ⓒ Ⓓ Ⓔ
127. Ⓐ Ⓑ Ⓒ Ⓓ Ⓔ
128. Ⓐ Ⓑ Ⓒ Ⓓ Ⓔ
129. Ⓐ Ⓑ Ⓒ Ⓓ Ⓔ
130. Ⓐ Ⓑ Ⓒ Ⓓ Ⓔ
131. Ⓐ Ⓑ Ⓒ Ⓓ Ⓔ
132. Ⓐ Ⓑ Ⓒ Ⓓ Ⓔ
133. Ⓐ Ⓑ Ⓒ Ⓓ Ⓔ
134. Ⓐ Ⓑ Ⓒ Ⓓ Ⓔ
135. Ⓐ Ⓑ Ⓒ Ⓓ Ⓔ
136. Ⓐ Ⓑ Ⓒ Ⓓ Ⓔ
137. Ⓐ Ⓑ Ⓒ Ⓓ Ⓔ
138. Ⓐ Ⓑ Ⓒ Ⓓ Ⓔ
139. Ⓐ Ⓑ Ⓒ Ⓓ Ⓔ
140. Ⓐ Ⓑ Ⓒ Ⓓ Ⓔ
141. Ⓐ Ⓑ Ⓒ Ⓓ Ⓔ
142. Ⓐ Ⓑ Ⓒ Ⓓ Ⓔ
143. Ⓐ Ⓑ Ⓒ Ⓓ Ⓔ
144. Ⓐ Ⓑ Ⓒ Ⓓ Ⓔ
145. Ⓐ Ⓑ Ⓒ Ⓓ Ⓔ

146. Ⓐ Ⓑ Ⓒ Ⓓ Ⓔ
147. Ⓐ Ⓑ Ⓒ Ⓓ Ⓔ
148. Ⓐ Ⓑ Ⓒ Ⓓ Ⓔ
149. Ⓐ Ⓑ Ⓒ Ⓓ Ⓔ
150. Ⓐ Ⓑ Ⓒ Ⓓ Ⓔ
151. Ⓐ Ⓑ Ⓒ Ⓓ Ⓔ
152. Ⓐ Ⓑ Ⓒ Ⓓ Ⓔ
153. Ⓐ Ⓑ Ⓒ Ⓓ Ⓔ
154. Ⓐ Ⓑ Ⓒ Ⓓ Ⓔ
155. Ⓐ Ⓑ Ⓒ Ⓓ Ⓔ
156. Ⓐ Ⓑ Ⓒ Ⓓ Ⓔ
157. Ⓐ Ⓑ Ⓒ Ⓓ Ⓔ
158. Ⓐ Ⓑ Ⓒ Ⓓ Ⓔ
159. Ⓐ Ⓑ Ⓒ Ⓓ Ⓔ
160. Ⓐ Ⓑ Ⓒ Ⓓ Ⓔ
161. Ⓐ Ⓑ Ⓒ Ⓓ Ⓔ
162. Ⓐ Ⓑ Ⓒ Ⓓ Ⓔ
163. Ⓐ Ⓑ Ⓒ Ⓓ Ⓔ
164. Ⓐ Ⓑ Ⓒ Ⓓ Ⓔ
165. Ⓐ Ⓑ Ⓒ Ⓓ Ⓔ
166. Ⓐ Ⓑ Ⓒ Ⓓ Ⓔ
167. Ⓐ Ⓑ Ⓒ Ⓓ Ⓔ
168. Ⓐ Ⓑ Ⓒ Ⓓ Ⓔ
169. Ⓐ Ⓑ Ⓒ Ⓓ Ⓔ
170. Ⓐ Ⓑ Ⓒ Ⓓ Ⓔ

171. Ⓐ Ⓑ Ⓒ Ⓓ Ⓔ
172. Ⓐ Ⓑ Ⓒ Ⓓ Ⓔ
173. Ⓐ Ⓑ Ⓒ Ⓓ Ⓔ
174. Ⓐ Ⓑ Ⓒ Ⓓ Ⓔ
175. Ⓐ Ⓑ Ⓒ Ⓓ Ⓔ
176. Ⓐ Ⓑ Ⓒ Ⓓ Ⓔ
177. Ⓐ Ⓑ Ⓒ Ⓓ Ⓔ
178. Ⓐ Ⓑ Ⓒ Ⓓ Ⓔ
179. Ⓐ Ⓑ Ⓒ Ⓓ Ⓔ
180. Ⓐ Ⓑ Ⓒ Ⓓ Ⓔ
181. Ⓐ Ⓑ Ⓒ Ⓓ Ⓔ
182. Ⓐ Ⓑ Ⓒ Ⓓ Ⓔ
183. Ⓐ Ⓑ Ⓒ Ⓓ Ⓔ
184. Ⓐ Ⓑ Ⓒ Ⓓ Ⓔ
185. Ⓐ Ⓑ Ⓒ Ⓓ Ⓔ

Directions: Complete each of the following questions with the best possible answer.

1. Diarrhea is most common with which of the following medications?

   (A) Allopurinol
   (B) Probenecid
   (C) Indomethacin
   (D) Acetaminophen
   (E) Colchicine

2. Which of the following statements regarding A1c is FALSE?

   (A) It is used to evaluate glycemic control in patients with diabetes.
   (B) It represents a time frame of approximately 30–45 days.
   (C) It can be inaccurate in cases of severe anemia.
   (D) The most commonly used normal reference range is 4–6%.
   (E) An A1c of 10% would indicate average blood sugar over 200 mg/dL.

3. Which of the following atypical antipsychotics requires rigorous monitoring of WBC and ANC?

   (A) Olanzapine
   (B) Risperidone
   (C) Quetiapine
   (D) Ziprasidone
   (E) Clozapine

4. What information should the doctor consider prior to initiating Mirapex in a patient with Parkinson's disease?

   I. Decrease the levodopa dose by 20–30% when initiating Mirapex.
   II. Patient must wear patch for 24 hours for efficacy.
   III. Monitor for serious cardiac side effects.

   (A) I only
   (B) III only
   (C) I and II only
   (D) II and III only
   (E) I, II, and III

5. A patient has been diagnosed with depression and will begin antidepressant therapy today. Which of the following is MOST appropriate, assuming the patient has no other health conditions?

   (A) Venlafaxine 37.5 mg PO BID
   (B) Lexapro 10 mg PO BID
   (C) Fluvoxamine 80 mg PO weekly
   (D) Nortriptyline 300 mg PO daily
   (E) Mirtazapine 10 mg PO Q a.m.

6. Which of the following counseling points is/are TRUE?

   I. NuvaRing should be inserted once every month.
   II. Ortho-Evra should be applied once every week for 3 weeks/month.
   III. Seasonale should result in menses approximately every 3 months.

   (A) I only
   (B) III only
   (C) I and II only
   (D) II and III only
   (E) I, II, and III

7. Which of the following key monitoring parameters is NOT correctly matched to its corresponding medication?

   (A) Blood glucose – prednisone
   (B) CBC – methotrexate
   (C) Ocular exam – hydroxychloroquine
   (D) Serum creatinine – Enbrel
   (E) Hepatic enzymes – leflunomide

8. Which of the following statements regarding serum creatinine is TRUE?

   (A) Serum creatinine is most commonly used to assess hepatic disease.
   (B) Serum creatinine is dependent upon the amount of iron consumed in the diet.
   (C) Serum creatinine is a more accurate measure in the very elderly than in young adults.
   (D) Serum creatinine is used in the Cockroft-Gault equation.
   (E) Serum creatinine is synonymous with microalbumin.

9. Which of the following statements regarding the use of natalizumab in multiple sclerosis is/are TRUE?

   I. Patients must enroll in the MS-TOUCH program prior to receiving.
   II. It should be reserved for those unresponsive to other medications.
   III. It should be added to other disease-modifying drugs when relapse occurs.

   (A) I only
   (B) III only
   (C) I and II only
   (D) II and III only
   (E) I, II, and III

10. Allopurinol is indicated for which of the following gout presentations?

    (A) Prophylaxis in patients with slightly elevated uric acid levels
    (B) Prophylaxis in patients with moderately elevated uric acid and uric acid overproduction
    (C) Prophylaxis in patients with uric acid excretion indicative of underexcretion
    (D) Treatment of acute gout
    (E) Treatment of asymptomatic hyperuricemia

11. Which of the following medication(s) require monitoring of serum drug concentrations?

    I. Lamotrigine
    II. Valproic acid
    III. Lithium

    (A) I only
    (B) III only
    (C) I and II only
    (D) II and III only
    (E) I, II, and III

12. Which of the following trade names is NOT correctly matched with its generic name?

    (A) Zyprexa – olanzapine
    (B) Risperdal – risperidone
    (C) Geodon – ziprasidone
    (D) Abilify – aripiprazole
    (E) Haldol – clozapine

13. Migraine prophylaxis could be achieved with which of the following medication classes?

    (A) ACE inhibitors
    (B) Acetaminophen
    (C) Antidepressants
    (D) H_2 antagonist
    (E) Anticholinergics

14. What is the MOST appropriate recommendation for a patient with osteoarthritis and stomach ulcers?

    (A) Aspirin 325 mg PO every 4–6 hours
    (B) Tramadol 25 mg PO every 4–6 hours
    (C) Diclofenac 50 mg PO BID
    (D) Daypro 600 mg PO daily
    (E) Mobic 7.5 mg PO daily

Questions 15–19 refer to the following patient profile.

Patient Name: Tamara Yates

Age: 40   **Height:** 5'2"
Sex: F   **Weight:** 90 lb

Allergies: Geodon

Diagnosis

    Primary:

       Hypertension
       Depression
       Schizophrenia

    Chief Complaint: tardive dyskinesia, dystonia

Lab/Diagnostic Tests

Date	Test/Result	
03/02	Sodium	133 mEq/L
(last week)	Potassium	3.5 mEq/L
	Serum creatinine	1.0 mg/dL
	Blood pressure	166/98 mmHg
	Heart rate	80 bpm

Medications

Date	Name and Strength	Route	Directions
02/20	HCTZ 25 mg	PO	1 tablet in the morning
	Citalopram 20 mg	PO	1 tablet daily
	Haloperidol 2 mg	PO	1 tablet BID

Additional Information

Date	Comment
03/02	Patient has been suspected of bulimia by her primary physician and dentist.

---

15. Which of the following is likely causing Ms. Yates's chief complaint?

    (A) Hydrochlorothiazide
    (B) Citalopram
    (C) Haloperidol
    (D) Hyponatremia
    (E) Uncontrolled blood pressure

16. What additional monitoring is needed to evaluate haloperidol?

    (A) Serum drug levels
    (B) A1c
    (C) Ejection fraction
    (D) Bone mineral density
    (E) CBC

17. Which of the following recommendations is/are appropriate to address Ms. Yates's chief complaint?

    I. Switch to the liquid formulation of haloperidol.
    II. Switch the haloperidol to ziprasidone.
    III. Switch the haloperidol to Risperdal.

(A) I only
(B) III only
(C) I and II only
(D) II and III only
(E) I, II, and III

18. What education should be provided to Ms. Yates concerning her antipsychotic medications?

(A) Medications for schizophrenia are absorbed better in an acidic environment and should be taken with orange juice or vitamin C.
(B) Medications for schizophrenia work quickly and should start to take effect within two to three doses.
(C) If side effects are bothersome, stop taking the medication.
(D) Alcohol should be avoided.
(E) If side effects are bothersome, cut the dose in half.

19. Ms. Yates was told by a friend that her citalopram is bad for her. Although you have tried to talk with her about it, she wants another antidepressant. Which of the following is the MOST appropriate recommendation?

(A) Bupropion 100 mg PO BID
(B) Alprazolam 1 mg PO TID
(C) Lexapro 10 mg PO daily
(D) Venlafaxine 37.5 mg PO BID
(E) Propranolol 80 mg PO daily

20. What is the purpose of adding carbidopa to levodopa in the treatment of Parkinson's disease?

    I. It prevents the peripheral degradation of levodopa.
    II. It allows for extended dosing intervals.
    III. It prevents some of the CNS side effects of levodopa from occurring.

(A) I only
(B) III only
(C) I and II only
(D) II and III only
(E) I, II, and III

21. Which of the following is first-line treatment for acute gout?

(A) Acetaminophen 1,000 mg PO PRN up to QID
(B) Colchicine 2 mg PO PRN
(C) Indomethacin 25 mg PO TID
(D) Allopurinol 100 mg PO daily
(E) Probenecid 250 mg PO BID

22. Which of the following medications is/are correctly matched with common side effects?

    I. Mirtazapine – somnolence
    II. Paroxetine – disorder of ejaculation/impotence
    III. Amitriptyline – weight gain

(A) I only
(B) III only
(C) I and II only
(D) II and III only
(E) I, II, and III

23. Phenytoin is available in which of the following dosage forms?

    I. Chewable tablets
    II. Oral suspension
    III. Parenteral solution

    (A) I only
    (B) III only
    (C) I and II only
    (D) II and III only
    (E) I, II, and III

24. What is the role of NSAIDs in rheumatoid arthritis?

    (A) NSAIDs function as a disease-modifying antirheumatic drug (DMARD).
    (B) NSAIDs are used for PRN symptomatic relief.
    (C) NSAIDs are used as adjunctive therapy in patients with refractory symptoms.
    (D) NSAIDs can prevent the flushing associated with biological injections.
    (E) NSAIDs must be given in combination with infliximab.

25. What abortive therapy would be appropriate for a patient who experiences severe nausea and vomiting every time a migraine occurs?

    I. Amerge oral tablets
    II. Relpax oral tablets
    III. Maxalt MLT

    (A) I only
    (B) III only
    (C) I and II only
    (D) II and III only
    (E) I, II, and III

26. Which of the following statements is TRUE?

    (A) Oxcarbazepine and lamotrigine both have a possibility of causing Stevens-Johnson syndrome.
    (B) Oxcarbazepine is the generic name for Tegretol.
    (C) Lithium has a significant drug interaction with beta-blockers.
    (D) Valproic acid is contraindicated in renal disease.
    (E) Lithium works by increasing GABA concentration in the brain.

27. Which of the following is/are contraindications to using bupropion?

    I. Current smoker
    II. Bulimia
    III. Seizure disorder

    (A) I only
    (B) III only
    (C) I and II only
    (D) II and III only
    (E) I, II, and III

28. Which of the following statements regarding methotrexate is FALSE?

    (A) It may cause folate deficiency.
    (B) It should be taken with food.
    (C) It is the first-line DMARD for treatment of rheumatoid arthritis.
    (D) The usual dose is 7.5 mg PO once weekly.
    (E) It requires ophthalmic exams every 3 months.

29. Which of the following statements regarding oxybutynin is/are TRUE?

    I. It is available in oral and transdermal patch formulations.
    II. It is an anticholinergic medication.
    III. Common side effects include dry mouth and dry eyes.

    (A) I only
    (B) III only
    (C) I and II only
    (D) II and III only
    (E) I, II, and III

30. Which of the following medication(s) can be used for both treatment and prevention of gout?

    I. NSAIDs
    II. Corticosteroids
    III. Colchicine

    (A) I only
    (B) III only
    (C) I and II only
    (D) II and III only
    (E) I, II, and III

Questions 31–35 apply to the following case.

Patient Name: Janelle Brown

Age: 21   **Height:** 5'2"
Sex: F   **Weight:** 120 lb

Allergies: Pollen

Diagnosis

    Primary:
      1. Acne vulgaris
      2. Migraine headaches

    Chief Complaint: Acne lesions and frequent migraine headaches

Lab/Diagnostic Tests

Date	Test/Result	
03/02	Sodium	134 mEq/L
(last week)	Potassium	3.5 mEq/L
	Serum creatinine	1.0 mg/dL
	Blood pressure	116/82 mmHg
	Heart rate	78 bpm

Medications

Date	Name and Strength	Route	Directions
02/20	Ovcon-50	PO	1 tablet daily utd
	Maxalt MLT 10 mg	PO	Take PRN

---

31. Which of the following side effects is MOST common with Ms. Brown's oral contraceptive?

    (A) Hot flushes
    (B) Decreased libido
    (C) Breast tenderness
    (D) Spotting
    (E) Dyspareunia

32. After talking with Ms. Brown, it seems she may be experiencing some side effects from her Ovcon-50. You call her physician, who provides you with a new prescription for Seasonale. Which of the following is/are the MOST appropriate counseling points for this medication?

    I. Take one tablet by mouth daily.
    II. Smoking while on this medication will increase your risk of serious side effects.
    III. Apply one patch each week.

    (A) I only
    (B) III only
    (C) I and II only
    (D) II and III only
    (E) I, II, and III

33. Ms. Brown is prescribed amoxicillin 500 mg PO TID for 1 week. Which of the following is the MOST appropriate counseling information for her?

    (A) There is no drug interaction present. Take the antibiotic three times daily as prescribed.
    (B) There is a drug interaction between the antibiotic and oral contraceptive, which renders the antibiotic less effective. Hold the contraceptive until the antibiotic regimen is complete.
    (C) There is a drug interaction between the antibiotic and oral contraceptive, which renders the oral contraceptive less effective. Do not take the antibiotics.
    (D) There is a drug interaction between the antibiotic and oral contraceptive, which renders the oral contraceptive less effective. Take two extra Seasonale tablets daily during the week of antibiotic therapy.
    (E) There is a drug interaction between the antibiotic and oral contraceptive, which renders the oral contraceptive less effective. Take both medications as prescribed and use a backup method of contraception for at least 7 days after finishing the antibiotic therapy.

34. Ms. Brown has several noninflammatory comedones on her face. She states that she has never tried therapy for her acne and requests a recommendation for a medication. Which of the following would be the MOST appropriate initial recommendation?

    (A) Tetracycline 500 mg PO QID
    (B) Isotretinoin 20 mg PO daily
    (C) Benzoyl peroxide 5% topical cream daily
    (D) Benzoyl peroxide 5% topical cream and tretinoin 0.1% gel applied daily
    (E) Isotretinoin 20 mg PO daily and tretinoin 0.1% gel applied daily

35. Ms. Brown asks for information about prophylactic migraine medications. She states that she is currently experiencing about four migraine headaches per week. Which of the following would be the MOST appropriate recommendation for migraine prophylaxis for Ms. Brown?

    (A) She is not a good candidate for migraine prophylaxis because she does not have headaches frequently enough.
    (B) Imitrex
    (C) Topiramate
    (D) Propranolol
    (E) Hydrocodone

36. Which of the following medications has no known drug interaction with oral contraceptives?

    (A) Neurontin
    (B) Carbamazepine
    (C) Valproic acid
    (D) Phenytoin
    (E) Phenobarbital

37. Which of the following trade names is correctly matched with its generic name?

    (A) Detrol – oxybutynin
    (B) Vesicare – tolterodine
    (C) Enablex – darifenacin
    (D) Ditropan – imipramine
    (E) Tofranil – solifenacin

38. When should biologics be initiated in rheumatoid arthritis?

    I. Within 3 months of a diagnosis
    II. For PRN symptom relief
    III. When DMARDs have been ineffective

    (A) I only
    (B) III only
    (C) I and II only
    (D) II and III only
    (E) I, II, and III

39. Which of the following statements regarding tricyclic antidepressants is/are TRUE?

    I. They may exhibit anticholinergic side effects.
    II. They are very dangerous and often fatal in overdosage.
    III. They have a significant drug–food interaction with aged cheese.

    (A) I only
    (B) III only
    (C) I and II only
    (D) II and III only
    (E) I, II, and III

40. A patient was started on a selegiline patch 3 days ago for major depression. The family states that it is not working. Which of the following is the MOST appropriate action to take at this time?

    (A) Add fluoxetine if the selegiline is still not working in 2 weeks.
    (B) Add duloxetine if he/she is not feeling better in 6–8 weeks.
    (C) Have the patient start a high caffeine intake so that the selegiline will be absorbed better.
    (D) Inform the family that the selegiline has not had time to work yet and may take 1–2 months.
    (E) Switch the patient to oral selegiline for better efficacy.

41. Which of the following products contains aspirin with butalbital and caffeine?

    (A) Fiorinal
    (B) Fioricet
    (C) Excedrin Migraine
    (D) Migranal
    (E) Amerge

42. A 15-year-old female patient is given a new prescription for Retin-A. Which of the following would be an appropriate counseling point for this patient?

    (A) This medication works best if combined with an astringent or abrasive soap.
    (B) This medication should result in rapid improvement within 1–2 days.
    (C) This medication should be used only as a "spot treatment" for blemishes.
    (D) It is important to use sunblock prior to sun exposure due to the risk of photosensitivity.
    (E) It is important to apply this product to wet skin immediately after washing the face.

Ship To:

Jacqueline Dickakian
1911 Pleasant Creek Drive
Kingwood, TX 77345-1658

Order ID: 105-1473197-3549825

Thank you for buying from Cherry_Books on Amazon Marketplace.

Shipping Address:	**Order Date:**	Nov 18, 2015
Jacqueline Dickakian	Shipping Service:	Standard
1911 Pleasant Creek Drive	Buyer Name:	Jacqueline Dickakian
Kingwood, TX 77345-1658	Seller Name:	Cherry_Books

Quantity	Product Details
1	**NAPLEX 2015 Strategies, Practice, and Review with 2 Practice Tests (Kaplan Medical Naplex) [Paperback] [2015] Brooks Pharm.D. BCPS CDE, Amie; Sanoski B.S. Pharm.D., Cynthia; Hajjar PharmD. BCPS BCACP CGP, Emily R.; Overholser PharmD FCCP, Brian R.** SKU: 1618657968SRZ ASIN: 1618657968 Listing ID: 1118PV49ENF Order Item ID: 01952272212602 Condition: Used - Like New Comments: In Perfect Condition. We do not ship to APO/FPO addresses.

Returning your item:
Go to "Your Account" on Amazon.com, click "Your Orders" and then click the "seller profile" link for this order to get information about the return and refund policies that apply.
Visit http://www.amazon.com/returns to print a return shipping label. Please have your order ID ready.

Thanks for buying on Amazon Marketplace. To provide feedback for the seller please visit www.amazon.com/feedback. To contact the seller, go to Your Orders in Your Account. Click the seller's name under the appropriate product. Then, in the "Further Information" section, click "Contact the Seller."

43. Which of the following is/are alternative treatment(s) for osteoporosis in patients who are unable to tolerate bisphosphonates?

    I. Zoledronic acid
    II. Calcitonin
    III. Raloxifene

(A) I only
(B) III only
(C) I and II only
(D) II and III only
(E) I, II, and III

44. Which of the following antianxiety medications takes 2–3 weeks to reach maximal efficacy?

(A) Xanax
(B) Librium
(C) Buspar
(D) Valium
(E) Vistaril

45. Common side effects of isotretinoin include which of the following?

    I. Cheilitis
    II. Pruritus
    III. Hypertrichosis

(A) I only
(B) III only
(C) I and II only
(D) II and III only
(E) I, II, and III

46. Which of the following is NOT a treatment option for psoriasis?

(A) Methotrexate
(B) Prednisone
(C) Coal tar
(D) Benzoyl peroxide
(E) Anthralin

47. In the TNM classification of cancer staging, N represents which of the following?

(A) The size of the tumor in centimeters
(B) The number of tumors
(C) The number of involved lymph nodes
(D) The number of involved organs
(E) The presence of distant metastases

48. Which of the following statements regarding neoadjuvant chemotherapy is/are TRUE?

    I. It is given prior to surgery.
    II. The goal is to reduce tumor burden.
    III. It is given to relieve symptoms and has no effect on survival.

(A) I only
(B) III only
(C) I and II only
(D) II and III only
(E) I, II, and III

49. Leucovorin should be given as rescue therapy to patients receiving _____, but will increase both the toxicity and the chemotherapeutic activity of _____.

(A) fluorouracil; methotrexate
(B) doxorubicin; fluorouracil
(C) fluorouracil; cytarabine
(D) methotrexate; fluorouracil
(E) methotrexate; doxorubicin

50. Which of the following statements regarding cytarabine is/are TRUE?

    I. Its main mechanism of action is inhibition of DNA polymerase.

    II. Patients should be monitored for neurotoxicity at each office visit.

    III. Pre- and posttreatment corticosteroid eye drops should be given to prevent conjunctivitis.

(A) I only
(B) III only
(C) I and II only
(D) II and III only
(E) I, II, and III

51. Which of the following is the MOST significant adverse effect of anthracyclines?

(A) Ototoxicity
(B) Infusion-related reactions
(C) Folate deficiency
(D) Cardiotoxicity
(E) Hand and foot syndrome

52. Which of the following is the trade name for bevacizumab?

(A) Gleevec
(B) Herceptin
(C) Avastin
(D) Tarceva
(E) Taxol

Questions 53–56 refer to the following patient profile.

Patient Name: Mary Jefferson

Age: 42   **Height:** 5'6"
Sex: F   **Weight:** 125 lb

Allergies: None known

Diagnosis
  Primary:
    1. Adenocarcinoma
    2. Asthma

Lab/Diagnostic Tests
  WBC 1×10^3 cells/mm^3; 50% segs
    10% bands 30% lymphs
    10% monos
  Hgb: 14.5 g/dL
  Blood pressure: 134/85 mmHg
  Heart rate: 75 bpm

---

53. What is Ms. Jefferson's absolute neutrophil count?

(A) 3,000
(B) 750
(C) 600
(D) 300
(E) 50

54. Ms. Jefferson's neutropenia would be considered

(A) transient.
(B) mild.
(C) moderate.
(D) severe.
(E) absent. This patient is not neutropenic, as the ANC is within normal range.

55. Which of the following will put patients with neutropenia at risk for developing infection?

    (A) Severe neutropenia
    (B) A rapid fall in ANC
    (C) Invasive procedures such as enemas, catheter placement, or dental procedures
    (D) Neutropenia lasting more than 7 days
    (E) All of the above

56. Which of the following medications would be appropriate for Ms. Jefferson?

    (A) Neupogen
    (B) Epogen
    (C) Procrit
    (D) Aranesp
    (E) None of the above

57. Gender and race are considered which of the following types of data?

    (A) Nominal
    (B) Ordinal
    (C) Interval
    (D) Ratio
    (E) Frequency

58. To increase the power of a study, the researchers could

    (A) decrease the sample size.
    (B) lengthen the duration of the study.
    (C) decrease the duration of the study.
    (D) increase the number of dependent variables being studied.
    (E) increase the sample size.

59. Which of the following statements regarding Type II errors is FALSE?

    (A) A Type II error occurs when a study fails to detect a difference between study groups but in fact a difference does exist.
    (B) Not achieving power in a study may increase the likelihood of Type II errors.
    (C) A Type II error means that the null hypothesis was accepted when it actually is false.
    (D) A Type II error occurs when researchers find a difference between study groups when no difference actually exists.
    (E) All of the above are true regarding Type II errors.

60. A clinical trial is evaluating whether there is a difference in the mean LDL cholesterol levels between adults in three different treatment groups. The data collected follows a normal distribution. Which of the following would be the MOST appropriate statistical test for this analysis?

    (A) Student's t-test
    (B) Paired t-test
    (C) Chi-square test
    (D) ANOVA
    (E) Mann-Whitney U test

61. You need to make 30 g of 0.4% w/w hydrocortisone ointment. You have 2.5% w/w hydrocortisone ointment in stock. How much of the 2.5% ointment must you mix with white petrolatum to make the appropriate quantity of 0.4% ointment?

    (A) 2.4 g
    (B) 2.5 g
    (C) 4.8 g
    (D) 9.6 g
    (E) 30 g

62. The formula for hydrophilic petrolatum USP is given below. How much white wax do you need to weigh out to compound 70 g of hydrophilic petrolatum?

Hydrophilic petrolatum:
   3% w/w cholesterol
   3% w/w stearyl alcohol
   8% w/w white wax
   86% w/w white petrolatum

(A) 2.1 g
(B) 8 g
(C) 5.6 g
(D) 60.2 g
(E) 70 g

63. How many 4-mg tablets of chlorpheniramine maleate would be required to compound 4 fluid ounces of a syrup containing 2 mg of chlorpheniramine maleate in every tablespoonful dose?

(A) 1
(B) 2
(C) 4
(D) 8
(E) 12

64. A 60-kg patient is to receive a constant IV infusion of dobutamine at a rate of 5 mcg/kg/min. The available solution has a concentration of 0.5 mg/mL. For what rate should the infusion pump be set?

(A) 0.6 mL/hr
(B) 3.6 mL/hr
(C) 18 mL/hr
(D) 36 mL/hr
(E) 600 mL/hr

65. A patient is given an IV bolus dose of 1 g of Drug A. The plasma level is measured shortly after administration and is found to be 0.2 mg/mL. The same patient is later given an IV bolus dose of Drug B. The plasma level of Drug B shortly after administration is 83 mcg/mL. On the basis of this data, which of the following statements is/are TRUE?

    I. Drug A has a smaller volume of distribution than Drug B.
    II. Drug A is better absorbed than Drug B.
    III. Drug A induced the metabolism of Drug B.

(A) I only
(B) III only
(C) I and II only
(D) II and III only
(E) I, II, and III

66. To treat preeclampsia, a patient receives an IV infusion of 40 mL of a 10% w/v solution of magnesium sulfate for injection. How many mEq of magnesium did she receive?
(MW $MgSO_4 \cdot (H_2O)_7 = 246.36$)

(A) 8.63 mEq Mg^{2+}
(B) 16.25 mEq Mg^{2+}
(C) 32.5 mEq Mg^{2+}
(D) 65 mEq Mg^{2+}
(E) 130 mEq Mg^{2+}

67. You receive a prescription for 240 mL of a potassium citrate solution with a concentration of 15 mEq/15 mL. How much potassium citrate must you weigh out to compound this prescription? (MW $C_6H_5K_3O_7$ = 306)

    (A) 2.72 g
    (B) 8.16 g
    (C) 24.48 g
    (D) 73.44 g
    (E) 367.2 g

68. You are considering adding HgbA1c monitoring services to your clinical pharmacy offerings and are evaluating an HgbA1c monitor to decide if it sufficiently precise and accurate to be used in your clinic. Using a test solution that produces a value of 7.5% on standardized laboratory tests, you perform 10 sample tests on the monitor. The values you obtain are:

    7.9
    8.1
    7.9
    8.0
    7.9
    7.9
    8.0
    8.1
    7.9
    8.0

    You would say that the monitor being evaluated produces readings that are

    (A) accurate but not precise.
    (B) precise but not accurate.
    (C) both precise and accurate.
    (D) neither precise nor accurate.
    (E) You do not have enough information to answer this question.

69. How much sodium chloride must be added to the prescription to make the solution isotonic?

    Rx: Tetracaine hydrochloride   0.5% w/v
            (E = 0.18)
          NaCl (0.9%)   qs
          Sterile water   add 30 mL

    M et ft isotonic eye drops

    (A) 0.027 g NaCl
    (B) 0.243 g NaCl
    (C) 0.27 g NaCl
    (D) 0.83 g NaCl
    (E) 0.9 g NaCl

70. Given the capsule recipe provided below, how much diphenhydramine must you weigh out to compound 60 capsules?

    Diphenhydramine hydrochloride: 0.5 g
    Acetaminophen: 6.5 g
    Lactose qs: M et div caps #10

    (A) 0.5 g
    (B) 3 g
    (C) 7 g
    (D) 30 g
    (E) 42 g

**Questions 71–74 refer to
the following patient information:**

AJ is a 70-kg male with a creatinine
clearance of 100 mL/min. You have
the following information about the
behavior of a particular drug in this
patient:

$CL = 400$ mL/min;
$\quad CLr = 25$ mL/min

$V_d = 140$ L

95% bound to plasma proteins

---

71. What is the filtration clearance of this
drug?

    (A)   0 mL/min
    (B)   1.25 mL/min
    (C)   5 mL/min
    (D)   20 mL/min
    (E)   95 mL/min

72. You can conclude that this drug is

    (A)   only filtered.
    (B)   both filtered and reabsorbed.
    (C)   both filtered and secreted.
    (D)   secreted and reabsorbed but not
          filtered.
    (E)   You do not have enough information
          to answer this question.

73. The half-life of this drug in this patient is

    (A)   4 hours.
    (B)   12 hours.
    (C)   24 hours.
    (D)   48 hours.
    (E)   60 hours.

74. What blood level would you expect after
    a single IV bolus dose of 250 mg of this
    drug?

    (A)   0.1 mg/dL
    (B)   0.13 mg/dL
    (C)   0.15 mg/dL
    (D)   0.18 mg/dL
    (E)   0.2 mg/dL

75. MT is being treated for a serious infection
    with *Pseudomonas aeruginosa*. After
    obtaining culture and sensitivity data,
    her physician starts her on tobramycin
    70 mg IV q8h. During her hospital stay,
    MT's serum creatinine increased from
    0.8 to 1.6 mg/dL. What pharmacokinetic
    parameters have been affected, and what
    modification should be made to MT's
    tobramycin therapy?

    (A)   The bioavailability for tobramycin
          is increased, resulting in kidney
          impairment. The tobramycin should
          be discontinued.
    (B)   The clearance for tobramycin has
          decreased, resulting in a longer
          half-life. MT may experience drug
          accumulation, so the tobramycin
          dose should be decreased.
    (C)   The clearance for tobramycin has
          increased, resulting in a shorter
          half-life. MT may experience
          subtherapeutic drug concentrations,
          so the tobramycin dose should be
          increased.
    (D)   The clearance for tobramycin has
          decreased, resulting in a longer
          half-life. MT may experience
          subtherapeutic drug concentrations,
          so the tobramycin dose should be
          increased.
    (E)   The V_d of tobramycin has increased,
          resulting in a longer half-life. MT
          may experience drug accumulation,
          so the tobramycin dose should be
          decreased.

76. Penicillin is a weakly acidic drug that is secreted by the kidney. Probenecid, also a weakly acidic drug, competes for the carrier system that is responsible for the secretion of penicillin. When penicillin and probenecid are administered together, what do you expect will happen to penicillin's clearance and steady-state plasma concentrations?

    (A) Clearance decreases and steady-state concentrations increase.
    (B) Clearance increases and steady-state concentrations increase.
    (C) Clearance increases and steady-state concentrations decrease.
    (D) Clearance decreases and steady-state concentrations decrease.
    (E) Clearance and steady-state concentrations are nearly unchanged.

77. Which of the following modifications to a drug will increase its aqueous solubility?

    (A) Convert anhydrous to trihydrate form.
    (B) Convert crystalline to amorphous form.
    (C) Add a lipophilic group.
    (D) Remove a hydroxyl group.
    (E) All of the above.

78. The pKa of a weak base is 8.4. What form will the drug be in at an intestinal pH of 7.4?

    (A) 75% un-ionized
    (B) Greater than 90% un-ionized
    (C) 75% ionized
    (D) Greater than 90% ionized
    (E) Approximately equal amounts ionized/un-ionized

79. Which dosage form would be the BEST option for a drug that is prone to first-pass metabolism?

    (A) Tablet
    (B) Syrup
    (C) Capsule
    (D) Rapid-dissolve strip
    (E) Transdermal patch

80. Structured vehicles form suspensions by what means?

    (A) Promoting loose aggregation of suspended particles
    (B) Increasing viscosity, thereby slowing sedimentation
    (C) Maximizing sedimentation volume
    (D) Reducing repulsive forces between particles
    (E) All of the above

81. Phenytoin is formulated in a cosolvent system. IV administration of this drug should occur slowly because

    (A) the onset of drug action will be faster.
    (B) slow injection will prevent precipitation of the drug from solution.
    (C) rapid infusion will lead to hemolysis.
    (D) it will prevent the drug from being metabolized too quickly.
    (E) the cosolvent system is too viscous for rapid administration.

82. Which of the following ophthalmic products must contain a preservative?

    I. Saline in a multiple-dose container

    II. Saline in a single-dose container

    III. Single-use rinse solution used in eye surgery

(A) I only
(B) III only
(C) I and II only
(D) II and III only
(E) I, II, and III

83. Medications may be administered rectally to provide local treatment for which of the following conditions?

(A) Nausea
(B) Chronic pain
(C) Ulcerative colitis
(D) Hormone replacement
(E) Migraines

84. Metronidazole leads to a disulfiram reaction when taken with alcohol. Which of the following liquid dosage forms would be the MOST appropriate way of delivering metronidazole?

(A) Spirit
(B) Elixir USP
(C) Tincture
(D) Suspension
(E) Fluid extract

85. A bottle of drug solution was left open in a dark room. After one day, the solution had changed from colorless to pink. An identical bottle, left capped, remained unchanged. The opened solution has undergone what type of degradation?

(A) Hydrolysis
(B) Photolysis
(C) Oxidation
(D) Sedimentation
(E) Polymorphism

86. Calamine lotion remains thick when sitting on the shelf, yet pours easily when shaken. What type of flow is calamine lotion exhibiting?

(A) Dilatant
(B) Newtonian
(C) Plastic
(D) Pseudoplastic
(E) Thixotropic

87. How many 50-mg phenytoin tablets should a 5-year-old child receive per day, given the following information?

$$V_{max} = 300 \text{ mg/day}$$
$$K_M = 6.5 \text{ mg/L}$$
$$C_{SS} \text{ (desired)} = 14 \text{ mg/L}$$

Salt factor for phenytoin tablets = 1

(A) 1 tablet
(B) 4 tablets
(C) 5 tablets
(D) 6 tablets
(E) 7 tablets

88. Which of the following tablet excipients would be MOST expected to decrease product bioavailability?

    (A) Starch
    (B) Microcrystalline cellulose
    (C) Lactose
    (D) Magnesium stearate
    (E) Mannitol

89. Poor metabolizers of CYP2D6 are most likely to receive therapeutic benefit from which of the following opioids?

    (A) Codeine
    (B) Morphine
    (C) Hydrocodone
    (D) Oxycodone
    (E) Dextromethorphan

90. Patients taking protease inhibitors should avoid drinking grapefruit juice because it

    (A) inhibits CYP3A, leading to toxic levels of the drug.
    (B) inhibits CYP3A, leading to subtherapeutic levels of the drug.
    (C) induces CYP3A, leading to toxic levels of the drug.
    (D) induces CYP3A, leading to subtherapeutic levels of the drug.
    (E) binds to the drug, preventing absorption.

91. You receive an order for 10 mL of epinephrine 1:10,000 solution. What is another way to express this concentration?

    (A) 10% w/v
    (B) 1% w/v
    (C) 0.1% w/v
    (D) 0.01% w/v
    (E) 0.001% w/v

92. You need to measure out 100 g of methyl salicylate to use in a compound. The specific gravity of methyl salicylate is 1.18. How much methyl salicylate should you measure, by volume, to deliver the appropriate amount?

    (A) 69.5 mL
    (B) 84.75 mL
    (C) 100 mL
    (D) 115.25 mL
    (E) 130.5 mL

Questions 93–97 refer to the following patient profile.

Patient Name: John Marx

Age: 70   **Height:** 5'10"
Sex: M   **Weight:** 198 lb
Race: Black

Allergies: NKDA

Diagnosis

Primary:
1. Hypertension
2. Dyslipidemia
3. Heart failure

Secondary:
1. MI (5 years ago)

Chief Complaint: Swelling in legs

Medications

Date	Name and Strength	Route	Directions
10/25	Aspirin 81 mg	PO	1 tablet daily
	Digoxin 0.125 mg	PO	1 tablet daily
	Furosemide 20 mg	PO	1 tablet in the morning
	Lisinopril 20 mg	PO	1 tablet daily
	Toprol XL 25 mg	PO	1 tablet daily
	Vytorin 40/10 mg	PO	1 tablet at bedtime

Lab/Diagnostic Tests

Date	Test/Result	
11/10	Sodium	145 mEq/L
	Potassium	3.9 mEq/L
	Serum creatinine	1.1 mg/dL
	Digoxin	0.8 ng/mL
	Blood pressure	122/80 mmHg
	Heart rate	70 bpm
	LVEF	35%

Additional Information

Date	Comment
11/10	Patient has gained 3 lb in the past week.

---

93. Vytorin is the brand name for which of the following combinations?

   (A) Atorvastatin and amlodipine
   (B) Atorvastatin and ezetimibe
   (C) Lovastatin and niacin
   (D) Simvastatin and ezetimibe
   (E) Simvastatin and lisinopril

94. Which of the following is/are appropriate nonpharmacological recommendations for Mr. Marx?

   I. Restrict fluid intake.
   II. Restrict sodium intake.
   III. Restrict vitamin K intake.

   (A) I only
   (B) III only
   (C) I and II only
   (D) II and III only
   (E) I, II, and III

95. Which of the following signs/symptoms is/are associated with digoxin toxicity?

   I. Anorexia
   II. Arrhythmias
   III. Visual disturbances

   (A) I only
   (B) III only
   (C) I and II only
   (D) II and III only
   (E) I, II, and III

96. Which of the following medications is contraindicated in Mr. Marx?

   (A) Aldactone
   (B) BiDil
   (C) Diovan
   (D) Calan SR
   (E) Inspra

97. Mr. Marx's furosemide is increased to 40 mg PO BID. The pharmacist should counsel the patient on which of the following?

   (A) He should separate both doses of furosemide from other medications by 2 hours.
   (B) He should take the second dose of furosemide before 5 p.m. each day.
   (C) He should take both doses of furosemide with food or milk.
   (D) He should take the second dose of furosemide at bedtime.
   (E) He should take both doses of furosemide on an empty stomach.

Questions 98–101 refer to the following patient profile.

Patient Name: Susan Brown

Age: 42   **Height:** 5'4"
Sex: F   **Weight:** 162 lb

Allergies: NKDA

Diagnosis

Primary:
    1. UTI
    2. DVT (secondary to oral contraceptive use)
    3. Hypertension

Chief Complaint: Pain with urination

Medications

Date	Name and Strength	Route	Directions
3/3	Depo-Provera 150 mg	IM	Every 3 months
5/5	Coumadin 5 mg	PO	1 tablet daily
	HCTZ 25 mg	PO	1 tablet daily
	Lisinopril 10 mg	PO	1 tablet daily

Lab/Diagnostic Tests

Date	Test/Result	
5/22	Urinalysis	pyuria, nitrite (+)
	Sodium	145 mEq/L
	Potassium	3.9 mEq/L
	Serum creatinine	0.9 mg/dL
	INR	2.3
	Blood pressure	125/72 mmHg
	Heart rate	71 bpm

Additional Information

Date	Comment
5/5	Patient contemplating smoking cessation
5/22	Patient prescribed Bactrim DS 1 tablet PO BID × 3 days, #6

---

98. Bactrim DS is MOST likely being used to treat which of the following microorganisms?

(A) *Chlamydia pneumoniae*
(B) *Clostridium difficile*
(C) *Enterococcus faecalis*
(D) *Escherichia coli*
(E) *Pseudomonas aeruginosa*

99. Which of the following lab alterations would you expect to see in Ms. Brown as a result of starting the Bactrim DS?

(A) Increased INR
(B) Decreased INR
(C) Increased potassium
(D) Decreased potassium
(E) Increased sodium

100. Bactrim DS is the brand name for which of the following medications?

(A) Amoxicillin and clavulanic acid
(B) Ciprofloxacin and doxycycline
(C) Imipenem and cilastatin
(D) Isoniazid and rifampin
(E) Trimethoprim and sulfamethoxazole

101. Lisinopril belongs to which of the following classes of drugs?

(A) Angiotensin-converting enzyme inhibitor
(B) Angiotensin II receptor blocker
(C) Aldosterone receptor antagonist
(D) Calcium channel blocker
(E) Potassium-sparing diuretic

102. A patient recently moved to the United States from England. She brings in her prescription bottle and asks the pharmacist if he carries the antibiotic that she has been taking for a UTI. Which of the following references could be used by the pharmacist to determine if there is an equivalent antibiotic available in the United States?

(A) Facts and Comparisons
(B) Martindale
(C) Merck Index
(D) PDR
(E) Red Book

103. A patient presents with a prescription for Xalatan. Xalatan is probably being used to treat which of the following disease states?

(A) Anxiety
(B) Asthma
(C) Depression
(D) Glaucoma
(E) Sepsis

104. Which of the following medications is/are classified as macrolide(s)?

I. Keflex
II. Keppra
III. Ketek

(A) I only
(B) III only
(C) I and II only
(D) II and III only
(E) I, II, and III

105. Patients taking sulfasalazine for inflammatory bowel disease should be counseled on which of the following?

    I. Take on an empty stomach.
    II. It may cause orange bodily fluids.
    III. Wear sunscreen and protective clothing.

  (A) I only
  (B) III only
  (C) I and II only
  (D) II and III only
  (E) I, II, and III

106. During a hospital stay for pneumonia, David Jones developed *Clostridium difficile*. Which of the following antibiotics would be the BEST treatment for Mr. Jones?

  (A) Amoxicillin
  (B) Azithromycin
  (C) Levofloxacin
  (D) Metronidazole
  (E) Tobramycin

107. A 22-year-old woman comes to the pharmacy to pick up her new prescription for an oral contraceptive. Which of the following references would be the MOST appropriate source of important counseling advice for this patient?

  (A) Harriet Lane Handbook
  (B) Index Nominum
  (C) Merck Index
  (D) USP-DI Volume I
  (E) USP-DI Volume II

108. Cytotec is the brand name of which of the following medications?

  (A) Cimetidine
  (B) Metoclopramide
  (C) Misoprostol
  (D) Olsalazine
  (E) Sucralfate

109. Which of the following medications would be an appropriate treatment for genital herpes?

  (A) Acyclovir
  (B) Indinavir
  (C) Lamivudine
  (D) Oseltamivir
  (E) Valganciclovir

110. Which of the following references is the BEST source for obtaining the cost information of medications?

  (A) Facts and Comparisons
  (B) The Harriet Lane Handbook
  (C) PDR
  (D) Red Book
  (E) USP-DI Volume I

111. Which of the following is/are potential side effects of niacin?

    I. Flushing
    II. Hyperglycemia
    III. Hyperuricemia

  (A) I only
  (B) III only
  (C) I and II only
  (D) II and III only
  (E) I, II, and III

112. Cosopt is the brand name for which of the following combinations?

    (A) Timolol and brimonidine
    (B) Timolol and dorzolamide
    (C) Latanoprost and carbachol
    (D) Pilocarpine and brinzolamide
    (E) Pilocarpine and carbachol

113. Which of the following medications could be used intravenously to treat an invasive *Aspergillus* infection?

    I. Voriconazole
    II. Linezolid
    III. Miconazole

    (A) I only
    (B) III only
    (C) I and II only
    (D) II and III only
    (E) I, II, and III

114. Which of the following is/are appropriate nonpharmacological recommendations for a patient with gastroesophageal reflux disease?

    I. Avoid chocolate
    II. Stop smoking
    III. Lose weight

    (A) I only
    (B) III only
    (C) I and II only
    (D) II and III only
    (E) I, II, and III

115. Which of the following IV medications should be protected from light?

    (A) Enalaprilat
    (B) Esmolol
    (C) Fenoldopam
    (D) Nitroglycerin
    (E) Nitroprusside

116. A patient presents to the pharmacy with prescriptions for Biaxin, Amoxil, and Nexium. The patient is probably being treated for which of the following infections?

    (A) *Helicobacter pylori*
    (B) *Haemophilus influenzae*
    (C) *Klebsiella pneumoniae*
    (D) *Moraxella catarrhalis*
    (E) *Neisseria meningitidis*

117. Trusopt belongs to which of the following classes of drugs?

    (A) Antihistamine
    (B) Beta-blocker
    (C) Carbonic anhydrase inhibitor
    (D) Cholinergic agonist
    (E) Prostaglandin analog

118. The Commission E Monographs provide information on which of the following?

    (A) Dietary supplements
    (B) Foreign drugs
    (C) Herbal products
    (D) Homeopathic products
    (E) Nonprescription drugs

119. Clotrimazole is available in which of the following dosage forms?

    I. Troche
    II. Capsule
    III. Powder

    (A) I only
    (B) III only
    (C) I and II only
    (D) II and III only
    (E) I, II, and III

120. Which of the following is/are the MOST appropriate monitoring recommendations for a patient receiving amiodarone?

    I. Chest x-ray should be performed every 6 months.
    II. Thyroid function tests should be performed annually.
    III. Liver function tests should be performed every 6 months.

(A) I only
(B) III only
(C) I and II only
(D) II and III only
(E) I, II, and III

121. A patient using ophthalmic preparations should be given which of the following counseling information?

(A) The preparations can be used safely with contact lenses.
(B) The dropper tip should be placed on the edge of the lower eyelid.
(C) The upper eyelid should be pulled outward to form a pocket in which the medication can be placed.
(D) The eyes should be rubbed after the eye drops are administered.
(E) The administration of different medications should be separated by intervals of at least 10 minutes.

122. Information on IV medication compatibility can be found in which of the following references?

    I. Facts and Comparisons
    II. Physician's Desk Reference
    III. Trissel's Handbook on Injectable Drugs

(A) I only
(B) III only
(C) I and II only
(D) II and III only
(E) I, II, and III

123. Tagamet belongs to which of the following classes of drugs?

(A) Aminosalicylate
(B) H_2 receptor antagonist
(C) Immunosuppressant
(D) Prostaglandin analog
(E) Proton pump inhibitor

124. A patient brings in a prescription for methotrexate for the treatment of Crohn's disease. Which of the following tests should be monitored in this patient?

    I. Electrocardiogram
    II. Complete blood count
    III. Liver function tests

(A) I only
(B) III only
(C) I and II only
(D) II and III only
(E) I, II, and III

125. Which of the following medications may result in hyperkalemia?

    I. Candesartan
    II. Eplerenone
    III. Triamterene

(A) I only
(B) III only
(C) I and II only
(D) II and III only
(E) I, II, and III

126. Which of the following medications can be administered via a nasogastric tube?

    I. Esomeprazole
    II. Lansoprazole
    III. Pantoprazole

(A) I only
(B) III only
(C) I and II only
(D) II and III only
(E) I, II, and III

127. A patient is prescribed felodipine for her hypertension. She should be counseled to do which of the following?

(A) Avoid drinking grapefruit juice.
(B) Avoid foods with tyramine.
(C) Take the felodipine with folic acid.
(D) Take the felodipine on an empty stomach.
(E) Take the felodipine 2 hours before taking other medications.

128. An otherwise healthy patient develops community-acquired pneumonia. Which of the following antibiotics would be the MOST appropriate empiric treatment option for this patient?

(A) Azithromycin
(B) Metronidazole
(C) Penicillin
(D) Rifampin
(E) Vancomycin

129. Amoxicillin is available in which of the following dosage forms?

    I. IV injection
    II. Oral suspension
    III. Capsule

(A) I only
(B) III only
(C) I and II only
(D) II and III only
(E) I, II, and III

130. Which of the following medications would be MOST appropriate to use for the treatment of hypertension in a pregnant patient?

(A) Doxazosin
(B) Lisinopril
(C) Methyldopa
(D) Metolazone
(E) Valsartan

131. A patient is prescribed Prevacid for his peptic ulcer disease. He should be counseled to take it

(A) 15 to 30 minutes before breakfast.
(B) 30 minutes after breakfast.
(C) 2 hours before taking other medications.
(D) with the first bite of a meal.
(E) with a high-fat meal.

132. Sporanox is the brand name for which of the following medications?

    (A) Aripiprazole
    (B) Fluconazole
    (C) Itraconazole
    (D) Lansoprazole
    (E) Rabeprazole

133. A patient presents to the pharmacy with a prescription for simvastatin 40 mg PO at bedtime and gemfibrozil 600 mg PO BID. Which of the following adverse reactions is this patient likely to experience?

    (A) Dyspnea
    (B) Edema
    (C) Headache
    (D) Insomnia
    (E) Myopathy

134. A patient presents with a new prescription for Synthroid. Which of the following medications might have contributed to her recent diagnosis of hypothyroidism?

    (A) Amiodarone
    (B) Bisoprolol
    (C) Dofetilide
    (D) Hydralazine
    (E) Propafenone

135. Levaquin belongs to which of the following classes of drugs?

    (A) Aminoglycosides
    (B) Cephalosporins
    (C) Fluoroquinolones
    (D) Macrolides
    (E) Tetracyclines

136. Which of the following statements regarding amiodarone is/are TRUE?

    I. It is only effective for the treatment of atrial arrhythmias.
    II. It does not undergo cytochrome P450 metabolism by the liver.
    III. If pulmonary fibrosis develops, the amiodarone should be discontinued.

    (A) I only
    (B) III only
    (C) I and II only
    (D) II and III only
    (E) I, II, and III

137. Which of the following drug classes is/are used in the treatment of inflammatory bowel disease?

    I. Aminosalicylates
    II. Corticosteroids
    III. Immunosuppressants

    (A) I only
    (B) III only
    (C) I and II
    (D) II and III
    (E) I, II, and III

138. Which of the following medications can be used in an appropriate combination regimen to treat *H. pylori*?

    I. Amoxicillin
    II. Lansoprazole
    III. Clarithromycin

    (A) I only
    (B) III only
    (C) I and II
    (D) II and III
    (E) I, II, and III

Questions 139–143 refer to the following patient profile.

Patient Name: William Boyd

Age: 56   **Height:** 5'8"
Sex: M   **Weight:** 148 lb

Allergies: Codeine, PCN, Sulfa

Diagnosis

Primary
1. Hypertension
2. Hypothyroidism
3. Type 2 diabetes mellitus × 5 years

Secondary
1. Heartburn

Chief Complaint: Fatigue, tiredness, cold fingers, feeling down

Medications

Date	Name and Strength	Route	Directions
7/10	Prilosec OTC 10 mg	PO	3 tablets daily
	Synthroid 100 mcg	PO	1 tablet daily
	Metformin 1,000 mg	PO	1 tablet TID
	Lisinopril 10 mg	PO	1 tablet daily
	Ferrous sulfate 325 mg	PO	1 tablet daily

Lab/Diagnostic Tests

Date	Test/Result	
7/9	Sodium	141 mEq/L
	Potassium	3.5 mEq/L
	Serum creatinine	0.9 mg/dL
	TSH	10 mIU/L
	AST	18 IU/L
	ALT	16 IU/L
	A1c	5.5%
	Blood pressure	139/80 mmHg
	Heart rate	90 bpm
	GDS	4

Additional Information

Date	Comment
7/10	Patient complains of fatigue and lack of energy.
3/9	Pharmacist advised patient to start taking Prilosec OTC.
3/9	Pharmacist counseled patient to check blood sugars.

139. Which of the following statements regarding the metformin is TRUE?

    (A) It should be discontinued due to the patient's A1c level.
    (B) The pharmacist should contact the patient's physician because the dose is too high.
    (C) The pharmacist should recommend increasing the dose.
    (D) It is not indicated in this patient.
    (E) There is a significant drug interaction with lisinopril.

140. Which of the following is/are appropriate recommendations for Mr. Boyd?

    I. Continue taking all medications as prescribed.
    II. Start taking a multivitamin for energy.
    III. Call the doctor regarding the patient's heartburn.

    (A) I only
    (B) III only
    (C) I and II only
    (D) II and III only
    (E) I, II, and III

141. Which of the following is/are MOST likely associated with Mr. Boyd's chief complaints?

    I. Undertreated hypothyroidism
    II. Hypoglycemia
    III. Untreated depression

    (A) I only
    (B) III only
    (C) I and II only
    (D) II and III only
    (E) I, II, and III

142. Lisinopril helps to do which of the following for this patient?

    (A) Improve blood sugars by inhibiting ACE
    (B) Block renin to lower blood pressure
    (C) Inhibit ACE, which blocks the angiotensin II receptor
    (D) Block ACE to vasodilate
    (E) Protect his kidneys by lowering bradykinin

143. Mr. Boyd's Synthroid was increased to 125 mcg PO daily by the medical resident. The pharmacist should counsel Mr. Boyd to

    (A) monitor his blood sugar, as the Synthroid may cause hypoglycemia.
    (B) avoid taking the Synthroid with ferrous sulfate at the same time.
    (C) take the Synthroid only in the evening.
    (D) avoid taking the Synthroid with metformin.
    (E) take the Synthroid with milk.

144. Nevirapine is the generic name of which brand drug, and belongs in which drug class?

    (A) Viramune; non-nucleoside reverse transcriptase inhibitors
    (B) Ziagen; non-nucleoside reverse transcriptase inhibitors
    (C) Kaletra; protease inhibitors
    (D) Videx; nucleoside reverse transcriptase inhibitors
    (E) Fuzeon; fusion inhibitors

145. When should antiviral therapy for HIV be initiated?

    I. When diagnosis is confirmed by Western blot
    II. When the CD4 cell count is less than 500 cells/mm^3
    III. When the patient has a history of an opportunistic infection

(A) I only
(B) III only
(C) I and II only
(D) II and III only
(E) I, II, and III

Questions 146–151 refer to the following patient profile.

Patient Name: Mary Christensen

Age: 75   **Height:** 5'4"
Sex: F   **Weight:** 183 lb

Allergies: NKDA

Diagnosis

  Primary
    1. Asthma
    2. Hypertension
    3. Osteoarthritis

  Chief Complaint: Thrush, dizziness, tachycardia,
                  nausea, and vomiting

Lab/Diagnostic Tests

Date	Test/Result	
7/9	Sodium	140 mEq/L
	Potassium	3.5 mEq/L
	Serum creatinine	0.9 mg/dL
	Personal best FEV_1	325 L/sec
	FEV1	300 L/sec
	Blood pressure	90/70 mmHg
	Heart rate	110 bpm
	Theophylline level	23 mcg/mL

Medications

Date	Name and Strength	Route	Directions
7/20	Advair	PO	1 puff BID
	Theophylline XR 600 mg	PO	1 tablet daily
	Albuterol MDI	PO	1–2 puffs TID PRN
	Metoprolol 50 mg	PO	1 tablet BID
	Aspirin 325 mg	PO	1 tablet daily
	Fish oil 1,000 mg	PO	1 capsule daily
	Hydrocodone/ APAP 5/325 mg	PO	1–2 tablets q6h for pain
	Tylenol Arthritis 325 mg	PO	2 tablets TID

Additional Orders

Date	Comment
5/10	Pharmacist counseled patient on swish and spit after Advair use.
6/15	Pharmacist counseled patient on use of peak flow meter.
7/2	Patient stated she got a new cat.

---

146. The patient's chief complaints are likely caused by which of the following?

    I. Theophylline toxicity
    II. Lack of swishing and spitting after Advair use
    III. Excessive metoprolol dose

(A) I only
(B) III only
(C) I and II only
(D) II and III only
(E) I, II, and III

147. Which of the following medications would you recommend discontinuing in this patient?

(A) Advair because of thrush
(B) Aspirin because of nausea
(C) Albuterol due to excessive use
(D) Theophylline because of toxicity
(E) Metoprolol because of tachycardia

148. What is/are the generic ingredient(s) of Advair?

(A) Fluticasone
(B) Salmeterol
(C) Fluticasone and salmeterol
(D) Flunisolide
(E) Flunisolide and salmeterol

149. What is the likely reason that this patient is taking fish oil?

(A) To reduce total cholesterol
(B) To reduce LDL cholesterol
(C) To increase HDL cholesterol
(D) To reduce HDL cholesterol
(E) To reduce triglycerides

150. Which of the following is the MOST appropriate action to take regarding the acetaminophen this patient is currently taking?

(A) Call her doctor.
(B) Discuss how much acetaminophen is appropriate per day.
(C) Discontinue the hydrocodone/acetaminophen.
(D) Discontinue the Tylenol Arthritis.
(E) Consider switching the Tylenol Arthritis to an aspirin-containing product.

151. What is/are the major difference(s) between Spiriva and Atrovent?

    I. Atrovent has fewer side effects.
    II. Spiriva is taken once daily.
    III. Spiriva is a dry powder inhaler.

(A) I only
(B) III only
(C) I and II only
(D) II and III only
(E) I, II, and III

152. Which of the following drugs is/are inhaled corticosteroids?

    I. Pulmicort Respules
    II. Singulair
    III. Zyflo

(A) I only
(B) III only
(C) I and II only
(D) II and III only
(E) I, II, and III

153. Which of the following is the mechanism of action of Zyban?

    (A) It inhibits reuptake of serotonin.
    (B) It inhibits reuptake of norepinephrine.
    (C) It inhibits reuptake of dopamine.
    (D) It inhibits reuptake of dopamine and norepinephrine.
    (E) It inhibits reuptake of serotonin, norepinephrine, and dopamine.

154. Which of the following drugs is NOT commonly used in the treatment of nonresistant tuberculosis?

    (A) Isoniazid
    (B) Rifampin
    (C) Pyrazinamide
    (D) Ethambutol
    (E) Streptomycin

155. Vitamin K can be used to reverse the effects of which of the following drugs?

    (A) Unfractionated heparin
    (B) Dabigatran
    (C) Enoxaparin
    (D) Warfarin
    (E) Clopidogrel

156. Flumazenil is used to treat an overdose of which of the following medications?

    (A) Benzodiazepines
    (B) Opioids
    (C) Methanol
    (D) Methotrexate
    (E) Cisplatin

157. Cytomel is the brand name for which of the following active ingredients?

    (A) Liothyronine
    (B) Levothyroxine
    (C) Dessicated thyroid
    (D) T4
    (E) TSH

158. Which of the following medications is/are considered pregnancy category X?

    I. Finasteride
    II. Isotretinoin
    III. Ramipril

    (A) I only
    (B) III only
    (C) I and II only
    (D) II and III only
    (E) I, II, and III

159. When counseling a patient about medroxyprogesterone, which of the following is/are important factors to discuss?

    I. Weight gain
    II. Osteoporosis
    III. Pulmonary embolism

    (A) I only
    (B) III only
    (C) I and II only
    (D) II and III only
    (E) I, II, and III

160. How long does it take for the fentanyl patch to begin working?

    (A) 12 hours
    (B) 24 hours
    (C) 48 hours
    (D) 72 hours
    (E) 84 hours

161. Which of the following is/are important points to discuss with a patient taking morphine for chronic pain?

    I. The need for a stimulant laxative
    II. The importance of not driving a vehicle
    III. Compliance

    (A) I only
    (B) III only
    (C) I and II only
    (D) II and III only
    (E) I, II, and III

162. A woman comes into the pharmacy and requests an over-the-counter medication for pain in her knee, though she can't remember what her physician told her to purchase. She informs you that she has kidney problems. Which of the following medications would be MOST appropriate for this patient?

    (A) Ibuprofen
    (B) Ketoprofen
    (C) Naproxen
    (D) Acetaminophen
    (E) Aspirin

163. A PPD should be performed on which of the following individuals?

    I. Healthcare worker
    II. HIV-infected patient
    III. Immigrant

    (A) I only
    (B) III only
    (C) I and II only
    (D) II and III only
    (E) I, II, and III

164. The doses of which of the following pain medications must be adjusted in patients with renal dysfunction?

    I. Morphine
    II. Codeine
    III. Oxycodone

    (A) I only
    (B) III only
    (C) I and II only
    (D) II and III only
    (E) I, II, and III

165. Which NSAID has a maximum dose of 1,500 mg per day?

    (A) Naprosyn
    (B) Ibuprofen
    (C) Relafen
    (D) Ketoprofen
    (E) Daypro

166. Which of the following is NOT a warning sign of stroke?

    (A) Numbness or weakness of the face, arm, or leg
    (B) Sudden confusion, trouble speaking or understanding
    (C) Sudden trouble seeing in one or both eyes
    (D) Sudden seizure for no known reason
    (E) Sudden trouble walking, dizziness, loss of balance

167. Folic acid is important in which of the following conditions?

    I. Methotrexate treatment
    II. Neural tube defects
    III. Iron deficiency anemia

    (A) I only
    (B) III only
    (C) I and II only
    (D) II and III only
    (E) I, II, and III

168. Which of the following is/are the MOST common side effects of long-term treatment with ferrous sulfate?

      I. Constipation
      II. Dark stools
      III. Discoloration of urine

(A) I only
(B) III only
(C) I and II only
(D) II and III only
(E) I, II, and III

169. A patient with osteomalacia would BEST be given a nutritional supplement high in

(A) pyridoxine.
(B) ascorbic acid.
(C) beta-carotene.
(D) nicotinic acid.
(E) cholecalciferol.

170. Iron deficiency anemia requires a minimum of how many months of treatment?

(A) 1 month
(B) 3 months
(C) 6 months
(D) 9 months
(E) 12 months

171. What is the mechanism of action of epoetin alfa?

(A) It induces reticulocytes to create more iron stores.
(B) It induces erythropoiesis and the release of reticulocytes.
(C) It stimulates granulocyte colony-stimulating factor to generate more reticulocytes.
(D) It is a thrombopoietic growth factor, which stimulates iron absorption in the gut.
(E) It stimulates colony-stimulating factor to generate more iron absorption.

172. A patient taking chronic doses of isoniazid should be supplemented with which of the following?

(A) Beta-carotene
(B) Ascorbic acid
(C) Cyanocobalamin
(D) Thiamine
(E) Pyridoxine

173. Which of the following organizations is responsible for the enforcement of controlled substances?

(A) Federal Drug Association
(B) Food and Drug Administration
(C) Drug Enforcement Administration
(D) National Provider Indicators
(E) State Patrol

174. Which of the following statements regarding lifestyle modifications is FALSE?

    (A) Smoking cessation for more than a year can lead to an improvement in lung function.
    (B) Avoidance of asthma triggers such as mold, pollen, dust, cockroaches, grass, and smoke can replace the need for a short-acting beta-2 agonist bronchodilator.
    (C) Six months of lifestyle modifications should be followed prior to starting cholesterol-lowering medications for the treatment of dyslipidemia in most cases.
    (D) Patients with heartburn may raise the head of the bed by 2–3 inches to relieve symptoms during sleeping hours.
    (E) Patients with hypertension should limit their salt intake to less than 2.4 g/day.

175. Which of the following statements regarding the Dietary Supplement Health and Education Act of 1994 is FALSE?

    (A) Manufacturers are not required to demonstrate safety, purity, or efficacy of supplements.
    (B) Labeling must include the FDA statement: "This drug is not evaluated by the FDA, and not intended to diagnose, treat, cure, or prevent disease."
    (C) Products cannot have specific claims on their labels or use phrases such as "helps boost/support/enhance."
    (D) The FDA requires certain standards for manufacturing practices.
    (E) Manufacturers are not required to demonstrate safety.

176. Which of the following herbal products does NOT have the potential to interact with anticoagulant/antiplatelet agents?

    (A) Ginkgo biloba
    (B) Ginseng
    (C) Garlic
    (D) Saw palmetto
    (E) Feverfew

177. Which of the following organisms would MOST likely be present in a patient with a community-acquired skin and soft tissue infection?

    (A) *Haemophilus influenzae*
    (B) *Escherichia coli*
    (C) *Staphylococcus aureus*
    (D) *Streptococcus pneumoniae*
    (E) *Pseudomonas aeruginosa*

178. Which of the following is NOT a setting within an insulin pump?

    (A) Basal insulin rate
    (B) Insulin to carbohydrate ratio
    (C) Insulin sensitivity factor
    (D) Rule of 1,800
    (E) Goal blood sugar

179. Doses of vitamin E over 400 IU are known to increase

    (A) cardiovascular events.
    (B) Alzheimer's disease.
    (C) hepatotoxicity.
    (D) kidney dysfunction.
    (E) gastrointestinal discomfort.

180. Compilations of information concerning parenteral drug solutions are found in

(A) Goodman and Gilman.
(B) Martindale.
(C) Merck Index.
(D) Remington.
(E) Trissel's Handbook on Injectable Drugs.

181. Solubility data for potassium gluconate will be found in which of the following?

    I. Merck Index
    II. USP-NF
    III. Remington

(A) I only
(B) III only
(C) I and II only
(D) II and III only
(E) I, II, and III

182. _____ are currently available on the market.

(A) Metformin 1,250-mg tablets
(B) Ferrous sulfate 5-grain tablets
(C) Synthroid 212-mcg tablets
(D) Coumadin 15-mg tablets
(E) Lisinopril 80-mg tablets

183. Which statin is equivalent to Lipitor 10 mg?

(A) Rosuvastatin 10 mg
(B) Simvastatin 20 mg
(C) Pravastatin 20 mg
(D) Simvastatin 80 mg
(E) None of the above

184. St. John's wort interacts with which of the following medications?

    I. Pravachol
    II. Sertraline
    III. Warfarin

(A) I only
(B) III only
(C) I and II only
(D) II and III only
(E) I, II, and III

185. A patient who is experiencing a runny nose, sneezing, headache, and watery eyes should be counseled to take which of the following OTC agents?

    I. Diphenhydramine
    II. Acetaminophen
    III. Pseudoephedrine

(A) I only
(B) III only
(C) I and II only
(D) II and III only
(E) I, II, and III

Full-Length Practice Test Answers & Explanations

1. E

Diarrhea is a possible side effect of nearly any medication including approximately 1–10% of patients taking allopurinol (A), indomethacin (C), and acetaminophen (D); and <5% of patients taking probenecid (B). However, up to 25% of patients taking colchicine will experience this common, limiting side effect.

2. B

A1c is the gold standard for monitoring glycemic control in patients with diabetes (A). Because A1c measures glycosylated hemoglobin, the time frame it represents correlates with the lifespan of a red blood cell (90–120 days). In patients with severe anemia, low hemoglobin (Hgb) values can make the A1c value inaccurate (C). The most common normal reference range is 4–6% (D) while an A1c of 10% correlates with blood sugar values averaging in excess of 200 mg/dL (E).

3. E

Clozapine requires rigorous monitoring of white blood cell (WBC) count and absolute neutrophil count (ANC) due to the possibility of clozapine-induced agranulocytosis or severe granulocytopenia. Counts for both parameters should be obtained at baseline and at least weekly for the first 6 months of treatment with clozapine. If counts remain stable, then the WBC and ANC can be monitored every other week for the next 6 months and monthly thereafter. Due to these frequent monitoring requirements, clozapine is used less than other atypical antipsychotics and is often used for refractory cases of schizophrenia. Agranulocytosis is not associated with olanzapine (A), risperidone (B), quetiapine (C), or ziprasidone (D).

4. A

When initiating a dopamine agonist such as Mirapex, the levodopa dose should be decreased by 20–30%. II is incorrect because Mirapex does not come in a patch, which eliminates answer choices (C), (D), and (E). The ergot-derivative bromocriptine must be monitored for the cardiac side effects (III), which is why the nonergot derivatives such as Mirapex are much more commonly used.

5. A

Venlafaxine is an appropriate antidepressant medication to initiate and the initial dose should be 37.5 mg PO twice daily. Lexapro is dosed once daily (B). Fluvoxamine should be dosed once daily and is more commonly used for the treatment of obsessive-compulsive disorder (C); fluoxetine can be dosed weekly. The maximum dose of nortriptyline is 150 mg/day (D). Mirtazapine does not come in a 10-mg formulation and should be dosed at bedtime due to somnolence (E).

6. E

NuvaRing should be inserted once per month and left in place for 3 weeks, then removed for 1 week (I); Ortho-Evra is applied once each week for 3 consecutive weeks followed by 1 patch-free week per month (II); and Seasonale is a continuous oral contraceptive that is taken as 84 active pills followed by 7 inactive pills, resulting in menses approximately once every 3 months (III).

7. D

Corticosteroids such as prednisone may increase blood glucose (A) and blood pressure. Methotrexate may cause a folate deficiency; therefore, a CBC must be monitored (B). Hydroxychloroquine may cause macular damage, corneal deposits, or retinopathy, so ocular exams must be performed every 3 months (C). The dose of Enbrel (etanercept) is not dependent on renal function and the drug does not cause nephrotoxicity; therefore, serum creatinine does not need to be monitored during therapy with this drug (D). Leflunomide is contraindicated in hepatic disease and may elevate liver enzymes, so alanine aminotransferase (ALT) must be monitored monthly for 6 months, then every 6–8 weeks thereafter.

8. D

Serum creatinine is most commonly used to assess renal function, not hepatic function (A). Serum creatinine is not dependent upon the amount of iron in the diet and is sometimes an inaccurate representation of renal function in the very elderly (B, C). Serum creatinine is commonly used in the Cockroft-Gault equation to calculate creatinine clearance (D). Microalbumin, a microscopic protein, is measured in the urine and is not synonymous with serum creatinine (E).

9. C

Natalizumab is reserved for patients that have not responded to other disease-modifying drugs (DMDs) (II). Natalizumab is available only through a restrictive prescribing program called MS-TOUCH, in which both prescribers and patients must enroll (I), eliminating choices (A) and (D). Natalizumab should be used only as monotherapy and not in combination with other DMDs (III), eliminating choices (B), (D), and (E). Using natalizumab with DMDs increases the risk of progressive multifocal leukoencephalopathy.

10. B

Allopurinol is indicated for prophylaxis of gout exacerbations in patients with moderately elevated serum uric acid levels and a history of nephrolithiasis, tophi, serum creatinine >2 mg/dL, or urinary uric acid excretion indicative of overproduction (B). If the serum uric acid levels are only slightly elevated, colchicine is used for prophylaxis (A). In patients who have urinary uric acid excretion levels indicative of underexcretion, uricosuric drugs (e.g., probenecid) are used for prophylaxis (C). Allopurinol should never be used to treat acute gout because it can actually worsen the symptoms (D). Asymptomatic hyperuricemia does not require therapy (E).

11. D

Lamotrigine (I) does not require monitoring of serum drug concentrations. Valproic acid (II) should be monitored to achieve serum drug concentrations of 50–100 mcg/mL. Therapeutic serum drug concentrations of lithium (III) are 0.6–1.5 mEq/L.

12. E

All of the trade/generic names are correctly matched except that Haldol is the trade name for haloperidol. Clozapine is the generic name for Clozaril.

13. C

Available prophylactic agents for migraines include beta-blockers (such as propranolol, atenolol, metoprolol), antidepressants (such as amitriptyline, paroxetine, fluoxetine, sertraline), and anticonvulsants (such as valproic acid, gabapentin, tiagabine, topiramate). Acetaminophen (B) is considered abortive treatment for migraines and is not taken for prophylaxis. Angiotensin-converting enzyme inhibitors (ACEIs) (A), H2 antagonists (D), and anticholinergics (E) have no role in the prevention of migraines.

14. B

Tramadol (B) is an oral analgesic that does not cause GI upset or bleeding. Aspirin (A) is a nonsteroidal anti-inflammatory drug (NSAID) that may cause GI bleeding. Diclofenac (C) and Daypro (oxaprozin; D) are both NSAIDs that may cause GI upset and bleeding. Although Mobic (meloxicam; E) is more COX-2–selective than traditional NSAIDs, it still possesses the potential to cause GI upset and stomach bleeding.

15. C

Haloperidol (C) is a first-generation antipsychotic. First-generation antipsychotics are known for their potential to cause extrapyramidal symptoms (EPS) such as tardive dyskinesia and dystonia. Hydrochlorothiazide (A) is a common antihypertensive that does not cause EPS. Citalopram (B) is a common antidepressant that does not cause EPS. Although low sodium (D) can be dangerous, it does not cause EPS. Uncontrolled blood pressure (E) may lead to organ damage but does not cause EPS.

16. E

Haloperidol (E) requires periodic monitoring of a CBC because of its potential to cause agranulocytosis. Serum drug levels (A) are not measured with haloperidol. Although a baseline electrocardiogram is recommended upon haloperidol initiation, monitoring of ejection fraction (C) is not necessary. A1c (B) could be monitored with atypical antipsychotics (such as olanzapine or ziprasidone) due to their likelihood of causing metabolic syndrome. Bone mineral density (D) is not routine monitoring for any antipsychotic.

17. B

Switching between formulations of haloperidol (I) would not provide any benefit with EPS. Changing the patient to an atypical antipsychotic would be the best option since atypicals have fewer extrapyramidal side effects. This patient is allergic to Geodon (ziprasidone) so (II) would not be appropriate. This leaves the atypical antipsychotic Risperdal (risperidone; III), which would be appropriate.

18. D

Alcohol should be avoided in combination with antipsychotics due to the excessive central nervous system (CNS) depression it may cause. An acidic environment is not required with antipsychotic medications and patients may take most of the medications with food if GI upset occurs (A). Medications for schizophrenia may take 2–4 weeks to work, so (B) is not correct. It is also important that these medications not be abruptly stopped (C) or self-adjusted (E). If bothersome side effects occur, physicians should be contacted to make adjustments and changes in the medications.

19. C

Alprazolam (B) is not used for depression but may be used in anxiety disorders. Propranolol (E) is a beta-blocker which may actually worsen depression. Although not contraindicated, venlafaxine (D) may not be the best option for this patient considering her uncontrolled blood pressure. Venlafaxine can increase blood pressure and should be monitored closely. Bupropion (A) is contraindicated if the patient actually has an eating disorder. Since this woman is suspected of having an eating disorder, bupropion is not the most appropriate recommendation. Lexapro (escitalopram; C) is a selective serotonin reuptake inhibitor (SSRI) similar to her current citalopram and would be an appropriate substitution.

20. A

Carbidopa is a dopa-decarboxylase inhibitor, which must be combined with levodopa to prevent the peripheral degradation of levodopa (I). If the levodopa is degraded in the periphery, it does not enter into the blood-brain barrier for site of action. The carbidopa does not extend the dosing interval (II) or prevent CNS side effects of levodopa from occurring (III), therefore eliminating answer choices (B)–(E).

21. C

NSAIDs such as indomethacin are the first-line treatment for acute gout. If the patient is unable to take NSAIDs, the time course of the event must be evaluated. If the symptoms have been present for less than 48 hours, colchicine (B) is recommended. If the symptoms have been present for >48 hours, a corticosteroid is recommended. Allopurinol (D) should never be used in the treatment of acute gout and can worsen the symptoms. Probenecid (E) is not useful in an acute exacerbation of gout and should be avoided as it may precipitate attacks. Acetaminophen (A) plays no role in the treatment of acute gout.

22. E

All of the medications are correctly matched with their common side effects. Mirtazapine is typically dosed at bedtime because of the somnolence it causes (I). All of the SSRIs (paroxetine) have the potential to cause ejaculation disorders or impotence (II). The tricyclic antidepressants (TCAs) (amitriptyline) have the potential to cause weight gain along with anticholinergic side effects (III).

23. E

Phenytoin is available in many dosage forms including chewable tablets (I), capsules, extended-release capsules, and oral suspension (II). Phenytoin can also be given intramuscularly (IM) or intravenously (IV), as it comes in a parenteral solution (III).

24. B

NSAIDs are used for symptomatic relief during the onset of disease-modifying antirheumatic drug (DMARD) therapy and as needed symptomatic relief (B). NSAIDs do not alter the disease progression of rheumatoid arthritis; therefore, they are not considered DMARDs (A). Although NSAIDs can be given along with DMARDs for symptoms, they are not considered adjunctive therapy for patients with refractory symptoms (C); that is the role of corticosteroids. The biologics are not known to cause flushing, (D) although NSAIDs could be used for PRN symptom relief with the biologics. Methotrexate must be given in combination with infliximab, not NSAIDs (E).

25. B

If a patient is experiencing severe nausea and vomiting whenever a migraine occurs, most likely he/she will not receive maximum benefit from a regular oral tablet (I and II) due to the emesis. Many other dosage forms are available within the triptan class of abortive therapies. Maxalt MLT (rizatriptan) (III) is a rapidly disintegrating tablet that is one possible option for treatment in these patients. Other triptan options for patients experiencing severe nausea and vomiting include Imitrex (sumatriptan) injection or nasal spray and Zomig (zolmitriptan) orally disintegrating tablet or nasal spray.

26. A

Oxcarbazepine and lamotrigine both have the potential to cause Stevens-Johnson syndrome (A), especially when lamotrigine is used in combination with valproic acid. Oxcarbazepine is the generic name for Trileptal (B). Lithium does not interact with beta-blockers (C); however, it does have significant drug interactions with ACEIs and diuretics. Lithium works by altering the sodium transport (E), which helps in understanding the interaction with ACEIs and diuretics; while valproic acid is thought to affect GABA. Valproic acid is contraindicated in hepatic dysfunction and requires baseline and periodic liver function tests (D).

27. D

Bupropion can be used for smoking cessation (I). Bupropion is contraindicated in patients with seizure disorders due to an increased risk of seizures (III). Bupropion is also contraindicated in patients with eating disorders such as bulimia or anorexia (II). A patient's medical history must be obtained before initiation of bupropion.

28. E

Methotrexate is first-line DMARD therapy for patients with rheumatoid arthritis (C). Patients may be supplemented with folic acid during treatment with methotrexate to decrease adverse effects and prevent folate deficiency (A). To lessen GI upset, methotrexate should be taken with food (B). The usual dosing for rheumatoid arthritis is 7.5 mg PO once weekly (D). Methotrexate does not require frequent ophthalmic exams; that is a requirement of hydroxychloroquine.

29. E

Oxybutynin is available in an oral form (Ditropan and Ditropan XL) as well as a transdermal form (Oxytrol patch) (I). It is also available as a topical gel (Gelnique). It is an anticholinergic medication used to treat overactive bladder (II). Common anticholinergic side effects of oxybutynin include dry mouth and dry eyes (III).

30. B

Colchicine can be used both for prophylaxis and treatment of gout (III). NSAIDs are used only for acute symptoms and do not prevent gout from occurring (I). Corticosteroids are used during acute gouty attacks when symptoms have been present for >48 hours (II).

31. C

Hot flushes (A), decreased libido (B), spotting (D), and dyspareunia (E) are all common side effects of estrogen deficiency. Since Ovcon-50 is a high estrogen-containing oral contraceptive, side effects of estrogen excess (such as breast tenderness) would be more common.

32. C

Seasonale is an oral contraceptive tablet and should be taken by mouth once daily (I). Smoking while on any oral contraceptive will increase the risk of thromboembolic events (II). Seasonale is not available in a transdermal patch formulation (III).

33. E

Oral antibiotics may inhibit the efficacy of oral contraceptive medications, so (A) and (B) are inaccurate. It would be inappropriate to advise a patient not to take an antibiotic (C) and it would also be inappropriate to advise a patient to double the dose of oral contraceptive during the use of the antibiotics (D); the safety and efficacy of this practice have not been established and this could pose harm to the patient. During the use of interacting antibiotics, it is important to advise a patient to adhere to a backup method of contraception during, for at least 7 days, and up to a full cycle after the completion of the antibiotic.

34. C

First-line therapy for comedonal acne is topical benzoyl peroxide (C). The use of oral antibiotics (A) would be recommended in pustular acne or in cases that were not responsive to topical therapy. Also, tetracycline would interact with Ms. Brown's oral contraceptive medication and would not be ideal. Isotretinoin (B and E) is reserved for severe cystic or refractory acne. Topical retinoid agents should not be initially combined with topical benzoyl peroxide (D) due to an increased risk of drying of the skin.

35. D

Ms. Brown's headaches are quite frequent, making her a candidate for prophylactic therapy (A). Imitrex (sumatriptan; B) is an abortive therapy medication and is not appropriate for prophylaxis. Topiramate (C) is used as prophylactic therapy, but would have a drug interaction with her oral contraceptive (may decrease efficacy).

Hydrocodone (E), an opioid analgesic, is used for the treatment of pain and would be inappropriate for migraine prophylaxis. Propranolol (D) is commonly used for migraine prophylaxis and would be the most appropriate of these options.

36. A

Patients taking oral contraceptives should be educated to consult their pharmacist or physician when starting any new medication because of the strong possibility of multiple drug interactions. Neurontin (gabapentin; A) does not have any known drug interactions. Carbamazepine (B), valproic acid (C), phenytoin (D), and phenobarbital (E) have a long list of drug interactions, decreasing the effectiveness of oral contraceptives.

37. C

Tolterodine is the generic name for Detrol, oxybutynin is the generic name for Ditropan, solifenacin is the generic name for Vesicare, and imipramine is the generic name for Tofranil.

38. B

When a diagnosis of rheumatoid arthritis is made, DMARDs should be initiated within 3 months to slow the progression of the disease (I, eliminating choices A, C, and E). Biologics should be initiated when methotrexate monotherapy has been ineffective and possibly other DMARDs have been tried and ineffective as well (III). Biologics would not provide PRN relief as they are given by injection at weekly or longer intervals, with the exception of anakinra, which is a daily injection (II, eliminating choice D). NSAIDs are used for PRN symptom relief.

39. C

TCAs often exhibit anticholinergic side effects (I). In overdose situations, these agents are very dangerous and often fatal (II); therefore, in patients with high suicidality, they should be used with caution. There is no drug–food interaction between aged cheese and TCAs; this interaction is with the monoamine oxidase inhibitors (MAOIs; III).

40. D

Antidepressants may take several weeks to show maximum efficacy. Neither SSRIs such as fluoxetine (A) nor serotonin norepinephrine reuptake inhibitors (SNRIs) such as duloxetine (B) should be used in combination with MAOIs (selegiline). Choice (C) is incorrect because caffeine should be avoided in combination with MAOIs because of the risk of hypertensive crisis. Although there is an oral formulation of selegiline (E), it is not indicated for depression (used for Parkinson's disease) and would not increase efficacy.

41. A

Fiorinal contains aspirin with butalbital and caffeine. Fioricet (B) contains acetaminophen with butalbital and caffeine. Excedrin Migraine (C) contains acetaminophen and aspirin with caffeine. Migranal (D) is a dihydroergotamine nasal spray. Amerge (E) is naratriptan.

42. D

Photosensitivity is a common side effect with Retin-A (tretinoin), and the use of sunblock prior to sun exposure is very important. Retinoids such as Retin-A should not be used with astringents or abrasive soaps due to the increased risk of excessive drying of the skin (A). Topical retinoids take significantly longer than 1–2 days to result in a benefit (B). Topical retinoids are not used as spot treatment (C) and should be applied sparingly over the face after the face has been allowed to dry fully (E) after cleansing.

43. D

Zoledronic acid (I) is an annual IV infusion for the treatment of osteoporosis but is a bisphosphonate, so it is not an alternative to bisphosphonate therapy. Calcitonin (II) is an endogenous hormone that is indicated for the treatment of osteoporosis; it is usually administered intranasally. Raloxifene (III) is a selective estrogen receptor modulator that is recommended as an alternative choice for the treatment of osteoporosis.

44. C

The benzodiazepines including Xanax (alprazolam; A), Librium (chlordiazepoxide; B), and Valium (diazepam; D) vary in their peak activity and duration of action, but all have an onset of effect of minutes to hours. Vistaril (hydroxyzine; E) also works within minutes to hours, while Buspar (buspirone; C) takes up to 2 to 3 weeks to reach maximal efficacy.

45. C

Cheilitis (chapped lips; I) is the most common side effect of isotretinoin therapy. Pruritus (itching; II) related to dry skin is also a very common side effect of isotretinoin therapy. Hypertrichosis, or excessive hair growth (III), is not a known side effect of this medication.

46. D

Topical agents such as coal tar (C) and anthralin (E) are commonly used in the treatment of psoriasis. Systemic agents such as antimetabolites (methotrexate; A) and corticosteroids (prednisone; B) are often used in combination with topical agents in the treatment of psoriasis. Benzoyl peroxide (D) is not an effective treatment option for psoriasis.

47. C

In the TNM classification, T represents the severity of the primary tumor, N represents the severity of lymph node involvement, and M represents the severity of distant metastases. Generally, N0 and M0 mean no nodal involvement and no metastases, respectively.

48. C

Adjuvant chemotherapy is chemotherapy given after surgical treatment to provide further reduction in tumor burden. Neoadjuvant chemotherapy is given prior to surgical treatment (I) to provide an initial decrease in tumor burden (II). Both adjuvant and neoadjuvant chemotherapy are expected to increase survival (III). Palliative chemotherapy is given to relieve symptoms without expectation of survival benefit.

49. D

Methotrexate inhibits dihydrofolate reductase. When administered at the appropriate time in a chemotherapy cycle, leucovorin permits healthy cells to continue DNA replication and RNA transcription by providing a folic acid source that is not dependent on the action of dihydrofolate reductase. 5-fluorouracil inhibits thymidylate synthase, as does leucovorin. The two agents therefore have a synergistic effect. Doxorubicin is an anthracycline that works as an intercalating agent, interrupting DNA synthesis. Cytarabine inhibits DNA polymerase. Leucovorin does not interact with the mechanism of action of doxorubicin or cytarabine.

50. E

The primary mechanism of action of cytarabine is inhibition of DNA polymerase (I). Common side effects of cytarabine treatment include conjunctivitis and neurotoxicity (II). Corticosteroid eye drops are recommended as prophylaxis of conjunctivitis before and after cytarabine treatment (III).

51. D

The most clinically important side effect of anthracyclines is cardiac damage, including acute arrhythmias and cardiomyopathy following prolonged exposure. The risk of cardiotoxicity increases with cumulative lifetime dose. Hand and foot syndrome (E), or palmar-plantar erythrodysesthesia, is more common with 5-fluorouracil. Ototoxicity (A) is rarely seen with anthracyclines, and is more commonly a side effect of platinum compounds and nitrogen mustards. Methotrexate can cause symptoms of folate deficiency (C). Infusion reactions (B) are more common with etoposide, platinum compounds, and mustard compounds.

52. C

Avastin is the brand name for bevacizumab (C). Gleevec (A) is imatinib, Herceptin (B) is trastuzumab, Tarceva (D) is erlotinib, and Taxol (E) is paclitaxel.

53. C

ANC = white blood cells × (% segs + % bands).

54. B

The ANC range for mild neutropenia is 500–1,000/mm^3. Moderate neutropenia (C) is 100–500/mm^3, while severe (D) is less than 100/mm^3. A normal ANC is 3,000–7,000/mm^3 (E).

55. E

Severe (A) or prolonged neutropenia (D) or a sudden drop in ANC (B) are all risk factors for infection. Invasive procedures, including dental procedures, catheter placement, and enemas, also increase the risk of infection (C).

56. E

None of the erythropoietin derivatives (Epogen, Procrit, and Aranesp) are indicated in this patient, as her hemoglobin level is normal at 14.5 g/dL. She is suffering mild neutropenia, which does not warrant treatment with a colony-stimulating factor (such as Neupogen [filgrastim]). Therefore, none of the listed drugs are appropriate and choice (E) is correct.

57. A

Nominal or categorical data are qualitative and have no implied order among the categories. These data can be answered by "yes" or "no" responses. Gender and race are considered nominal data. Ordinal data (B) are ordered categories where the differences between categories cannot be considered equal. Satisfaction surveys and pain scales are examples of ordinal data. With interval data (C), there is an equal distance between the numeric values; however, there is an arbitrary zero point. The Celsius temperature scale is an example of interval data. With ratio data (such as weight or blood pressure; D), there is an equal distance between values and the zero point is meaningful. Frequency (E) refers to a proportion and not a type of data.

58. E

Power depends on sample size and variation within groups. The easiest way to increase power is to increase the sample size of a study. Altering the duration of the study (B, C) or decreasing the sample size (A) will not increase power. Increasing the number of dependent variables being studied (D) will also not increase the power of the study.

59. D

Type II errors occur when it is stated that there is no difference when a difference actually exists. The null hypothesis is the hypothesis that there is no difference between study groups; not detecting a true difference between groups will lead to a Type II error. Insufficient study power may mean that a difference between groups will not be discovered or will not be found to be statistically significant. Therefore, choices (A), (B), and (C) are all true statements about Type II errors. Type I errors occur when a difference between groups is detected that does not actually exist. Because the question is asking for which statement regarding Type II errors is false, the answer is (D).

60. D

ANOVA is the only test listed that is appropriate for such data (D). A student's T-test (A) and a paired t-test (B) are appropriate only when studying two groups. The Mann-Whitney U (E) is a nonparametric test appropriate for ordinal data. Chi-square tests (C) are used on nominal data.

61. C

$$0.12\,g \times \frac{100\,g\,ung}{2.5\,g\,HC} = 4.8\,g\,ung$$

$$30\,g\,ung \times \frac{0.4\,g\,HC}{100\,g\,ung} = 0.12\,g\,HC\,required$$

4.8 g of the 2.5% ointment is required to deliver the correct amount of hydrocortisone.

62. C

$$70\,g\,HPet \times \frac{8\,g\,WW}{100\,g\,HPet} = 5.6\,g\,WW$$

63. C

$$4\,fl\,oz \times \frac{30\,mL}{1\,fl\,oz} \times \frac{1\,tbsp}{15\,mL} \times \frac{2\,mg}{1\,tbsp} \times \frac{1\,tab}{4\,mg} = 4\,tabs$$

64. D

$$60\,kg \times \frac{5\,mcg}{kg \times \min} \times \frac{1\,mg}{1000\,mcg} \times$$

$$\frac{1\,mL}{0.5\,mg} \times \frac{60\,\min}{1\,hr} = 36\,\frac{mL}{hr}$$

65. A

The initial concentration (C_0) will be obtained by drawing blood very soon after administration. Using the equation $V_d = \dfrac{dose}{C_0}$, we can see that for equal doses, V_d will vary inversely with C_0. Drug A has a higher C_0 than Drug B (0.2 mg/mL > 83 mcg/mL); therefore, Drug A has a smaller volume of distribution.

66. C

$$40\,mL\,so\ln \times \frac{10\,g\,MgSO_4}{100\,mL\,so\ln} \times \frac{1000\,mg}{1\,g} \times$$

$$\frac{1\,mmol\,MgSO_4}{246.36\,mg\,MgSO_4} \times \frac{1\,mmol\,Mg^{2+}}{1\,mmol\,MgSO_4} \times$$

$$\frac{2\,mEq\,Mg^{2+}}{1\,mmol\,Mg^{2+}} = 32.5\,mEq\,Mg^{2+}$$

67. C

$$240\,mL \times \frac{15\,mEq}{15\,mL} \times \frac{1\,mmol\,K^+}{1\,mEq\,K^+} \times$$

$$\frac{1\,mmol\,C_6H_5K_3O_7}{3\,mmol\,K^+} \times \frac{1\,mol}{1000\,mmol} \times$$

$$\frac{306\,g\,C_6H_5K_3O_7}{1\,mol\,C_6H_5K_3O_7} = 24.48\,g\,C_6H_5K_3O_7$$

68. B

Accuracy refers to how closely test values approach the true value. Precision refers to how closely test values approach each other. Because the test values given are tightly grouped (8.0 ± 0.1) but differ significantly from the true value given (7.5), it can be said the values are precise but not accurate.

69. B

$$\frac{0.9\,g\,NaCl}{100\,mL} \times 30\,mL = 0.27\,g\,NaCl$$

needed to make volume isotonic

$$30\,mL \times \frac{0.5\,g\,TetHCl}{100\,mL} \times \frac{0.18\,g\,NaCl(Eq)}{1\,g\,TetHCl} = 0.027\,g$$

NaCl equivalent present

0.27 g – 0.027 g = 0.243 g NaCl needed to make the solution isotonic

70. B

The recipe makes 10 capsules (M et div caps #10). Therefore each capsule contains (0.5/10) or 0.05 g diphenhydramine. Then, $0.05 \times 60 = 3$ g.

71. C

fup = 1 – (fraction bound to proteins) = 0.05

Filtration clearance = fup × CLcr =
   0.05 × 100 mL/min = 5 mL/min

72. C

CLr = amount filtered + amount secreted –
   amount reabsorbed

All molecules small enough to pass through the glomerular membrane, which includes most nonprotein-bound small molecule drugs, are filtered.

If CLr > filtration clearance, some drug must be secreted. (Some reabsorption may also occur, but less is reabsorbed than secreted.)

If CLr < filtration clearance, some drug must be reabsorbed. (Some secretion may also occur, but less is secreted than is reabsorbed.)

Because CLr = 25 mL/min, while filtration clearance is only 5 mL/min, the drug must be secreted as well as filtered.

73. **A**

$$k = \frac{CL}{V_d} = \frac{400\,mL\,/\,min}{140\,L} \times \frac{1\,L}{1000\,mL} \times$$

$$\frac{60\,min}{hr} = 0.171\,hr^{-1}$$

$$t_{1/2} = \frac{0.693}{k} = \frac{0.693}{0.171\,hr^{-1}} = 4.04\,hr$$

74. **D**

$$C_{peak} = \frac{dose}{V_d} = \frac{250\,mg}{140\,L} = 1.79\,mg\,/\,L = 0.179\,mg\,/\,dL$$

75. **B**

Tobramycin is predominantly cleared by the kidneys. The increase in serum creatinine concentration indicates a decrease in creatinine clearance, which in turn implies a decrease in tobramycin clearance. Therefore, choices (C) and (E) are wrong. The bioavailability of any drug given IV is 1; therefore, choice (A) is wrong. When clearance decreases, the half-life and serum concentration will increase, leading to drug accumulation. Therefore, choice (D) is wrong and (B) is correct.

76. **A**

Because penicillin and probenecid compete for the same saturable excretion pathway, administration of probenecid will decrease the secretion and therefore the overall clearance of penicillin. Choices (B), (C), and (E) are incorrect. When clearance decreases, the steady-state plasma concentration of the drug will increase, so choice (D) is incorrect and (A) is the right answer.

77. **B**

Amorphous compounds are more soluble in water than their crystalline counterparts. Hydrates are less soluble in water than anhydrous drugs (A). Adding lipophilic groups (C)

and removing hydroxyl groups (D) will also decrease water solubility.

78. **D**

For weak bases, when pH < pKa the drug will be mostly ionized.

79. **E**

All medication given by mouth is subject to first-pass metabolism. Only medications given by routes that bypass the gastrointestinal tract can escape first-pass metabolism. Syrups (B), tablets (A), and capsules (C) are all swallowed, and their contents undergo first-pass metabolism. The rapid-dissolve strip (D) is also an oral product; the strip dissolves in the mouth, and the resultant solution is swallowed. Do not confuse a rapid-dissolve strip with a sublingual or buccal tablet—in these latter two dosage forms, the drug is absorbed across the oral mucosa, escaping the first-pass effect. Of the choices listed, only the transdermal patch is given by a nonoral route. Therefore (E) is the only choice that is not subject to first-pass metabolism.

80. **B**

Maximizing sediment volume (C) and promoting loose aggregation of suspended particles (A) are functions of controlled flocculation, not structured vehicles. Reducing repulsion between particles (D) will lead to increased sediment density, causing caking. Only slowing sedimentation by increasing viscosity is a behavior of structured vehicles, so (B) is correct.

81. **B**

The cosolvent system for phenytoin injection contains water, propylene glycol, and alcohol. The cosolvent system is necessary to keep phenytoin in solution, as phenytoin has only limited aqueous solubility. Rapid infusion would dilute the cosolvents, creating a super-saturated concentration of drug in a primarily aqueous environment, leading to precipitation. Onset of action will not be faster as a result of slow injection (A). Rapid injection is unlikely to lead to hemolysis (C); this is a complication of hypertonic solutions. The cosolvent system would have no effect on drug metabolism (D). The viscosity of the solution is not high enough to prevent rapid injection (E).

82. **A**

Ophthalmic products must contain preservative if they are in multiple-use containers to limit the possibility of severe eye infections. They do not require preservative when packaged in single-dose containers (II), or when being used as rinse solutions in eye surgery or trauma (III).

83. **C**

Ulcerative colitis is a local condition of the intestinal tract; medications administered rectally are providing treatment at the site of action. Nausea (A), chronic pain (B), hormone deficiency (D), and migraines (E) may be treated with medications administered rectally; however, these drugs are absorbed into the systemic circulation to act at distant sites of action.

84. **D**

The disulfiram reaction results from the inhibition of acetaldehyde dehydrogenase. Ethanol consumption leads to the buildup of acetaldehyde, causing nausea, vomiting, and severe discomfort. Tinctures (C), spirits (A), fluid extracts (E), and Elixir USP (B) all contain ethanol, and will trigger this reaction if taken in combination with metronidazole. Suspensions do not customarily contain ethanol and would be an appropriate way to deliver metronidazole.

85. **C**

Hydrolysis (A) results when the drug reacts with water in the dosage form. Because the reaction occurred in only one of the two bottles, this is unlikely. Photolysis (B) is chemical breakdown caused by light exposure; however, the drug was stored in a dark room. Sedimentation (D) and polymorphism (E) are physical changes, rather than chemical changes, and there was no difference in conditions between the capped and uncapped bottles that would explain a difference in the occurrence of these changes. Because only the open bottle was affected, while the capped bottle did not change color, the oxygen in the atmosphere likely caused the degradation.

86. **E**

Dilatant substances (A) become more viscous on agitation, and thin at rest. Newtonian substances (B) do not change viscosity when stirred or agitated. Plastic flow (C) occurs when a substance is thick at rest and remains thick until it receives sufficiently vigorous agitation, after which it behaves in a Newtonian manner. Pseudoplastic flow (D) is similar to plastic flow, but the material continues to thin if agitated more vigorously. Thixotropy is the property where a suspension remains thick until agitated, and then becomes easily pourable.

87. **B**

$$DR = \frac{V\max Css}{Km + Css} = \frac{(300)(14)}{6.5 + 14} =$$
$$205 mg / day = 4 \ tablets$$

88. **D**

Magnesium stearate is a lubricant, and at high concentration has a tendency to waterproof particles, preventing them from dissolving. Starch (A), microcrystalline cellulose (B), lactose (C), and mannitol (E) would not be expected to affect bioavailability.

89. B

Morphine is the only one of these products not metabolized by CYP2D6. Codeine (A), hydrocodone (C), and oxycodone (D) require metabolism by CYP2D6 in order to be activated to a therapeutically useful form. While structurally related to codeine, dextromethorphan (E) is not considered an opioid. This cough suppressant also requires metabolism via CYP2D6 to produce its active form.

90. A

Grapefruit juice inhibits CYP3A, the enzyme that metabolizes protease inhibitors. Therefore, choices (C), (D), and (E) can be eliminated. Inhibition of CYP3A will decrease clearance of drugs metabolized by that enzyme, leading to increased serum concentrations. Increased serum concentration will lead to toxic, rather than subtherapeutic (B), levels.

91. D

$$1:10,000 = \frac{1\,g}{10,000\,mL} = \frac{0.01\,g}{100\,mL} = 0.01\%\,w/v$$

92. B

$$SG = \frac{density_{substance}}{density_{water}}$$

$$SG \times density_{water} = density_{substance}$$

$$1.18 \times 1\,g/mL = 1.18\,g/mL$$

$$100\,g \times \frac{1\,mL}{1.18\,g} = 84.75\,mL$$

93. D

Simvastatin and ezetimibe combined are called Vytorin. The combination of atorvastatin and amlodipine (A) is called Caduet. The combination of atorvastotin and ezetimibe (B) is called Liptruzet. The combination of lovastatin and niacin (C) is called Advicor. There is no combination of simvastatin and lisinopril (E).

94. C

Nonpharmacological therapies that can be recommended to patients with heart failure include restricting fluid intake (<2 L/day) (I) and restricting sodium intake (≤3 g/day) (II). There is no specific reason why a patient with heart failure needs to restrict vitamin K in the diet (III).

95. E

Anorexia (I), arrhythmias (II), and visual disturbances (III) are all associated with digoxin toxicity.

96. D

Calan SR (verapamil) is a nondihydropyridine calcium channel blocker that is contraindicated in patients with heart failure with reduced ejection fraction (HFrEF) (left vertricular ejection fraction [LVEF] ≤40%). Aldactone (spironolactone; A) and Inspra (eplerenone; E), which are both aldosterone receptor antagonists, as well as the angiotensin receptor blocke (ARB), Diovan (valsartan; C), would be safe to use in a patient with heart failure. In addition, BiDil (B), the combination of hydralazine and isosorbide dinitrate, would also be appropriate to use in a patient with heart failure.

97. B

The second dose of furosemide should be taken before 5 p.m. to minimize nocturia. Furosemide does not need to be separated from other medications (A), does not need to be taken with food or milk (C), and does not need to be taken on an empty stomach (E). The second dose should not be taken at bedtime, as this will likely result in increased nocturia (D).

98. D

Bactrim DS (sulfamethoxazole/trimethoprim) is most likely being used to treat *Escherichia coli*, a common cause of urinary tract infections (UTIs). Bactrim DS does not cover the other bacteria listed.

99. A

The combination of Bactrim DS and Coumadin (warfarin) may lead to a significant drug interaction that would result in an increase in Ms. Brown's international normalized ratio (INR). Bactrim DS has no effect on plasma sodium or potassium concentrations.

100. E

The combination of trimethoprim and sulfamethoxazole is called Bactrim DS. The combination of amoxicillin and clavulanic acid (A) is called Augmentin, and the combination of imipenem and cilastatin (C) is called Primaxin. There are no combinations of ciprofloxacin and doxycycline (B), or of isoniazid and rifampin (D).

101. A

Lisinopril is an ACEI.

102. B

Martindale is the only reference that contains foreign drug information.

103. D

Xalatan (latanoprost) is an ophthalmic prostaglandin analog used to treat glaucoma.

104. B

Ketek (telithromycin; III) is a macrolide antibiotic. Keflex (cephalexin; I) is a first-generation cephalosporin antibiotic, and Keppra (levetiracetam; II) is an anticonvulsant.

105. D

Sulfasalazine may cause bodily fluids (e.g., urine, tears) to turn orange (II) and may cause photosensitivity (III). Sulfasalazine should be taken with food rather than on an empty stomach (I).

106. D

Metronidazole is the only option listed that can be used to treat *Clostridium difficile*.

107. E

USP-DI Volume II contains information for the patient in lay language. The other choices are all references for the healthcare professional.

108. C

Cytotec is the brand name for misoprostol. Cimetidine (A) is Tagamet. Metoclopramide (B) is Reglan. Olsalazine (D) is Dipentum. Sucralfate (E) is Carafate.

109. A

Acyclovir is an appropriate treatment for genital herpes. Indinavir (B) and lamivudine (C) are used to treat human immunodeficiency virus (HIV). Oseltamivir (D) is used to treat influenza. Valganciclovir (E) is used to treat cytomegalovirus.

110. D

The Red Book is the only choice listed that contains cost information.

111. E

Potential side effects of niacin include flushing (I), hyperglycemia (II), and hyperuricemia (III).

112. B

The combination of timolol and dorzolamide is called Cosopt. The combination of timolol and brimonidine (A) is called Combigan. There are no combinations of latanoprost and carbachol (C), pilocarpine and brinzolamide (D), or pilocarpine and carbachol (E).

113. A

Voriconazole is an antifungal that could be used to treat an invasive *Aspergillus* infection. Voriconazole can be administered either IV or orally. While miconazole (III) is also an antifungal drug, it is available only in topical formulations and as a buccal tablet and is used to treat superficial fungal infections. Linezolid (II) is used to treat gram-positive bacterial infections, such as methicillin-resistant *Staphylococcus aureus* or vancomycin-resistant *Enterococcus faecium*.

114. E

Avoiding chocolate (I), smoking cessation (II), and weight loss (III) are all appropriate non-pharmacological recommendations for a patient with GERD.

115. E

Nitroprusside should be protected from light. None of the other IV medications listed need to be protected from light.

116. A

The three-drug combination regimen of Biaxin (clarithromycin), Amoxil (amoxicillin), and Nexium (esomeprazole) would be used to treat a *Helicobacter pylori* infection.

117. C

Trusopt (dorzolamide) is an ophthalmic carbonic anhydrase inhibitor used in treating glaucoma.

118. C

The Commission E monographs provide information on herbal products.

119. A

Clotrimazole is available as a troche (I), topical cream, vaginal cream, and topical solution. However, it is not available as a capsule (II) or powder (III).

120. B

In patients receiving amiodarone, liver function tests should be performed every 6 months (III) to monitor for potential hepatotoxicity. A chest x-ray should be performed every 12 months (not 6 months) to monitor for pulmonary toxicity (I). Thyroid function tests (II) should be performed every 6 months (not every 12 months) to monitor for hyper- or hypothyroidism.

121. E

Patients should separate the administration of different ophthalmic preparations by intervals of at least 10 minutes. Contact lenses should be removed before using ophthalmic products (A). Patients should not touch the tip of the dropper to any part of the eye (B). Patients should pull out the lower eyelid (not the upper eyelid) to form a pocket for the medication to be placed (C). Patients should not rub their eyes after administration of ophthalmic preparations (D).

122. B

Trissel's (III) contains information on IV drug compatibility. Facts and Comparisons (I) and the Physician's Drug Reference (II) contain general drug information and do not contain IV drug compatibility information.

123. B

Tagamet (cimetidine) is an H_2 receptor antagonist.

124. D

Patients taking methotrexate should have a CBC (II) monitored for potential bone marrow suppression, and their liver function tests (III) monitored for potential hepatotoxicity. It is not necessary to have an electrocardiogram (I) performed while taking methotrexate.

125. E

Candesartan (ARB; I), eplerenone (aldosterone receptor antagonist; II), and triamterene (potassium-sparing diuretic; III) may all result in hyperkalemia.

126. E

For esomeprazole (I), the capsules can be opened and mixed with water in a syringe or the granules for oral suspension can be mixed with water in a syringe prior to administration via nasogastric tube. For lansoprazole (II), the capsules can be opened and mixed with apple juice or the orally disintegrating tablets can be mixed with water in a syringe prior to administration via nasogastric tube. The pantoprazole (III) granules for suspension can be mixed with apple juice in a syringe prior to administration via nasogastric tube.

127. A

A patient who is taking felodipine should avoid drinking grapefruit juice because grapefruit juice inhibits CYP3A4, which would result in increased concentrations of felodipine. Tyramine-containing foods (B) should be avoided in patients taking MAOIs. Felodipine does not cause folate deficiency, and therefore does not to be administered with folic acid (C). Felodipine does not need to be taken on an empty stomach (D), and does not need to be separated from other medications (E).

128. A

Azithromycin is the best option, as it will cover the most likely bacteria that would cause community-acquired pneumonia in this patient (*Streptococcus pneumoniae, Mycoplasma pneumoniae, Haemophilus influenzae*). The other antibiotic choices would not cover the appropriate bacteria.

129. D

Amoxicillin is available as an oral suspension (II) or a capsule (III), but not as an IV injection (I). A related antibiotic, ampicillin, can be administered IV.

130. C

Antihypertensives that can be used safely in pregnancy are methyldopa, a calcium channel blocker, and labetalol. ACEIs (such as lisinopril; B) and ARBs (such as valsartan; E) are contraindicated in pregnancy. Diuretics (such as metolazone; D) and α_1-receptor antagonists (such as doxazosin; A) are not recommended in pregnant patients.

131. A

Proton pump inhibitors (PPIs) should be taken 15–30 minutes before breakfast.

132. C

Sporanox is the brand name for itraconazole. Abilify is the brand name of aripiprazole (A). Diflucan is the brand name of fluconazole (B). Prevacid is the brand name of lansoprazole (D). Aciphex is the brand name of rabeprazole (E).

133. E

Simvastatin plus gemfibrozil is likely to result in myopathy (and possibly rhabdomyolysis). In fact, if a fibric acid derivative must be used

134. A

Amiodarone contains iodine and may potentially cause hyper- or hypothyroidism. The other listed medications do not cause hypothyroidism.

135. C

Levaquin (levofloxacin) is a fluoroquinolone.

136. B

Amiodarone-induced pulmonary fibrosis is a potentially life-threatening condition. Therefore, if this adverse effect occurs in a patient taking amiodarone, this antiarrhythmic must be discontinued. Amiodarone undergoes significant CYP450 metabolism (II) and is a substrate of the CYP3A4 isozyme. It is also an inhibitor of the CYP1A2, CYP2C9, CYP2D6, and CYP3A4 isozymes. Amiodarone is effective for the treatment of both ventricular and atrial arrhythmias (I).

137. E

Aminosalicylates (I), corticosteroids (II), and immunosuppressants (III) can all be used to treat inflammatory bowel disease.

138. E

All three of the drugs listed can be used in a 3-drug combination regimen to treat *H. pylori*. A 3-drug combination regimen for *H. pylori* consists of 2 antibiotics and a PPI.

139. B

The maximum daily dose of metformin is 2,550 mg/day. This patient's dose (3,000 mg/day) exceeds this, so the doctor should be contacted. Choice (A) is incorrect because this patient has controlled blood sugars based on

A1c less than 7%. The dose of metformin should not be increased (C), because it already exceeds the maximum recommended daily dose. Choice (D) is incorrect because the American Diabetes Association recommends metformin as the drug of choice in newly diagnosed patients with type 2 diabetes and this patient has no contraindications such as heart failure, renal disease, or age greater than 80 years. Lisinopril does not interact with metformin (E). In fact, there truly are no major drug interactions with metformin.

140. B

Choice (B) is the best answer because this patient is taking more than the recommended daily dose of Prilosec OTC: 20 mg daily × 14 days, which can be repeated in 4 months. Mr. Boyd has continued the treatment longer than the recommended 14 days for Prilosec OTC. A multivitamin (II) is not a bad option for any patient in any circumstances; however, Mr. Boyd's complaint of fatigue that he is experiencing is likely due to the symptoms of hypothyroidism.

141. A

Hypothyroidism (I) is the best answer because Mr. Boyd's thyroid-stimulating hormone (TSH) concentration is well out of the normal range (0.3–6 mIU/L). His symptoms are very consistent with hypothyroidism: weakness, fatigue, depression, cold feeling, weight gain. Hypoglycemia (II) is incorrect because he is taking metformin only, which does not cause hypoglycemia in monotherapy. Depression (III) is incorrect because his general depression score (GDS) was not greater than 7 and the hypothyroidism must be ruled out first.

142. D

Inhibition of ACE blocks the conversion of angiotensin I to angiotensin II. Angiotensin II is the most potent vasoconstrictor in the body; therefore, decreasing concentrations of angiotensin II results in vasodilation (D). Current literature does not support ACEIs lowering blood sugars (A). ACEIs do not inhibit renin (B). ARBs, not ACEIs, block the angiotensin II receptor (C). ACEIs lead to increased, not decreased, concentrations of bradykinin by preventing its breakdown (E).

143. B

Mr. Boyd should avoid taking the Synthroid (levothyroxine) at the same time as the ferrous sulfate, which will bind to the levothyroxine and prevent it from being absorbed. This interaction can be avoided by taking these medications at least 4 hours apart. Synthroid does not cause hypoglycemia (A). Taking Synthroid only in the evening (C) is possible, but the patient must be informed not to take it with the ferrous sulfate, so (B) is still the best option. There is no drug interaction with metformin (D), so Mr. Boyd could take the Synthroid at the same time as the metformin. Synthroid should not be taken with dairy products, as the calcium will bind to levothyroxine and prevent it from being absorbed (E).

144. A

There are only four drugs in the nonnucleoside reverse transcriptase inhibitor class, nevirapine, efavirenz, etravirine, and rilpivirine. The brand name of nevirapine is Viramune. Nearly all the protease inhibitors end in "-navir," which leaves the remaining drugs to be nucleoside reverse transcriptase inhibitors (NRTIs). Ziagen (abacavir) is an NRTI (B). Kaletra (lopinavir/ritonavir) is a protease inhibitor (C). Videx (didanosine) is an NRTI (D). Fuzeon (enfuvirtide) is the only fusion inhibitor (E).

145. D

Patients diagnosed with HIV will need to have a Western blot performed (I); however, starting highly active antiretroviral therapy is not recommended because of the long-term side effects and because some patients' viral load and CD4 rise and drop differently. However, when the CD4 cell count drops to less than 500 cells/mm^3 (II), it is recommended to start therapy. In addition, if patients have a history of an opportunistic infection regardless of their CD4 cell count (III), antiviral therapy should be initiated as well as treatment for the opportunistic infection.

146. C

Thrush is a common side effect of inhaled corticosteroids (II). The classic toxicity symptoms for theophylline include tachycardia, nausea, and vomiting, along with a theophylline level that exceeds the normal range of 5–15 mcg/mL (I). The metoprolol dose is well within the normal range, and this patient has tachycardia, not bradycardia (III).

147. D

The Advair does not need to be discontinued (A). Thrush must be treated with nystatin and the patient must be counseled to swish and spit after each use of Advair. The patient's nausea is likely due to the theophylline toxicity, and not the aspirin (B). There is not enough information to assess whether the patient is using the albuterol excessively (C). Theophylline should be discontinued due to toxicity symptoms. Metoprolol (E) does not cause tachycardia; it would cause bradycardia.

148. C

Fluticasone and salmeterol combined are called Advair. Fluticasone alone (A) is called Flovent, Flonase, or Veramyst. Salmeterol alone (B) is called Serevent and is available only as a dry powder inhaler. Flunisolide alone (D) is the ingredient of Aerospanor Nasalide. There are no combinations of flunisolide and salmeterol (E).

149. E

Fish oil targets triglyceride reduction. It is available over-the-counter and as a prescription product (Lovaza, Epanova, Omtryg, Vascepa). Fish oil is thought to inhibit acylCA:1,2 diacylglycerol acyltransferase and to increase hepatic beta-oxidation, causing a reduction in the hepatic synthesis of triglycerides or an increase in plasma lipoprotein lipase activity. Fish oils have only modest effects on the other lipid profiles, so choices (A), (B), (C), and (D) are incorrect.

150. B

The maximum daily dose of acetaminophen is 4,000 mg per day. The patient could potentially take 4,550 mg/day by taking 2 hydrocodone/acetaminophen tablets every 6 hours and the Tylenol 650 mg 3 times daily. Choice (B) is the best option because the pharmacist can easily educate the patient on the 4,000-mg guideline and help develop a plan of administration. There is no need to call the doctor (A); and the patient can have the flexibility to decide if she needs over-the-counter acetaminophen or the combination product with hydrocodone for more severe pain, so choices (C) and (D) are also incorrect. Aspirin is not a good option because she is already taking 325 mg/day of aspirin and this could increase her risk of bleeding (E).

151. D

Spiriva (tiotropium) and Atrovent (ipratropium) both block the action of acetylcholine at parasympathetic sites at the M3 receptor located on bronchial smooth muscle, causing bronchodi-

lation. Ipratropium is a metered-dose inhaler used 4 times per day and tiotropium is a dry powder inhaler (DPI) (III) administered with the HandiHaler device once daily (II). DPIs are breath-actuated, lessening the need for hand and breath coordination and allowing for better lung deposition. Tiotropium is longer-acting due to structural differences from ipratropium allowing for higher affinity to the M3 receptor. Ipratropium and tiotropium have virtually the same side effect profile, so (I) is incorrect.

152. A

Pulmicort Respules (budesonide; I) is the only nebulized inhaled corticosteroid available on the market. Singulair (montelukast; II) is a leukotriene receptor antagonist and Zyflo (zileuton; III) is a 5-lipoxygenase inhibitor.

153. D

The active ingredient in Zyban is bupropion. Bupropion is indicated both as an antidepressant and smoking cessation agent. It is not a serotonergic inhibitor (A); as a result, bupropion does not cause sexual dysfunction like most serotonergic antidepressants. Bupropion inhibits both norepinephrine and dopamine; therefore, choices (B) and (C) are incorrect. Effexor (venlafaxine) inhibits serotonin, norepinephrine, and dopamine (E).

154. E

Streptomycin is used only as a substitute for ethambutol and for drug-resistant tuberculosis. The other choices are commonly used in combination for treatment of tuberculosis.

155. D

Vitamin K is used to reverse the anticoagulant effects of warfarin. Protamine is used to reverse the effects of unfractionated heparin (A), and it may be used to partially reverse the effects of low molecular weight heparins, such as enoxaparin (C). Dabigatran (B) does not currently have an antidote. Clopidogrel (E) is an antiplatelet agent and does not have an antidote.

156. **A**

Flumazenil is the antidote for benzodiazepines. Choice (B) is incorrect because there are several antidotes for opioids, including naloxone and naltrexone. The antidote for methanol (C) or ethylene glycol toxicity is fomepizole. The antidote for an overdose of methotrexate (D) is leucovorin. Amifostine is used to prevent nephrotoxicity associated with repeated administration of cisplatin (E).

157. **A**

Liothyronine is called Cytomel. Levothyroxine (B) has multiple brand name products, including Levothyroid, Levoxyl, Synthroid, Tirosint, and Unithroid. Choice (C) is the natural animal thyroid which is desiccated from pig or cow and is called Armour Thyroid. T4 (D) is the abbreviated name for levothyroxine. TSH (E) is not an active ingredient in any drug.

158. **C**

ACEIs (ramipril; III) decrease placental blood flow, lower birth weight, cause fetal hypotension, and cause preterm delivery but as a class are not category X drugs. They are pregnancy category D. Finasteride (I) causes abnormalities of external male genitalia; and isotretinoin (II) causes major fetal abnormalities, both internal and external. Both drugs are pregnancy category X.

159. **E**

Weight gain (I), osteoporosis (II), and pulmonary embolism (III) are all potential side effects of medroxyprogesterone and should be discussed with the patient.

160. **B**

During the initial application, the absorption of transdermal fentanyl requires 12 to 24 hours to reach plateau. Therefore, transdermal fentanyl is inappropriate for management of acute pain. Choice (D) is misleading, as the patch needs to be changed every 72 hours.

161. **E**

For a patient who is taking morphine, it is highly recommended that a stimulant laxative be started to minimize the risk of constipation (I). Due to possible sedation, it is not recommended that antihistamines or other pain medications be used, as these can add to morphine's sedative effects. Likewise, it is not recommended that the patient drive a motorized vehicle (II). Compliance (III) is important for the treatment of chronic pain so the patient is able to prevent and stay ahead of the pain.

162. **D**

This question is designed to assess whether you know that choices (A), (B), (C), and (E) are all forms of NSAIDs. NSAIDs inhibit prostaglandins, which normally help to keep the afferent arterioles of the kidneys open. As a result, a recommendation other than acetaminophen (D) could compromise the patient's kidney function.

163. **E**

A PPD is a tuberculin test for tuberculosis. Tuberculosis results in individuals becoming sensitized to certain antigenic components of the *M. tuberculosis* organism. Healthcare workers (I) are at risk for being exposed to patients with tuberculosis. HIV-infected patients (II) are immunocompromised, which allows for easier inoculation and growth of the organism. Immigrant workers (III) have a higher rate of infection and lack of access to healthcare.

164. C

The doses of morphine (I) and codeine (II) should be reduced to 75% of the normal dose in patients with a creatinine clearance of 10–50 mL/min. When the creatinine clearance is less than 10 mL/min, the doses of these drugs should be reduced by 50%. Morphine has a metabolite, morphine-6-glucuronide, which can accumulate in renal insufficiency. The dose of oxycodone should be adjusted in patients with hepatic dysfunction (III); however, the dose does not need to be adjusted in renal impairment.

165. A

Naprosyn's (naproxen's) maximum daily dose is 1,500 mg. Other maximum daily doses are: ibuprofen (B), 3,200 mg/day; nabumetone (C), 2,000 mg/day; and ketoprofen (D), 300 mg/day. Daypro's (oxaprozin; E) maximum daily dose is 1,200 mg/day in patients who weigh less than 50 kg and 1,800 mg/day in patients who weigh more than 50 kg.

166. D

There are four warning signs for stroke. Of the five answer choices, only sudden seizure for no reason (D) is not considered common with stroke. Regardless, a patient should be rushed to the emergency room for care if a seizure occurred. The four warning signs for stroke (choices A, B, C, and E) are important in helping patients to receive treatment as soon as possible.

167. C

Folic acid is used with methotrexate treatment (I) because methotrexate is a folate antimetabolite that inhibits DNA synthesis. Methotrexate

irreversibly binds to dihydrofolate reductase and inhibits the formation of reduced folates. Use of folic acid is important in preparation for pregnancy to prevent neural tube defects (II). Iron deficiency anemia (IDA) (III) is a deficiency of iron. Folate deficiency is found in megaloblastic (macrocytic) anemias.

168. E

All three of these side effects are common with ferrous sulfate. It is important to recommend a stool softener to prevent constipation (I) and to counsel patients regarding the dark stools (II) and discoloration of urine (III).

169. E

Cholecalciferol is vitamin D3 and can be used for the treatment of vitamin D deficiency. Pyridoxine (A) is used for vitamin B6 deficiency or acute toxicity from isoniazid. Ascorbic acid (B) is used for prevention and treatment of scurvy and to acidify the urine. Beta-carotene (C) is used for prophylaxis and treatment of polymorphous light eruption, and for erythropoietic protoporphyria. Nicotinic acid (D) is used for dyslipidemia.

170. C

One of the problems with treating IDA is the side effects associated with treatment. Patients are often unable to tolerate the side effects, which limits the length of therapy. The minimum length of therapy with the lowest rates of relapsing IDA is 6 months.

171. B

The mechanism of action of epoetin alfa is inducing erythropoiesis and releasing reticulocytes, which are immature red blood cells. Choices (A), (C), (D), and (E) are all combinations of other drug mechanisms of actions.

172. E

Pyridoxine is used to prevent neurological toxicities associated with isoniazid therapy. The other options are not used with isoniazid treatment.

173. C

The Drug Enforcement Administration is the organization that is ultimately responsible for controlling and regulating controlled substances. The Federal Drug Association (A) is not a known association. The Food and Drug Administration (FDA) (B) is in charge of approving drugs for particular indications. The National Provider Indicators (D) is a group that assigns a national provider number to all healthcare professionals. The State Patrol (E) is often called on to arrest or investigate persons involved in drug diversion.

174. C

Choices (A), (B), (D), and (E) are all correct lifestyle modifications for their respective diseases. Choice (C) is incorrect (and thus the correct answer) because the most recent cholesterol guidelines recommend that cholesterol-lowering medications be started at the same time as heart-healthy lifestyle modifications.

175. D

Choices (A), (B), and (C) are all correct statements within the Dietary Supplement Health and Education Act of 1994. Choice (D) is not written into that act and has created much debate and controversy; the FDA is considering making a change but, to date, has not.

176. D

Saw palmetto has very few drug interactions. This is important because its prescription counterparts finasteride and dutasteride do interact with warfarin. Choices (A), (B), (C), and (E) all interact with warfarin by increasing INR levels by inhibiting CYP450 enzymes 1A2, 2D6, and 3A4. These herbal products may also increase the risk of bleeding when used with antiplatelet drugs, such as aspirin.

177. C

The most common organisms causing community-acquired skin and soft tissue infections are the Gram-positive organisms, *Staphylococcus aureus* (especially methicillin-resistant strains) (C) and *Streptococcus pyogenes* (not *Streptococcus pneumoniae* [D]). Gram-negative organisms, such as *Escherichia coli* (B) and *Pseudomonas aeruginosa* (E), are more likely to be found in nosocomial skin and soft tissue infections. *Haemophilus influenzae* (A) does not cause skin and soft tissue infections.

178. D

The most modern insulin pumps have basal insulin rates (A) that typically run for 24 hours per day, providing a small amount of continuous insulin. Insulin-to-carbohydrate ratio settings (B) are used for bolus injections during carbohydrate intake, and insulin sensitivity factor settings (C) are used for elevated blood sugars that are not related to food intake. The goal blood sugar setting (E) is used to determine how tightly controlled the patient should be. The rule of 1,800 (D) is used to determine the insulin sensitivity factor but is not within the insulin pump.

179. A

It has been suggested that vitamin E has several benefits, including serving as an antioxidant and preventing Alzheimer's disease. However, a recent meta-analysis suggests that doses greater than 400 IU can increase the risk for cardiovascular events.

180. E

Trissel's provides a compilation of all currently available stability information on drugs in compounded oral, enteral, topical, and IV formulations. Goodman and Gilman (A) focuses on drug pharmacology. Martindale (B) contains foreign drug information. The Merck Index (C) focuses on precise, comprehensive information on chemicals, drugs, and biologicals, whereas the Merck Manual focuses on diseases. Remington (D) is considered the pharmacy encyclopedia for pharmacology, theoretical science, sterilization, and practical pharmacy practice.

181. E

All three options provide solubility data on potassium gluconate. USP-NF (II) has official monographs for drug structure, solubilities, assays, and therapeutic category, but provides limited information on dosage and dosage forms. The other two options are described in the previous question.

182. B

Ferrous sulfate 5-grain tablets (B) are equivalent to 325 mg and are available on the market. Metformin tablets are available in 500-mg, 850-mg, and 1,000-mg, strengths; 1,250-mg tablets (A) are not available. The highest dosage form of Synthroid (levothyroxine) (C) is 300 mcg; however, a 212-mcg tablet is not available. The highest dosage form of Coumadin (warfarin) (D) is 10 mg; 15-mg tablets are not commercially available. Lisinopril's highest dosage form (E) is 40 mg.

183. B

Simvastatin is half as potent as Lipitor (atorvastatin), so simvastatin 20 mg is the correct answer. Rosuvastatin (A) is twice as potent as Lipitor. Pravastatin (C) is one-fourth as potent at atorvastatin and would require 40 mg to be equivalent.

184. D

St. John's wort is commonly used by patients for mild to moderate depression. However, it is associated with numerous drug interactions. It is a strong inducer of the CYP3A4 enzyme. Warfarin (III) is metabolized by 3A4; therefore, concomitant use with St. John Wort may lead to a reduction in warfarin concentrations, which may place a patient at risk for thromboembolic events. Sertraline (II) interacts with St. John's wort because both inhibit the reuptake of serotonin, which could result in serotonin syndrome. Pravachol (I) is the only statin not metabolized by 3A4; in fact, pravastatin is not metabolized at all via the CYP450 enzyme system.

185. C

This is a classic NAPLEX question which guides you to assess each complaint of the patient. There is no need to overtreat with an unneeded medication such as pseudoephedrine (III); the patient is not experiencing any congestion. Diphenhydramine (I) is used for the runny nose and sneezing, and the acetaminophen (II) is for the pain of the headache.

INDEX

Page numbers followed by *f* and *t* indicate figures and tables respectively.